Comparative Oncology

Michael W. Nolan • Damon R. Reed
Ryan D. Roberts • Audrey Ruple
Laura E. Selmic • Heather Wilson-Robles
Editors

Comparative Oncology

Springer

Editors
Michael W. Nolan
Department of Clinical Sciences,
College of Veterinary Medicine
North Carolina State University
Raleigh, NC, USA

Damon R. Reed
Department of Pediatrics
Memorial Sloan Kettering Cancer
Center
New York, NY, USA

Ryan D. Roberts
Nationwide Children's Hospital
Columbus, OH, USA

Audrey Ruple
Department of Population Health
Sciences
Virginia-Maryland College of Veterinary
Medicine, Virginia Tech
Blacksburg, VA, USA

Laura E. Selmic
Department of Veterinary Clinical
Sciences
The Ohio State University
Columbus, OH, USA

Heather Wilson-Robles
Ethos Discovery
San Diego, CA, USA

ISBN 978-3-032-04453-2 ISBN 978-3-032-04454-9 (eBook)
https://doi.org/10.1007/978-3-032-04454-9

This Springer imprint is published by the registered company Springer Nature Switzerland AG
The registered company address is: Gewerbestrasse 11, 6330 Cham, Switzerland

To the patients—both human and animal—who inspire our work every day.
To the families and caregivers who walk beside them with courage and hope.
And to the clinicians, researchers, and students who believe in the power of collaboration across species to transform the future of cancer care.
This book is for you.

Preface

Comparative oncology—the study of cancers across species—represents one of the most promising frontiers in both veterinary and human medicine. As we confront the complexity of cancer in people and animals alike, the need for collaborative, cross-disciplinary approaches has never been more apparent. Despite the clear intersections between veterinary and human oncology, no comprehensive resource has existed to unify these perspectives—until now.

This book was born from the shared vision of veterinary medical, radiation, and surgical oncologists alongside medical oncologists, all of whom recognized the power of comparative oncology to drive meaningful advances in cancer diagnosis, treatment, and prevention. Our goal is to bridge the existing gap by bringing together foundational knowledge, clinical insights, and translational research from both fields in a single, authoritative reference.

By examining the biologic similarities and differences of cancer across species, we can better understand tumor behavior, therapeutic response, and mechanisms of resistance. Companion animals, particularly dogs, often develop spontaneous cancers that closely mirror those seen in humans. Their shorter lifespans and intact immune systems create unique opportunities for translational research, where findings can inform both veterinary treatment protocols and human clinical trial design.

This book is designed to serve a broad audience, including veterinary and human oncologists, researchers, pathologists, clinicians, and students interested in the rapidly evolving field of comparative oncology. It includes contributions from leaders in veterinary and human medicine who provide not only a synthesis of current knowledge but also a roadmap for future collaboration.

We hope this work inspires continued dialogue and partnership across disciplines. By learning from each other and our patients—human and animal—we can accelerate progress against one of medicine's most formidable challenges.

Michael W. Nolan
Damon R. Reed
Ryan D. Roberts
Audrey Ruple
Laura E. Selmic
Heather Wilson-Robles

Acknowledgments

This textbook is the result of the collective efforts of a diverse and dedicated group of professionals who share a passion for advancing cancer care through collaboration across species. We extend our deepest gratitude to the contributors—veterinary and human medical, surgical, and radiation oncologists—who generously shared their expertise, clinical insight, and time to bring this vision to life.

We are especially thankful to our colleagues and mentors in both veterinary and human oncology who have long championed the field of comparative oncology, paving the way for this work. Your pioneering research and commitment to translational medicine continue to inspire and guide us.

To the institutions, hospitals, and research centers that supported our contributors and provided the infrastructure for the science and clinical care discussed in these pages—thank you. Your commitment to interdisciplinary collaboration made this book possible.

We also wish to acknowledge the editorial and production teams who helped shape this manuscript into its final form with care and precision. Your support throughout this process has been invaluable.

Finally, we are profoundly grateful to the patients—animal and human—whose lives and stories are at the heart of comparative oncology. Your resilience drives our pursuit of better outcomes, deeper understanding, and a shared future in which cancer care knows no species boundaries.

Contents

Background in Comparative Oncology

Introduction 3
Heather Wilson-Robles, Audrey Ruple, and Laura E. Selmic

Benefits of Comparative Oncology for Human Populations 13
Ryan D. Roberts and Damon R. Reed

Comparative Oncology: Evaluation of Oncology Across Nondomestic Species 23
Tara M. Harrison

Comparative Immunology 31
Shay Bracha and Seth Pollack

Comparative Cancer Diagnosis and Treatment

Comparative Pathology 55
Shane Sills

Comparative Radiobiology and Radiation Therapy 69
Charles A. Maitz and Ravi Patel

Comparative Aspects of Chemotherapy and Targeted Therapy: How Different Species Process Drugs 103
Luke A. Wittenburg and Ai-Ming Yu

Intraoperative Image Guidance in Human and Veterinary Surgical Oncology 123
Joanne Tuohy, William C. Eward, and John Rossmeisl

Comparative Oncology by Tumor Type

Osteosarcoma 143
Camille A. McAloney, Timothy M. Fan, and Ryan D. Roberts

Lymphoma 159
William C. Kisseberth, Walter Hanel, and Davis M. Seelig

Invasive Urinary Bladder Cancer 205
Deborah W. Knapp, Noah M. Hahn, Christopher M. Fulkerson, and Deepika Dhawan

Melanoma 245
Philip J. Bergman and Jedd D. Wolchok

Head and Neck Cancer 271
Pooja Karukonda, Ashlyn Rickard, Katherine Gonzalez, Yvonne M. Mowery, and Michael. W. Nolan

Central Nervous System Malignancies 301
Christopher L. Mariani, Lucas P. Wachsmuth, and Peter Fecci

Soft Tissue Sarcoma 329
Laura E. Selmic, William C. Kisseberth, and John Alexander

Utilizing Comparative Oncology Approaches

Organizing and Conducting Comparative Oncology Clinical Trials 361
Amy LeBlanc, Christina Mazcko, Erika Berger, and Jessica Beck

Clinical Investigation for Developing Imaging Technology 381
Brian Flesner, Maureen Griffin, and Amy LeBlanc

Integrating Comparative Oncology into the Translational Workflow 399
Suzanne Bartholf DeWitt, Heather L. Gardner, Nicole Cantor, Nicole Levine, Isabelle McMullen, Joanne Tuohy, Beatrice Schleupner, Veronica Colmenares, William C. Eward, and Jason A. Somarelli

Contributors

John Alexander Division of Musculoskeletal Oncology, Department of Orthopaedics, The Ohio State University Wexner Medical Center, Columbus, OH, USA

Frank H. Bassett III Department of Orthopaedic Surgery, Duke University Medical Center, Durham, NC, USA

Jessica Beck Comparative Oncology Program, Center for Cancer Research, National Cancer Institute, National Institutes of Health, Bethesda, MD, USA

Erika Berger Frederick National Laboratory for Cancer Research in the Comparative Oncology Program, National Cancer Institute, National Institutes of Health, Bethesda, MD, USA

Philip J. Bergman Adjunct Associate Faculty, Memorial Sloan-Kettering Cancer Center, New York, NY, USA

Veterinary Program, Focused Ultrasound Foundation, Charlottesville, VA, USA

Shay Bracha Department of Veterinary Clinical Sciences, College of Veterinary Medicine, The Ohio State University, Columbus, OH, USA

Nicole Cantor School of Osteopathic Medicine, Campbell University, Lillington, NC, USA

Veronica Colmenares Department of Medicine, University of Louisville, Louisville, KY, USA

Suzanne Bartholf DeWitt Centre for Cooperative Research in Biomaterials, Gipuzkoa, Spain

Deepika Dhawan Department of Veterinary Clinical Sciences, College of Veterinary Medicine, Purdue University, West Lafayette, IN, USA

William C. Eward Department of Orthopaedic Surgery, Duke University Medical Center, Durham, NC, USA

Timothy M. Fan Department of Veterinary Clinical Medicine, Cancer Center at Illinois, University of Illinois at Urbana-Champaign, Urbana, IL, USA

Peter Fecci Department of Neurosurgery, University of Colorado Anschutz Medical Campus, Aurora, CO, USA

Brian Flesner Mission Veterinary Emergency & Specialty, Mission, KS, USA

Department of Clinical Sciences & Advanced Medicine, University of Pennsylvania School of Veterinary Medicine, Philadelphia, PA, USA

Christopher M. Fulkerson Department of Veterinary Clinical Sciences, College of Veterinary Medicine, Purdue University, West Lafayette, IN, USA

Purdue University Institute for Cancer Research, West Lafayette, IN, USA

Katherine Gonzalez Department of Head and Neck Surgery & Communication Sciences, Duke University, Durham, NC, USA

Maureen Griffin Department of Clinical Sciences & Advanced Medicine, University of Pennsylvania School of Veterinary Medicine, Philadelphia, PA, USA

Noah M. Hahn Department of Oncology and Urology, Johns Hopkins University School of Medicine, Sidney Kimmel Comprehensive Cancer Center, Baltimore, MD, USA

Walter Hanel Division of Hematology, Department of Medicine, The Ohio State University Wexner Medical Center, Columbus, OH, USA

Tara M. Harrison North Carolina State University, College of Veterinary Medicine, Raleigh, NC, USA

Pooja Karukonda Department of Radiation Oncology, Duke Cancer Institute, Duke University, Durham, NC, USA

William C. Kisseberth Department of Veterinary Clinical Sciences, College of Veterinary Medicine, The Ohio State University, Columbus, OH, USA

Division of Hematology, Department of Medicine, The Ohio State University Wexner Medical Center, Columbus, OH, USA

Deborah W. Knapp Department of Veterinary Clinical Sciences, College of Veterinary Medicine, Purdue University, West Lafayette, IN, USA

Purdue University Institute for Cancer Research, West Lafayette, IN, USA

Amy LeBlanc Comparative Oncology Program, Center for Cancer Research, National Cancer Institute, National Institutes of Health, Bethesda, MD, USA

Nicole Levine Department of Orthopaedics, Duke University Medical Center, Durham, NC, USA

Charles A. Maitz College of Veterinary Medicine, University of Missouri, Columbia, MI, USA

Christopher L. Mariani Department of Small Animal Clinical Sciences, North Carolina State University, Raleigh, NC, USA

Christina Mazcko Comparative Oncology Program, Center for Cancer Research, National Cancer Institute, National Institutes of Health, Bethesda, MD, USA

Camille A. McAloney Charles River Laboratories, Mattawan, MI, USA

Isabelle McMullen College of Veterinary Medicine, North Carolina State University, Raleigh, NC, USA

Yvonne M. Mowery Department of Radiation Oncology, UPMC Hillman Cancer Center, Pittsburgh, PA, USA

Michael W. Nolan Department of Clinical Sciences, College of Veterinary Medicine, North Carolina State University, Raleigh, NC, USA

Ravi Patel UPMC Hillman Cancer Center, Pittsburg, PA, USA

Seth Pollack Division of Hematology and Oncology, Feinberg School of Medicine, Northwestern University, Chicago, IL, USA

Damon R. Reed Department of Pediatrics, Memorial Sloan Kettering Cancer Center, New York, NY, USA

Ashlyn Rickard Department of Radiation Oncology, UPMC Hillman Cancer Center, Pittsburgh, PA, USA

Ryan D. Roberts Nationwide Children's Hospital, Columbus, OH, USA

Steven T. Rosen Division of Hematology and Oncology, Feinberg School of Medicine, Northwestern University, Chicago, IL, USA

John Rossmeisl Department of Small Animal Clinical Sciences, Virginia-Maryland College of Veterinary Medicine, Virginia Polytechnic Institute and State University, Blacksburg, VA, USA

Audrey Ruple Department of Population Health Sciences, Virginia-Maryland College of Veterinary Medicine, Virginia Tech, Blacksburg, VA, USA

Beatrice Schleupner Department of Medicine, Duke University Medical Center, Durham, NC, USA

Davis M. Seelig Department of Veterinary Clinical Sciences, College of Veterinary Medicine, University of Minnesota, St. Paul, MN, USA

Laura E. Selmic Department of Veterinary Clinical Sciences, The Ohio State University, Columbus, OH, USA

Shane Sills Department of Veterinary Biosciences, College of Veterinary Medicine, The Ohio State University, Columbus, OH, USA

Jason A. Somarelli Department of Medicine, Duke University Medical Center, Durham, NC, USA

Joanne Tuohy Virginia-Maryland College of Veterinary Medicine, Virginia Polytechnic Institute and State University, Blacksburg, VA, USA

Heather Wilson-Robles Ethos Discovery, San Diego, CA, USA

Luke A. Wittenburg Department of Surgical and Radiological Sciences, Center for Companion Animal Health, School of Veterinary Medicine, University of California, Davis, Davis, CA, USA

Jedd D. Wolchok Meyer Director of the Sandra and Edward Meyer Cancer Center, Weill Cornell Medical College, Cornell University, New York, NY, USA

Ai-Ming Yu Department of Biochemistry and Molecular Medicine, School of Medicine, University of California, Davis, Sacramento, CA, USA

Background in Comparative Oncology

Introduction

Heather Wilson-Robles, Audrey Ruple,
and Laura E. Selmic

1 What Is the Value of Comparative Oncology?

The field of oncology in companion animals has expanded tremendously in the last few decades. Cancer risk has been shown to be the largest health concern among pet owners [1] and for good reason. Cancer is the leading cause of death in pet dogs over the age of 10 [1, 2]. Cancer is also a leading cause of death in people, with the lifetime risk of cancer reported as 38.5% in developed countries, with men and women at similar risk of developing cancer (26.27% and 23.96%, respectively) [3]. Cancer, as a health concern, is agnostic of species, and common themes exist among affected mammals.

Comparative oncology is a field of study adapted to investigate naturally and spontaneously developing cancers in nonhuman species as a model for human disease [4–10]. This field of study allows scientists to identify and take advantage of commonly perturbed molecular pathways or genomic aberrations to better understand the driving forces behind cancer and its progression as well as identify the most clinically relevant and druggable therapeutic targets. Cancer-associated pathways that are altered across species are likely to be the most important to study and the most clinically relevant.

The field of comparative oncology spawned from the need for more predictive clinical drug development models. Many of the novel drugs that enter human clinical trials never achieve approval due to the inability of many preclinical models to truly predict the efficacy or toxicity of these therapeutics [8, 11]. These frequent failures often result as a consequence of the limitations of each model. It is necessary to design models that can answer the complex questions necessary to move a drug forward through the development pathway [8, 12]. Unfortunately, there is no one model that is sufficient. Indeed, even humans fail to serve as effective models for cancer research as evidenced by the large number of drugs that advance from phase II to phase III clinical trials that never achieve approval. The huge amount of investment to promote a drug into phase III human clinical trials only to have it fail to receive approval can and does drive up the cost of the few that do receive approval.

In vitro *models* often utilize human tumor cell lines for the purposes of studying highly controlled conditions to study very specific

H. Wilson-Robles (✉)
Ethos Discovery, CA, USA

United Veterinary Care, Springfield, VA, USA
e-mail: heather.wilson-robles@tosvets.com

A. Ruple
Department of Population Health Sciences, Virginia-Maryland College of Veterinary Medicine, Virginia Tech, Blacksburg, VA, USA

L. E. Selmic
Department of Veterinary Clinical Sciences,
The Ohio State University, Columbus, OH, USA

M. W. Nolan et al. (eds.), *Comparative Oncology*, https://doi.org/10.1007/978-3-032-04454-9_1

scientifically directed questions. These studies are efficient, easy to conduct, fast, and cost-effective. While in vitro modeling is necessary for the early development of most anticancer therapies and is generally the first essential step for defining mechanisms of action and biomarkers of efficacy, these models lack the general complexity to efficiently predict efficacy in human patients [4]. The artificial environment in which these cells are grown selects for clones that thrive in conditions quite foreign to their natural environment. Additionally, more recent studies have highlighted the role that the microenvironment plays in cancer development and progression [13, 14]. These studies are unable to answer questions regarding drug metabolism and distribution within the host, toxicity, pharmacokinetics, and pharmacodynamics [8, 12]. Without these host–tumor interactions, one cannot hope to effectively predict a true response in a clinical patient.

The first human xenograft grown successfully in a murine model was reported in 1969 by Rygaard and Povlsen [15]. They used a nude mouse model with recessive thymic aplasia to grow xenografts generated from a 74-year-old woman with advanced colon cancer [15]. Since then, major advancements in the genetic engineering of murine models have made the mouse a fundamental part of cancer research. While more costly and time-consuming than in vitro work, the mouse has provided a model whereby tumors can be grown in three-dimensional architecture with stromal components and blood supply. These mice often grow tumors quickly that can be easily measured or assessed in the flank or mammary fat pad. Compared to human clinical trials, these studies are markedly faster and cheaper. These models can also better predict tumor responses and toxicity for cytotoxic drugs when a cytotoxic agent shows activity across xenograft models regardless of histology [16, 17]. However, when a single histology is evaluated, these models often fall short of predicting which drugs will demonstrate clinical efficacy in human patients [18–20]. Recent advances utilizing newer technologies such as the development of patient-derived xenograft (PDX) models and CRISPR-Cas9 technologies have made these models more relevant and improved their utility in cancer research [18, 21]; however, these models are not without their own pitfalls. Over time, the patient stroma is replaced with mouse stroma, and the immunosuppression needed to grow a xenograft still leads to an altered microenvironment. Additionally, as each PDX represents a single patient's disease, these results are hard to apply to the population as a whole and can be time-consuming and expensive. CRISPR-Cas9 technology has been revolutionary for the study of cancer pathogenesis and progression; however, redundancies in vital pathways can often impair interpretation of results in murine models using this technology.

Comparative oncology has the opportunity to add to advances made in both in vitro and murine models of disease (Fig. 1). While companion animals cannot replace these models, they can bridge a large gap between these models and the human patients in need of new therapies.

In most cases, comparative oncology focuses on cancer in companion canines as a model for human disease. Dogs are more similar to humans both genetically and physiologically [23]. Additionally, many of the sequences for cancer-associated genes of interest are more similar between the dog and human than the mouse and human [11]. Unlike xenograft murine models, companion canines develop spontaneous cancers in the face of an intact immune system and under similar environmental conditions as pet owners. In fact, this shared environment can be leveraged to elucidate the environmental components that are part of the etiology of cancers that occur in both humans and dogs. Investigations into environmental causes of cancer in dogs have considered both ecological-level indicators of contamination within the environment, such as industrial activity [24, 25], and exposure to specific agents known to be carcinogenic in human populations such as asbestos, pesticides, herbicides, and household chemicals [24–31].

Further, pet dogs are often treated with the same or similar chemotherapy drugs as humans which promotes similar processes of cancer progression, drug resistance, and metastasis [8].

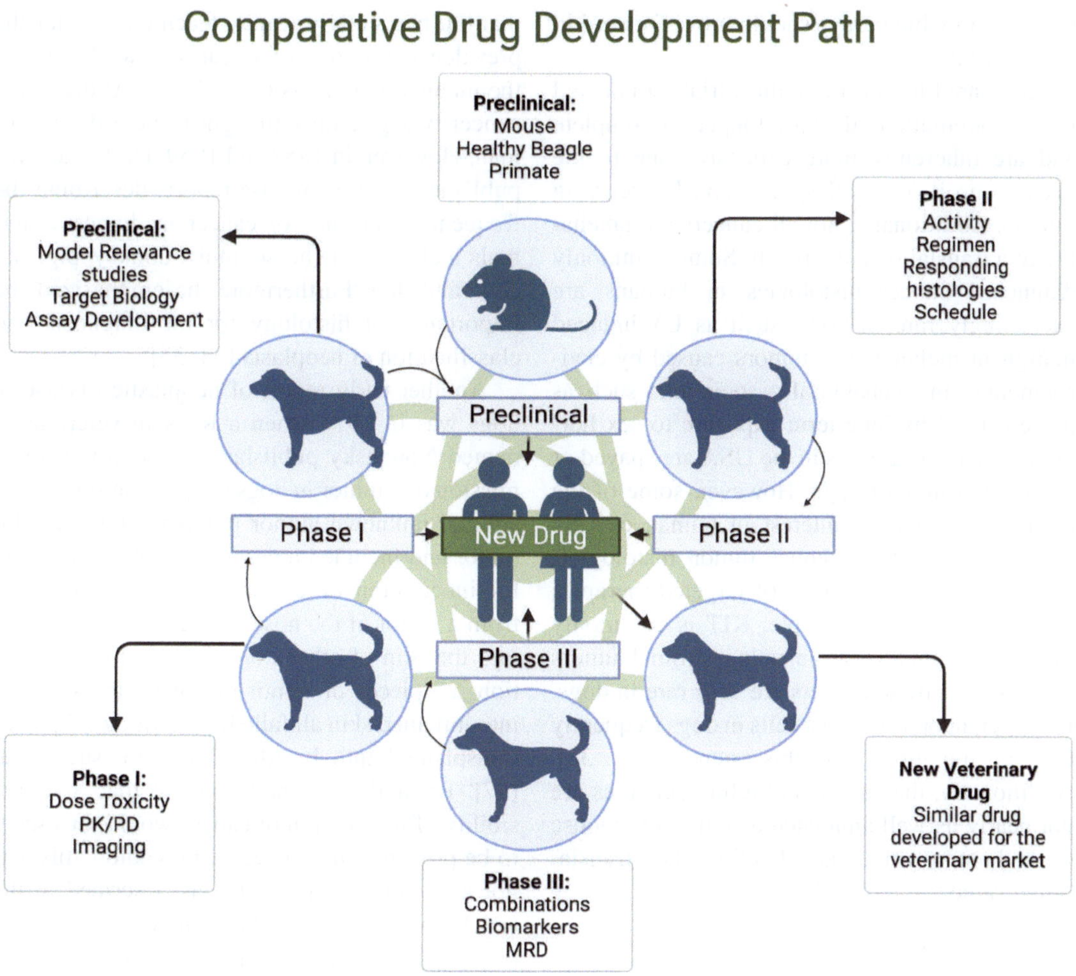

Fig. 1 Representation of a comparative oncology drug pathway to approval utilizing murine, canine, and human data [22]

Dogs also have a large body size, are genetically diverse, and process drugs in a very similar way to humans. Finally, a paucity of recognized standards of care therapies for specific diseases in dogs makes it possible to evaluate novel therapeutics up front in the naïve disease setting rather than in heavily pretreated and end-stage cancer patients. This can allow researchers to determine the utility of novel therapies in the adjuvant setting rather than in the gross disease setting, where they may be of greatest benefit to the patient population of highest need, those at risk for developing metastasis.

The use of mouse models for preclinical cancer research continues to be an important part of the field. Genetically engineered mice have allowed researchers to investigate the role of a single gene in cancer development, progression, or treatment responses. Xenograft studies lay the groundwork for treatment response to cytotoxic drugs and possible toxicities. Mouse studies can be completed rapidly and for a fraction of the cost of studies in larger mammals or humans. However, these studies tend to be biased toward false positive results as responses in a specific tumor type in mice are not predictive of a similar response in humans with the same tumor type [20]. Rather, pet dogs with spontaneous cancers can provide a necessary intermediary step between early and late phase studies in humans to best inform which drugs should move forward in clinical trials.

Compared to murine studies, trials conducted in dog populations do take longer to complete and are inherently more expensive due to the need to enroll dogs with spontaneously occurring tumors. Additionally, not all cancers are amenable to a translational approach. Some commonly diagnosed cancer histologies in humans are exceedingly rare in dogs, such as UV-induced malignant melanoma or tumors caused by environmental and behavioral associations such as those caused by long-term exposure to sex hormones as most pet dogs in the USA are spayed or neutered at an early age. However, some of the molecular targets of interest in human cancers may exist in other canine tumor histologies, allowing for investigations of targeted therapies in these cases. For example, KIT is commonly mutated in human gastrointestinal stromal tumors (GISTs), but these cancers are very rare in dogs. However, neoplastic mast cells in dogs frequently exhibit mutations in this gene [32, 33]. Additionally, the canine and feline genomes are not nearly as well annotated as either the mouse or the human which may also limit their translational value.

2 The History of Comparative Oncology

The concept of using animals as a model for disease, particularly infectious disease, is centuries old (Pastuer, Koch, Salmon). But perhaps the birthplace of the concept of comparative oncology is in London in 1802 when a member of the Medical Committee of the Society for Investigating the Nature and Cure of Cancer named Everard Home, an Examiner at the London Veterinary College, postulated whether "brute creatures are subject to any disease resembling cancer in the human body?" The group went on to publish an explanatory note associated with this query in which they asked, "what class of animals is chiefly subject to cancer: the wild or domesticated…This investigation may lead to much philosophical amusement and useful information; particularly it may teach us how far the prevalence or frequency of cancer may depend on the manner and habits of life" [33]. At that time, cancer was generally thought to be a disease of man. However, in 1858 and 1859, Dr. U. Leblanc published a series of case reports describing the frequent occurrence of cancer in domestic animals including the horse, mule, donkey, pig, cat, cow, and dog. Furthermore, he emphasized the importance of histology for the diagnosis and classification of neoplasia [34, 35].

Another early report of neoplastic disease in dogs was in 1876 when a Russian veterinarian named Nowinsky published on the coital transmission of a tumor in dogs [36]. In the same year, another unknown author published on a similar tumor and included a description of the successful inoculation of cancer in dogs using tissue from a tumor of the nose in one dog transplanted into the skin of other dogs [37]. In this description, 27 pieces of tumor that were transplanted into inflamed skin all failed, but 2 of the 15 pieces transplanted into healthy skin were successful [37]. The author's conclusion was that "the possibility of inoculation of cancer would thus seem to be proven." Of course, we now know this was not a medullary carcinoma, as described in the article, but a transmissible venereal tumor. It is one of the few tumors in mammals that can be transmitted horizontally. Professor Theobald Smith remarked "the most conspicuous investigators of human pathology have always had a yearning towards the rich fields of animal pathology" in his address to the Pathological Society of Philadelphia in 1900 [33]. Indeed, over the next 100 years, we find a smattering of publications highlighting the similarities and comparative aspects of cancers in domestic animals to those in humans, mostly from an epidemiology and pathology perspective rather than a modeling or novel therapeutics perspective [38–47].

There was very little growth in the concept of comparative oncology in the first half of the twentieth century as is echoed by Dr. W.H. Feldman in 1932: "The urge of other matters of greater pedagogic and economic interest, together with an almost invariable shortage of funds, have retarded the development of really comprehensive collections of tumours for teaching and museum purposes. Furthermore, interest in microscopic pathology is not particularly great amount many comparative pathologists."

One of the first comparative therapeutic studies published was in 1960 by Allen et al. describing the use of temporary local ligation to treat cutaneous, mammary, and testicular tumors in dogs as a method to possibly employ in humans with difficult-to-resect tumors [43]. This was followed by a 1978 study in dogs with soft tissue sarcomas of the limbs using isolated perfusion, intra-arterial infusion, and venous infusions of doxorubicin with the goal of applying the isolated perfusion model to humans in order to achieve higher therapeutic doses [48].

As a discipline, comparative oncology is relatively young, with the first publications published nearly 50 years ago [49, 50], which focused mostly on viral causes of cancer in domestic animals. In 1976, Professor E. Cotchin gave a Presidential Address to the Royal Society of Medicine entitled, "Comparative Oncology: The Veterinary Contribution," wherein he describes the history of veterinary oncology and the growing need to study a spontaneous disease model for human cancers by creating comparative oncology as a discipline [33]. Cotchin goes on to state, "I believe there is a justification for a graduate course in comparative oncology and I would not be surprised if a journal of comparative oncology were to be established" [33]. Just such a journal entitled *Veterinary and Comparative Oncology* was established in the early 2000s, with its inaugural issue published in March of 2003 under the guidance of editors Dr. David Argyle and Dr. Bruce Madewell. As recently as 35 years ago, Dr. E.G. MacEwen published one of the first articles truly focused on domestic animals as a model to study cancer biology and novel therapies [51]. This article described the biologic behavior of several common cancers in cats and dogs as well as comparative similarities between these cancers and their human counterparts. Ten years later, Dr. David Vail partnered with Dr. E.G. MacEwen to outline the advantages of studying dogs as a model for human cancers specifically. They highlighted lymphoma, osteosarcoma, soft tissue sarcomas, melanoma, and mammary tumors as models with the highest comparative interest for humans [52].

In 2003, the discipline of comparative oncology made a large leap forward with the launch of the Comparative Oncology Trials Consortium (COTC) by the National Cancer Institute (NCI) under the guidance of Dr. Chand Khanna to provide desperately needed infrastructure and resources to the cooperative efforts of several academic institutions with interest in this field [7]. This program, for the first time, provided oversight and management as well as open communication between the NCI's Comparative Oncology Program, pharmaceutical companies, nongovernmental groups, and 20 extramural academic comparative oncology groups to allow for multicenter case recruitment nationally. They also provided a pharmacodynamic core for the assessment of pharmacodynamic, biological, and pharmacokinetic end points within the COTC trials. Since their inception, the COTC has completed 15 large-scale multicenter trials with 4 additional trials ongoing and over 30 publications as a result of this research.

In 2004, the NCI also launched the Canine Comparative Oncology Genomics Consortium (CCOGC) research project in an effort to create a biospecimen repository of canine cancer, blood, urine, and tissue [53]. Tissues from the most common and translationally relevant cancer histologies were collected from multiple institutions across the USA and remain available for research use to this day.

In 2008, the LUPA project was established by the European Commission to use dogs as models for complex diseases of humans, including cancer. This project represents the collaborative efforts of 22 veterinary research centers across Europe [54]. One of the key successes of this project was the identification of key loci associated with disease susceptibility for several complex diseases that have been identified. Additionally, well-structured collaborations between veterinarians and geneticists have been generated as a result of this work [55, 56].

There have been a number of translational successes that have emerged from studies conducted in companion animals. These include the utility of L-MTP-PE for the treatment of metastatic osteosarcoma, the development of tomotherapy for advanced conformal radiation therapy delivery, the first DNA vaccine to be approved by the USDA for use in animals—ONCEPT (hCSPG4 CAR T cell therapy research is ongoing in human melanoma patients), Tanovea (rabacfosadine) for the treatment of lymphoma, as well as the use of small molecule inhibitors such as toceranib and its related compound sunitinib for the human market [32, 57–61].

3 The Future of Comparative Oncology

Compared to 20 years ago, there is an increased general awareness across all areas of medicine that species other than humans develop a variety of similar diseases spontaneously and that those animals may be a useful resource for knowledge and research that is mutually beneficial to all. However, there are still many hurdles to clear before we can actualize the full potential of Comparative Oncology.

While the annotation of the canine genome has improved significantly over the last 2 decades, it is far from complete [62]. Many of the regulatory elements such as enhancers, promoters, and transcription starting sites are still uncharacterized. While resources such as BarkBase provide an unparalleled epigenomic annotation resource for up to 27 tissue types in the dog, the atlas is far from complete for many important tissues [63]. Until the canine (and feline) genomic databases are on par with those of the mouse or human, there will always be limitations to what we can do from a comparative aspect, especially for diseases that are inherently genetic, such as cancer.

Another factor that limits comparative oncology is the difference in the comprehensiveness of medicine commonly practiced between human and veterinary species. These differences are inclusive of early detection programs that are often successful in humans, such as at-home colon cancer screening, PSA monitoring in men, and mammography in women which are virtually nonexistent in veterinary species to the level of disease staging between the two species, and finally, the level of therapeutic intervention. Veterinary patients are often diagnosed with disease once they are symptomatic for the disease. Additionally, PET scans and repeated CT scans are uncommon in veterinary patients due to cost and the need for heavy sedation or anesthesia, limiting the degree of staging that is typically done for veterinary oncology patients.

Finally, there is limited availability and access to the most specialized of veterinary oncology care, limiting our ability to make true comparisons for the dog as a model of disease. A primary example of this is metastatic disease. Many canine trials involving therapy for metastatic disease are performed in a gross disease setting rather than post metastasectomy as they often are applied in humans. Another example is the lack of canonized monoclonal antibody therapies in dogs, limiting the comparative research for many immunotherapeutic applications. Currently, these therapies are in their infancy in veterinary oncology. As they develop, our ability to thoroughly evaluate dogs (or cats) as a model for human disease will improve exponentially.

In order to push the boundaries of comparative oncology and to grow the field, we will need to continue and expand collaboration and integration of progressive veterinary programs (academic, private, and nonprofit) with progressive medical programs. While this has traditionally been limited to academic centers, there is a growing interest within private and nonprofit organizations to expand the capabilities and resources of comparative oncology through direct funding and support of clinical trial networks. With these expansions have come new advanced training programs in genomics, surgical oncology, interventional radiology, and others. These advanced training programs will help bolster research and specialized medicine programs, making them common rather than an exception in the field.

Finally, it is important to enhance communication between human and veterinary researchers through conferences and collaborations. Support for this work can be enhanced by granting agencies providing funding for collaborative comparative research as well as national and international conferences and working groups working together to solve the most important health questions for both species.

References

1. Foundation, Morris Animal (1998 and 2005) Animal health survey. News, Companion Animal, Englewood, CO
2. Fleming JM, Creevy KE, Promislow DEL (2011) Mortality in north american dogs from 1984 to 2004: an investigation into age-, size-, and breed-related causes of death. J Vet Intern Med 25(2):187–198
3. Zheng R, Wang S, Zhang S, Zeng H, Chen R, Sun K et al (2023) Global, regional, and national lifetime probabilities of developing cancer in 2020. Sci Bull (Beijing) 68(21):2620–2628
4. Oh JH, Cho JY (2023) Comparative oncology: overcoming human cancer through companion animal studies. Exp Mol Med 55(4):725–734
5. About the Comparative Oncology Program. https://ccr.cancer.gov/comparative-oncology-program/about. National Institutes of Health
6. Schiffman JD, Breen M (2015) Comparative oncology: what dogs and other species can teach us about humans with cancer. Philos Trans R Soc Lond B Biol Sci [Internet] 370(1673) Available from: https://www.ncbi.nlm.nih.gov/pubmed/26056372
7. Gordon I, Paoloni M, Mazcko C, Khanna C (2009) The comparative oncology trials consortium: using spontaneously occurring cancers in dogs to inform the cancer drug development pathway. PLoS Med 6(10):e1000161
8. Gordon IK, Khanna C (2010) Modeling opportunities in comparative oncology for drug development. ILAR J 51(3):214–220
9. Khanna C, Fan TM, Gorlick R, Helman LJ, Kleinerman ES, Adamson PC et al (2014) Toward a drug development path that targets metastatic progression in osteosarcoma. Clin Cancer Res 20(16):4200–4209
10. LeBlanc AK, Breen M, Choyke P, Dewhirst M, Fan TM, Gustafson DL et al (2016) Perspectives from man's best friend: national academy of medicine's workshop on comparative oncology. Sci Transl Med 8(324):324ps5
11. Paoloni M, Khanna C (2008) Translation of new cancer treatments from pet dogs to humans. Nat Rev Cancer 8(2):147–156
12. Riccardo F, Aurisicchio L, Impellizeri JA, Cavallo F (2015) The importance of comparative oncology in translational medicine. Cancer Immunol Immunother 64(2):137–148
13. Reinecke JB, Gross AC, Cam M, Garcia LJ, Cannon MV, Dries R et al (2024) Aberrant activation of wound healing programs within the metastatic niche facilitates lung colonization by osteosarcoma cells. bioRxiv [Internet]. Available from: https://www.ncbi.nlm.nih.gov/pubmed/38260361
14. Binnewies M, Roberts EW, Kersten K, Chan V, Fearon DF, Merad M et al (2018) Understanding the tumor immune microenvironment (TIME) for effective therapy. Nat Med 24(5):541–550
15. Rygaard J, Povlsen CO (1969) Heterotransplantation of a human malignant tumour to "nude" mice. Acta Pathol Microbiol Scand 77(4):758–760
16. Kelland LR (2004) Of mice and men: values and liabilities of the athymic nude mouse model in anticancer drug development. Eur J Cancer 40(6):827–836
17. Bibby MC (2004) Orthotopic models of cancer for preclinical drug evaluation: advantages and disadvantages. Eur J Cancer 40(6):852–857
18. Aslani S, Saad MI (2024) Patient-derived xenograft models in cancer research: methodology, applications, and future prospects. Methods Mol Biol 2806:9–18
19. Yadav R, Mahajan S, Singh H, Mehra NK, Madan J, Doijad N et al (2024) Emerging in vitro and in vivo models: Hope for the better understanding of cancer progression and treatment. Adv Biol (Weinh) 8:e2300487
20. Schuh JC (2004) Trials, tribulations, and trends in tumor modeling in mice. Toxicol Pathol 32(Suppl 1):53–66
21. Fitzmaurice C, Abate D, Abbasi N, Abbastabar H, Abd-Allah F, Abdel-Rahman O et al (2019) Global, regional, and National Cancer Incidence, mortality, years of life lost, years lived with disability, and disability-adjusted life-years for 29 cancer groups, 1990 to 2017: a systematic analysis for the global burden of disease study. JAMA Oncol 5(12):1749–1768
22. Wilson-Robles H (2025) In: BioRender (ed) Comparative oncology drug development path. https://BioRender.com/3lgs2p1
23. Goodstadt L, Ponting CP (2006) Phylogenetic reconstruction of orthology, paralogy, and conserved synteny for dog and human. PLoS Comput Biol 2(9):e133
24. Hayes HM Jr, Hoover R, Tarone RE (1981) Bladder cancer in pet dogs: a sentinel for environmental cancer? Am J Epidemiol 114(2):229–233
25. Gavazza A, Presciuttini S, Barale R, Lubas G, Gugliucci B (2001) Association between canine malignant lymphoma, living in industrial areas, and use of chemicals by dog owners. J Vet Intern Med 15(3):190–195
26. Glickman LT, Domanski LM, Maguire TG, Dubielzig RR, Churg A (1983) Mesothelioma in pet dogs associated with exposure of their owners to asbestos. Environ Res 32(2):305–313
27. Glickman LT, Raghavan M, Knapp DW, Bonney PL, Dawson MH (2004) Herbicide exposure and the risk of transitional cell carcinoma of the urinary bladder in Scottish terriers. J Am Vet Med Assoc 224(8):1290–1297
28. Glickman LT, Schofer FS, McKee LJ, Reif JS, Goldschmidt MH (1989) Epidemiologic study of

insecticide exposures, obesity, and risk of bladder cancer in household dogs. J Toxicol Environ Health 28(4):407–414
29. Takashima-Uebelhoer BB, Barber LG, Zagarins SE, Procter-Gray E, Gollenberg AL, Moore AS et al (2012) Household chemical exposures and the risk of canine malignant lymphoma, a model for human non-Hodgkin's lymphoma. Environ Res 112:171–176
30. Backer LC, Coss AM, Wolkin AF, Flanders WD, Reif JS (2008) Evaluation of associations between lifetime exposure to drinking water disinfection by-products and bladder cancer in dogs. J Am Vet Med Assoc 232(11):1663–1668
31. Backer LC, Grindem CB, Corbett WT, Cullins L, Hunter JL (2001) Pet dogs as sentinels for environmental contamination. Sci Total Environ 274(1–3):161–169
32. London CA, Malpas PB, Wood-Follis SL, Boucher JF, Rusk AW, Rosenberg MP et al (2009) Multi-center, placebo-controlled, double-blind, randomized study of oral toceranib phosphate (SU11654), a receptor tyrosine kinase inhibitor, for the treatment of dogs with recurrent (either local or distant) mast cell tumor following surgical excision. Clin Cancer Res 15(11):3856–3865
33. Cotchin E, Presidential address. (1976) Comparative oncology: the veterinary contribution. Proc R Soc Med 69(9):649–656
34. Leblanc U (1858) Recherches sur le concer des animaux. Rec med vet 35:769–93, 902–916
35. Leblanc U (1859) Recherches sur le cancer des animaux. Rec Med vet 36:25–41
36. Nowinsky M (1876) Zur Frage uber die Impfung der krebsigen Geschwulste. Centralbl F D med 14:790–791
37. Unknown (1877) Successful inoculation of cancer in dogs, 7th edn. Edinb Med J, Edinburgh, p 654
38. Jenny J (1946) On the comparative pathological anatomy of primary lung cancer, taking into account a case in horses and dogs. Schweiz Z Pathol Bakteriol 9(6):618–643
39. Scully RE, Coffin DL (1952) Canine testicular tumors with special reference to their histogenesis, comparative morphology, and endocrinology. Cancer 5(3):592–605
40. Worley G, Gorham JR (1954) The comparative pathology of rhabdomyosarcoma with a report of a case in a dog. Am J Pathol 30(4):837–849
41. Schulz LC (1958) Comparative observations on the incidence of sarcoma in man and dogs; etiology of traumatic osteogenic sarcoma. Z Krebsforsch 62(3):278–290
42. Orkin M, Schwartzman RM (1959) A comparative study of canine and human dermatology. II. Cutaneous tumors; the mast cell and canine mastocytoma. J Invest Dermatol 32(3):451–466
43. Allen FM, Kaplan MM, Meranze DR, Gradess M (1960) Treatment of spontaneous tumours by temporary local ligation. A comparative study in dogs. Bull World Health Organ 23(6):727–737
44. Mulligan RM (1963) Comparative pathology of human and canine cancer. Ann N Y Acad Sci 108:642–690
45. Owen LN (1967) Comparative aspects of bone tumours in man and dog. Proc R Soc Med 60(12):1309–1310
46. Dorn CR (1972) Comparative oncology: dogs, cats, and man. Perspect Biol Med 15(4):507–519
47. Lingeman CH, Garner FM (1972) Comparative study of intestinal adenocarcinomas of animals and man. J Natl Cancer Inst 48(2):325–346
48. Didolkar MS, Kanter PM, Baffi RR, Schwartz HS, Lopez R (1978) Comparison of regional versus systemic chemotherapy with adriamycin. Ann Surg 187(3):332–336
49. Immunity Against Cancer (1974) Use of spontaneous tumors of domestic animals as models for research: 1. Bull World Health Organ 50(6):537–548
50. Immunity Against Cancer (1974) Use of spontaneous tumors of domestic animals as models for research: 2. Bull World Health Organ 50(6):549–558
51. MacEwen EG (1990) Spontaneous tumors in dogs and cats: models for the study of cancer biology and treatment. Cancer Metastasis Rev 9(2):125–136
52. Vail DM, MacEwen EG (2000) Spontaneously occurring tumors of companion animals as models for human cancer. Cancer Investig 18(8):781–792
53. Mazcko C, Thomas R (2015) The establishment of the Pfizer-canine comparative oncology and genomics consortium biospecimen repository. Vet Sci 2(3):127–130
54. Lequarré AS, Andersson L, André C, Fredholm M, Hitte C, Leeb T et al (2011) LUPA: a European initiative taking advantage of the canine genome architecture for unravelling complex disorders in both human and dogs. Vet J 189(2):155–159
55. Vaysse A, Ratnakumar A, Derrien T, Axelsson E, Rosengren Pielberg G, Sigurdsson S et al (2011) Identification of genomic regions associated with phenotypic variation between dog breeds using selection mapping. PLoS Genet 7(10):e1002316
56. Berglund J, Nevalainen EM, Molin AM, Perloski M, André C, Zody MC et al (2012) Novel origins of copy number variation in the dog genome. Genome Biol 13(8):R73
57. Anderson P (2006) Liposomal muramyl tripeptide phosphatidyl ethanolamine: ifosfamide-containing chemotherapy in osteosarcoma. Future Oncol 2(3):333–343
58. Grosenbaugh DA, Leard AT, Bergman PJ, Klein MK, Meleo K, Susaneck S et al (2011) Safety and efficacy of a xenogeneic DNA vaccine encoding for human tyrosinase as adjunctive treatment for oral malignant melanoma in dogs following surgical excision of the primary tumor. Am J Vet Res 72(12):1631–1638
59. Forrest LJ, Mackie TR, Ruchala K, Turek M, Kapatoes J, Jaradat H et al (2004) The utility of megavoltage computed tomography images from a helical tomotherapy system for setup verification purposes. Int J Radiat Oncol Biol Phys 60(5):1639–1644

60. Vail DM, Thamm DH, Reiser H, Ray AS, Wolfgang GH, Watkins WJ et al (2009) Assessment of GS-9219 in a pet dog model of non-Hodgkin's lymphoma. Clin Cancer Res 15(10):3503–3510
61. Kropp KN, Fatho M, Huduti E, Faust M, Lübcke S, Lennerz V et al (2023) Targeting the melanoma-associated antigen CSPG4 with HLA-C*07:01-restricted T-cell receptors. Front Immunol 14:1245559
62. Wang C, Wallerman O, Arendt ML, Sundström E, Karlsson Å, Nordin J et al (2021) A novel canine reference genome resolves genomic architecture and uncovers transcript complexity. Commun Biol 4(1):185
63. Megquier K, Genereux DP, Hekman J, Swofford R, Turner-Maier J, Johnson J et al (2019) BarkBase: Epigenomic annotation of canine genomes. Genes (Basel) [Internet] 10(6) Available from: https://www.ncbi.nlm.nih.gov/pubmed/31181663

Benefits of Comparative Oncology for Human Populations

Ryan D. Roberts and Damon R. Reed

1 History of Comparative Oncology in the Study of Human Cancer

Scientists have long used animals as models of human diseases. Indeed, the modern biomedical scientific enterprise depends heavily on research that uses laboratory mice and rats, occasionally dogs and primates, and even fish as surrogates for humans when studying human diseases. We manipulate the genes of mice to study development and the interactions of specific genes and pathways. We grow tumors—sometimes human tumors—in mice so that we may test responses to candidate therapies. The screening of drugs for signs of toxicity in multiple species, often rodent and larger animals, before giving these agents to humans is not only commonplace but required.

These laboratory models of human biology and disease have proven powerful for research where many elements that cause variability can be tightly controlled. In most of these models, we control the environment, diet, treatment, and genetic background. In some systems, we can impose gene expression or eliminate gene expression, limit the manipulation of specific genes to specific tissues, and control their expression or suppression over time. The level of control that today's scientists can impose on these systems is impressive and powerful, driving many impactful discoveries.

However, these are not real-world conditions. Most of these models recapitulate very poorly the heterogeneity of human malignancies, the natural history of the disease, the variable timing of diagnosis, a microenvironment that reacts and at times unknowingly contributes throughout the process of oncogenesis, or the variable environments that surround our human patients. These shortcomings have led doctors and scientists studying human cancers to revisit comparative oncology as a mechanism for evaluating therapeutic and biological concepts in companion animals. This approach can, in many ways, correct the shortcomings of our laboratory models. After all, our pets represent a diverse population of creatures that share our diverse environments and are affected by a similar array of illnesses and diseases, including cancer, for whom we seek care from specialists when affected. Thus, wherever diseases affect both us and our animals, there exist opportunities to create systems in which we can learn from the care our animals receive, just like we do in human clinical trials.

Indeed, some aspects of malignancy can be studied more easily/effectively in dogs and other companion animals. These include the study of

R. D. Roberts (✉)
Nationwide Children's Hospital,
Columbus, OH, USA
e-mail: ryan.roberts@nationwidechildrens.org

D. R. Reed
Memorial Sloan Kettering Cancer Center,
New York, NY, USA

M. W. Nolan et al. (eds.), *Comparative Oncology*, https://doi.org/10.1007/978-3-032-04454-9_2

cancers that are prevalent in animals but rare in humans, pharmacodynamics of agents where specific toxicities are of significant concern, biology that requires manipulations not feasible in human populations such as repeat biopsies and short durations of therapy introduced prior to resection, and research that requires spontaneously arising tumors and/or intact immune systems. In each of these areas, trials completed in companion animals have informed our understanding of human disease and the development of interventions for human cancers.

While the concepts underlying comparative oncology are not new [1], research and technologies that have improved our understanding of the relationship between canine and human cancers, infrastructure that has enhanced our capacity to perform large-scale trials in veterinary patients, and improving collaboration between veterinary and human oncologists and scientists have reinvigorated interest and investment in research that integrates work being done in both human and animal species. Two landmark developments that evidence the evolution in our thinking about integrative/comparative research are the NIH-led research investment in comparative oncology and the National Academy of Medicine workshop that focused on comparative oncology.

In the early 2000s, the National Cancer Institute formally established a Comparative Oncology Program [2], tasked with promoting the study of naturally occurring cancers in dogs and other companion animals. This represented a significant investment in the concept that knowledge gained in the pursuit of biological mechanisms of and responses to therapy in canines diagnosed with cancer could inform our understanding of the human disease. This initiative drove science that created an increasingly robust foundation of information validating this integrative/comparative model. Early efforts focused largely on sarcomas, where leaders of that program saw obvious opportunities to accelerate discovery and drug development by using canine models.

The successes of the NIH program and those emerging within several academic veterinary medical centers drove interest and awareness within veterinary and human research enterprises alike. However, while the science suggested clear opportunities for comparative oncology, many struggled to figure out exactly how comparative clinical trials could best be used to improve and accelerate the process of drug development. Uncertainties about how regulatory agencies would view multiple types of data coming from canine clinical trials made those leading development efforts wary of engaging veterinary colleagues. Funding sources struggled with the potential value of applications proposing canine trials. And, few conduits existed for collaborations involving scientists and clinicians studying human diseases and those studying diseases arising in animals. This flurry of interest and environment of uncertainty prompted the US National Academy of Medicine's National Cancer Policy Forum to convene a workshop in 2015 to establish the state of the then-current science and define the most important barriers to progress in the involvement of companion animals with naturally occurring cancers in clinical trials [3]. The results of that workshop became a roadmap for accelerating and enhancing the incorporation of canine clinical trials in the drug development process.

2 Establishing Clinical Research, Regulatory, and Cross-Disciplinary Infrastructure

2.1 Comparative Oncology Trials Consortium

One early success of the NCI's Comparative Oncology Program was to establish a network of academic veterinary centers that could bring highly structured, coordinated trials to a more expansive population of animals diagnosed with cancer, mirroring the activities of the cooperative groups already established within the NCI for the conduct of human clinical trials. Some early successes, such as the completion of the first three arms of the osteosarcoma study originally funded by the Morris Animal Foundation [4, 5] established the ability of this network to design and conduct clinical research in animals that would accrue rapidly and follow standards on par with the rigor applied to human clinical trials. These successes caught the interest of several human-facing organizations, especially within pediatric oncology groups, and opened the door to an era of increased cooperation between veterinarians and human oncologists.

2.2 Inclusion of Veterinary Experts

The growth of this veterinary clinical enterprise and the recognition of its potential prompted the inclusion of veterinary oncologists in program project groups, national and international meetings, and on boards, governing bodies, and granting agencies throughout the cancer research enterprise. This was especially evident within the pediatric and sarcoma cancer research communities, where several observations suggested particularly attractive opportunities for collaboration. These included (1) specific similarities between childhood tumors and sarcomas and their canine orthologs, where these entities are rare in humans but much more common in dogs, (2) seemingly reduced barriers to research in terms of regulatory burden and cost, (3) potential flexibility in the types of trials that might be accomplished, given a less established standard of care in canines at least partially due to what owners are willing to endure. This variability allows for clever trial options such as window therapies and other differences in what types of procedures and schedules of systemic therapy deviations might be ethically acceptable in a dog versus a child, and (4) the ability to do some biological and discovery work with animals that had spontaneously arising malignancies and intact immune systems. Thus, with the emergence of organized consortia that augmented the number of potential patients and provided centralized leadership teams that could facilitate collaboration, several cooperative relationships emerged.

The efforts of several visionary organizations, foundations, and regulatory agencies helped to accelerate these collaborations. Meetings brokered by groups like the Animal Cancer Foundation and the Canines-n-Kids Foundation facilitate discussions between the multiple stakeholders, including human and veterinary clinical specialists, biologists, pharmaceutical industry representatives, regulatory entities, and philanthropic funding entities to discuss the potential of integrative drug development models and the barriers to using them. This series of meetings culminated in the National Academies of Medicine workshop, which produced the most comprehensive report on the potential of comparative oncology and identified several potential barriers preventing more wide-scale implementation of integrative development. Key statements emerging from these meetings included guidance from representatives of the Food and Drug Administration, which allayed some concerns from industry about the risks assumed when choosing to include studies exposing client-owned animals to a drug as part of a drug development plan and declarations regarding the ethics of some trial designs, which emphasized how clinical trials in animal species created ways for these animals to receive treatments that they might otherwise never be able to access.

2.3 Cancer Moonshot

One program that significantly boosted these efforts was the NIH solicitation of canine immunotherapy trials as part of the Cancer Moonshot. While the actual funding provided was not exponentially greater than those available prior to the Moonshot, the earmarking of funds for comparative oncology trials accelerated activity in the field and represented both a formal recognition of the potential for this approach to impact human disease and an endorsement of the validity of such approaches. Indeed, the resulting awards organized under the PRECINCT collaborative (PRE-medical Cancer Immunotherapy Network Canine Trials) served to advertise this overlooked resource to a much broader community of oncologists and scientists.

3 Enabling Work

While many of these large-scale efforts have accelerated the use of comparative oncology, they were only possible because of the groundwork laid by a long string of dedicated veterinary oncologists and scientists. Indeed, the concept of comparative oncology dates to Virchow, although the deliberate incorporation of (first laboratory) canines into cancer research pipelines came much later—first in the development of limb-sparing surgical procedures [6] and later in the testing of chemotherapies, beginning with nitrogen mustards [7].

More recent efforts have focused on the integration of clinical trials in companion animals with spontaneously occurring cancers (rather than laboratory-based studies using research animals where the cancer is iatrogenic) into the drug development process. These studies, however, didn't gain momentum until the early 2000s, when a large body of work documenting the similarities between canine and human cancers began to mature, and shared mechanisms of malignancy started to become clear [7]. This research continues to mature and has been critical to the incorporation of canine studies within overall drug development strategies.

3.1 Genetic Tools and Reference Datasets

Perhaps the most influential tool facilitating integrative drug development has been the ever-increasing depth and quality of genetic sequencing and genomic annotation within the canine reference datasets. These data have shown far smaller evolutionary distances between dogs and humans than between either species and the mouse [8]. The growing breadth and quality of these data have facilitated the identification of shared drivers, comparison of characteristics between species both at baseline and within the somatic mutation landscapes of their respective malignancies, and the development of research tools such as microarrays, probe sets, and analytic pipelines for diverse sequencing-based approaches. While efforts to improve the annotation of the canine genome continue and the final product remains incomplete, modern versions have become far more informative and usable, facilitating work not only within the canine species but also comparative work evaluating the similarities and differences between species. These resources have been crucial, for instance, in the elucidation of both similarities and differences between dogs and humans in key immune response mechanisms [9], the discovery of cancer susceptibility genes [10], and the identification of shared drivers in some cancer subtypes [11].

3.2 Comparative Pathology and Identification of Shared Drivers

Widespread efforts have begun to more rigorously define the similarities and differences between canine and human cancers. Driven by shared interests among veterinary and human researchers, early efforts focused on comparative analyses of specific cancer types, like osteosarcoma [12, 13], non-Hodgkin's lymphoma [14], and rare soft tissue sarcomas [15]. These efforts were inspired by apparent clinical and histological similarities in the corresponding human and canine entities, and the comparative analysis showed a high degree of genetic similarity, effectively credentialing the dog as a viable clinical/preclinical model for research.

Subsequent efforts have taken a more comprehensive, structured approach to the harmonization of human and veterinary diagnostic models. Led by coalitions of veterinary and anatomic pathologists, projects intended to clarify the relationships between the diagnostic hierarchies employed by pathologists treating both species have been undertaken for brain tumors [16, 17], soft tissue sarcomas [15], melanomas [18], and other malignancies [19]. These studies have generally revealed clear similarities across the universe of malignant entities that affect both species. However, variances in the overall incidence of cancer types and specific driver mutations leading to many of these entities certainly exist. That said, there are high-level similarities in the collection of tumor suppressor and oncogene drivers between the two species, and the histological and clinical behaviors of these entities tend to suggest common underlying biologies.

3.3 Unique Characteristics of Canine Populations

Some of the features that distinguish canine malignancies from their human counterparts can be leveraged to facilitate the study of shared diseases. The most obvious of these is the differential prevalence of cancer subtypes. While many cancer types affecting both canines and humans show a high degree of similarity, the prevalence of these entities can vary dramatically between species. This is perhaps best documented in the markedly high incidence of pediatric-type cancers and soft tissue sarcomas, which are rare within human populations but much more common in dogs. For instance, the greater numbers of canine patients with osteosarcoma and angiosarcoma coming through veterinary clinics make clinical investigations focused on canine patients have a much lower theoretical (and sometimes practical) activation energy, which has, in part, fueled the focus on these and similar diseases in the comparative oncology enterprise. This is a logical and meaningful approach since focusing on diseases more prevalent in dogs than humans can accelerate discovery that may lead to improved care for humans while maximizing the benefits that the work might have for canines, the species most impacted by the disease.

Another characteristic of canines that has facilitated discovery relevant to humans is the existence of well-established breeds with well-documented pedigrees and variable predispositions for certain cancers. This remains an active area of research, facilitated by well-documented family histories in breeds with diverse baseline risks for specific malignancies. Perhaps the most expansive effort supporting this work has been the Dog10K Project, an international consortium aiming to generate a massive database of well-annotated whole-genome sequencing from 10,000 individual canines [20]. As of 2022, this collaborative had published more than 2000 sequenced and annotated genomes, making it one of the largest resources for genotype-phenotype and evolutionary discovery. One of the established subprojects in this collaborative is focused on elucidating the genomic features that drive breed-related cancer predisposition. This project has also fueled the development of a more robust canine reference genome with more detailed and rigorous annotation [21], which facilitates many aspects of comparative oncology.

Finally, the study of similar cancers across multiple species has presented significant opportunities for identifying true drivers of disease. One phenomenon that has facilitated this type of cross-species discovery has been that, while mammals share most genes in their genomes, evolution has reorganized the genes of each species across different numbers of chromosomes, each arranged differently. This variability in genomic organization has proven useful in identifying the true driver genes in several different diseases [22, 23].

4 Clinical Trials

The impacts that research leveraging comparative oncology has had on human medicine have been both concrete and conceptual. These impacts range from canine clinical trials that have supported New Drug Applications to clinical trials that have addressed questions related to sequencing, pharmacodynamics, and combinatorial toxicities to conceptual innovations that have advanced our understanding of biological mechanisms common to both species. Many of those impacts are detailed in subsequent chapters of this work, but a few examples include:

4.1 Internal Prostheses

Many of the orthopedic techniques and technologies utilized today to preserve functional limbs while removing large tumors were pioneered and optimized in veterinary clinics [6], where smaller bodies reduce mechanical stresses, and regulatory timelines can be significantly shorter.

4.2 Biologic Therapies

Several lines of foundational work leveraging innovative biologic therapies for cancer treatment have found their start in comparative oncology trials. For instance, veterinary oncology studies reporting prolonged disease-free survival in dogs receiving postresection muramyl tripeptide (MTP-PE, a macrophage-activating compound isolated from bacterial cell walls) for hemangiosarcoma [24], osteosarcoma [25], and melanoma [26] prompted a series of large, multinational human trials that ultimately led to EMA approval [27]. More recently, veterinary oncologists reported significant activity for an attenuated listeria preparation engineered to express a tumor antigen [28] in the treatment of dogs with osteosarcoma. This prompted the development of much larger clinical trials in both dogs [29] and humans. These trials are informing ongoing development of the preparation.

4.3 Immuno-Oncology Approaches

While a series of expansive developments in the realm of immuno-oncology have transformed care for patients with many diseases, accurate laboratory models facilitating the mechanistic study of these immune-related phenomena and of novel combinations and treatment approaches have been challenging to develop since many laboratory models of human cancers require the use of immune-deficient mice. Comparative oncology presents a powerful tool for studying these immune-dependent therapeutics. Through collaborative efforts like PRECINCT, veterinary and medical scientists have evaluated immune therapies for osteosarcoma [30], diffuse large B cell lymphoma [31], glioblastoma [32], and generalized NK-cell therapies [33]. These projects have informed ongoing development, with successor trials in human patients now active for most of these approaches.

4.4 Targeted Therapeutics

Growing numbers of clinical trials utilizing canine companion animals diagnosed with spontaneously occurring malignancies have evaluated small molecule inhibitors during the preclinical and clinical development process. These have included clinical trials of KIT inhibitors [5], BTK inhibitors [34], HSP90 inhibitors [35], and XPO1 inhibitors [36], among others. The results of these trials have informed ongoing development decisions that ultimately led to definitive human trials and, in many cases, FDA approval.

5 Limitations

There remain limitations in the extent to which spontaneously occurring malignancies in canines and other animals can be used as models of human disease. Most obviously, not all canine malignancies have clear human disease orthologs, nor do all human diseases have obvious canine correlates. Indeed, as many of the above efforts begin to address these similarities and differences more rigorously and comprehensively, it has become clear that there can be caveats to the conclusions that may be drawn from comparative studies. While these studies often provide insights, they should be interpreted with caution. Dogs are not four-legged humans, and comparative trials will never replace human trials.

One important way in which clinical trial results may differ between species emerges from the fact that very similar tumor types arising in humans and dogs often exhibit both shared and divergent drivers and modifiers of malignant behavior. Indeed, even the physiologically normal wiring of cellular processes can differ in subtle but important ways. While responses to targeting agents are usually similar between species, these differences can sometimes lead to unanticipated divergence in the response to targeted therapeutics.

These differences are perhaps most obvious in the realm of immuno-oncology. While canine and human immune systems are, at a very high level, almost identical, the specific mediators of some intercellular interactions and the biology of checkpoint systems do differ between species. As is evident in the trials mentioned above and detailed in subsequent chapters, this does not preclude the utility of comparative oncology, though an understanding of the similarities and differences is essential to the accurate interpretation of results.

While our understanding of the biological similarities and differences between dogs and humans has improved dramatically over the last decade, the larger efforts to date have (appropriately) focused largely on the identification of similarities between species, seeking to justify comparative approaches. In the next generation, a more sophisticated research agenda focused on elucidating the nuances inherent to both the similarities and distinctions of species- and tumor-specific biology will be essential if we are to realize the true potential of comparative oncology.

Even when disease drivers and signaling pathways are identical between species, subtle differences in the structures and sequences of target genes can dramatically affect the way that drugs bind those targets (or don't). Combined with frequent interspecies variability in the pharmacokinetics of individual drugs, this can create challenges in modeling how a drug might behave in a human versus a canine and can complicate the interpretation of concepts like target coverage and therapeutic window. Examples of cases where these differences created significant problems abound, but an obvious example is MDM2 inhibitors, where the agents' enhanced engagement of their target in humans (relative to dogs and mice) led to the late recognition of a profound dose-limiting thrombocytopenia, which was not wholly appreciated in the preclinical studies [37].

Sometimes, the limitations of comparative oncology are more practical. This is most evident in the different capacities of our veterinary and medical care systems to provide supportive care. Culturally, we will tolerate the increased risk and cost associated with providing treatments that require prolonged hospitalizations or expensive supportive interventions for the treatment of humans much more readily than for the treatment of companion animals. Indeed, many standard-of-care therapies are difficult to translate directly to the realm of veterinary medicine simply because the intensive resources needed to provide the associated supportive care are not readily available or accepted by owners.

6 Conclusions

Comparative oncology leverages naturally occurring cancers in companion animals, particularly dogs, to bridge the gap between traditional laboratory models and real-world clinical trials in humans with cancer. By integrating veterinary clinical trials into the cancer research pipeline, scientists have gained valuable insights into tumor biology, drug responses, and immunotherapy, accelerating the development of many novel treatments. Programs like the NCI's Comparative Oncology Program and other emerging collaborative networks are facilitating this approach, leading to advancements in targeted therapies and immuno-oncology while fostering partnerships between veterinary and human oncologists.

Despite its promise, comparative oncology faces challenges, including species-specific differences in some cancer genetics and nuanced differences in the biology of immune responses, as well as regulatory and ethical complexity. While comparative oncology cannot replace human clinical trials, strengths include the ability to leverage these naturally occurring malignancies as a tool that enhances our understanding and, in certain cases, can speed up drug development. Continued investment, enhanced collaboration, establishment of more sophisticated resources, and refinement of methodologies will be crucial to realizing the potential of this approach for improving cancer treatment for humans—and for dogs.

References

1. LeBlanc AK et al (2016) Perspectives from man's best friend: National Academy of medicine's workshop on comparative oncology. Sci Transl Med 8:324ps5
2. Khanna C et al (2009) Guiding the optimal translation of new cancer treatments from canine to human cancer patients. Clin Cancer Res 15(18):5671–5677
3. Nass SJ et al (2015) The role of clinical studies for pets with naturally occurring tumors in translational cancer research
4. Leblanc AK et al (2021) Adjuvant Sirolimus does not improve outcome in pet dogs receiving standard-of-care therapy for appendicular osteosarcoma: a prospective, randomized trial of 324 dogs. Clin Cancer Res 27(11):3005–3016
5. Mason NJ et al (2024) Immunological responses and clinical outcomes in pet dogs with osteosarcoma receiving standard of care therapy and a recombinant Listeria vaccine expressing HER2/neu. Mol Ther 33:1674
6. Forriol F (2016) History of surgery for limb bone tumors. Springer International Publishing, pp 1–26
7. Hansen K, Khanna C (2004) Spontaneous and genetically engineered animal models: use in preclinical cancer drug development. Eur J Cancer 40(6):858–880
8. Kirkness EF et al (2003) The dog genome: survey sequencing and comparative analysis. Science 301(5641):1898–1903
9. Mason NJ (2020) Comparative immunology and immunotherapy of canine osteosarcoma. In: Current advances in the science of osteosarcoma: research perspectives: tumor biology, organ microenvironment, potential new therapeutic targets, and canine models, pp 199–221
10. Hédan B et al (2021) Identification of common predisposing loci to hematopoietic cancers in four dog breeds. PLoS Genet 17(4):e1009395
11. Rodrigues L et al (2023) Shared hotspot mutations in oncogenes position dogs as an unparalleled comparative model for precision therapeutics. Sci Rep 13(1)
12. Gardner HL et al (2019) Canine osteosarcoma genome sequencing identifies recurrent mutations in DMD and the histone methyltransferase gene SETD2. Commun Biol 2(1)
13. Paoloni M et al (2009) Canine tumor cross-species genomics uncovers targets linked to osteosarcoma progression. BMC Genomics 10:625
14. Ito D, Frantz AM, Modiano JF (2014) Canine lymphoma as a comparative model for human non-Hodgkin lymphoma: recent progress and applications. Vet Immunol Immunopathol 159(3–4):192–201
15. Milovancev M et al (2015) Comparative pathology of canine soft tissue sarcomas: possible models of human non-rhabdomyosarcoma soft tissue sarcomas. J Comp Pathol 152(1):22–27
16. Koehler JW et al (2018) A revised diagnostic classification of canine glioma: towards validation of the canine glioma patient as a naturally occurring preclinical model for human glioma. J Neuropathol Exp Neurol 77(11):1039–1054
17. Leblanc AK et al (2016) Creation of an NCI comparative brain tumor consortium: informing the translation of new knowledge from canine to human brain tumor patients. Neuro-Oncology 18(9):1209–1218
18. Simpson RM et al (2014) Sporadic naturally occurring melanoma in dogs as a preclinical model for human melanoma. Pigment Cell Melanoma Res 27(1):37–47
19. Avallone G et al (2021) Review of histological grading systems in veterinary medicine. Vet Pathol 58(5):809–828
20. Meadows JRS et al (2023) Genome sequencing of 2000 canids by the Dog10K consortium advances the understanding of demography, genome function and architecture. Genome Biol 24(1)
21. Jagannathan V et al (2021) Dog10K_Boxer_Tasha_1.0: a long-read assembly of the dog reference genome. Genes 12(6):847
22. Shapiro SG et al (2015) Canine urothelial carcinoma: genomically aberrant and comparatively relevant. Chromosom Res 23(2):311–331
23. Thomas R et al (2009) 'Putting our heads together': insights into genomic conservation between human and canine intracranial tumors. J Neuro-Oncol 94:333–349
24. Vail DM, MacEwen EG, Kurzman ID, Dubielzig RR, Helfand SC, Kisseberth WC, London CA, Obradovich JE, Madewell BR, Rodriguez CO Jr (1995) Liposome-encapsulated muramyl tripeptide phosphatidylethanolamine adjuvant immunotherapy for splenic hemangiosarcoma in the dog: a randomized multi-institutional clinical trial. Clin Cancer Res 1(10):1165–1170
25. Kurzman ID et al (1995) Adjuvant therapy for osteosarcoma in dogs: results of randomized clinical trials using combined liposome-encapsulated muramyl tripeptide and cisplatin. Clin Cancer Res 1(12):1595–1601
26. MacEwen EG et al (1999) Adjuvant therapy for melanoma in dogs: results of randomized clinical trials using surgery, liposome-encapsulated muramyl tripeptide, and granulocyte macrophage colony-stimulating factor. Clin Cancer Res 5(12):4249–4258
27. Meyers PA et al (2005) Osteosarcoma: a randomized, prospective trial of the addition of Ifosfamide and/or Muramyl tripeptide to cisplatin, doxorubicin, and high-dose methotrexate. J Clin Oncol 23(9):2004–2011
28. Mason NJ et al (2016) Immunotherapy with a HER2-targeting listeria induces HER2-specific immunity

and demonstrates potential therapeutic effects in a phase I trial in canine osteosarcoma. Clin Cancer Res 22(17):4380–4390
29. Mason NJ et al (2025) Immunological responses and clinical outcomes in pet dogs with osteosarcoma receiving standard of care therapy and a recombinant listeria vaccine expressing HER2/neu. Mol Ther 33:1674
30. Regan DP et al (2022) Losartan blocks osteosarcoma-elicited monocyte recruitment, and combined with the kinase inhibitor Toceranib, exerts significant clinical benefit in canine metastatic osteosarcoma. Clin Cancer Res 28(4):662–676
31. McLinden GP et al (2024) Safety and biologic activity of a canin anti-CD20 monoclonal antibody in dogs with diffuse large B-cell lymphoma. J Vet Intern Med 38(3):1666–1674
32. Chambers MR et al (2020) The one health consortium: design of a Phase I clinical trial to evaluate M032, a genetically engineered HSV-1 expressing IL-12, in combination with a checkpoint inhibitor in canine patients with sporadic high grade gliomas. Front Surg 7
33. Razmara AM et al (2024) Preclinical evaluation and first-in-dog clinical trials of PBMC-expanded natural killer cells for adoptive immunotherapy in dogs with cancer. J Immunother Cancer 12(4):e007963
34. Honigberg LA et al (2010) The Bruton tyrosine kinase inhibitor PCI-32765 blocks B-cell activation and is efficacious in models of autoimmune disease and B-cell malignancy. Proc Natl Acad Sci 107(29):13075–13080
35. London CA et al (2011) Phase I evaluation of STA-1474, a prodrug of the novel HSP90 inhibitor Ganetespib, in dogs with spontaneous cancer. PLoS One 6(11):e27018
36. London CA et al (2014) Preclinical evaluation of the novel, orally bioavailable selective inhibitor of nuclear export (SINE) KPT-335 in spontaneous canine cancer: results of a phase I study. PLoS One 9(2):e87585
37. Wang W et al (2024) MDM2 inhibitors for cancer therapy: the past, present, and future. Pharmacol Rev 76(3):414–453

Comparative Oncology: Evaluation of Oncology Across Nondomestic Species

Tara M. Harrison

Neoplasia has been diagnosed in a wide range of species, and the fossil record provides evidence that cancer as a disease complex dates back at least 75 million years (Ekhtiari et al. [68] The Lancet Oncology). Nonetheless, little is known about neoplasia in nondomestic species.

Information on cancer in nondomestic animals has previously existed solely as case reports, case series, or single institution or laboratory summaries. While this information is valuable, the current state of knowledge essentially exists as a collection of anecdotes devoid of a systematic approach to research, and the data have not been gathered and analyzed in a manner which allows broad interpretation and generalization. For many species, the epidemiology, natural history, biology, and clinical behavior of neoplasia are truly unknown. Further, many of these neoplasms, treatments, and survival expectations are extrapolated from treatment doses and survival times determined in domestic animals. In fact, a true species-specific constant (K in the Meeh's formula) to establish proper body surface area is not even known for many nondomestic species and is estimated based on other animal species [31]. Additionally, pharmacokinetic and pharmacodynamic studies have not been performed in most species, and as such, the choices for treatment are typically based on experiences in domestic animals or humans.

As a general observation of the published literature describing disease in nondomestic animals, reports of neoplasia are more common in mammals than nonmammalian species. This is unsurprising and similar to the clinical experience in veterinary medicine as it is far more common for owners of mammalian pets to seek veterinary care. Likewise, in zoological and aquarium institutions, there historically has been an apparent bias toward focusing diagnostic resources (including performing necropsies) on mammals. Also contributing to the relative infrequency of reporting neoplasia in reptiles, amphibians, birds, and fish could be that cancer is more challenging to diagnose in these species (e.g., because their bodies are prone to becoming rapidly autolyzed—with that often happening before a full necropsy can be performed). That said, many institutions and even private/pet owners have shifted toward performing more routine examinations on reptiles, amphibians, birds, and fish than previously, and these exams frequently include advanced diagnostic procedures which can lead to earlier diagnosis of neoplasia. Additionally, with many nondomestic animals, infectious disease previously had been a major cause of death, and with increased preventive medicine and routine medical care, it has allowed animals to live longer lives and develop other

T. M. Harrison (✉)
North Carolina State University, College of Veterinary Medicine, Raleigh, NC, USA
e-mail: tmharri7@ncsu.edu

M. W. Nolan et al. (eds.), *Comparative Oncology*, https://doi.org/10.1007/978-3-032-04454-9_3

conditions that were previously unreported, such as neoplasia.

Multiple studies have focused on specific neoplasms in animals, with many attempting to determine the prevalence and frequency of neoplasia in domesticated species [15, 42, 54]. More recently, interest has grown in evaluating the evolutionary aspects of neoplasia across species. One prominent theory, first proposed by Peto in 1977, suggests that cancer risk is linked to an animal's number of cells and lifespan [48]. However, further research has shown that the prevalence of neoplasia does not necessarily increase with body size and lifespan, a phenomenon now known as "Peto's paradox" [44]. Perhaps the best-known example of this paradox is found in elephants, where the prevalence of malignant neoplasia appeared to be remarkably low despite their large body size and long lifespan [1]. This resistance to cancer was attributed to their 20 copies (40 alleles) of the TP53 gene, which plays a crucial role in tumor suppression [1]. However, a recent paper has reported a higher prevalence of neoplasia in elephants, yet research on elephant TP53 is continuing [69].

Many studies on comparative oncology in nondomestic species face challenges related to limited data availability, small sample sizes, and inconsistency. Additionally, researchers often lack access to entire populations, leading to generalizations about the most common neoplasms in a species based solely on data from specific laboratories or institutions. While some ongoing studies aim to conduct population-wide evaluations, data accessibility remains a significant challenge.

1 Comparative Oncology

There have been reports that certain species such as naked mole rats and sharks do not develop cancer [46, 50, 55]. These reports have been proven to not be entirely accurate as these animals do develop cancer, but perhaps at different rates than expected [4, 28, 57]. Turtles are another species with a notably low reported prevalence of neoplasia [8]. A large-scale study examining cancer prevalence across approximately 1000 animal species found that cancer was more common in squamates and mammals, while turtles exhibited remarkably low rates of neoplasia [8]. However, no current studies have explored potential links between turtle physiology and human cancer.

Among nonhuman species, primates share the most genetic similarity with humans, making them particularly relevant for comparative oncology research. Despite this, some cancers, such as carcinomas, appear to be less frequently reported in chimpanzees, our closest relatives [36, 61]. Beyond traditional models like mice and domestic dogs, researchers are increasingly investigating zoological species with similarities to human cancers. For example, ovarian cancer in jaguars and liver cancer in lemurs are being studied for their potential relevance to human oncology [12, 19]. Additional research is underway to evaluate cancer prevalence across species using necropsy records for 16,049 individual animals and 292 species as it is suspected that there may be additional models for cancer that are housed within zoological and aquarium institutions. Recent research has found that neoplasia but not malignancy prevalence increased with the weight of the animal as an adult but decreased with longer gestation time; it also found that mammals had greater prevalence of neoplasia than birds, reptiles, and amphibians [11] (Fig. 1). The findings in Compton et al. contrast with Peto's paradox in observing that larger and longer-lived animals do get neoplasia, which is also confirmed with Bulls et al.'s study as well [8, 11]. These comparative evaluations of neoplasia are important to gain a better understanding of the evolution of neoplasia as well as the overall prevalence of neoplasia across species and may aid in discovering additional animal models for human cancers.

Treatment of neoplasia across species has been challenging for zoo, aquatic, and exotic animal veterinarians. In many instances, there has been extrapolation of the cancer biology, treatment dosing, and regimens from work done in the field of domestic canine and feline oncology [20]. This is not ideal as treatments for neoplasia are not equal across species, and some medications, such as cisplatin, are toxic in some domestic

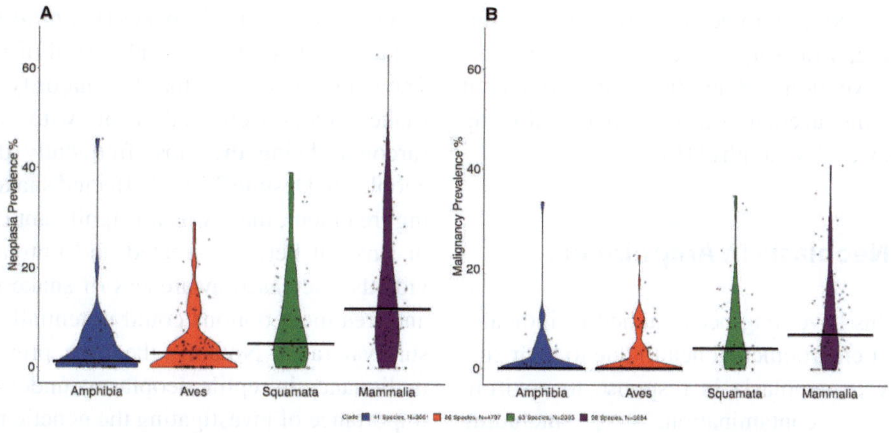

Fig. 1 Distributions of neoplasia (**a**) and malignancy (**b**) prevalences across four clades of animals, Amphibia, Aves, Squamata, and Mammalia [11]

species but an effective form of therapy in other animals [33]. As such, a greater understanding of which treatments can be tolerated and the appropriate dosage range for nondomestic species is warranted.

Further, most chemotherapy dosing has been calculated using body surface area calculations. As mentioned previously, the K constant for the body surface area equation does not exist for many nondomestic species. K constants are being developed for amphibians, bearded dragons, snakes, ferrets, and stingrays to improve calculations for chemotherapy medications and to improve appropriate dosing of medications, but much work is left to be done [9, 25, 30, 31].

2 Neoplasia in Fish

Comparative neoplasia research in fish has been studied in laboratory settings for some time [6, 10, 38]. More recently, research on naturally occurring neoplasia in fish has expanded, particularly through enhanced preventive medicine programs in aquarium facilities [16, 67]. Diagnosing and treating neoplastic disease in aquatic species presents unique challenges, as these animals are often housed in group exhibits or within shared water systems. While some facilities have designated medical pools or separate treatment areas, relocating an individual fish to an independent system is not always feasible. Additionally, biosecurity concerns may limit the use of chemotherapy.

Neoplasia prevalence in fish has been evaluated in several studies. A single-aquarium study examining 62 fish (37 species, including two elasmobranchs) found that freshwater fish had a higher incidence of neoplasia compared to saltwater species, with elasmobranchs being the least affected [67]. Similarly, a laboratory study reported a low cancer prevalence of 0.4% in elasmobranchs [17]. In the Wright et al. study, most fish neoplasms were malignant, with lymphoma being the most common diagnosis—half of those cases occurred in tropical freshwater fish. Additionally, iridophoromas (pigment cell tumors) were frequently reported, consistent with previous findings in reptiles [40, 66].

A broader study by Ferraro et al. examined neoplasia prevalence across multiple institutions and laboratories, identifying 455 cases across 178 fish species [16]. Koi (*Cyprinus rubrofuscus*) and goldfish (*Carassius auratus*) were the most commonly affected species. The average age at diagnosis was 8.25 years, with soft tissue sarcomas being the most frequently reported neoplasm. The eye was the most common tumor site. Among cases where sex was reported, 19.3% were female and 17.8% male, with the remaining fish having an unreported sex. Regarding treatment, only 2.86% of cases in the Ferraro et al.

study received chemotherapy, surgery, or supportive care, with surgery being the most common intervention. Regardless of treatment modality, the average survival time following diagnosis was 8.8 months [16].

3 Neoplasia in Amphibians

Amphibians have long been studied as indicator species for environmental health due to their susceptibility to neoplasia in response to environmental contamination, including chemotherapeutic exposure [34]. In fact, amphibians have been a primary focus of research on neoplasms in lesser vertebrates [32, 39]. While their relevance to human neoplasia is recognized, the understanding of naturally occurring neoplasia in amphibians has been limited until recently.

A review of the literature identified 50 cases of naturally occurring neoplasms in amphibians, with an average age at diagnosis of 5.7 years [27]. The study found that amphibians had an average survival time of 6.6 months post-diagnosis, with females affected more frequently than males. Neoplasia was most commonly reported in African clawed frogs (*Xenopus laevis*) and axolotls (*Ambystoma mexicanum*), with chromatophoromas and lymphoma/leukemia being the most frequently diagnosed neoplasms [27]. Improving the understanding of naturally occurring amphibian neoplasia may provide valuable insights and potential correlations to human cancers, fostering further research in comparative oncology.

4 Neoplasia in Reptiles

Neoplasia is reported in reptiles, with snakes being the most frequently affected group [8, 14]. One study reported on neoplasia in 133 snakes across 65 species, identifying common or northern watersnakes (*Nerodia sipedon*), eastern diamond-backed rattlesnakes (*Crotalus adamanteus*), and timber rattlesnakes (*Crotalus horridus*) as having the highest prevalence of disease [14]. The study also found that the majority (87%) of snake tumors were malignant, with soft tissue sarcomas being the most frequently diagnosed neoplasm. Despite 27% of affected snakes receiving treatment, there was no significant difference in survival between treated and untreated individuals. Increased awareness of snake neoplasia and treatment options could potentially improve survival rates. Notably, the high prevalence of malignancy in reptile neoplasms underscores the importance of investigating the genetic mutations that may predispose these animals to cancer, which could have implications for human oncology.

Lizards are also commonly affected by neoplasia. A study analyzing a cancer database and literature reports documented 55 cases in a database and 219 cases from published studies [66]. This study found that Komodo dragons and Savannah monitors had a higher likelihood of mortality due to neoplasia compared to other species. Additionally, leukemia and islet cell carcinoma were significantly associated with neoplasia-related deaths, whereas chondrosarcoma, myxosarcoma, osteosarcoma, and squamous cell carcinoma were more commonly associated with non-neoplastic-related deaths [66]. Similar to snakes, lizards had a higher proportion of malignant neoplasia than benign cases. Furthermore, treatment outcomes indicated that animals receiving surgery or radiation therapy alone were significantly more likely to die from non-neoplastic-related causes [66].

Although the proportion of benign neoplasia in lizards was higher than in snakes, the prevalence of malignant neoplasia remains significant [14]. To date, reptile neoplasia has not been explored for comparative oncology research. Given the high prevalence of malignancy in both snakes and lizards, further investigation into reptile cancers could provide valuable insights into tumor biology and potential translational applications in human medicine.

5 Neoplasia in Avians

With advancements in husbandry and infectious disease prevention, neoplasia is becoming a growing concern in avian patients [51]. Unsurprisingly, psittacines—particularly budgerigars—are most commonly diagnosed with neoplasia, likely due to their popularity as pet birds, which may contribute to submission bias [51]. Further, budgerigars are most often kept in human homes, and this link with neoplasia should be further explored.

Although avian neoplasia has not been a major focus in comparative oncology, some research explores shared avian and human infections, such as malaria, as potential models for human brain cancer [56, 65]. Additionally, chickens have been studied as models for spontaneous ovarian cancer in humans, showing comparable gene expression patterns [43, 56]. Expanding oncology research beyond poultry could provide further insights, as many pet birds live in close proximity to humans, share dietary habits, and can live for 50 years or more, exposing them to similar environmental risk factors over long periods of time. Thus, pet birds may well be the new “canaries in the coal mine” in that they may serve as indicator organisms for modern-day life.

6 Neoplasia in Nondomestic Mammals

Neoplasia is most commonly reported in mammalian species [11], likely because exotic and nontraditional mammals are more frequently examined and treated in preventive veterinary care compared to other exotic species. Among mammals, marine species tend to have fewer reported tumors than their land-dwelling counterparts, though cases of squamous cell carcinoma have been documented in dolphins [3].

Among terrestrial mammals diagnosed with neoplasia, felids are overrepresented, with big cats—such as lions, jaguars, and tigers—being the most commonly affected [11, 41]. Lymphoma is the most frequently reported neoplasm in big cats, and when diagnosed early, treatment can be effective, with reported survival times exceeding 1 year [21, 22]. Other commonly affected mammals include opossums and domestic ferrets [11]. In fact, ferrets are one of the most frequently treated zoological companion animals in private clinical practice for neoplasia, with common tumor types including insulinoma, adrenal neoplasia, and lymphoma [53]. In contrast, chinchillas are the least likely zoological companion animals to develop cancer [26].

Among small mammals, rats most commonly develop benign mammary fibroadenomas, which have been linked to pituitary adenomas [62]. While deslorelin implants have been tested as a treatment, early ovariohysterectomy appears to be the most effective preventive measure [63]. Small mammals have long been used as models for induced neoplasia in oncologic research [37, 45, 60, 64]. However, limitations exist in studying specific cancer types and advanced cancer conditions such as cancer cachexia, and naturally occurring cancers. Expanding research to include a broader range of species with spontaneous neoplasia could improve cancer modeling and lead to more effective treatments [18, 23, 29, 35, 47, 59].

7 Summary

Neoplasia is widely reported across nondomestic species, though diagnosis and treatment remain less common and less advanced compared to domestic animals. Ongoing research, including efforts by Exotic Species Cancer Research Alliance (ESCRA), is improving our understanding of neoplasia prevalence and advancing effective therapies in exotic species, helping to raise awareness and encourage continued treatment. While the true prevalence of neoplasia across species is still being investigated, these insights contribute to the development and refinement of spontaneous cancer models for comparative oncology research—building on existing models in zebrafish, chickens, rabbits, and elephants.

References

1. Abegglen LM, Caulin AF, Chan A, Lee K, Robinson R, Campbell MS, Kiso WK, Schmitt DL, Waddell PJ, Bhaskara S, Jensen ST, Maley CC, Schiffman JD (2015) Potential mechanisms for cancer resistance in elephants and comparative cellular response to DNA damage in humans. JAMA 314:1850–1860
2. Abegglen LM, Harrison TM, Moresco A, Fowles JS, Troan BV, Kiso WK, Schmitt D, Boddy AM, Schiffman JD (2022) Of elephants and other mammals: a comparative review of reproductive tumors and potential impact on conservation. Animals (Basel) 12:2005
3. Alves-Motta MR, Luz-Carvalho V, Nunes-Pinheiro DCS, Groch KR, Gonçalves-Pereira L, Sánchez-Sarmiento AM, Sacristán C, Catão-Dias JL, Díaz-Delgado J (2020) Facial squamous cell carcinoma and abdominal peripheral nerve sheath tumour with Rhabdomyoblastic differentiation in a rough-toothed dolphin (Steno bredanensis). J Comp Pathol 176:122–127
4. Archer KR, Groll T, Harvey RJ, Thornton SM, Stidworthy MF, Denk D (2023) Case series: lymphoid neoplasia in three elasmobranch species. J Fish Dis 46:273–279
5. Beck J, Ren L, Huang S, Berger E, Bardales K, Mannheimer J, Mazcko C, Leblanc A (2022) Canine and murine models of osteosarcoma. Vet Pathol 59:399–414
6. Berghmans S, Murphey RD, Wienholds E, Neuberg D, Kutok JL, Fletcher CD, Morris JP, Liu TX, Schulte-Merker S, Kanki JP, Plasterk R, Zon LI, Look AT (2005) tp53 mutant zebrafish develop malignant peripheral nerve sheath tumors. Proc Natl Acad Sci USA 102:407–412
7. Browning HM, Gulland FM, Hammond JA, Colegrove KM, Hall AJ (2015) Common cancer in a wild animal: the California Sea lion (Zalophus californianus) as an emerging model for carcinogenesis. Philos Trans R Soc Lond Ser B Biol Sci 370:20140228
8. Bulls SE, Platner L, Ayub W, Moreno N, Arditi JP, Dreyer S, McCain S, Wagner P, Burgstaller S, Davis LR (2022) Cancer prevalence is related to body mass and lifespan in tetrapods and remarkably low in turtles. *bioRxiv*, 2022.07. 12.499088
9. Calcagno JN, Nelson NC, Duke EG, Harrison TM (2023) Defining a species-specific K constant in American bullfrogs (Lithobates catesbeianus) through use of computed tomography. Am J Vet Res 84:1
10. Choorapoikayil S, Kuiper RV, De Bruin A, Den Hertog J (2012) Haploinsufficiency of the genes encoding the tumor suppressor Pten predisposes zebrafish to hemangiosarcoma. Dis Model Mech 5:241–247
11. Compton ZT, Mellon W et al (2024) Cancer prevalence across vertebrates. *bioRxiv*, 2023.02.15.527881
12. Corner S, Parys M, Moresco A, Yuzbasiyan-Gurkan V, Agnew D (2017) TMEM-020: ovarian adenocarcinoma in jaguars (Panthera ONCA): a naturally-occurring model of human inherited ovarian cancer? In: Proceedings of the 11th biennial ovarian cancer research symposium, Seattle
13. Cutler DC, Shiomitsu K, Liu CC, Nevarez JG (2016) Comparison of calculated radiation delivery versus actual radiation delivery in military macaws (Ara militaris). J Avian Med Surg 30:1–7
14. Duke EG, Harrison SH, Moresco A, Trout T, Troan BV, Garner MM, Smith M, Smith S, Harrison TM (2022) A multi-institutional collaboration to understand neoplasia, vol 12. Treatment and Survival of Snakes, Animals (Basel), p 12
15. Edmunds G, Beck S, Kale KU, Spasic I et al (2023) Associations between dog breed and clinical features of mammary epithelial neoplasia in bitches: an epidemiological study of submissions to a single diagnostic pathology Centre between 2008-2021. J Mammary Gland Biol Neoplasia 28:6
16. Ferraro E, Harrison SH, Duke E, Troan B, Boddy A, Abegglen LM, Harrison TM (2024) Retrospective study of the prevalence, histopathology, therapy, and survival time of neoplastic disease in fish. Animals 14:464
17. Garner M (2013) A retrospective study of disease in elasmobranchs. Vet Pathol 50:377–389
18. Giles ED, Wellberg EA (2020) Preclinical models to study obesity and breast cancer in females: considerations, caveats, and tools. J Mammary Gland Biol Neoplasia 25:237–253
19. Gunady EF, Ware KE, Hoskinson Plumlee S, Devos N, Corcoran D, Prinz J, Misetic H, Ciccarelli FD, Harrison TM, Thorne JL, Schopler R, Everitt JI, Eward WC, Somarelli JA (2022) Exome sequencing of hepatocellular carcinoma in lemurs identifies potential cancer drivers: a pilot study. Evolution Medicine Public Health 10:221–230
20. Harrison TM, Kitchell BE (2017) Principles and applications of medical oncology in exotic animals. Vet Clin Exot Anim Pract 20:209–234
21. Harrison TM, McKnight CA, Sikarskie JG, Kitchell BE, Garner MM, Raymond JT, Fitzgerald SD, Valli VE, Agnew D, Kiupel M (2010) Malignant lymphoma in african lions (panthera leo). Vet Pathol 47:952–957
22. Harrison TM, Sikarskie J, Kitchell B, Rosenstein DS, Flaherty H, Fitzgerald SD, Kiupel M (2007) Treatment of malignant lymphoma in an African lion (Panthera leo). J Zoo Wildl Med 38:333–336
23. Heishima K, Aketa N, Heishima M, Kawachi A (2023) Hemangiosarcoma in dogs as a potential non-rodent animal model for drug discovery research of angiosarcoma in humans. Front Oncol 13:1250766
24. Hinkle D, Eshar D, Ambar N, Schneider S, Azuma C (2022) Successful radiation treatment of undertail fibrosarcoma in a Major Mitchell's cockatoo (Lophochroa leadbeateri). J Am Vet Med Assoc 260:1–4
25. Hinkle DG, Nelson NC, Duke EG, Harrison TM (2024) Calculation of body surface area of corn snakes (Pantherophis guttatus) utilizing computed tomography. Am J Vet Res 85

26. Hocker SE, Eshar D, Wouda RM (2017) Rodent oncology: diseases, diagnostics, and therapeutics. Vet Clin North Am Exot Anim Pract 20:111–134
27. Hopewell E, Harrison SH, Posey R, Duke EG, Troan B, Harrison T (2020) Analysis of published amphibian neoplasia case reports. J Herpetol Med Surg 30:148–155
28. Huveneers C, Klebe S, Fox A, Bruce B, Robbins R, Borucinska JD, Jones R, Michael Z (2016) First histological examination of a neoplastic lesion from a free-swimming white shark, Carcharodon carcharias L. J Fish Dis 39:1269–1273
29. Jarvis S, Koumadoraki E, Madouros N, Sharif S, Saleem A, Khan S (2021) Non-rodent animal models of osteosarcoma: a review. Cancer Treat Res Commun 27:100307
30. Jones KL, Granger LA, Kearney MT, Da Cunha AF, Cutler DC, Shapiro ME, Tully TN, Shiomitsu K (2015) Evaluation of a ferret-specific formula for determining body surface area to improve chemotherapeutic dosing. Am J Vet Res 76:142–148
31. Keeney CMH, Nelson NC, Harrison TM (2021) Use of computed tomography to determine a species-specific formula for body surface area in bearded dragons (Pogona vitticeps). Am J Vet Res 82:629–633
32. Khudoley VV (1977) Tumor induction by carcinogenic agents in anuran amphibian Rana temporaria. Arch Geschwulstforsch 47:385–399
33. Knapp DW, Richardson RC, Denicola DB, Long GG, Blevins WE (1987) Cisplatin toxicity in cats. J Vet Intern Med 1:29–35
34. Leblanc GA, Bain LJ (1997) Chronic toxicity of environmental contaminants: sentinels and biomarkers. Environ Health Perspect 105(Suppl 1):65–80
35. Li L, Wazir J, Huang Z, Wang Y, Wang H (2024) A comprehensive review of animal models for cancer cachexia: implications for translational research. Genes Dis 11:101080
36. Lovstad JN, Gamble K, Sullivan M, Akroush M, Terio KA (2023) Prospective postmortem assessment of the incidence of mammary neoplasia in chimpanzees (pan troglodytes). J Zoo Wildl Med 54:428–434
37. Ma S (2023) Experimental models for preclinical cancer research. Exp Cell Res 429:113643
38. Machotka SV (1992) Hepatocellular neoplasia in fish, rats and man: a selected comparative review. In Vivo 6:339–347
39. Mizgireuv IV, Flax NL, Borkin LJ, Khudoley VV (1984) Dysplastic lesions and abnormalities in amphibians associated with environmental conditions. Neoplasma 31:175–181
40. Monahan CF, Garner MM, Kiupel M (2022) Chromatophoromas in reptiles. Vet Sci 9
41. Moresco A, Muñoz KE, Gutiérrez F, Arias-Bernal L, Yarto-Jaramillo E, Teixeira RHF, Peña-Stadlin J, Troan BV (2020) Taxonomic distribution of neoplasia among non-domestic felid species under managed care. Animals (Basel) 10:10
42. Nam Y, White M, Karlsson EK, Creevy KE, Promislow DEL, McClelland RL (2024) Dog size and patterns of disease history across the canine age spectrum: results from the dog aging project. PLoS One 19:e0295840
43. Niebora J, Data K, Domagatimes newa D, Józkowiak M, Barrett S, Norizadeh Abbariki T, Bryja A, Kulus M, WoŹniak S, Ziemak H, Piotrowska-Kempisty H, Antosik P, Bukowska D, Mozdziak P, Dzięgiel P, Kempisty B (2024) Avian models for human carcinogenesis-recent findings from molecular and clinical research. Cells 13
44. Nunney L, Maley CC, Breen M, Hochberg ME, Schiffman JD (2015) Peto's paradox and the promise of comparative oncology. Philos Trans R Soc B Biol Sci 370(1673):20140177
45. Olivier M, Hollstein M, Hainaut P (2010) TP53 mutations in human cancers: origins, consequences, and clinical use. Cold Spring Harb Perspect Biol 2:a001008
46. Ostrander GK, Cheng KC, Wolf JC, Wolfe MJ (2004) Shark cartilage, cancer and the growing threat of pseudoscience. Cancer Res 64:8485–8491
47. Perleberg C, Kind A, Schnieke A (2018) Genetically engineered pigs as models for human disease. Dis Model Mech 11
48. Peto R (2016) Epidemiology, multistage models, and short-term mutagenicity tests. Int J Epidemiol 45:621–637
49. Petritz O, Womble M, Gruber E, Thompson A, Harrison T (2023) Clinicopathologic, gross necropsy, and hisopathologic effects of repeated glycocorticoid administration in domestic pigeons *(Columbia livia)*. Proc ExoticsCon
50. Piersigilli A, Meyerholz DK (2016) The "naked truth": naked mole-rats do get cancer. Vet Pathol 53:519–520
51. Robat CS, Ammersbach M, Mans C (2017) Avian oncology: diseases, diagnostics, and therapeutics. Vet Clin North Am Exot Anim Pract 20:57–86
52. Ryman-Tubb T, Lothion-Roy JH, Metzler VM, Harris AE, Robinson BD, Rizvanov AA, Jeyapalan JN, James VH, England G, Rutland CS, Persson JL, Kenner L, Rubin MA, Mongan NP, De Brot S (2022) Comparative pathology of dog and human prostate cancer. Vet Med Sci 8:110–120
53. Schoemaker NJ (2017) Ferret oncology: diseases, diagnostics, and therapeutics. Vet Clin North Am Exot Anim Pract 20:183–208
54. Schwartz SM, Urfer SR, White M, Megquier K, Shrager S, Ruple A (2022) Lifetime prevalence of malignant and benign tumours in companion dogs: cross-sectional analysis of dog aging project baseline survey. Vet Comp Oncol 20:797–804
55. Shepard A, Kissil JL (2020) The use of non-traditional models in the study of cancer resistance – the case of the naked mole rat. Oncogene 39:5083–5097
56. Song G, Han JY (2011) Avian biomodels for use as pharmaceutical bioreactors and for studying human diseases. Ann N Y Acad Sci 1229:69–75
57. Taylor KR, Milone NA, Rodriguez CE (2017) Four cases of spontaneous neoplasia in the naked mole-rat

(Heterocephalus glaber), a putative cancer-resistant species. J Gerontol A Biol Sci Med Sci 72:38–43
58. Tollis M, Ferris E, Campbell MS, Harris VK, Rupp SM, Harrison TM, Kiso WK, Schmitt DL, Garner MM, Aktipis CA, Maley CC, Boddy AM, Yandell M, Gregg C, Schiffman JD, Abegglen LM (2021) Elephant genomes reveal accelerated evolution in mechanisms underlying disease defenses. Mol Biol Evol 38:3606–3620
59. Ton MN, Keitley D, Theeuwes B, Guibentif C, Ahnfelt-Rønne J, Andreassen TK, Calero-Nieto FJ, Imaz-Rosshandler I, Pijuan-Sala B, Nichols J, Benito-Gutiérrez È, Marioni JC, Göttgens B (2023) An atlas of rabbit development as a model for single-cell comparative genomics. Nat Cell Biol 25:1061–1072
60. Tosti E, Srivastava N, Edelmann W (2023) Vaccination and microbiota manipulation approaches for colon cancer prevention in rodent models. Cancer Prev Res (Phila) 16:429–438
61. Varki NM, Varki A (2015) On the apparent rarity of epithelial cancers in captive chimpanzees. Philos Trans R Soc Lond Ser B Biol Sci 370: 20140225
62. Vergneau-Grosset C, Keel MK, Goldsmith D, Kass PH, Paul-Murphy J, Hawkins MG (2016) Description of the prevalence, histologic characteristics, concomitant abnormalities, and outcomes of mammary gland tumors in companion rats (Rattus norvegicus): 100 cases (1990-2015). J Am Vet Med Assoc 249:1170–1179
63. Vergneau-Grosset C, Peña L, Cluzel C, Hawkins MG, Maccolini E, Sinclair K, Graham J, Sadar MJ, Guzman DS-M, Lair S, Langlois I, Paul-Murphy J (2019) Evaluation of deslorelin implant on subsequent mammary tumors of rats (Rattus norvegicus). J Exot Pet Med 31:108–116
64. Wang Z, Cormier RT (2022) Golden Syrian hamster models for cancer research. Cells 11
65. Ward M, Benelli G (2017) Avian and simian malaria: do they have a cancer connection? Parasitol Res 116:839–845
66. Willig F, Torpy FJ, Harrison SH, Duke EG, Troan B, Boddy AM, Abegglen LM, Harrison TM (2024) Evaluation of neoplasia, treatments, and survival in lizard species. Animals (Basel) 14
67. Wright SE, Pawlik M, Snyman HN, Haulena M (2024) Review of neoplasia in fish at a large display aquarium, 2005-2021. J Vet Diagn Invest 36:362–367
68. Ekhtiari S, K Chibae, S Popovicb, R Crowtherf, G Wohlc, A Kin On Wongg, DH Tankeh, DM Dufault, OD Geenb, N Parasud, MA Crowtherb, Evans DC (2020) First case of osteosarcoma in a dinosaur: a multimodal diagnosis. The Lancet Oncology, 21(8):1021–1022
69. Boddy AM, Abegglen LM, Pessier AP, Aktipis A, Schiffman JD, Maley CC, Witte C (2020) Lifetime cancer prevalence and life history traits in mammals. Evolution, medicine, and public health. 2020 (1):187–195

Comparative Immunology

Shay Bracha and Seth Pollack

1 Introduction

Evading immune destruction is a recognized hallmark of cancer and has been a major research focus, driving significant advancements in the development of novel therapies over the past two decades [1]. The immune system's ability to either promote or inhibit tumor development is known as immune editing, a process that progresses through three distinct phases: elimination, equilibrium, and escape [2, 3]. The elimination phase is the equivalent to the Macfarlane Burnet's theory of cancer immunosurveillance that relates to the capacity of immune cells to identify and eliminate cancer cells [4]. Malignant cells that evade eradication by the innate or adaptive immune systems progress to the equilibrium phase, where selective pressures favor the survival of cells with reduced immunogenicity [5]. During the equilibrium phase, the overall tumor size remains unchanged; however, high cell turnover and selective pressures ultimately promote immune tolerance [5]. Once these tolerant populations survive the equilibrium phase, a progression to escape phase follows, that is characterized by a clinically detectable disease. Immune editing is not restricted to tumor genesis and is evident during intervention with immunotherapy which can promote equilibrium and even eradication of the tumor by unleashing the immune system.

Harnessing immunity for cancer therapy was described more than a century ago by Dr. William B. Coley who noticed spontaneous remissions in cancer patients with surgical site infections [6]. Following these observations, Coley inoculated cancer patients with intralesional injections of *Streptococcus pyrogens* and *Serratia marcescens* which led to various degrees of remission in some patients with solid and hematological cancers [6, 7]. Due to the crudeness of this approach and harsh side effects leading to sepsis and death in many of these cases, Coley's method in its rudimentary form was stalled. However, reports of lengthy remissions following unanticipated infections have been reported in veterinary and human medicine, providing a basis for the research of immuno-oncology [8, 9]. More than a decade after Coley's experiment, a deeper understanding of immunotherapy mechanisms has led to the development of safer and effective novel immunotherapies.

The tumor microenvironment (TME) is complex and often dictates the response to immunotherapies. Tools like immune scoring were

S. Bracha (✉)
Department of Veterinary Clinical Sciences, College of Veterinary Medicine, The Ohio State University, Columbus, OH, USA
e-mail: bracha.2@osu.edu

S. Pollack
Division of Hematology and Oncology, Feinberg School of Medicine, Northwestern University, Chicago, IL, USA

M. W. Nolan et al. (eds.), *Comparative Oncology*, https://doi.org/10.1007/978-3-032-04454-9_4

developed to identify which patients are most likely to benefit from immunotherapy and determine the optimal combination of treatments. The immune score is determined based on the immune contexture, considering the type, quantity, and spatial arrangement of immune cells infiltrating the tumor [10]. This scale is a key predictor for the patient outcome, with high score being associated with favorable prognosis [11, 12]. As such, tumors with high immune score, demonstrate higher infiltration of immune cells often driven by the increased tumor mutational burden (TMB), and the frequent microsatellite instabilities (MSI) due to existing mismatch repair deficiencies [11, 12]. In addition, some of these tumors have tertiary lymphoid structures (TLS), made of a B- and T cell centers with dendritic cells and macrophages. These TLS can induce an efficient antitumor immune response that is associated with improved prognosis in many of the solid tumors [11–14]. In contrast, tumors with low TMB and MSI, generally do not exhibit a significant proliferation of immune cells or TLS formation [14].

Immune score can be categorized to distinct immune signatures characterized by parameters that include the expression of certain genes, the type of immune infiltrates, and cytokines released [11]. A prognostic signature is often calculated prior to therapy and helps with the prediction of therapeutic response by characterizing the type of tumor-infiltrating lymphocytes (TILs), the expression of programed death one (PD1) receptor and its ligand (PDL1) among other factors [11, 15]. Tumor-associated macrophages are critical for predicting patients outcome and can be classified as polarized M1 or M2 cells. Through the secretion of interleukins and cytokines the M1 cells promote the activation and proliferation of Th1 cells resulting a proinflammatory TME, while M2 cells are anti-inflammatory and activate Th2 cells to drive an immunosuppressive contexture [16]. A "technical" immune signature pertains to the specific changes induced by an explicit therapy (chemotherapy, radiotherapy, targeted or immunotherapy), and includes additional factors such as the expression of major histocompatibility complex (MHCI), formation of damage-associated molecular patterns (DAMPs), and more. Escape signature is characterized as a reduction of immune favoring component in relapsing patients. This signature often include markers associated with resistance to PD1 blockade, lost expression of MHC I, or mutation in IFNγ-related genes [17].

Common immunotherapies such as checkpoint inhibitors, adoptive cell therapies, bacterial and tumor vaccines, and oncolytic viruses are among the strategies that have proven effective and are used to benefit patients at all stages of the disease. Regardless of the therapeutic agent, the complexity of the immune response and the TME makes identifying a relevant preclinical model a significant challenge for many researchers. In this chapter, we will discuss some of the most common immunotherapies and explore the differences between animal models used to investigate and validate the growing array of immunotherapies.

2 Current and Developing Immunotherapies

2.1 Immune Checkpoint Inhibitors

Cellular checkpoints are key regulators of the immune response and prevention of autoimmunity. These checkpoints expressed in healthy tissues and are often hijacked by cancer cells in their effort to evade the host immunity, underscoring their potential as therapeutic targets. There are currently three approved checkpoint inhibitors for clinical use by the FDA and many more are in different clinical trial phases and in the pharmaceutical research pipeline. These molecules became the focus of several successful immunotherapies and are targeted in a wide variety of therapeutic settings.

An anticipated activation of T cells is primarily triggered by the binding of an antigen presenting cell (APC), MHC region to T cell receptor (TCR). The response to such a trigger is fine-tuned by a costimulation of the CD28 and the cytotoxic T lymphocyte-associated protein 4

(CTLA-4) that can both bind to the B7–1 and BF-2 (CD80 and CD86 correspondingly) ligands expressed by the antigen presenting cells (APC) [18, 19]. Binding of the CD28 receptor to the B7 ligands will promote activation, proliferation, and differentiation of T cells. However, CTLA-4 expression on the cell surface will also be activated by the binding of CD28, with a higher affinity to the B7 ligand, and once the ratio exceeds the CD28 binding it will induce anergy rather than T cell activation [18, 20]. Intracellularly, CTLA4 can impair T cell signaling such as NF-Kb, MAPK, ERK, and ultimately cripple IL-2 production [21–23].

The promotion of anergy is advantageous to cancer cells, and expression of B7 on malignant cells is a known mechanism of immune evasion. Ipilimumab, a monoclonal drug designed to block the inhibitory effect of CTLA-4 and thus promote T cell activation, was approved by the FDA for clinical use [24]. A pooled analysis of early trials in patients with advanced melanoma, revealed survival rates plateau at three years with 26% for treatment-naive patients and 20% for previously treated patients [25]. Since it was first introduced, another version of Ipilimumab was created and the indication for Ipilimumab was broadened to malignant pleural mesothelioma, renal cell carcinoma (RCC), colorectal cancer, non-small cell lung cancer (NSCLC), and hepatocellular carcinoma, and many other cancers as a sole or multiagent therapy [26–29].

Following the signaling induced by the binding of the APC and T cells through MHC-TCR and CD28 binding to CD80 and or CD86, there is an upregulation of the suppressor receptor PD1 on the T cells. Other than T cells, PD1 is expressed on B cells, NK cells, and myeloid cells and can bind to PDL1 and PDL2 [30–32]. PDL1 is primarily expressed at the TME and the malignant cells, and with the expression of PD1 that is upregulated on T cells and promote the proliferation of T regulatory. Upregulation and mutations of pathways such as JAK/STAT, mitogen-activated protein kinase (MAPK), phosphatase and tensin homolog (PTEN) were all associated with upregulation of PDL1 expression in malignant cells [21, 33–35]. In addition, mutation of the *9p24.1* chromosome in Epstein-Barr virus-positive Hodgkin lymphoma, and disruption of the PDL1 3'-UTR in various cancers were shown to induce the expression of PDL1 in malignant cells and promote immune evasion [21, 36, 37].

A blockade of the PD1 and PDL1 binding with a monoclonal antibody, prevent their inhibitory signal and will reactivate anergic T cells to induce a durable antitumor response. The approval of Pembrolizumab (Keytruda) in 2014 was the first anti-PD1 to be approved by the FDA for patients with advanced or unresectable melanoma and was followed by the approval of other agents such as Nivolumab (Opdivo) and Cemiplimab (Libtayo) for several cancers including NSCLC, malignant pleural mesothelioma, RCC, squamous cell carcinoma of the head and neck (SCCHN), Hodgkin's lymphoma, and carcinomas of the gastrointestinal tract [38–41]. Atezolizumab (Tecentriq), Avelumab (Bavencio), and Durvalumab (Imfinzi) are used for PDL1 blockade and have been approved for treating variety of cancers. These monoclonal antibodies have been prescribed as monotherapies, but combination with radiation, chemotherapy and other targeted therapies are being developed. In an attempt to increase the efficacy and reduce toxicity, combinations of anti PD1/PDL1 with anti CTLA4 therapies have been tested and resulted improved outcomes with lower toxicities when compared to monotherapies in melanoma, RCC and colorectal cancer patients [42–45]. This effect is likely due to the proliferation of inducible costimulator (ICOS)-expressing T helper 1-like cells, an increase in active CD4 and CD8 effector cells, and a reduction in exhausted CD8 cells within the TME that these combinations promote [46–48].

As mentioned earlier in this chapter, research in recent years identified tumor biomarkers and scoring systems that can significantly predict response to checkpoint inhibitors. One of these markers is the tumor proportion score (TPS) which factors the immunostaining percentage of the malignant PDL1 positive cells in the tumor and was directly correlated with immune checkpoint inhibitors (ICI's) therapeutic response [49–51]. In comparison, the combined positive score (CPS) account for the expression of PDL1 on the tumor's inflammatory cells in addition to the malignant cells, and can more accurately predict response to therapy in bladder cancer, cervical carcinoma, esophageal and gastric carcinomas, while showing an equivalent predictive value to TPS in NSCLC [52]. The TMB is another robust and independent predictor and defined as the number of somatic mutations per tumor DNA mega base [53]. Higher TMB can be caused by environmental factors such as cigarette smoke, and ionizing radiation, and is associated with a favorable clinical response to checkpoint inhibitor therapies [53, 54]. Microsatellite instability promotes high TMB but is also a standalone predictive factor for therapy. Some solid tumors such as colorectal, gastric, ovarian, prostatic, and pancreatic carcinomas that bear high microsatellite instability and faulty DNA mismatch repair mechanism exhibit direct correlation to ICI response [55, 56].

While the expression of PD1 and PDL1 are a strong prognostic indicator for ICI therapies, other factors that are associated with resistance to these drugs should be considered. Signaling pathways of TGF-β were associated with resistance to ICI, likely due to the up regulation the WNT, KRAS, and IGF pathways and the negation of cytotoxic T and NK cells activity [57, 58]. The expression of TGF-β in the TME was correlated with poor prognosis and resistance to ICI in several cancers such as gynecological malignancies, urothelial and esophageal carcinomas [57–59]. In addition, inflammation of some TME can induce resistance to ICI therapies, the high microsatellite instability exhibited in tumors such colorectal, melanoma and head and neck cancer patients [60, 61]. In an in vivo model of fibrosarcoma, and in patients with NSCLC, tumor burden showed an inverse correlation with response to immune ICI therapy, with advanced disease or larger baseline tumor sizes being less responsive [62, 63]. In addition, increased tumor hypoxia, and as a result angiogenic factors such as the vascular endothelial growth factor-A and hypoxia-inducible factors (HIF1α) that promote immunosuppression by upregulating the expression of PD1 and CTLA4 on cytotoxic T cells, hamper maturation and infiltration of immune cells, thus diminishing the therapeutic potential of ICIs [64, 65].

2.2 Adoptive Cellular Therapies

2.2.1 CART Cells

The premise of adoptive T cell therapies is the re-infusion of autologous or allogenic T cells obtained from peripheral blood or tumor-infiltrating lymphocytes (TILs) to overcome immune tolerance and trigger antitumor response [66]. Isolation of TILs allows the ex vivo activation and expansion of these cells with interleukins and cytokines prior to reinfusing it to the patient. When the using peripheral blood, T cells are isolated via leukapheresis, and processed with natural recognition of the desired antigen via their TCR or transduced with a synthetic receptor such as a chimeric antigen receptor (CAR) [66]. The selected cells are than expanded and cleaned prior to reinfusion.

When using TILs, the cells isolation and selection is based on their capacity for recognizing tumor antigens when co cultured with the patient's own tumor or with human leukocyte antigen matched cancer cell lines [67]. The selected cells are than cultured and expanded with a high concentration of IL-2. The reinfusion of TILs was one of the first adoptive therapies and used primarily for treating advanced stage melanoma [68, 69]. In early studies using TILs, better, but short-lived, response in melanoma patients was reported; however, these remissions were greatly improved by depleting the natural lymphocyte population of the patient using high dose of chemotherapy prior to the TIL's infusion [67]. Lymphodepletion allowed an effective repopulation of the expanded TILs and induced objective response rates of up to 72% and complete remission in 22% of the patients with metastatic disease, although the majority of these patients (95%) failed other therapies [67].

The genetic engineering of T cells has particularly induced exceptional outcomes in patients with hematological cancers. T cells for CAR therapies are primarily collected from the patient and engineered to target specific tumor antigens to induce cytolytic and inflammatory response against the cancer cell. The first products were approved by the FDA in 2017 (Kymriah®-tisagenlecleucel) for treating refractory/relapsed pediatric acute lymphoblastic leukemias (ALL), and more products have been approved for large B cell lymphoma (LBCL) since, including diffuse large B cell lymphoma (DLBCL) follicular and mantle cell lymphomas in adult patients [70–73]. The targeting of CD19 on B cell lymphoma or leukemia cells, by the CAR T cells has shown to be extremely effective in the eradication of leukemia and lymphoma with overall response rates that exceeded 80% [70, 71]. The durability of the response correlates with the in vivo expansion capacity of the cells and their persistence in circulation which can be prolonged with selective cell preparation [74].

T cell engineering is primarily conducted using viral vectors, such as lentivirus, to modify the natural TCR to recognize antigens presented by the cancer's MHC [75]. A more advanced preparation includes the addition of a CAR to the surface of the cell, that has the advantage recognizing any surface proteins, and not only the ones expressed by the MHCs. The first CAR generation had a simplistic structure made of a chimeric monoclonal antibody domains with an external heavy and light chains, fused to a hinge domain, transmembrane domain (i.e., CD8a, CD28) and a T cell signaling domain (CD3ζ) [76]. The structures of second generation included the addition of a costimulatory domain with CD28 or 4–1 BB, to improve the proliferation, durability and activation of the cells, while the third generation of CAR T included both (CD28 and 4–1 BB) [77, 78]. The latest generations (four and five) contain an addition of a cytokine release domain such as IL-12 (fourth generation) or an IL-2 receptor beta chain domain (IL-2Rβ) (fifth generation) to promote the trafficking of innate immune cells to tumor [79]. Fifth-generation CAR T cells were also designed with STAT3/5 binding site to further promote their proliferation and sustainability [79].

The persistence of CAR T cells after reinfusion can be constrained by various factors that may limit their durability and ability to eradicate the tumor. Assuming the CAR T expansion was robust and sufficient number of cells were injected to the patient, it is still possible that these allogenic cells will be rejected by the host immunity due to recognition of the CAR construction [80]. As other immune therapies, the TME contexture is critical for treatment success and a highly immunosuppressive environment can hinder the CAR T activity [81]. Continued triggering of the CAR T cells can exhaust the cells and reduce their efficacy, and on the other hand, the reduction or complete elimination of the target maybe too low to maintain a dividing population of the CAR T cells [82]. While not common in CAR T therapy, it is possible that the expression of the target by healthy cells will outcome an immunotolerance that will prevent the attack of the tumor cells [82]. Lastly, like other T cells of the immune system, CAR T cells may be subjected to activation-induced cell death (AICD) due to hyper or auto-activation through a Fas/FasL apoptotic pathway, reducing the cell number needed for antitumor effect [83].

The capacity of CAR T cells to proliferate and self-renew is critical for their sustained efficacy. Naïve and subtypes of memory T cells at early differentiation stages are more likely to sustain their proliferative capacity and likely to persist longer [84]. Persistence of CAR T cells may also be determined by the costimulatory domain that impacts the cell metabolic pathways and the selective expansion of distinct T cell subtypes. The 4-1BB domain can promote mitochondrial biogenesis and induce proliferation of early differentiated cells, with the induction of central memory and persistence of 4 years in comparison to the CD28 costimulatory domain that induce glycolytic metabolic pathway with expansion of differentiated cells, exhibiting persistence for 30 days [85]. Other interventions have been suggested to improve CAR T persistence by the simultaneous use of ICI, use of small molecule inhibitors and epigenetic modifications [86–88].

One potentially dangerous side effect for CAR T therapy is cytokine release syndromes (CRS) that can manifest within the first several days in patients treated with CAR therapies and is usually characterized by plethora of symptoms including fever, hypotension, and lethargy. While mild CRS is generally characterized by only mild symptoms with fever, in some cases CRS can be life threatening. This syndrome typically induces a substantial increase of circulating IL-6 that can be treated with Tocilizumab, an IL-6 antibody. Neurological toxicities such as seizures, dizziness, hallucinations and impaired cognitive skills are also relatively common adverse effects seen in CAR-treated patients and are generally treated with supportive care and steroids.

2.3 Natural Killer Cells

Natural killer (NK) cells are one of first lines of defense against cancer and have caught the attention of many investigators for their potential as adoptive immunotherapies. Natural killer cells are 5–10% of all circulating white blood cells and their infiltration to tumor cells directly correlates with prognosis [89, 90]. While these cells share many similarities with CD8+ T cells, the activation and regulatory mechanisms between these cells are different and thus have distinct therapeutic amplitudes [91]. Natural killer cells offer broad safety and efficacy profiles as adoptive therapy, along with relatively easy manufacturing and potential for "off-the-shelf" use [92]. In addition, these cells can exert their antitumor effect directly, with, or without prior activation and can even generate NK cell memory for lasting immunity [91, 93–96].

A direct activation of NK cells is induced by recognition of malignant cells by several specific mechanisms. One of the most efficient activation pathways is the "missing self," characterized by low, or absent MHC I as described in malignant and poorly differentiated cells [94, 95, 97, 98]. The low expression of MHC I will remove the restraining signal of the inhibitory receptors group, i.e., killer inhibitory receptor family (KIRs), killer cell lectin-like receptors, and the leukocyte immunoglobulin-like receptors (LILRs) [99–102]. The NKG2D receptor of NK cells activates a critical mechanism that can identify the MHC I chain-related molecules (MIC A and MIC B). These molecules are often expressed on malignant cells and are upregulated following DNA damage from low-dose chemotherapy or radiation and targeted for elimination by the immune surveillance of NK cells [103].

The NKp46 receptor is a natural cytotoxic receptors (NCR) that is continuously expressed on NK cells and play a significant role in recognition and elimination of malignant cells [104]. Another effective mechanism of activation for NK cells is the recognition of antibodies bound to the target cells. These antibodies are recognized by CD16 expressed on the membrane of the NK cells and activate them [105]. Once a malignant cell is recognized, the triggering of cytotoxicity by NK cells will be fine-tuned by activating and inhibitory signals that will orchestrate a direct attack on the cancer cells with perforins and granzymes, or indirectly through the secretion of cytokines [96, 106]. Broadly, there are two distinct NK cells phenotypes, the potent cytokine release cells characterized by $CD56^{bright}$, $CD16^{weak/-}$, and the cytotoxic phenotype with $CD56^{weak/-}$ $CD16^{bright}$ markings; however, a more detailed classification describes further distinct functional phenotypes [96–98]. The apoptosis of malignant cells by NK cells is mediated by the expression of death receptors such as the FasL/Fas, and the TNF-related apoptosis-inducing ligand (TRAIL) pathways [106].

Natural Killer cells can be harvested for therapeutic use from peripheral blood or umbilical cord. Because a large amount of cells is required for infusion, collection of NK cells from cell lines is favored in many cases and allows an "off the shelf use" [107]. An expansion and differentiation of the cells is often promoted by feeder cells and cytokines, after which the cells are sorted by flow cytometry to confirm their purity [107, 108].

3 Bacterial-Derived Immunotherapies

Inoculation of tumors and their microenvironment with bacteria, wild or modified was shown to overcome immune evasion and promote immunosurveillance. These affects were investigated in several cancers that were inoculated with certain species of *Staphylococcus aureus, E. coli*, and listeria that induced a lytic effect of the malignant cells leading to a general immune response that include antitumor properties and the cross presentation of neoantigens with more specific targeting [109–111]. Bacterial components such as bacterial cyclic dinucleotides, flagellin, beta-glucan, muramyl, and bacterial lipopolysaccharides can promote tumor immunity by recognition of a Toll-like receptor (TLR) or nucleotide binding oligomerization domain 1(NOD1)-mediated mechanism and priming of CD8+ T cells [112]. In addition, certain bacterial metabolites such as toxins, transforming growth factor-b1 (TGF-b1), and Monophosphorylate lipid A (MPL) can induce antitumor effect that is primarily T-cell dependent [112, 113]. Other immune cells including macrophages and neutrophils infiltrate the TME following treatments with bacterial components and promote immunity even in "cold" tumors.

A commonly used bacterial product is the Bacillus Calmette-Guerin (BCG), a live-attenuated tuberculosis vaccine that is commonly used for early stages of urothelial cell carcinoma (UCC) [114]. BCG is primarily used in patients intravesicularly and can exert a direct effect on cancer cells inducing necrosis or through the activation of caspases 8 and 9, ultimately resulting apoptosis [115–117]. BCG was also shown to upregulate the tumor necrosis factor-related apoptotic ligand (TRAIL), that induce a selective apoptosis in malignant cells while sparing the healthy cells [118]. UCC can internalize the attenuated bacteria effectively where BCG can induce intracellular oxidative stress damaging the DNA and cell death through apoptosis [119]. In addition to its direct effect, BCG can also induce an effective immune response against cancer cells through the TLR or NOD1 recognition, and the secretion of several cytokines, including IL-2, IL-8, IFN-γ, and TNF-α to activate immune cells in the TME [120–122]. The direct lytic cytotoxic effect in addition to the cytokine release and immune cell infiltration can induce a sustained and specific antitumor immune response.

Bioengineering of certain bacteria has been utilized for the induction of a broad inflammatory response or triggering immunity for a specific target. These modifications can eliminate the bacterial virulent capacity, modify their cytotoxic properties, and even change their cargo to include desired immunomodulatory factors. A specific triggering mechanism designed to allow a targeted release of an anticipated cargo to the tumor environment by sensing specific cues such as hypoxia, or pH changes to prevent an off-target effect and increase efficacy [123, 124]. The use of tools such as the PROT3EcT (probiotic type 3 secretion *E. coli* therapeutic) that allow an accurate release of predesigned nanobodies to the extracellular space of tumors has been greatly improved in the recent years and broaden the use of bacterial agents for immunotherapies [125].

Gram positive and negative bacteria produce membrane bound particles named bacterial extracellular vesicles (BEV). These particles contain proteins, RNA, lipopolysaccharides, enzymes, and peptidoglycans in their cargo which is used for intercellular communication. These vesicles also contain bacterial membrane derivatives with pathogen-associated molecular patterns (PAMPS) that are similar to the bacteria of origin, and after being intake intracellularly are recognized by NOD to start the activation of efficient immune cascade [127, 128]. BEVs have several advantages as therapies, they are noninfectious, their small size allowing accumulation in the TME, and their cargo can be easily modified [126]. The recognition of BEVs induces the release of cytokine and chemokines such as G-CSF, interferon-β (IFNβ), IL-6, IL-7, IL-8, and IL-13 and ultimately induces the activation of neutrophils, macrophages, and T cells [129–131]. The induction of effective immunity against a BEV expressing a desired tumor antigen, can be used for the design of cancer vaccines [132].

4 Conventional Animal Models (Existing Conventional/ Rodent Models)

4.1 Overview

Animal models are essential for immunotherapy research, yet in vivo murine models occasionally fail to capture the complex interplay of tumor biology, including environmental, genetic, and epigenetic factors [133]. These challenges are further amplified in immunotherapy research, where models must reflect the TME in relation to the host immune responses, despite interspecies differences. For example, syngeneic murine models, often use carcinogens, have provided fundamental insights into cancer immunology; however, it often lacks critical characteristics of spontaneous tumors in humans [134, 135]. Other models such as patient-derived xenograft (PDX) models have been instrumental in developing many targeted therapies and can be valuable for adoptive cellular therapies, and they may have limited applicability for immunomodulatory treatments such as ICI [136]. Humanized murine models resolve some of the deficiencies mentioned before but still lack certain human elements and can be cumbersome to use [137]. Here, we review the important considerations regarding commonly used murine models in cancer for immunotherapy applications.

4.2 Syngeneic Models

Syngeneic models are some of the most commonly used models in immunotherapy. These are immunocompetent models that have the advantage of rapid growth. They are generally easy to breed using one of the common systems (such as BALB/c, C57/BL7, or FVB). Because these mice can often be implanted from cell lines in culture they are easily manipulated in a highly reproducible way. Some of these tumors were initially identified through inducible systems, as discussed below. For example, MCA-induced murine fibrosarcoma can be harvested and developed into cell lines, which can later be implanted to create a reproducible tumor model [138].

Because murine tumor lines can be studied in vitro, before in vivo analysis, aspects of tumor biology can be investigated independently from their interactions with host immunity. However, it is important to note that although implanted syngeneic models are immune-competent, the tumors do not develop within a native TME [139]. This contrasts with human tumors, where cancer evolves under the natural selective pressure of host immunity, a process that some genetically engineered models replicate effectively. For certain tumors, phenotype may vary based on the site of engraftment, which is not necessarily a barrier but a factor that should be taken into account [140]. The lack of heterogeneity which makes these models so attractive for their reproducibility is also in a sense a potential weakness as true cancers have a high degree of variability. Some investigators have attempted to account for this by using multiple mice injected simultaneously which does reflect certain aspects of human tumor biology [141].

4.3 Induced Models

Chemicals induce a wide variety of tumor models both through direct alterations in DNA or through manipulation of epigenetics [142, 143]. When chemicals are administered directly to mice, it can create a highly natural TME because the tumor and immune response coevolve. However, there can be significant heterogeneity among mice with induced tumors, as they may exhibit entirely different mutational profiles and distinct driver mutations. Syngeneic models can be developed from induced models by establishing a tumor line. However, as mentioned above, while implanted syngeneic models offer high reproducibility, they do not necessarily coevolve with the immune response within TME.

Because cancers formed from chemically-induced alterations in the DNA, they are by definition highly mutated, these tumors are generally inflammatory and well suited to studies of PD1 manipulations or TILs. Some of the best examples in immunotherapy research have developed by directly mimicking carcinogens responsible for the cancer in human disease biology. For example, a number of key studies have arisen from mice exposed to inhaled tobacco smoke to model tobacco-related human lung cancer allowing analysis of immunotherapies including ICI [144, 145]. These sorts of studies enable detailed analysis of the TME, notably helping to allow recognition of the importance of the functions of neutrophils and other myeloid populations [146, 147]. To be sure, some similar studies have added tobacco elements, notably nicotine, to isolate its impact on implantable immunocompetent models [148, 149]. A similar approach has been taken to model UV induced melanoma which allowed for detailed profiling that might not otherwise be possible [150, 151]. Similarly asbestos induced mesothelioma models have been critical for the investigation of the disease biology [152].

A wide variety of cancers may be induced using different chemical agents and these models can be powerful even if the human cancer biology is not related to the chemical inducer. Historically methylcholanthere (MCA) has been one of the most examined, particularly as many MCA induced tumor lines are excellent for use in syngeneic models [153–155]. This powerful mutagenic agent has led to multiple models and revealed critical insights particularly with relation to the mutation specific T cell repertoire [156, 157].

Other common chemical inducers used for inducing cancers includes: Azoxymethane for the induction of colon cancer in mice that has a mutational profile similar to human tumors, generally with activated KRAS signaling and a similar pattern of metastasis including lymphogenic spread [158]. Dextran sulfate sodium also induces colon cancer but through a different mechanism involving chronic colonic inflammation, that is comparable to some human colon cancers [159, 160]. Similarly, pancreatic cancer can be induced using cerulein that induces the cancer through chronic inflammation [161]. Diethylnitrosamine causes direct DNA damage to hepatocytes leading to p53, beta-catenin, and MET mutated hepatocellular carcinoma [162, 163]. DMBA is a known environmental carcinogen that induces a variety of breast cancer phenotypes in mice [164]. The hamster cheek pouch has also been studied with respect to a number of inducible carcinogens to model squamous cell head and neck cancers [165, 166].

4.4 Xenograft Models

Xenograft models may be established either from established human cell lines or recently resected tumor as in the case of patient derived xenografts (PDX). These models offer both significant advantages as well as severe disadvantages over other model systems. The great disadvantage is that naturally and by definition, these are severely immunocompromised models. Often, xenograft models use mice with severe combined immunodeficiency (SCID mice) or that have *RAG-1* or *RAG-2* knocked out. Athymic nude mice, or those with knock outs in various cytokines or knock outs of their receptors can also be used for implantable tumors [167, 168]. Most commonly, xenografts are placed into mice with more than one alteration leading to immunodeficiency, such as the NOD/SCID with Rag 1 or 2 knock out, and/or mutated *IL2rγ or NSG mice (*NOD. Cg-*Prkdc*^{scid} *Il2rg*^{tm1Wjl}/SzJ).

The biggest advantage of these models is that they use actual human cancer cells. However, there are naturally significant differences with human tumors as these cancers lack a true human TME. They do develop a stroma often including infiltrating host myeloid cells, but this is necessarily murine [160, 169]. When these limitations are carefully considered in experimental design, xenograft models can be very powerful. These models have been some of the most important for the development of adoptive cellular therapy using engineered human T cells to expressed tumor specific CAR or TCRs [170]. Although studies using established lines and TILs are challenging due to the need for HLA matching, TILs can be effectively paired with PDX models in highly impactful ways [171]. Natural killer cell studies benefit from not being HLA-restricted, making studies using established cell lines in xenografts a promising approach [172]. These models have been further developed and were used for adoptive macrophage transfer [173].

4.5 Humanized Models

Recently, humanized models have been utilized in order to better model human TMEs. These models primarily use an established human cell line, though humanized PDX models have been made [174]. To make a humanized model, human CD34+ cells taken from cord blood are administered to NSG mice to populate human immune lineages including T cells. These tumors can experience graft versus tumor effect and can even be susceptible to PD-1 targeting [175]. More sophisticated humanized models are continuing to move the field forward such as the MSTR-G mice which express thrombopoietin, granulocyte/macrophage colony-stimulating factor, either with or without IL-3, thus enabling long-term engraftment of human immune elements [176].

4.6 Genetically Engineered Mouse Models (GEMM)

GEMMs are one of the best ways to create immunocompetent systems, often in a way that evolves to overcome a natural endogenous immune response [177]. These are probably the best models for working with standard sets of reproducible genetic alterations such as translocations. To be sure, these are generally the less immunogenic, more immunologically "quiet" tumor types but are still important for immune studies. Practical challenges can impact the utilization of these models for example some of these models have a relatively low penetrance and many mice need to be followed to form one tumor. In some cases, it may take many months for these tumors to grow. These models include KRAS in pancreatic cancer [178], *MYC* oncogenes in breast cancer [179], or APC in colon cancer [180].

5 Companion Animal Models

5.1 Overview

As mentioned above, murine models are critical for cancer research and advanced the investigation of novel therapies in a controlled environment, with genetically modified animals to fit a wide variety of research goals. However, the successes seen in preclinical trials with murine models have often failed to translate to human patients, primarily due to differences in genetics, environmental factors, tumor biology, and drug metabolism between these species. Several key differences in murine immunity, including the ratios of circulating immune cells, variations in activation and priming of innate and adaptive immunity, and distinct gene expression profiles of MHC, TCR, and TLR, impact the translation of findings to human models [181–183]. Other limiting factors such as the specific pathogen free environment husbandry, that is used in some mouse models, does not reflect the complexities between the tumor the host biome and the immune system [184].

Companion animals, and primarily dogs, have been recognized as a reliable model for clinical trials in cancer research. The goal of using client owned dogs, is to expedite the approval of potential therapeutics from preclinical studies, by examining their toxicity and efficacy in animals with naturally occurring disease [185]. The similar etiologies, histological appearances, mutational signatures, and pathways between the two species were all identified as advantageous for the canine model [185–187]. Although the exact number is not yet determined, it is estimated that the lifetime incidence of cancer in dogs is comparable to that in humans [186]. However, some cancers that are considered relatively rare in human, such as osteosarcoma, soft tissue sarcomas and mucosal melanomas have higher prevalence in dogs and thus allow an efficient platform for clinical trials [186, 187]. Furthermore, the chemotherapy drugs and protocols used in dogs are identical to their human companions, allowing similar points for comparison and the design of combinatorial drug trials.

Having an intact immune system in dogs with spontaneous disease is key advantage of this model as it is more likely to reflect the TME and immune contexture of human tumors [188, 189]. The exposure to similar environmental stressors such as toxins, bacterial and viral infections, constantly reshape the tumor and host immunity, and is essential for the assessment of potential immunotherapies. Among these factors, the host microbiome has become a recent research focus due to its role in immune modulation and its relevance to the effectiveness of immunotherapies [190]. While the role significance of the biome in relation to canine immunotherapy has not been determined thus far, an overlap between the gut biome of the two species has been described [191]. Several studies have shown that dogs and humans share a similar microbial phylogeny and functionality, with dietary changes inducing comparable effects in both species [191, 192]. Furthermore, the similarities between the canine and human biome exceeded other species like the mouse and pig [191].

5.2 Tumor Contexture in Natural Occurring Tumors of Companion Animal

The configuration of the tumor contexture was researched in several canine tumors such as osteosarcoma, glioma, and oral melanoma and was correlated to the tumor grade and prognosis [193–195]. Similar to findings in humans, these tumors were also categorized by their immune contexture: "hot tumors" with favorable outcomes and "cold tumors" with less favorable outcomes [194, 196]. The immune contexture was also investigated in canine UCC with a gene set variation analysis (GSVA) performed on the tumors exome revealing subsets of genetically "hot" and "cold" tumors; however, there was no correlation with prognosis in this study [195].

5.3 Tumor-Infiltrating Lymphocytes

In a comparative study, Lenz et al. found that high T cell density in archived tissues obtained from histiocytic sarcoma patients, was directly correlated with better outcome [197]. Estrela-Lima et al. examined IHC for CD4 and CD8 on tissues from fifty one dogs with mammary tumors, and reported that of CD8+ cells were increased in nonmetastatic mixed tumors, while a high CD4+/CD8+ ratio was significantly increased in dogs with metastatic disease [198]. The authors of this article suggested that the CD4 cells exhibit an inhibitory effect on immunity; however, specific markers for regulatory cells were not used, and this assumption could not be confirmed [198]. When TILs were evaluated in canine osteosarcoma, it was found that there was no proliferation of CD8+ cells in the majority of these tumors; in some cases, however, the cells were proliferating in the tumor margins as described in other excluded tumors [199]. Similar assessment of TILs in oral melanoma revealed an improved survival for patients with a high TIL's score and increased tumoral expression of CD8+ cells, while the expression of Tregs was identified primarily in tumors with a low TIL score [194].

The molecular landscape of tumors often drives the proliferation of TILs and dictates its immunophenotypic signature. For example, $BRAF^{V595E}$ mutation in canine is an autologous for the human $BRAF^{600}$ mutation that induced the proliferation of Tregs in canine UCC [200]. The $BRAF^{V595E}$ mutation mediated proliferation of Tregs through the increased secretion of the CCL17 chemokine by the malignant cells and its binding to the CCR4 receptor on Tregs [200, 201]. Patients with a high tumor Tregs proliferation, and elevated concentration of the CCL17 in their urine experienced a less favorable prognosis. Chemokine driven migration of Tregs in canine glioma cell lines was also demonstrated in vitro when CCL2 was shown to increase this process while a blocked of the CCL2-CCR4 axis prevented it [202]. In canine UCC tumors that were considered immunologically hot based on exome analysis, there was an increased expression of gene clusters associated with response to IFNα and IFNγ, allograph rejection and cell cycle checkpoints demonstrating the variable factors associated with the reshaping of the TME [203].

5.4 Tumor-Associated Macrophages

Similar to the classification in human, macrophage-associated tumors in canine can be classified as M1 or M2 phenotype, and while polarized M1 macrophages are proinflammatory the proliferation of polarized M2 macrophages is considered immunosuppressive [204]. In human, murine and the canine model, an increased ratio of M2/M1 in the TME of several tumors was consistent with decreased disease-free intervals and poor prognosis. An IHC analysis of 73 canine gliomas identified a robust proliferation of T cell microglia and macrophages in the tumor. Interestingly, the staining of FOXP3 was consistent through all gliomas regardless of grade suggesting an overall presence of Tregs. In addition, the expression of CD163+ used as a marker for M2 macrophages, was prominent in gliomas and directly correlated with tumor grade [193]. A significantly higher Infiltration of CD163+, CD204+, and MAC387+ cells was described in the TME of dogs with oral melanoma when compared to dogs with oral melanocytoma, the number of CD163+ cells alone was associated with increased metastases and poor prognosis [205].

The increased infiltration of CD204+ in the primary tumors of dogs with osteosarcoma was associated with improved prognosis, suggesting a more complex etiology of the immune contexture in this disease [195]. A follow-up study by the same group identified an increase of CD204+ cells in osteosarcoma lung metastatic sites, in addition to the infiltration of T and B cells [195, 206]. Dogs diagnosed with pulmonary adenocarcinomas and UCC that had high infiltration of CD204 cells in the TME, experienced a significantly shorter overall survival [204]. In a different study, CD204 was used in visceral hemangiosarcoma as a universal marker for all canine macrophages, while CD206 was used as a marker for M2 cells. The examined splenic and cardiac tumors reveled a significant proliferation of M2 cells in the tumors in comparison to their surrounding tissues but did not reveal a significant difference between the two visceral sites [207].

5.5 Immunotherapies in Companion Animals

5.5.1 Cell Checkpoint Inhibitors

The tremendous success of ICI in human medicine inspired the research of these factors in veterinary medicine, and for the development of similar therapies. Although several monoclonal antibodies have been tried, at this time there are no extensive studies that fully assessed the efficacy of ICI in companion animals. The expression of PDL1 was identified in several canine cancers including lymphoma, melanoma, osteosarcoma, hemangiosarcoma, mammary adenocarcinoma, and prostatic adenocarcinomas [208, 209]. The expression of PDL1 was identified also in canine cell lines of lymphoma, melanoma, and osteosarcoma; furthermore, the coincubation with Interferon Gamma induced the expression of PDL1 in cell lines that did not express it initially [208]. When the levels of circulating PD1 and PDL1 were compared between dogs diagnosed with cancer versus healthy controls, the levels of PDL1 and PD1 were elevated in the cancer cohort, with most significant increase of PDL1 in lymphoma patients and of PD1 in dogs with epithelial malignancies [210].

Examination of canine osteosarcomas revealed expression of PDL1, HEVA, and B7H3 in these tumors, and a contexture that matched excluded tumor or an immune desert, characterized by the proliferation of T cells on the tumor margins but not in the tumor [199]. The lung metastatic sites at the same study had high expression of all three checkpoints, consistent with an immunosuppressive contexture [199]. The infiltration of CD8+ PD1+ cells was found to be significantly increased in the urine of dogs diagnosed with UCC which suggests it is a relevant target for these patients [211].

A safety study on the use of a chimeric, caninized, anti-PD1 monoclonal antibody in dogs showed that 63% of dogs experienced adverse effects, most of these were low grade with only 6% of dogs experiencing toxicities higher than grade 3. While the study was not designed to assess clinical outcome, it was reported that 4/15 patients with lung metastasis of oral melanoma experienced an objective clinical response [212]. The use of PDL1 monoclonal antibody in dogs with oral melanoma resulted a relatively low overall response of 7.7%; however, some dogs with lung metastasis experienced a durable remissions, and the overall survival time was longer in the treated group when compared to historical control cases [213].

The expression of CTLA4 was detected in canine oral melanoma by RT-qPCR and immunohistochemistry, and was associated with unfavorable prognosis [214]. CTLA4 was also found to be expressed on canine T helpers, cytotoxic T cells, and T regulatory cells, and its blockade with monoclonal antibody has induced the expression of IFNγ [215]. When the caninized monoclonal CTLA4 antibody was tested in vitro, it had high binding rate to its target and prevented the binding to CD80/CD86 [216]. There are ongoing clinical trials that aim to identify the efficacy of anti CTLA4 monoclonal antibodies in dogs to assess its potential use in the canine model.

5.6 Adaptive T Cell Therapies in the Canine Model

5.6.1 CART Cells

Preclinical trials with CART cells have often failed to predict efficacy and often resulted life risking toxicities [217]. This is primarily to the use of murine xenograft models that did not reflect severity and extent of cytokine release syndrome, graft versus host disease, cardiotoxicities and neurotoxicities that were later reported in humans [218–220]. The development of CART cell therapy in canines offers a spontaneous and relevant model that can effectively predict clinical response and adverse events related to this line of therapy [221]. The design of CART cells in canines is similar to the human therapies, which includes cell stimulation with anti-CD3, and anti-CD28 used for cell engineering with the addition of IL-2 and IL-21 to induce cell proliferation, the transduction of the cells with a retrovirus or insertion of mRNA with electroporation were used for target expression [222, 223].

A canine CD20-CART cell was designed to treat B cell non-Hodgkin lymphoma in dogs. After testing several constructs, the most efficient production was demonstrated by cells stimulated with a single anti-CD3 domain, and coincubation with recombinant human IL-2 and IL-21 that induced a robust proliferation. For the insertion of a specific target, electroporation of mRNA for CD20 was used, which induced only a transient infection of the cells [222]. When these cells were further examined, the specific and efficient secretion of IFNγ for lytic activity against CD20+ was demonstrated [222]. A study of 4 dogs treated with a CD20-CART cells that were engineered with a lentivirus vector for transduction and with CD28ζ domain exhibited a good safety profile; however, three of the four patients experienced a disease progression within one month [224].

A canine-specific B7H3-CART cell was designed to target canine sarcomas that express the B7H3 target. The stimulation of the canine CART cells with canine anti CD3 and canine anti CD28 showed a 100-fold expansion that was augmented to 300-fold once the cells were coincubated with rhIL2 and a B7H3, human antibody (MGA271) was used for this construct [225]. The cells were injected to two healthy, purposely bred dogs that were lymphodepleted with fludarabine and cyclophosphamide. These dogs experienced a low-grade adverse events following the treatment and an increase concentration of IFNγ, IL-6, TNFα, IL-2, IL-8, MCP1, and IL-10 in circulation [225]. The design of HER2-CART canine cells, secreted IFNγ and induced cell lysis when incubated with osteosarcoma cell lines that expresses HER2 [223]. In a different study, the use of humanized IL13Rα-CART exhibited a specific cell lysis capacity against canine osteosarcoma and glioma cells in vitro and was effective in eliminating the disease in an orthotopic mouse model [226].

5.7 NK Cells

The exact characterizing phenotype of NK cells in canines remains a topic of debate and is a significant challenge for advancing comparative clinical trials. Canine NK cells were characterized as CD4-, CD21- in addition to a low CD5 ($CD5^{dim}$) [227, 228]. The expression of NKp46, along with other activation markers such as NKp30, NKp44, CD16, and CD94, has been observed in canine NK cells upon IL-2 activation. Additionally, these cells form granules, upregulate granzyme and perforin expression, and demonstrate cytotoxic capacity [229]. Although canine NK cells lack the T cell marker CD4, a subset with an NK-like phenotype can express CD8 [229–231]. When $CD5^{dim}$, CD3+, and CD21- cells were examined overtime, they have lost NK markers such as NKG2D and NKp30 and had lower secretion of IFNγ and granzyme B [232]. Prolonged culture of these cells promoted the proliferation of non-T, non-B cells with a predominant phenotype of $CD5^{dim}$, CD3-, and CD21- and were further characterized as CD4-, CD8+, TCRαβ− TCRγδ− CD11c+/− CD11d− [232]. The role of CD3 in canine NK cells is not fully understood and warrants further investigation. Cells with a CD3- NKp46+ phenotype exhibit higher cytotoxicity compared to NK cells without this phenotype. These cells can be efficiently expanded in the presence of feeder cells and secrete IFN-γ, TNF-α, IL-8, and IL-10 [233].

The use of NK cells in dogs has been tested in several small studies and was shown to be safe. Natural killer cells ($CD5^{dim}$, CD3-) were harvested from the PBMCs of healthy dogs. Following their expansion and activation, the NK cells proved cytotoxic against the canine osteosarcoma cell lines and in a PDX model [234]. An infusion of autologous NK cells to 10 osteosarcoma dogs showed homing of the cells to the primary tumor after palliative radiation treatment [234]. Six of the ten dogs treated with this protocol had no signs of lung metastasis for at least six months from diagnosis [234]. In another study, dogs with lung metastasis of osteosarcoma and oral melanoma received autologous NK cells that were expended with irradiated feeder cells and rhIL-2. In addition to the autologous NK infusions, these dogs also received nebulization of IL-15 vapor twice daily. A stable disease was documented in one dog, and a partial response in another, while no severe adverse events reported for this cohort [235]. The same study also described the infusion of allogenic NK cells in dogs with oral melanoma that were treated with a palliative course of radiation. While efficacy could not be concluded due to the small cohort size, no severe adverse effects were reported in these dogs suggesting that the use of allogenic NK cells in dogs is safe [235].

6 Conclusion

The advancement of immunotherapies has created a crucial need for relevant models that can be efficiently translated to the clinic. While traditional murine models remain essential for early-stage discovery and preclinical trials, the canine model, as discussed in this chapter, provides a valuable intermediate step in the drug development process. With their genetic diversity, naturally occurring tumors, and intact immune systems that closely resemble those of humans, dogs offer unique insights into the efficacy and safety of novel treatments. As research progresses, the integration of canine cancer models into immunotherapy trials will continue to enhance translational success, ultimately improving outcomes for both human and veterinary patients.

References

1. Fridman WH et al (2012) The immune contexture in human tumours: impact on clinical outcome. Nat Rev Cancer 12(4):298–306
2. Dunn GP, Old LJ, Schreiber RD (2004) The immunobiology of cancer immunosurveillance and immunoediting. Immunity 21(2):137–148
3. Dunn GP et al (2002) Cancer immunoediting: from immunosurveillance to tumor escape. Nat Immunol 3(11):991–998
4. Burnet M (1957) Cancer—a biological approach. I. The processes of control. II. Sign Somatic Mutat 1(5022):779–786
5. Quezada SA et al (2011) Shifting the equilibrium in cancer immunoediting: from tumor tolerance to eradication. Immunol Rev 241(1):104–118
6. Coley WB (1914) The treatment of malignant inoperable tumors with the mixed toxins of erysipelas and bacillus prodigiosus. Weissenbruch
7. Coley WB, Coley BL (1927) Primary malignant tumors of the long bones: end results in one hundred and seventy operable cases. Arch Surg 14(1):63–141
8. Lascelles BDX et al (2005) Improved survival associated with postoperative wound infection in dogs treated with limb-salvage surgery for osteosarcoma. Ann Surg Oncol 12(12):1073–1083
9. Jeys LM et al (2007) Post operative infection and increased survival in osteosarcoma patients: are they associated? Ann Surg Oncol 14(10):2887–2895
10. Galon J et al (2012) Cancer classification using the Immunoscore: a worldwide task force. J Transl Med 10(1):1–10
11. Bruni D, Angell HK, Galon J (2020) The immune contexture and Immunoscore in cancer prognosis and therapeutic efficacy. Nat Rev Cancer 20(11):662–680
12. Kirilovsky A et al (2016) Rational bases for the use of the Immunoscore in routine clinical settings as a prognostic and predictive biomarker in cancer patients. Int Immunol 28(8):373–382
13. Bindea G et al (2013) Spatiotemporal dynamics of intratumoral immune cells reveal the immune landscape in human cancer. Immunity 39(4):782–795
14. Di Caro G et al (2015) Tertiary lymphoid tissue in the tumor microenvironment: from its occurrence to immunotherapeutic implications. Int Rev Immunol 34(2):123–133
15. Tumeh PC et al (2014) PD-1 blockade induces responses by inhibiting adaptive immune resistance. Nature 515(7528):568–571
16. Mantovani A et al (2002) Macrophage polarization: tumor-associated macrophages as a paradigm for polarized M2 mononuclear phagocytes. Trends Immunol 23(11):549–555
17. Sun J-Y et al (2020) Resistance to PD-1/PD-L1 blockade cancer immunotherapy: mechanisms, predictive factors, and future perspectives. Biomark Res 8(1):35
18. Chambers CA et al (2001) CTLA-4-mediated inhibition in regulation of T cell responses: mechanisms and manipulation in tumor immunotherapy. Annu Rev Immunol 19:565–594
19. Parry RV et al (2005) CTLA-4 and PD-1 receptors inhibit T-cell activation by distinct mechanisms. Mol Cell Biol 25(21):9543–9553
20. Fallarino F, Fields PE, Gajewski TF (1998) B7-1 engagement of cytotoxic T lymphocyte antigen 4 inhibits T cell activation in the absence of CD28. J Exp Med 188(1):205–210
21. Menter T, Tzankov A (2018) Mechanisms of immune evasion and immune modulation by lymphoma cells. Front Oncol 8:54
22. Fraser JH et al (1999) CTLA4 ligation attenuates AP-1, NFAT and NF-kappaB activity in activated T cells. Eur J Immunol 29(3):838–844
23. Brunner MC et al (1999) CTLA-4-mediated inhibition of early events of T cell proliferation. J Immunol 162(10):5813–5820
24. Fong L, Small EJ (2008) Anti-cytotoxic T-lymphocyte antigen-4 antibody: the first in an emerging class of immunomodulatory antibodies for cancer treatment. J Clin Oncol 26(32):5275–5283
25. Schadendorf D et al (2015) Pooled analysis of long-term survival data from phase II and phase III trials of Ipilimumab in Unresectable or metastatic melanoma. J Clin Oncol 33(17):1889–1894
26. Saung MT et al (2021) FDA approval summary: Nivolumab plus Ipilimumab for the treatment of patients with hepatocellular carcinoma previously treated with Sorafenib. Oncologist 26(9):797–806
27. Nakajima EC et al (2022) FDA approval summary: Nivolumab in combination with Ipilimumab for the treatment of Unresectable malignant pleural mesothelioma. Clin Cancer Res 28(3):446–451
28. Vellanki PJ et al (2021) FDA approval summary: Nivolumab with Ipilimumab and chemotherapy for metastatic non–small cell lung cancer, a collaborative project Orbis review. Clin Cancer Res 27(13):3522–3527
29. Lipson EJ, Drake CG (2011) Ipilimumab: an anti-CTLA-4 antibody for metastatic melanoma. Clin Cancer Res 17(22):6958–6962
30. Kundra A et al (2013) Programmed cell death receptor (PD-1), PD-1 ligand (PD-L1) expression and myeloid derived suppressor cells (MDSC) in myeloid neoplasms implicate the mechanism of IMiD treatment of myelofibrosis. Blood 122(21):2837
31. Thibult ML et al (2013) PD-1 is a novel regulator of human B-cell activation. Int Immunol 25(2):129–137
32. Quatrini L et al (2020) The immune checkpoint PD-1 in natural killer cells: expression, function and targeting in tumour immunotherapy. Cancers (Basel) 12(11)
33. Doi T et al (2017) The JAK/STAT pathway is involved in the upregulation of PD-L1 expression in pancreatic cancer cell lines. Oncol Rep 37(3):1545–1554

34. Atefi M et al (2014) Effects of MAPK and PI3K pathways on PD-L1 expression in melanoma. Clin Cancer Res 20(13):3446–3457
35. Xu C et al (2014) Loss of Lkb1 and Pten leads to lung squamous cell carcinoma with elevated PD-L1 expression. Cancer Cell 25(5):590–604
36. Shiraiwa S et al (2022) 9p24.1 genetic alteration and PD-L1 expression are characteristic of De novo and methotrexate-associated Epstein-Barr virus-positive Hodgkin lymphoma, but not methotrexate-associated Hodgkin-like lesions. Am J Surg Pathol 46(8):1017–1024
37. Chen Z et al (2023) The 3' non-coding sequence negatively regulates PD-L1 expression, and its regulators are systematically identified in pan-cancer. Genes (Basel) 14(8)
38. Motzer RJ et al (2015) Nivolumab for metastatic renal cell carcinoma: results of a randomized phase II trial. J Clin Oncol 33(13):1430–1437
39. Chung CH et al (2022) Phase II multi-institutional clinical trial result of concurrent Cetuximab and Nivolumab in recurrent and/or metastatic head and neck squamous cell carcinoma. Clin Cancer Res 28(11):2329–2338
40. Baas P et al (2021) First-line nivolumab plus ipilimumab in unresectable malignant pleural mesothelioma (CheckMate 743): a multicentre, randomised, open-label, phase 3 trial. Lancet 397(10272):375–386
41. Ansell SM (2017) Nivolumab in the treatment of Hodgkin lymphoma. Clin Cancer Res 23(7):1623–1626
42. Larkin J et al (2015) Combined nivolumab and ipilimumab or monotherapy in untreated melanoma. N Engl J Med 373(1):23–34
43. Overman MJ et al (2018) Durable clinical benefit with nivolumab plus ipilimumab in DNA mismatch repair-deficient/microsatellite instability-high metastatic colorectal cancer. J Clin Oncol 36(8):773–779
44. Motzer RJ et al (2018) Nivolumab plus ipilimumab versus sunitinib in advanced renal-cell carcinoma. N Engl J Med 378(14):1277–1290
45. Rotte A (2019) Combination of CTLA-4 and PD-1 blockers for treatment of cancer. J Exp Clin Cancer Res 38(1):255
46. Wei SC et al (2019) Combination anti-CTLA-4 plus anti-PD-1 checkpoint blockade utilizes cellular mechanisms partially distinct from monotherapies. Proc Natl Acad Sci USA 116(45):22699–22709
47. Alspach E et al (2019) MHC-II neoantigens shape tumour immunity and response to immunotherapy. Nature 574(7780):696–701
48. Sharma P, Allison JP (2020) Dissecting the mechanisms of immune checkpoint therapy. Nat Rev Immunol 20(2):75–76
49. Mok TSK et al (2019) Pembrolizumab versus chemotherapy for previously untreated, PD-L1-expressing, locally advanced or metastatic non-small-cell lung cancer (KEYNOTE-042): a randomised, open-label, controlled, phase 3 trial. Lancet 393(10183):1819–1830
50. Sul J et al (2016) FDA approval summary: pembrolizumab for the treatment of patients with metastatic non-small cell lung cancer whose tumors express programmed death-ligand 1. Oncologist 21(5):643–650
51. Liu J et al (2021) Automated tumor proportion score analysis for PD-L1 (22C3) expression in lung squamous cell carcinoma. Sci Rep 11(1):15907
52. De Marchi P et al (2021) PD-L1 expression by tumor proportion score (TPS) and combined positive score (CPS) are similar in non-small cell lung cancer (NSCLC). J Clin Pathol 74(11):735–740
53. Goodman AM et al (2017) Tumor mutational burden as an independent predictor of response to immunotherapy in diverse cancers. Mol Cancer Ther 16(11):2598–2608
54. Klempner SJ et al (2020) Tumor mutational burden as a predictive biomarker for response to immune checkpoint inhibitors: a review of current evidence. Oncologist 25(1):e147–e159
55. Malapelle U et al (2021) Evaluation of micro satellite instability and mismatch repair status in different solid tumors: a multicenter analysis in a real world setting. Cells 10(8)
56. Eng C et al (2019) Atezolizumab with or without cobimetinib versus regorafenib in previously treated metastatic colorectal cancer (IMblaze370): a multicentre, open-label, phase 3, randomised, controlled trial. Lancet Oncol 20(6):849–861
57. Wang L et al (2018) EMT-and stroma-related gene expression and resistance to PD-1 blockade in urothelial cancer. Nat Commun 9(1):3503
58. Ni Y et al (2021) High TGF-β signature predicts immunotherapy resistance in gynecologic cancer patients treated with immune checkpoint inhibition. Npj Preci Oncol 5(1):101
59. Chen X et al (2018) Dual TGF-β and PD-1 blockade synergistically enhances MAGE-A3-specific CD8+ T cell response in esophageal squamous cell carcinoma. Int J Cancer 143(10):2561–2574
60. Sui Q et al (2022) Inflammation promotes resistance to immune checkpoint inhibitors in high microsatellite instability colorectal cancer. Nat Commun 13(1):7316
61. Ayers M et al (2017) IFN-γ–related mRNA profile predicts clinical response to PD-1 blockade. J Clin Invest 127(8):2930–2940
62. Yang YF et al (1997) Enhanced induction of antitumor T-cell responses by cytotoxic T lymphocyte-associated molecule-4 blockade: the effect is manifested only at the restricted tumor-bearing stages. Cancer Res 57(18):4036–4041
63. Katsurada M et al (2019) Baseline tumor size as a predictive and prognostic factor of immune checkpoint inhibitor therapy for non-small cell lung cancer. Anticancer Res 39(2):815–825
64. Schaaf MB, Garg AD, Agostinis P (2018) Defining the role of the tumor vasculature in antitumor immunity and immunotherapy. Cell Death Dis 9(2):115
65. Ribatti D (2022) Immunosuppressive effects of vascular endothelial growth factor. Oncol Lett 24(4):369

66. Zhang Y, Zhang Z (2020) The history and advances in cancer immunotherapy: understanding the characteristics of tumor-infiltrating immune cells and their therapeutic implications. Cell Mol Immunol 17(8):807–821
67. Rosenberg SA et al (2011) Durable complete responses in heavily pretreated patients with metastatic melanoma using T-cell transfer immunotherapy. Clin Cancer Res 17(13):4550–4557
68. Rosenberg SA et al (1988) Use of tumor-infiltrating lymphocytes and interleukin-2 in the immunotherapy of patients with metastatic melanoma. A preliminary report. N Engl J Med 319(25):1676–1680
69. Rosenberg SA et al (1994) Treatment of patients with metastatic melanoma with autologous tumor-infiltrating lymphocytes and interleukin 2. JNCI J Natl Cancer Inst 86(15):1159–1166
70. Rives S et al (2022) S112: tisagenlecleucel in pediatric and young adult patients (PTS) with relapsed/refractory (R/R) B-cell acute lymphoblastic leukemia (B-ALL): final analyses from the Eliana study. HemaSphere 6:13–14
71. Schuster SJ et al (2021) Long-term clinical outcomes of tisagenlecleucel in patients with relapsed or refractory aggressive B-cell lymphomas (JULIET): a multicentre, open-label, single-arm, phase 2 study. Lancet Oncol 22(10):1403–1415
72. Awasthi R et al (2023) Kymriah® (tisagenlecleucel) – an overview of the clinical development journey of the first approved CAR-T therapy. Hum Vaccin Immunother 19(1):2210046
73. Abramson JS et al (2023) Lisocabtagene maraleucel as second-line therapy for large B-cell lymphoma: primary analysis of the phase 3 TRANSFORM study. Blood 141(14):1675–1684
74. Porter DL et al (2015) Chimeric antigen receptor T cells persist and induce sustained remissions in relapsed refractory chronic lymphocytic leukemia. Sci Transl Med 7(303):303ra139-303ra139
75. Ghassemi S et al (2022) Rapid manufacturing of non-activated potent CAR T cells. Nature Biomed Eng 6(2):118–128
76. Bridgeman JS et al (2010) The optimal antigen response of chimeric antigen receptors harboring the CD3ζ transmembrane domain is dependent upon incorporation of the receptor into the endogenous TCR/CD3 complex. J Immunol 184(12):6938–6949
77. Imai C et al (2004) Chimeric receptors with 4-1BB signaling capacity provoke potent cytotoxicity against acute lymphoblastic leukemia. Leukemia 18(4):676–684
78. López-Cantillo G et al (2022) CAR-T cell performance: how to improve their persistence? Front Immunol 13:878209
79. Kagoya Y et al (2018) A novel chimeric antigen receptor containing a JAK-STAT signaling domain mediates superior antitumor effects. Nat Med 24(3):352–359
80. Jallouk AP et al (2023) Cellular mechanisms affecting allogeneic CAR T cell expansion and rejection in large B-cell lymphoma. Blood 142(Supplement 1):4832–4832
81. Kankeu Fonkoua LA et al (2022) CAR T cell therapy and the tumor microenvironment: current challenges and opportunities. Mol Ther Oncoly 25:69–77
82. Shah NN, Fry TJ (2019) Mechanisms of resistance to CAR T cell therapy. Nat Rev Clin Oncol 16(6):372–385
83. Huan T et al (2022) Activation-induced cell death in CAR-T cell therapy. Hum Cell 35(2):441–447
84. Tantalo DG et al (2021) Understanding T cell phenotype for the design of effective chimeric antigen receptor T cell therapies. J Immunother Cancer 9(5)
85. Kawalekar OU et al (2016) Distinct signaling of Coreceptors regulates specific metabolism pathways and impacts memory development in CAR T cells. Immunity 44(3):712
86. Fraietta JA et al (2018) Disruption of TET2 promotes the therapeutic efficacy of CD19-targeted T cells. Nature 558(7709):307–312
87. McGowan E et al (2020) PD-1 disrupted CAR-T cells in the treatment of solid tumors: promises and challenges. Biomed Pharmacother 121:109625
88. Cao X et al (2023) Small-molecule compounds boost CAR-T cell therapy in hematological malignancies. Curr Treat Options in Oncol 24(3):184–211
89. Cherrier DE, Serafini N, Di Santo JP (2018) Innate lymphoid cell development: AT cell perspective. Immunity 48(6):1091–1103
90. Cózar B et al (2021) Tumor-infiltrating natural killer cells. Cancer Discov 11(1):34–44
91. Sun JC, Lanier LL (2011) NK cell development, homeostasis and function: parallels with CD8+ T cells. Nat Rev Immunol 11(10):645–657
92. Page A et al (2024) Development of NK cell-based cancer immunotherapies through receptor engineering. Cell Mol Immunol 21(4):315–331
93. Cerwenka A, Lanier LL (2016) Natural killer cell memory in infection, inflammation and cancer. Nat Rev Immunol 16(2):112–123
94. Gidlund M et al (1981) Natural killer cells kill tumour cells at a given stage of differentiation. Nature 292(5826):848–850
95. Ljunggren H-G, Kärre K (1990) In search of the 'missing self': MHC molecules and NK cell recognition. Immunol Today 11:237–244
96. Carreira-Santos S et al (2023) Enhanced expression of natural cytotoxicity receptors on cytokine-induced memory-like natural killer cells correlates with effector function. Front Immunol 14:1256404
97. Wu S-Y et al (2020) Natural killer cells in cancer biology and therapy. Mol Cancer 19(1):120
98. Fu B, Tian Z, Wei H (2014) Subsets of human natural killer cells and their regulatory effects. Immunology 141(4):483–489
99. Portale F, Di Mitri D (2023) NK cells in cancer: mechanisms of dysfunction and therapeutic potential. Int J Mol Sci 24(11):9521
100. Screpanti V et al (2005) Impact of FASL-induced apoptosis in the elimination of tumor cells by NK cells. Mol Immunol 42(4):495–499

101. Takeda K et al (2002) Critical role for tumor necrosis factor–related apoptosis-inducing ligand in immune surveillance against tumor development. J Exp Med 195(2):161–169
102. Smyth MJ et al (2001) Tumor necrosis factor-related apoptosis-inducing ligand (TRAIL) contributes to interferon gamma-dependent natural killer cell protection from tumor metastasis. J Exp Med 193(6):661–670
103. Dhar P, Wu JD (2018) NKG2D and its ligands in cancer. Curr Opin Immunol 51:55–61
104. Arnon TI et al (2004) The mechanisms controlling the recognition of tumor- and virus-infected cells by NKp46. Blood 103(2):664–672
105. Capuano C et al (2021) Harnessing CD16-mediated NK cell functions to enhance therapeutic efficacy of tumor-targeting mAbs. Cancers (Basel) 13(10)
106. Topham NJ, Hewitt EW (2009) Natural killer cell cytotoxicity: how do they pull the trigger? Immunology 128(1):7–15
107. Lapteva N et al (2014) Clinical grade purification and expansion of natural killer cells. Crit Rev Oncog 19(1–2):121–132
108. Du N et al (2021) NK cell therapy: a rising star in cancer treatment. Cancers (Basel) 13(16)
109. Liu C-C et al (2024) Characterization of immunomodulating agents from Staphylococcus aureus for priming immunotherapy in triple-negative breast cancers. Sci Rep 14(1):756
110. Wei B et al (2021) Polarization of tumor-associated macrophages by nanoparticle-loaded Escherichia coli combined with immunogenic cell death for cancer immunotherapy. Nano Lett 21(10):4231–4240
111. Ding YD et al (2023) Listeria monocytogenes: a promising vector for tumor immunotherapy. Front Immunol 14:1278011
112. Zhou M et al (2023) Bacteria-based immunotherapy for cancer: a systematic review of preclinical studies. Front Immunol 14:1140463
113. Gregg KA et al (2017) Rationally designed TLR4 ligands for vaccine adjuvant discovery. MBio **8**(3):10.1128/mbio.00492-17
114. Redelman-Sidi G, Glickman MS, Bochner BH (2014) The mechanism of action of BCG therapy for bladder cancer—a current perspective. Nat Rev Urol 11(3):153–162
115. Yu D-S et al (2015) Bacille Calmette-Guerin can induce cellular apoptosis of urothelial cancer directly through toll-like receptor 7 activation. Kaohsiung J Med Sci 31(8):391–397
116. Holla S et al (2014) Mycobacterium bovis BCG promotes tumor cell survival from tumor necrosis factor-α-induced apoptosis. Mol Cancer 13(210):1–13
117. Sandes E et al (2007) Cathepsin B is involved in the apoptosis intrinsic pathway induced by bacillus Calmette-Guerin in transitional cancer cell lines. Int J Mol Med 20(6):823–828
118. Rosevear HM et al (2009) The role of neutrophils and TNF-related apoptosis-inducing ligand (TRAIL) in bacillus Calmette–Guérin (BCG) immunotherapy for urothelial carcinoma of the bladder. Cancer Metastasis Rev 28(3):345–353
119. Ryk C et al (2015) Outcome after BCG treatment for urinary bladder cancer may be influenced by polymorphisms in the NOS2 and NOS3 genes. Redox Biol 6:272–277
120. Ibarra C et al (2019) BCG-induced cytokine release in bladder cancer cells is regulated by ca(2+) signaling. Mol Oncol 13(2):202–211
121. Miyazaki J et al (2006) Uroepithelial cells can directly respond to Mycobacterium bovis bacillus Calmette-Guérin through toll-like receptor signalling. BJU Int 97(4):860–864
122. Kardoust Parizi M et al (2021) Value of tumour-infiltrating immune cells in predicting response to intravesical BCG in patients with non-muscle-invasive bladder cancer: a systematic review and meta-analysis. BJU Int 127(6):617–625
123. Jahanban-Esfahlan R et al (2018) Modulating tumor hypoxia by nanomedicine for effective cancer therapy. J Cell Physiol 233(3):2019–2031
124. Ryan R et al (2009) Bacterial delivery of a novel cytolysin to hypoxic areas of solid tumors. Gene Ther 16(3):329–339
125. Lynch JP et al (2023) Engineered Escherichia coli for the in situ secretion of therapeutic nanobodies in the gut. Cell Host Microbe 31(4):634–649.e8
126. Zhao M et al (2024) Bacterial protoplast-derived nanovesicles carrying CRISPR-Cas9 tools re-educate tumor-associated macrophages for enhanced cancer immunotherapy. Nat Commun 15(1):950
127. Kaparakis M et al (2010) Bacterial membrane vesicles deliver peptidoglycan to NOD1 in epithelial cells. Cell Microbiol 12(3):372–385
128. Chatterjee D, Chaudhuri K (2013) Vibrio cholerae O395 outer membrane vesicles modulate intestinal epithelial cells in a NOD1 protein-dependent manner and induce dendritic cell-mediated Th2/Th17 cell responses. J Biol Chem 288(6):4299–4309
129. Galka F et al (2008) Proteomic characterization of the whole secretome of legionella pneumophila and functional analysis of outer membrane vesicles. Infect Immun 76(5):1825–1836
130. Lapinet JA et al (2000) Gene expression and production of tumor necrosis factor alpha, interleukin-1β (IL-1β), IL-8, macrophage inflammatory protein 1α (MIP-1α), MIP-1β, and gamma interferon-inducible protein 10 by human neutrophils stimulated with group B meningococcal outer membrane vesicles. Infect Immun 68(12):6917–6923
131. Kaparakis-Liaskos M, Ferrero RL (2015) Immune modulation by bacterial outer membrane vesicles. Nat Rev Immunol 15(6):375–387
132. Cheng K et al (2021) Bioengineered bacteria-derived outer membrane vesicles as a versatile antigen display platform for tumor vaccination via plug-and-display technology. Nat Commun 12(1):2041
133. Chulpanova DS et al (2020) Mouse tumor models for advanced cancer immunotherapy. Int J Mol Sci 21(11)

134. Zamora AE et al (2015) Models to study NK cell biology and possible clinical application. Curr Protoc Immunol 110:14 37 1–14 37 14
135. Dhar P et al (2021) Tumor-derived NKG2D ligand sMIC reprograms NK cells to an inflammatory phenotype through CBM signalosome activation. Commun Biol 4(1):905
136. Liu Y et al (2023) Patient-derived xenograft models in cancer therapy: technologies and applications. Signal Transduct Target Ther 8(1):160
137. Chuprin J et al (2023) Humanized mouse models for immuno-oncology research. Nat Rev Clin Oncol 20(3):192–206
138. Uno T et al (2006) Eradication of established tumors in mice by a combination antibody-based therapy. Nat Med 12(6):693–698
139. Olson B et al (2018) Mouse models for cancer immunotherapy research. Cancer Discov 8(11):1358–1365
140. He M et al (2020) Preclinical mouse models for immunotherapeutic and non-immunotherapeutic drug development for pancreatic ductal adenocarcinoma. Ann Pancreat Cancer:3
141. Calbo J et al (2011) A functional role for tumor cell heterogeneity in a mouse model of small cell lung cancer. Cancer Cell 19(2):244–256
142. Sewduth RN, Georgelou K (2024) Relevance of carcinogen-induced preclinical cancer models. J Xenobiot 14(1):96–109
143. Liu Y et al (2015) Mammalian models of chemically induced primary malignancies exploitable for imaging-based preclinical theragnostic research. Quant Imaging Med Surg 5(5):708–729
144. Stabile LP et al (2021) Syngeneic tobacco carcinogen-induced mouse lung adenocarcinoma model exhibits PD-L1 expression and high tumor mutational burden. Insight 6(3)
145. Witschi H et al (2002) A mouse lung tumor model of tobacco smoke carcinogenesis. Toxicol Sci 68(2):322–330
146. Houghton AM et al (2010) Neutrophil elastase-mediated degradation of IRS-1 accelerates lung tumor growth. Nat Med 16(2):219–223
147. Liu CH et al (2021) Lipopolysaccharide-mediated chronic inflammation promotes tobacco carcinogen-induced lung cancer and determines the efficacy of immunotherapy. Cancer Res 81(1):144–157
148. Davis R et al (2009) Nicotine promotes tumor growth and metastasis in mouse models of lung cancer. PLoS One 4(10):e7524
149. Busch SE et al (2016) Lung cancer subtypes generate unique immune responses. J Immunol 197(11):4493–4503
150. Day CP et al (2017) Mouse models of UV-induced melanoma: genetics, pathology, and clinical relevance. Lab Investig 97(6):698–705
151. Leonard MK et al (2021) Comprehensive molecular profiling of UV-induced metastatic melanoma in Nme1/Nme2-deficient mice reveals novel markers of survival in human patients. Oncogene 40(45):6329–6342
152. Seastedt KP, Pruett N, Hoang CD (2021) Mouse models for mesothelioma drug discovery and development. Expert Opin Drug Discov 16(6):697–708
153. Lauder SN et al (2021) Using methylcholanthrene-induced fibrosarcomas to study tumor immunology. Methods Cell Biol 163:59–75
154. Ligtenberg MA et al (2015) Methylcholanthrene-induced sarcomas develop independently from NOX2-derived ROS. PLoS One 10(6):e0129786
155. Swann JB et al (2008) Demonstration of inflammation-induced cancer and cancer immunoediting during primary tumorigenesis. Proc Natl Acad Sci USA 105(2):652–656
156. Schreiber TH, Podack ER (2009) A critical analysis of the tumour immunosurveillance controversy for 3-MCA-induced sarcomas. Br J Cancer 101(3):381–386
157. Sultan H et al (2024) Neoantigen-specific cytotoxic Tr1 CD4 T cells suppress cancer immunotherapy. Nature 632:182
158. Chen J, Huang XF (2009) The signal pathways in azoxymethane-induced colon cancer and preventive implications. Cancer Biol Ther 8(14):1313–1317
159. Hoffmann M et al (2018) A refined and translationally relevant model of chronic DSS colitis in BALB/c mice. Lab Anim 52(3):240–252
160. Sato Y et al (2023) Inflammatory bowel disease and colorectal cancer: epidemiology, etiology, surveillance, and management. Cancers (Basel) 15(16)
161. Ahmadi A et al (2016) An optimised mouse model of chronic pancreatitis with a combination of ethanol and cerulein. Cent Eur J Immunol 41(1):54–63
162. Schulien I, Hasselblatt P (2021) Diethylnitrosamine-induced liver tumorigenesis in mice. Methods Cell Biol 163:137–152
163. Memon A et al (2020) A modified protocol of Diethylnitrosamine Administration in Mice to model hepatocellular carcinoma. Int J Mol Sci 21(15)
164. Stewart MK et al (2015) Cx26 knockout predisposes the mammary gland to primary mammary tumors in a DMBA-induced mouse model of breast cancer. Oncotarget 6(35):37185–37199
165. Monti-Hughes, A., et al., The hamster cheek pouch model for field cancerization studies. Periodontol 2000, 2015. 67(1): p. 292–311
166. Wani MK et al (2001) Cancer induction in the DMBA hamster cheek pouch: a modified technique using a promoter. Laryngoscope 111(2): 204–206
167. Hasgur S et al (2016) Generation of Immunodeficient mice bearing human immune systems by the engraftment of hematopoietic stem cells. Methods Mol Biol 1438:67–78
168. Walsh NC et al (2017) Humanized mouse models of clinical disease. Annu Rev Pathol 12:187–215
169. Tuxhorn JA et al (2002) Stromal cells promote angiogenesis and growth of human prostate tumors in a differential reactive stroma (DRS) xenograft model. Cancer Res 62(11):3298–3307

170. Duncan BB, Dunbar CE, Ishii K (2022) Applying a clinical lens to animal models of CAR-T cell therapies. Mol Ther Methods Clin Dev 27:17–31
171. Gitto SB et al (2020) An autologous humanized patient-derived-xenograft platform to evaluate immunotherapy in ovarian cancer. Gynecol Oncol 156(1):222–232
172. Liu S et al (2021) NK cell-based cancer immunotherapy: from basic biology to clinical development. J Hematol Oncol 14(1):7
173. Anderson NR et al (2021) Macrophage-based approaches for cancer immunotherapy. Cancer Res 81(5):1201–1208
174. Steinkamp MP et al (2023) Humanized patient-derived xenograft models of disseminated ovarian cancer recapitulate key aspects of the tumor immune environment within the peritoneal cavity. Cancer Res Commun 3(2):309–324
175. Wang M et al (2018) Humanized mice in studying efficacy and mechanisms of PD-1-targeted cancer immunotherapy. FASEB J 32(3):1537–1549
176. Saito Y et al (2016) Peripheral blood CD34(+) cells efficiently engraft human cytokine knock-in mice. Blood 128(14):1829–1833
177. Kersten K et al (2017) Genetically engineered mouse models in oncology research and cancer medicine. EMBO Mol Med 9(2):137–153
178. Laney V et al (2024) MR molecular image guided treatment of pancreatic cancer with targeted ECO/miR-200c nanoparticles in immunocompetent mouse tumor models. Pharm Res 41:1811
179. Sinn E et al (1987) Coexpression of MMTV/v--ha-ras and MMTV/c-myc genes in transgenic mice: synergistic action of oncogenes in vivo. Cell 49(4):465–475
180. Shibata H et al (1997) Rapid colorectal adenoma formation initiated by conditional targeting of the Apc gene. Science 278(5335):120–123
181. Bahram S (2001) MIC genes: from genetics to biology. In: Dixon FJ (ed) Advances in immunology. Academic Press, pp 1–60
182. Rehli M (2002) Of mice and men: species variations of toll-like receptor expression. Trends Immunol 23(8):375–378
183. Mestas J, Hughes CCW (2004) Of mice and not men: differences between mouse and human immunology. J Immunol 172(5):2731–2738
184. Dobson GP et al (2019) Specific pathogen-free (SPF) animal status as a variable in biomedical research: have we come full circle? EBioMedicine 41:42–43
185. Paoloni M, Khanna C (2008) Translation of new cancer treatments from pet dogs to humans. Nat Rev Cancer 8(2):147–156
186. Gardner HL, Fenger JM, London CA (2016) Dogs as a model for cancer. Annu Rev Anim Biosci 4:199–222
187. Schiffman JD, Breen M (2015) Comparative oncology: what dogs and other species can teach us about humans with cancer. Philosoph Trans Royal Soc B: Biol Sci 370(1673):20140231
188. Dow S (2019) A role for dogs in advancing cancer immunotherapy research. Front Immunol 10:2935
189. Von Rueden SK, Fan TM (2021) Cancer-immunity cycle and therapeutic interventions- opportunities for including pet dogs with cancer. Front Oncology 11:11
190. Gopalakrishnan V et al (2018) Gut microbiome modulates response to anti–PD-1 immunotherapy in melanoma patients. Science 359(6371):97–103
191. Coelho LP et al (2018) Similarity of the dog and human gut microbiomes in gene content and response to diet. Microbiome 6(1):72
192. Pinto C, Aluai-Cunha C, Santos A (2023) The human and animals' malignant melanoma: comparative tumor models and the role of microbiome in dogs and humans. Melanoma Res 33(2):87–103
193. Krane GA et al (2021) Immunohistochemical evaluation of immune cell infiltration in canine gliomas. Vet Pathol 58(5):952–963
194. Yasumaru CC et al (2021) Intratumoral T-lymphocyte subsets in canine Oral melanoma and their association with clinical and histopathological parameters. Vet Pathol 58(3):491–502
195. Withers SS et al (2019) Association of macrophage and lymphocyte infiltration with outcome in canine osteosarcoma. Vet Comp Oncol 17(1):49–60
196. Modiano JF et al (2012) Inflammation, apoptosis, and necrosis induced by neoadjuvant fas ligand gene therapy improves survival of dogs with spontaneous bone cancer. Mol Ther 20(12):2234–2243
197. Lenz JA et al (2022) Increased tumor-infiltrating lymphocyte density is associated with favorable outcomes in a comparative study of canine histiocytic sarcoma. Cancer Immunol Immunother 71(4):807–818
198. Estrela-Lima A et al (2010) Immunophenotypic features of tumor infiltrating lymphocytes from mammary carcinomas in female dogs associated with prognostic factors and survival rates. BMC Cancer 10(1):256
199. Cascio MJ et al (2021) Canine osteosarcoma checkpoint expression correlates with metastasis and T-cell infiltrate. Vet Immunol Immunopathol 232:110169
200. Maeda S et al (2021) BRAFV595E mutation associates CCL17 expression and regulatory T cell recruitment in urothelial carcinoma of dogs. Vet Pathol 58(5):971–980
201. Maeda S et al (2019) CCR4 blockade depletes regulatory T cells and prolongs survival in a canine model of bladder cancer. Cancer Immunol Res 7(7):1175–1187
202. Panek WK et al (2024) The CCL2-CCR4 axis promotes regulatory T cell trafficking to canine glioma tissues. J Neuro-Oncol 169(3):647–658
203. Cronise KE et al (2022) Characterizing the molecular and immune landscape of canine bladder cancer. Vet Comp Oncol 20(1):69–81
204. Yokota S et al (2023) CD204⁺ tumor-associated macrophages are associated with clinical outcome in

canine pulmonary adenocarcinoma and transitional cell carcinoma. Vet J 296-297:105992
205. Porcellato I et al (2022) Tumor-associated macrophages in canine Oral and cutaneous melanomas and Melanocytomas: phenotypic and prognostic assessment. Front Veter Sci 9:9
206. Withers SS et al (2019) Metastatic immune infiltrates correlate with those of the primary tumour in canine osteosarcoma. Vet Comp Oncol 17(3):242–252
207. Kerboeuf M et al (2024) Tumor-associated macrophages in canine visceral hemangiosarcoma. Vet Pathol 61(1):32–45
208. SHOSU K et al (2016) Programmed cell death ligand 1 expression in canine cancer. In Vivo 30(3):195–204
209. Maekawa N et al (2016) Immunohistochemical analysis of PD-L1 expression in canine malignant cancers and PD-1 expression on lymphocytes in canine oral melanoma. PLoS One 11(6):e0157176
210. Song DW, Ro WB, Park HM (2021) Evaluation of circulating PD-1 and PD-L1 as diagnostic biomarkers in dogs with tumors. J Vet Sci 22(5):e75
211. Pinard CJ et al (2022) Evaluation of lymphocyte-specific programmed cell death protein 1 receptor expression and cytokines in blood and urine in canine urothelial carcinoma patients. Vet Comp Oncol 20(2):427–436
212. Igase M et al (2020) A pilot clinical study of the therapeutic antibody against canine PD-1 for advanced spontaneous cancers in dogs. Sci Rep 10(1):18311
213. Maekawa N et al (2021) PD-L1 immunohistochemistry for canine cancers and clinical benefit of anti-PD-L1 antibody in dogs with pulmonary metastatic oral malignant melanoma. Npj Prec Oncol 5(1):10
214. Porcellato I et al (2021) FoxP3, CTLA-4, and IDO in canine melanocytic tumors. Vet Pathol 58(1):42–52
215. Marable J et al (2021) Nanobody-based CTLA4 inhibitors for immune checkpoint blockade therapy of canine cancer patients. Sci Rep 11(1):20763
216. Mason NJ et al (2021) Development of a fully canine anti-canine CTLA4 monoclonal antibody for comparative translational research in dogs with spontaneous tumors. MAbs 13(1):2004638
217. Maude SL et al (2014) Managing cytokine release syndrome associated with novel T cell-engaging therapies. Cancer J 20(2):119–122
218. Linette GP et al (2013) Cardiovascular toxicity and titin cross-reactivity of affinity-enhanced T cells in myeloma and melanoma. Blood 122(6):863–871
219. Morgan RA et al (2013) Cancer regression and neurological toxicity following anti-MAGE-A3 TCR gene therapy. J Immunother 36(2):133–151
220. Brudno JN, Kochenderfer JN (2016) Toxicities of chimeric antigen receptor T cells: recognition and management. Blood 127(26):3321–3330
221. Mata M, Gottschalk S (2016) Man's best friend: utilizing naturally occurring tumors in dogs to improve chimeric antigen receptor T-cell therapy for human cancers. Mol Ther 24(9):1511–1512
222. Panjwani MK et al (2016) Feasibility and safety of RNA-transfected CD20-specific chimeric antigen receptor T cells in dogs with spontaneous B cell lymphoma. Mol Ther 24(9):1602–1614
223. Mata M et al (2014) Toward immunotherapy with redirected T cells in a large animal model: ex vivo activation, expansion, and genetic modification of canine T cells. J Immunother 37(8):407–415
224. Panjwani MK et al (2020) Establishing a model system for evaluating CAR T cell therapy using dogs with spontaneous diffuse large B cell lymphoma. Onco Targets Ther 9(1):1676615
225. Zhang S et al (2022) B7-H3 specific CAR T cells for the naturally occurring, spontaneous canine sarcoma model. Mol Cancer Ther 21(6):999–1009
226. Yin Y et al (2018) Checkpoint blockade reverses Anergy in IL-13Rα2 humanized scFv-based CAR T cells to treat murine and canine gliomas. Mol Ther Oncol 11:20–38
227. McDonough SP, Moore PF (2000) Clinical, hematologic, and immunophenotypic characterization of canine large granular lymphocytosis. Vet Pathol 37(6):637–646
228. Lin CS et al (2018) Activating natural killer (NK) cytotoxicity of canine CD5(−)CD21(−) cells requires low surface CD5 density NK cells. Iran J Vet Res 19(2):87–95
229. Huang Y-C et al (2008) CD5-low expression lymphocytes in canine peripheral blood show characteristics of natural killer cells. J Leukoc Biol 84(6):1501–1510
230. Lin C et al (2018) Activating natural killer (NK) cytotoxicity of canine CD5− CD21− cells requires low surface CD5 density NK cells. Iranian J Vet Res 19(2):87
231. Lin Y-C et al (2010) Canine CD8 T cells showing NK cytotoxic activity express mRNAs for NK cell-associated surface molecules. Vet Immunol Immunopathol 133(2–4):144–153
232. Lee S-H et al (2018) Comparison of phenotypic and functional characteristics between canine non-B, non-T natural killer lymphocytes and CD3+CD5dimCD21− cytotoxic large granular lymphocytes. Front Immunol 9
233. Foltz JA et al (2016) NCR1 expression identifies canine natural killer cell subsets with phenotypic similarity to human natural killer cells. Front Immunol 7
234. Canter RJ et al (2017) Radiotherapy enhances natural killer cell cytotoxicity and localization in preclinical canine sarcomas and first-in-dog clinical trial. J Immunother Cancer 5(1):98
235. Razmara AM et al (2024) Preclinical evaluation and first-in-dog clinical trials of PBMC-expanded natural killer cells for adoptive immunotherapy in dogs with cancer. J Immunother Cancer 12(4):e007963

Comparative Cancer Diagnosis and Treatment

Comparative Pathology

Shane Sills

1 Introduction

Cancer is a heterogeneous group of diseases defined by dysregulated and uncontrolled cellular growth and a leading cause of morbidity and mortality in the human population. In the United States alone, there are almost 2 million new cases each year, with over 600,000 deaths [1]. Due to the genetic and molecular complexity of cancer, and neoplasia in general, treatment selection and outcome are widely variable, and seldom does one cancer respond precisely as another to any treatment regimen.

Animal models are vital to basic science and clinical research [2, 3]. They add to our understanding of cancer biology and help to develop or refine new treatment modalities. Experimental studies using laboratory animals, particularly rodents, are the most commonly utilized [2, 4]. These studies have provided invaluable information on the underlying cellular and molecular mechanisms of cancer development and metastasis in a highly controlled environment. In this instance, "environment" not only reflects the environment of the animal, but the environment of the cancer itself, namely, the animal tissues. Rodent models are often inbred lines or genetically modified, critical for experimental control. These studies are critical for not only basic cancer biology studies, but also for preclinical safety and assessment studies in drug development [5].

Another source of highly valuable in vivo information comes from spontaneous models of cancer [6]. In particular, the pet dog is an underutilized model for neoplasia and a potential goldmine of information [7]. There more than 89 million pet dogs in the United States alone. These beloved pets share similar environments to their human family, living in the same homes, outdoors, towns and cities. Similar phenotypes of cancer have been observed in dogs as in humans for a variety of different cancers, including cutaneous, hematopoietic, intestinal, mammary, and others [8]. Importantly, these similar phenotypes manifest spontaneously in dogs, and often at similar life stages. In dogs, diffuse large B cell lymphoma is the most common nodal lymphoma, just as it is in humans, and occurs at a similar life stage [9]. Gene expression studies have even shown overlap in affected molecular pathways, with similar transcriptional subtypes between humans and dogs [10]. In some cases, there are distinct and peculiar differences in canine neoplasia when compared to the human counterpart, which may in itself offer clues to the underlying disease processes. For example, canine osteosarcoma has very similar histologic features to humans, but occurs in older, large

S. Sills (✉)
Department of Veterinary Biosciences, The Ohio State University, College of Veterinary Medicine, Columbus, OH, USA
e-mail: sills.36@osu.edu

M. W. Nolan et al. (eds.), *Comparative Oncology*, https://doi.org/10.1007/978-3-032-04454-9_5

breed dogs most commonly; in humans, osteosarcoma is typically considered a childhood cancer. As we grow to understand canine cancer, we develop an understanding of human cancer as well. Dogs are very important from a drug development perspective as well. Large animals are required as preclinical safety assessment models for drug development. Clinical trials in canine patients can also provide much needed data on efficacy in a live patient as well [5, 11].

Beyond the powerful utility as a model for spontaneous neoplasia in humans, a deeper understanding of cancer in dogs serves its own purpose: improving the quality of life for our canine companions. Pet dogs are living longer than ever before, and the incidence of neoplasia, as our canine population ages, also rises. In this regard, the concept of One Health truly shines. As we study canine cancer, we learn more about cancer biology and the human disease, which leads to further development of powerful treatment modalities and diagnostic tools. These treatments can then be back translated from humans to dogs, ultimately benefiting both human and veterinary patients alike.

2 Comparative Pathology in Cancer Research

The term "*neoplasia*" literally translates as "new growth" and describes a mass of tissue composed principally of *irreversibly* altered cells that grow in an excessive, un-coordinated, and dysregulated manner. Importantly, this excessive, abnormal growth will persist even after the initiating stimulus is removed, and the genetic alterations are permanent, passing along to the daughter cells. Neoplasia is, fundamentally, a genetic disease. Genetic alterations promote alterations in molecular pathways affecting cell growth, regulation, replication, and metabolism. Neoplastic tumors arise from the clonal expansion of these initial neoplastic cells. The number and type of molecular pathways altered, as well as the degree of alteration, affect whether and how the cell will become neoplastic, how rapidly it will manifest, the extent of its growth and spread of disease, how the body will respond, and potentially affect clinical assessment and treatment.

The "hallmarks of malignancy" are a heuristic approach to categorize the myriad cellular and molecular phenomena that lead to the development of cancer [12, 13]. Initially described as six acquired characteristics of neoplasms in 2000 by Hanahan and Weinberg, the hallmarks now consist of 14 features that enable the neoplastic transformation of cells, as well as the persistence and spread of the neoplasm. The current hallmarks of malignancy include:

- Sustained proliferative signaling.
- Genome instability and mutation.
- Enabling replicative immortality.
- Resisting cell death.
- Evading growth suppressors.
- Evading immune destruction.
- Tumor-promoting inflammation.
- Inducing or accessing vasculature.
- Activation of invasion and metastasis.
- Deregulated cellular metabolism.
- Unlocking phenotypic plasticity.
- Cellular senescence.
- Polymorphic microbiomes.
- Epigenetic reprogramming.

Figure 1 highlights the hallmarks of malignancy in the context of where they may impact a given neoplasm, from alterations in the genetic code to the complex interactions within the tumor microenvironment. Importantly, the hallmarks are not necessarily discrete, monolithic categories. Rather, each hallmark may encompass multiple neoplastic features from the genetic to the systemic level; conversely, a single feature, such as a mutation, may fit multiple hallmarks of malignancy, depending on the severity of the change and the downstream impact. Distinguishing benign from malignant neoplasia is among the first steps of tumor evaluation, and is often assessed with routine histopathology and clinical examination, as in Fig. 2. However, in human medicine and increasingly so in veterinary medicine, characterization of neoplasia goes beyond morphology and must include careful genetic and molecular evaluation as well.

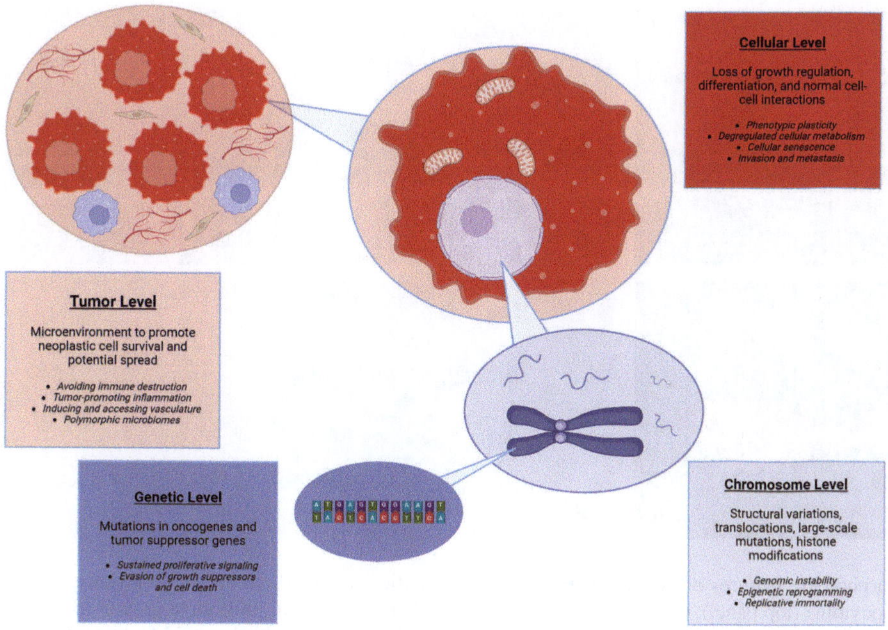

Fig. 1 The hallmarks of malignancy can be observed at various levels, from the tissue to the genetic level. Importantly, these are not static categories, and some hallmarks may span multiple levels and vice versa. (Created in BioRender. Sills, S. (2025) https://BioRender.com/lq8pqt9)

The genetic basis of cancer in humans and companion animals shares remarkable similarities. The human and canine genomes share approximately 85% homology, with even higher similarity among cancer-related genes [14]. Many cancer-driving mutations are shared between dogs and humans, such as the c-Kit gene mutation found in both human gastrointestinal stromal tumors and canine mast cell tumors [15].

Several cancer types show striking similarities between humans and companion animals. Osteosarcoma in dogs and children is almost indistinguishable at the microscopic level [16]. Canine and human breast cancers share many pathological and molecular similarities, including estrogen receptor positivity and common tumor phenotypes (luminal A, luminal B, and triple-negative) [8, 17]. Lymphomas, particularly diffuse large B cell lymphomas (DLBCL), show similar incidence rates and tumor behaviors in dogs and humans [8]. Here, we will highlight a few key examples of histopathological similarities and differences in common tumors between humans and domestic animals. Extensive comparisons of these tumors will be discussed in individual chapters within this book.

3 Tumors of Connective Tissue

Osteosarcoma (OS) is the most common bone tumor of both humans and dogs [18]. OS is considered to one of the most translatable diseases of dogs and humans and there have been numerous publications highlighting the similarities of this disease between the species [16, 18–21]. In both species, these tumors characterized as malignant spindle cell tumors with production of osteoid matrix by tumor cells [19]. Both species share common subtypes of OS including osteoblastic, chondroblastic, fibroblastic, and telangiectatic [22]. The osteoblastic subtype predominates in both, accounting for over 50% cases in both species [19]. However, the frequency of the other subtypes varies between the species [23]. Vascular invasion is also common in both species with up to 70% of primary tumors displaying this feature [23]. More recently, research has

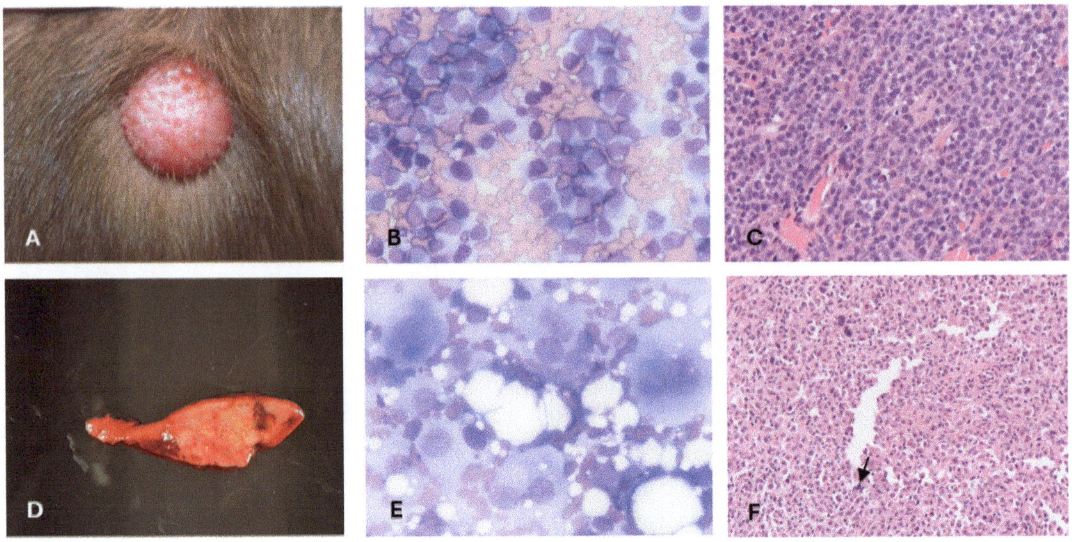

Fig. 2 Morphologic features of neoplasia. Benign cutaneous histiocytoma (top panel): Grossly, the mass is well-demarcated, expansile, and smooth (**a**). Cytologically, the cells have typical histiocytoid features, including pale cytoplasm, occasional vacuoles, and oval to round nuclei. The cells are monomorphic with minimal atypia (**b**). Histologically, the cells have similar features as in (**b**) and form sheets and cords (**c**). Malignant pulmonary histiocytic sarcoma (bottom panel): grossly, the mass is poorly demarcated with infiltrative growth (**d**). On cytology, the cells have some histiocytoid features, but are much more pleomorphic, with anisokaryosis and multinucleation (**e**). Similar histologic features show marked cellular and nuclear atypia with bizarre mitotic figures (arrow) (**f**). (Image credits: R. Jennings, B. Bessemer, S. Neal, S. Sills)

identified three distinct tumor microenvironmental subtypes in canine OS based on the composition of the cell present. These include immune enriched, immune enriched dense extracellular matrix-like, and immune desert. These subtypes are conserved in humans and can predict progression-free survival outcomes [24].

Sarcomas of soft tissues are much more common in dogs than in humans, but have many shared features. Canine soft tissue sarcomas (STS) are a group of morphologically and molecularly heterogeneous neoplasms, similar to human STS. Location and grade bear significant prognostic significance in both species [25]. Histologically, canine STS typically bears a close resemblance to human spindle cell sarcomas, myxoid sarcomas, and undifferentiated pleomorphic sarcomas [26]. Genomic and transcriptomic studies have shown a propensity for important fusion events as a recurring mutation type in both canine and human STSs [27].

4 Lymphoid Tumors

Lymphoma is the most common cancer diagnosed in pet dogs and the most common hematopoietic tumor of humans. Lymphoma is a term used to describe a spectrum of disorders characterized by a malignant monoclonal proliferation of lymphoid cells [28]. While there are many more subtypes of lymphoma identified in humans, many of the most common subtypes have also been identified in dogs. Extensive molecular analysis for the purpose of subtyping lymphoid malignancies in dogs has not yet been performed; however, ongoing research is continuously adding to our knowledge of this common disease.

The most commonly diagnosed lymphoma in humans and pet dogs is diffuse large B cell lymphoma (DLBCL) [29]. This disease is characterized by an expansion of large lymphoid cells with vesicular nuclei, prominent nucleoli and varying amounts of cytoplasm in both species. Severe cellular pleomorphism can also be observed in both species. Necrosis and varying numbers of mitotic cells are common in both species as well. Other shared subtypes include follicular lymphoma, mantle cell lymphoma and peripheral T cell lymphoma, not otherwise specified. Immunophenotyping via immunohistochemistry or flow cytometry is commonly used in both species and can provide both diagnostic and prognostic information.

5 Tumors of the Mammae and Reproductive Tracts

Comparative pathology has been utilized to draw comparisons between human breast cancer and canine mammary tumors. There are many similarities but also many differences between dogs and humans. Both human breast and canine mammary tumors display similar histological patterns, including ductal and lobular carcinomas [30]. They also have similar phenotypes including luminal A, luminal B, and triple-negative (basal-like) carcinomas [31]. Furthermore, approximately 60% of human breast cancers and 45% of canine mammary tumors are estrogen receptor positive [30]. This finding, however, highlights one of the main differences between human and canine tumors of the mammary gland, at least within the continental United States, as most female dogs are spayed before reaching sexual maturity significantly decreasing the role hormones play in the development of these tumors in dogs. Consequently, hormone receptor modulators are rarely used therapeutically in spayed female dogs. Even in intact female dogs, they average only two estrus cycles per year with a prolonged luteal phase with high progesterone levels which may influence tumor development differently than humans [30, 32, 33]. Evidence also suggests that there is a histological continuum from benign to malignant tumors in both humans and dogs [34].

While there are many similarities, there are also several differences between these species. Dogs have five pairs of mammae and will frequently develop tumors in multiple sites that may vary in histology. In general, canine tumors possess a more complex morphology with myoepithelial cell proliferation that is an uncommon feature in breast cancer in humans [35, 36].

The similarities between human and canine mammary tumors make dogs valuable models for studying breast cancer biology and testing new therapies [37]. However, the differences highlight the need for caution when extrapolating results between species. The spontaneous occurrence of mammary tumors in dogs, combined with their shared living environment with humans, provides unique opportunities for studying environmental and genetic factors in cancer development [37].

Another tumor of interest to comparative oncologists is prostatic carcinoma. This tumor is extremely common in men and cancer researchers have long searched for a comparative model for this disease. While the dog does develop prostatic carcinoma, there are some key differences making this a challenging model for the most common forms of prostatic cancer in men. One main difference is that the canine prostate has a uniform morphology without distinct zones while the human prostate is divided into zones [38]. The canine prostate also has a discontinuous basal cell layer, which differs from the human prostate structure [38]. Another major difference is the androgen dependence of these tumors in dogs and humans. In humans, androgens provide a driving source for malignant transformation, while canine prostatic carcinoma is often androgen independent [38, 39].

While dogs do have a much lower incidence of prostate cancer than humans, castration has been associated with a higher risk of developing prostate cancer in this species [39]. Neutered dogs also tend to have more aggressive disease with higher metastatic rates than intact dogs with prostatic cancer. In dogs, metastasis at the time of diagnosis has been reported to be as high as 80%, typically to regional lymph nodes [40, 41]. This is much higher than what is reported in humans at diagnosis. Though it should be noted that widespread routine screening using PSA levels in humans often leads to a much earlier diagnosis in humans than dogs.

While these similarities support the use of canine models in cancer research, it's important to note that some differences exist, such as the frequency of specific tumor morphologies and hormonal influences. The comparative histology between canine and human tumors provides valuable insights for developing new diagnostic techniques and treatment strategies that can benefit both species.

6 Comparative Aspects of Molecular Diagnostics in Oncology: Animals and Humans

Molecular diagnostics have revolutionized the field of oncology in both human and veterinary medicine. Here, we explore the comparative aspects of molecular diagnostic techniques used in cancer detection, prognosis, and treatment planning for animals and humans.

6.1 Fundamentals of Molecular Diagnostics in Oncology

Molecular diagnostics in oncology involve the analysis of DNA, RNA, and proteins to detect genetic alterations associated with cancer. These techniques provide valuable insights into tumor biology, enabling more precise diagnosis, prognosis, and treatment selection.

6.2 Shared Techniques

Both human and veterinary oncology utilize similar molecular diagnostic techniques:

- Polymerase chain reaction (PCR) and its variants (qPCR, RT-PCR, Multiplex PCR).
- Next-generation sequencing (NGS).
- Immunohistochemistry (IHC).
- Flow cytometry (FC).
- Fluorescent in situ hybridization (FISH).

These methods allow for the detection of specific genetic mutations, gene expression profiles and protein biomarkers associated with various cancer types,

Polymerase chain reaction (*PCR*) has become a cornerstone of molecular diagnostics in oncology, offering unparalleled sensitivity and specificity for detecting cancer-associated genetic alterations. Its ability to identify even minute quantities of nucleic acids makes it an indispensable tool for diagnosing cancers at early stages, monitoring disease progression, and guiding personalized treatment strategies. PCR can be used to detect known cancer-specific mutations such as point mutations, deletions and translocations with excellent sensitivity. In humans, for example, it is used to detect mutations in genes such as *TP53, KRAS,* and *EGFR* in both lung and colorectal cancers [42–45]. These mutations can help determine prognosis or drive treatment decisions [43–45]. Quantitative PCR techniques have been used to measure HER2 gene amplification in breast cancer tissues to guide targeted therapies [46]. In veterinary medicine, PCR is frequently used to diagnose urothelial cell carcinoma (UCC). A *BRAF p.V595E* mutation can be detected in the urine of dogs with both UCC and prostatic carcinoma [47, 48]. Interestingly, in humans, this same BRAF mutation is commonly observed in melanoma. In canine melanoma, this mutation is not common; however, canine melanomas do demonstrate upregulation of the MAPK pathway and therefore may have overlapping features with BRAF-independent human melanoma [49]. PCR has also been used to determine clonality within lymphoid populations to diagnose lymphoma [47, 50]. Additionally, PCR has been used to detect *cKIT* mutations in canine mast cell tumors, which can help guide treatment and also have prognostic value [47, 51].

NGS utilizes ultra-low passage whole-genome sequencing to identify large alterations in the DNA of cancer cells. Deeper sequencing techniques can be used to identify specific genetic mutations that may represent druggable targets with the tumor itself. Comprehensive genomic profiling of tumors is increasingly used in human oncology to guide treatment decisions. While not as advanced in veterinary oncology, similar approaches are being developed for companion animals. In humans, many of the common genetic alterations in specific cancers have been interrogated for their utility as druggable target. For example, primary lung tumors in humans are often sequenced to identify mutations in EGFR or MET. Drugs targeting these pathways have been developed and have shown significant clinical benefit [52]. It is important to understand that only 10% of the human genome contains druggable targets and that only half of these are actually disease relevant [53]. This is an important concept to grasp as veterinary medicine ventures into its own genetic age. While many tumors have multiple mutations that may have a corresponding therapeutic, many of them will not have driver roles in the tumor. This means that targeting them will have no or even a deleterious effect [54]. While NGS analysis of tumors is commercially available for veterinary species, the data demonstrating which of these identified targets are actually disease relevant in specific cancers is lacking and use of these panels to drive clinical decision making should be done with extreme caution.

Immunohistochemistry (IHC) is a histologic technique for visualizing the expression of a select protein in tissue sections. IHC is most commonly performed on formalin-fixed, paraffin-embedded tissue, although snap-frozen sections are also possible [55]. Protein expression is identified using antibodies directed at the antigen of interest, and expression is visualized using a chromogenic reaction, or fluorescence (*immunofluorescence*, IF) [56, 57]. IHC methods may be direct (primary antibody only) or indirect (primary and secondary antibodies). Primary antibodies are developed for the particular antigen of interest, such as CD45 for leukocytes, vimentin for mesenchymal tissues, or various cytokeratins for different epithelial populations. In severely anaplastic neoplasms, IHC is necessary to even determine whether the neoplasm is epithelial or mesenchymal, as demonstrated in Fig. 3 [56, 57]. Other biomarkers may have prognostic potential. IHC is often employed to assess the proliferative activity of neoplastic cells, which is commonly associated with increased malignant potential. Biomarkers such as antigen Kiel 67 (Ki-67) or proliferating cell nuclear antigen (PCNA) are more sensitive than traditional mitotic counts, because they are expressed in a broader range of the cell cycle. Cells within the proliferative pool that may not have entered the M phase are not visible as mitotic figures but can be visualized by their expression of these markers. Other biomarkers may have prognostic implications for more specific neoplasms [58]. In humans, breast cancers are routinely subtyped based on the profile of their expression of estrogen and progesterone receptors, as well as human epidermal growth factor receptor 2 (HER2) [59, 60]. Breast cancers that lack expression of all three of these markers ("triple-negative breast cancer") carries a poorer prognosis than other subtypes and identifying them is critical information for treatment. Notably, recent molecular analysis of canine mammary malignancies has shown that mammary carcinoma of dogs most closely resembles triple-negative breast cancer in humans, including overlapping signaling pathways and histomorphology [61]. As mentioned above, identification of the stem cell factor receptor c-kit has prognostic significance in cutaneous mast cell tumors [62]. IHC is especially useful in this case, because the distribution of the c-kit protein is an important feature. Normally expressed on the cell membrane, c-kit can be detectable in the cytoplasm or even nucleus of neoplastic mast cells, and nuclear expression is associated with a poorer prognosis. IHC has also been utilized to detect potential therapeutic targets, such as the immune checkpoint molecules PD1 and its ligand, PD-L1 [63]. By inhibiting these checkpoints with antibodies, the immune system "brakes" are disrupted, allowing a more robust immune response within the tumor microenvironment. PD1 and PD-L1 are often targets of IHC to evaluate their expression in a neoplasm prior to administering immune checkpoint blockade, and have been demonstrated and targeted for therapy in human and canine cases [63–65].

Flow cytometry is another technology for detecting protein biomarkers. Identification of antigens with flow cytometry is similar to IHC; that is, antigen-antibody recognition, although flow cytometry typically uses fluorescent tags.

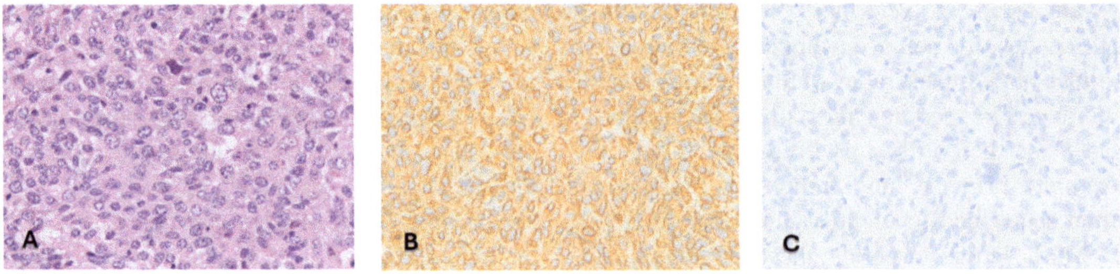

Fig. 3 Utility of immunohistochemistry in phenotyping (400× magnification). This malignant neoplasm is severely anaplastic, hindering identification on H&E (**a**). Using IHC staining, the neoplastic cells exhibit robust cytoplasmic labeling for vimentin (**b**) and no labeling for pancytokeratin (**c**). This expression pattern indicates a mesenchymal cell origin, supporting a diagnosis of sarcoma. (Image credits: S. Sills, K. Sarkan)

Flow cytometry does not typically provide in situ information unless an imaging cytometer is used. Instead of visualization on a tissue slide, flow cytometry is conducted on single-cell suspensions [66]. In cancer biology and oncology, solid tumor samples can be dissociated and brought into suspension, or cell aspirates can be suspended. The suspension is then stained with a cocktail of fluorescent-conjugated antibodies directed at a number of cell surface antigens. Within the cytometer, the cells are hydrodynamically forced into a single-file line, where each passes through a laser set perpendicular to the flow line. Light transmitted through the cells, as well as fluorescence emitted from the conjugated antibodies, are then recorded by various detectors [66]. Flow cytometry has wide applications in human and canine oncology. It is especially useful in characterizing lymphoproliferative and myeloproliferative diseases, as these neoplasms are typically easily brought into single-cell suspension, and have numerous cell-surface molecules that act as phenotyping and prognostic targets, particularly the various cluster of differentiation (CD) molecules used to describe leukocytic lineages [66–68]. Flow cytometry has also been heavily utilized in cancer immunology, to extensively characterize the tumor microenvironment and immune response in humans and dogs [69, 70].

In some cases, it may be more useful to visualize gene expression rather than protein expression. While molecular techniques such as polymerase chain reaction (PCR) are the gold standard for quantifying a particular gene or set of genes, observing where in the cell, and where in the tumor, a particular gene is expressed may be preferable. Moreover, in some instances, detecting a protein product using IHC or flow cytometry may be particularly difficult, particularly if translation or expression of a protein is rare. It may be more valuable to detect the RNA transcript of a gene instead. For this, pathologists increasingly rely on RNA in situ hybridization [71]. This technique works in a similar fashion to IHC; it provides a color change to visualize expression of a molecule of interest in FFPE tissue. Instead of direct or indirect antibodies, specific probes designed to hybridize with key segments of an RNA transcript are attached to a chromogenic or fluorescent probe. This is especially powerful when paired with PCR, as the probes for RNA in situ hybridization are often similar to, if not identical to, the primers used in a PCR reaction. PCR, much like flow cytometry, provides more quantifiable data to complement the spatial information provided by in situ hybridization. RNA in situ hybridization has seen increased usage in cancer diagnostics, in both humans and dogs [71, 72].

Cytogenetic studies, such as basic and spectral karyotyping and DNA fluorescent in situ hybridization (FISH), allow visualizations of genomic segments or entire chromosomes, to detect structural variations such as large-scale duplications or deletions, translocations, inversions, or aneuploidy. For example, although located on different chromosomes in dogs and humans, a translocation resulting in fusion of the BCR and ABL genes is detectable in chronic myeloid leukemia of both species [73]. This translocation is readily observed using FISH, as the two genes of interest are stained with distinct fluorescent probes; the aberrant juxtaposition of the two probes in close proximity is indicative of translocation and fusion, and is appreciable on fluorescent microscopy. As technology advances, it has become increasingly cost-effective for DNA sequencing of human and canine cancers. These next-generation techniques allow for identification of somatic and germline mutations across the entire exome (protein-coding portion) or even genomes of cancers, identifying key mutations and the possible impact on the biological behavior of a given neoplasm.

6.3 Cancer Detection

Diagnostic biomarkers play a crucial role in cancer diagnosis for both humans and animals. In veterinary oncology, diagnostic biomarkers are used to primarily to identify or confirm the presence of a tumor and determine its type [47]. However, in human oncology, molecular biomarkers have expanded importance and have also become essential for tumor classification and subtyping. For example, in canine lymphoma, immunophenotyping using flow cytometry for markers such as CD79a and CD3 can be used to diagnose and subtype lymphoma [47]. Additional biomarkers, such as MHC class II expression have been shown to have prognostic significance for canines [47]. In humans, the approach to diagnosing lymphomas includes a multifaceted approach, including immunophenotyping (by flow cytometry and/or IHC), as well as cytogenetics and mutational profiling. For example, human DLBCL is typically further classified into germinal center B cell (GCB) and activated B cell (ABC) subtypes. Assignment of these subtypes has important prognostic significance, as ABC subtypes have a poorer prognosis and response to treatment [74]. This assessment can be done through RNA profiling, but is also often accomplished through IHC algorithms, comparing expression of markers such as CD10, MUM1, FoxP1, and BCL6 [75]. In dogs, similar molecular features in DLBCL have been shown [10]; however, the IHC expression pattern differs from humans, and the prognostic significance has not been elucidated in dogs.

Liquid biopsy is an emerging technology to characterize neoplasia through minimally invasive techniques, such as blood draw or urinalysis. Genetic and molecular characteristics can be gleaned from circulating tumor cells (CTC), cell-free DNA (cfDNA), and even extracellular vesicles (EV), and their utility are summarized in Fig. 4 [76]. Liquid biopsy techniques have been successfully applied in human and veterinary medicine through several commercial offerings. Screening of large presumably healthy populations using tests such as Cologuard®, have improved the early detection of colorectal cancer (CRC) in humans [77]. The sensitivity of this test for detecting CRC directly is low; however, its ability to identify a subset of patients who benefit from enhanced screening from colonoscopy or advanced imaging has led to improved outcomes and a decreased risk of mortality due to CRC [77, 78].

Liquid biopsy tests for the purpose of cancer detection are becoming more commonplace in human medicine. In a 2020 study by Liu et al., the authors demonstrated the utility of a multi-cancer detection assay using methylation signatures in cfDNA to detect and identify the tissue of origin of cancer cells in the blood [79]. This test has been shown to detect more than 50 types of cancer, most of which are uncommon and do not have existing screening protocols. This work lead to the pivotal PATHFINDER study published by Nadauld et al. in 2021. In this study, test results were provided to the clinicians for "real-world" assessment utilizing this tool. In this study of more than 6000 participants, 34 (0.5%) received a positive result without a diagnosis of cancer. Of the patients with an identifiable cancer diagnosis, just under half of them had early stage cancers detected and 71% of the cancers detected were cancers that do not have standard screening protocols [80]. The sensitivity of this test for all cancers detected was just over 50%. As expected, sensitivity increased with tumor burden and the presence of systemic disease (stage I—16.8%,

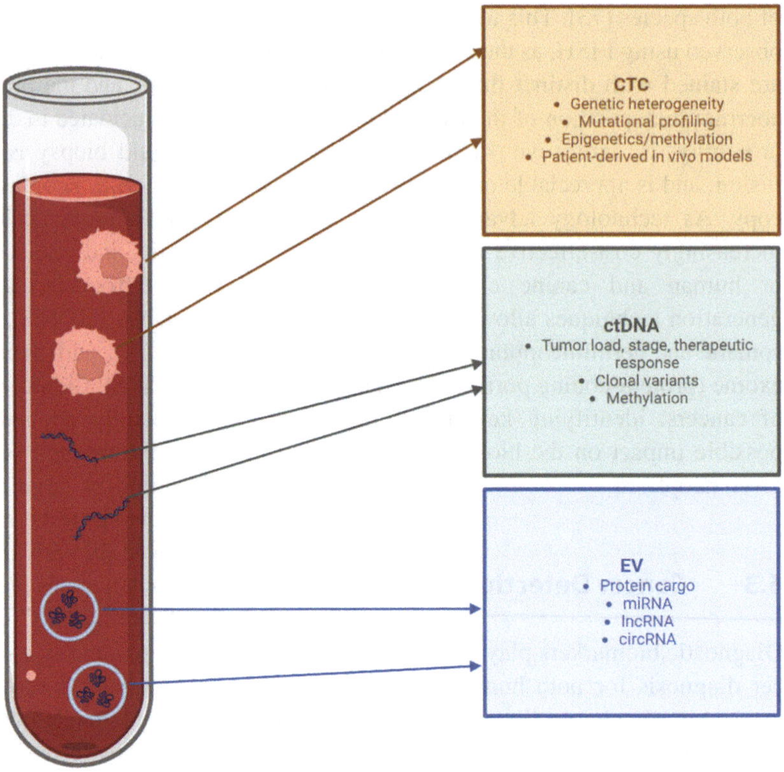

Fig. 4 Applications of liquid biopsy in human and canine medicine. Neoplasia-associated factors, including circulating tumor cells (CTC), circulating tumor DNA (ctDNA), and tumor-associated extracellular vesicles (EV), can be isolated from patient blood, allowing for deep characterization, diagnosis, and prognostication of neoplasia from minimally invasive blood draws. (Created in BioRender. Sills, S. (2025) https://BioRender.com/2hlm4ba)

stage II—40.4%, stage III—77.0%, and stage IV—90.1%) [81].

For veterinary patients, there are a few commercially available screening tests. Adoption by general practitioners has been slow but awareness is improving with time. The first of these tests is the Cancer Risk Assessment™ (CRA) score available through VDI laboratories which first launched in 2013 [82]. This test uses a dual biomarker algorithm to create a score of cancer risk using C-reactive protein (CRP) and thymidine kinase 1 (TK1). The Pet Preferred Early Cancer Screening Test is available for dogs and cats and uses serum concentrations of onconeural antibodies to assess patients for a risk of a variety of cancers and neurological diseases. The Nu.Q Cancer Test quantifies the amount of circulating nucleosomes in the blood of dogs as a surrogate of cfDNA levels and cancer risk. This test has been used to identify up to 18 different histologic types of cancer with varying levels of performance, but works best for lymphoma, hemangiosarcoma and histiocytic sarcoma [83].

7 Conclusions

Accurate diagnosis of neoplasia is essential for prognostics and treatment. Understanding the vocabulary of neoplasia ensures accurate communication between colleagues and disciplines. Proper communication and coordination between clinicians and pathologists allow for a more refined diagnostic approach. This includes margin evaluations, grading, staging, and selection of ancillary diagnostics to provide the most pertinent information for diagnosis and treatment. Cancer is a heterogeneous disease but has many overlapping features between individuals, be they canine or human, and a comparative approach to cancer research and diagnostics will be beneficial to both human and veterinary medical care.

References

1. American Cancer Society (2022) Cancer facts & figures 2022. American Cancer Society, Atlanta
2. Li Z, Zheng W, Wang H, Cheng Y, Fang Y, Wu F et al (2021) Application of animal models in cancer research: recent progress and future prospects. Cancer Manag Res 13:2455–2475
3. Onaciu A, Munteanu R, Munteanu VC, Gulei D, Raduly L, Feder R-I, Pirlog R, Atanasov AG, Korban SS, Irimie A et al (2020) Spontaneous and induced animal models for cancer research. Diagnostics 10(9):660
4. Nance RL, Sajib AM, Smith BF (2022) Chapter 3 – canine models of human cancer: bridging the gap to improve precision medicine. In: Tao Y-X (ed) Progress in molecular biology and translational science, vol 189. Academic Press, pp 67–99
5. Ruggeri BA, Camp F, Miknyoczki S (2014) Animal models of disease: pre-clinical animal models of cancer and their applications and utility in drug discovery. Biochem Pharmacol 87(1):150–161
6. Pinho SS, Carvalho S, Cabral J, Reis CA, Gartner F (2012) Canine tumors: a spontaneous animal model of human carcinogenesis. Transl Res 159(3):165–172
7. Gardner HL, Fenger JM, London CA (2016) Dogs as a model for cancer. Annu Rev Anim Biosci 4:199–222
8. Oh JH, Cho JY (2023) Comparative oncology: overcoming human cancer through companion animal studies. Exp Mol Med 55:725–734
9. Valli VE, Kass PH, San Myint M, Scott F (2013) Canine lymphomas: association of classification type, disease stage, tumor subtype, mitotic rate, and treatment with survival. Vet Pathol 50(5):738–748
10. Richards KL, Motsinger-Reif AA, Chen H-W, Fedoriw Y, Fan C et al (2013) Gene profiling of canine B-cell lymphoma reveals germinal center and postgerminal center subtypes with different survival times, modeling human DLBCL. Cancer Res 73(16):5029–5039
11. Lucroy MD, Suckow MA (2020) Predictive modeling for cancer drug discovery using canine models. Expert Opin Drug Discov 15(6):731–738
12. Hanahan D, Weinberg RA (2011) Hallmarks of cancer: the next generation. Cell 144(5):646–674
13. Hanahan D (2022) Hallmarks of cancer: new dimensions. Cancer Discov 12(1):31–46
14. Chibuk J, Flory A, Kruglyak KM, Leibman N, Nahama A, Dharajiya N et al (2021) Horizons in veterinary precision oncology: fundamentals of cancer genomics and applications of liquid biopsy for the detection, characterization, and management of cancer in dogs. Front Vet Sci. 8:664718
15. Roskoski R (2018) The role of small molecule kit protein-tyrosine kinase inhibitors in the treatment of neoplastic disorders. Pharmacol Res 133:35–52
16. Khanna C, Fan TM, Gorlick R, Helman LJ, Kleinerman ES, Adamson PC et al (2014) Toward a drug development path that targets metastatic progression in osteosarcoma. Clin Cancer Res 20(16):4200–4209
17. Paoloni MC, Khanna C (2007) Comparative oncology today. Vet Clin North Am Small Anim Pract 37(6):1023–1032. v
18. Paoloni M, Davis S, Lana S, Withrow S, Sangiorgi L, Picci P et al (2009) Canine tumor cross-species genomics uncovers targets linked to osteosarcoma progression. BMC Genomics 10:625
19. Mueller F, Fuchs B, Kaser-Hotz B (2007) Comparative biology of human and canine osteosarcoma. Anticancer Res 27(1A):155–164
20. Gordon I, Paoloni M, Mazcko C, Khanna C (2009) The comparative oncology trials consortium: using spontaneously occurring cancers in dogs to inform the cancer drug development pathway. PLoS Med 6(10):e1000161
21. Paoloni MC, Mazcko C, Fox E, Fan T, Lana S, Kisseberth W et al (2010) Rapamycin pharmacokinetic and pharmacodynamic relationships in osteosarcoma: a comparative oncology study in dogs. PLoS One 5(6):e11013
22. Nagamine E, Hirayama K, Matsuda K, Okamoto M, Ohmachi T, Kadosawa T et al (2015) Diversity of histologic patterns and expression of cytoskeletal proteins in canine skeletal osteosarcoma. Vet Pathol 52(5):977–984
23. Culp WT, Rebhun RB, Alvarez EM, Malogolowkin MM, Randall RL, Thorpe SW (2020) Canine osteosarcoma: where human and canine research intersect. Ann Joint 5
24. Patkar S, Mannheimer J, Harmon SA, Ramirez CJ, Mazcko CN, Choyke PL et al (2024) Large-scale comparative analysis of canine and human osteosarcomas uncovers conserved clinically relevant tumor microenvironment subtypes. Clin Cancer Res 30(24):5630–5642
25. Dell'Anno F, Giugliano R, Listorti V, Razzuoli E (2024) A review on canine and human soft tissue sarcomas: new insights on prognosis factors and treatment measures. Vet Sci 11(8):362
26. Milovancev M, Hauck M, Keller C, Stranahan LW, Mansoor A et al (2015) Comparative pathology of canine soft tissue sarcomas: possible models of human non-rhabdomyosarcoma soft tissue sarcomas. J Comp Pathol 152(1):22–27
27. Das S, Idate R, Lana SE, Regan DP, Duval DL (2023) Integrated analysis of canine soft tissue sarcomas identifies recurrent mutations in TP53, KMT genes and PDGFB fusions. Sci Rep 13:10422
28. Ito D, Frantz AM, Modiano JF (2014) Canine lymphoma as a comparative model for human non-Hodgkin lymphoma: recent progress and applications. Vet Immunol Immunopathol 159(3–4):192–201
29. Aresu L, Ferraresso S, Marconato L, Cascione L, Napoli S, Gaudio E et al (2019) New molecular and therapeutic insights into canine diffuse large B-cell lymphoma elucidates the role of the dog as a model for human disease. Haematologica 104(6):e256–e2e9
30. Ektefaie Y, Yuan W, Dillon DA, Lin NU, Golden JA, Kohane IS et al (2021) Integrative multiomics-

histopathology analysis for breast cancer classification. NPJ Breast Cancer 7(1):147
31. Chocteau F, Abadie J, Loussouarn D, Nguyen F (2019) Proposal for a histological staging system of mammary carcinomas in dogs and cats. Part 1: canine mammary carcinomas. Front Vet Sci 6:388
32. Fillmore CM, Gupta PB, Rudnick JA, Caballero S, Keller PJ, Lander ES et al (2010) Estrogen expands breast cancer stem-like cells through paracrine FGF/Tbx3 signaling. Proc Natl Acad Sci USA 107(50):21737–21742
33. Rueda JR, Porto CD, Franco RP, da Costa IB, Bueno LMC, Girio RJS et al (2024) Mammary neoplasms in female dogs: clinical, diagnostic and therapeutic aspects. Vet Med (Praha) 69(4):99–114
34. Sorenmo KU, Kristiansen VM, Cofone MA, Shofer FS, Breen AM, Langeland M et al (2009) Canine mammary gland tumours; a histological continuum from benign to malignant; clinical and histopathological evidence. Vet Comp Oncol 7(3):162–172
35. Rosen PP (1987) Adenomyoepithelioma of the breast. Hum Pathol 18(12):1232–1237
36. Visan S, Balacescu O, Berindan-Neagoe I, Catoi C (2016) In vitro comparative models for canine and human breast cancers. Clujul Med 89(1):38–49
37. Bhutta ZA, Choi KC (2025) Canine mammary tumors as a promising adjunct preclinical model for human breast cancer research: similarities, opportunities, and challenges. Arch Pharm Res 48(1):43–61
38. Nascente EP, Amorim RL, Fonseca-Alves CE, de Moura VMBD (2022) Comparative pathobiology of canine and human prostate cancer: state of the art and future directions. Cancers (Basel) 14(11)
39. Ryman-Tubb T, Lothion-Roy JH, Metzler VM, Harris AE, Robinson BD, Rizvanov AA et al (2022) Comparative pathology of dog and human prostate cancer. Vet Med Sci 8(1):110–120
40. Cannon CM, Allstadt SD (2015) Lower urinary tract cancer. Vet Clin North Am Small Anim Pract 45(4):807–824
41. Langdon SP (2012) Animal modeling of cancer pathology and studying tumor response to therapy. Curr Drug Targets 13(12):1535–1547
42. Raj GV, Moreno JG, Gomella LG (1998) Utilization of polymerase chain reaction technology in the detection of solid tumors. Cancer 82(8):1419–1442
43. Netter J, Lehmann-Che J, Lambert J, Tallet A, Lourenco N, Soliman H et al (2015) Functional TP53 mutations have no impact on response to cytotoxic agents in metastatic colon cancer. Bull Cancer 102(2):117–125
44. Das S, Samaddar S (2025) Recent advances in the clinical translation of small-cell lung cancer therapeutics. Cancers (Basel) 17(2)
45. Hosamani KR et al (2024) Pyrazole, Pyrazoline, and fused Pyrazole derivatives: new horizons in EGFR-targeted anticancer agents. Chem Biodivers 21(11):e202400880
46. El Hadi H, Abdellaoui-Maane I, Kottwitz D, El Amrani M, Bouchoutrouch N, Qmichou Z et al (2017) Development and evaluation of a novel RT-qPCR based test for the quantification of HER2 gene expression in breast cancer. Gene 605:114–122
47. Aupperle-Lellbach H, Kehl A, de Brot S, van der Weyden L (2024) Clinical use of molecular biomarkers in canine and feline oncology: current and future. Vet Sci 11(5)
48. Thomas R, Wiley CA, Droste EL, Robertson J, Inman BA, Breen M (2023) Whole exome sequencing analysis of canine urothelial carcinomas without BRAF V595E mutation: short in-frame deletions in BRAF and MAP2K1 suggest alternative mechanisms for MAPK pathway disruption. PLoS Genet 19(4):e1010575
49. Mochizuki H, Breen M (2015) Comparative aspects of BRAF mutations in canine cancers. Vet Sci 2(3):231–245
50. Hwang MH, Darzentas N, Bienzle D, Moore PF, Guscetti F, Morrison J et al (2019) A review of canine B cell clonality assays and primer set optimization using large-scale repertoire data. Vet Immunol Immunopathol 209:45–52
51. Alvarez-Twose I, Gonzalez de Olano D, Sanchez-Munoz L, Matito A, Esteban-Lopez MI, Vega A et al (2010) Clinical, biological, and molecular characteristics of clonal mast cell disorders presenting with systemic mast cell activation symptoms. J Allergy Clin Immunol 125(6):1269–78 e2
52. Garcia-Robledo JE, Rosell R, Ruíz-Patiño A, Sotelo C, Arrieta O, Zatarain-Barrón L et al (2022) KRAS and MET in non-small-cell lung cancer: two of the new kids on the 'drivers' block. Ther Adv Respir Dis 16:17534666211066064
53. Cheng AC, Coleman RG, Smyth KT, Cao Q, Soulard P, Caffrey DR et al (2007) Structure-based maximal affinity model predicts small-molecule druggability. Nat Biotechnol 25(1):71–75
54. López-Cortés A, Cabrera-Andrade A, Echeverría-Garcés G, Echeverría-Espinoza P, Pineda-Albán M, Elsitdie N et al (2024) Unraveling druggable cancer-driving proteins and targeted drugs using artificial intelligence and multi-omics analyses. Sci Rep 14(1):19359
55. Ella-Tongwiis P, Makanga A, Shergill I, Hughes SF (2021) Optimisation and validation of immunohistochemistry protocols for cancer research. Histol Histopathol 36(4):415–424
56. Ramos-Vara JA, Miller MA (2014) When tissue antigens and antibodies get along: revisiting the technical aspects of immunohistochemistry – the red, brown, and blue technique. Vet Pathol 51(1):42–87
57. Ramos-Vara JA (2005) Technical aspects of immunohistochemistry. Vet Pathol 42(4):405–426
58. Jurikova M, Danihel L, Polak S, Varga I et al (2016) Ki67, PCNA, and MCM proteins: markers of proliferation in the diagnosis of breast cancer. Acta Histochem 118(5):544–552
59. Bonacho T, Rodrigues F, Liberal J (2020) Immunohistochemistry for diagnosis and progno-

sis of breast cancer: a review. Biotech Histochem 95(2):71–91
60. Yaghoobi V, Martinez-Morilla S, Liu Y, Charette L, Rimm DL, Harigopal M (2020) Advances in quantitative immunohistochemistry and their contribution to breast cancer. Expert Rev Mol Diagn 20(5):509–522
61. Namagerdi AA, d'Angelo D, Ciani F, Iannuzzi CA, Napolitano F et al (2020) Triple-negative breast cancer comparison with canine mammary tumors from light microscopy to molecular pathology. Front Oncol 10:563779
62. Webster JD, Yuzbasiyan-Gurkan V, Kaneene JB, Miller RA, Resau JH, Kiupel M (2006) The role of c-KIT in tumorigenesis: evaluation in canine cutaneous mast cell tumors. Neoplasia 8(2):104–111
63. Taube JM, Akturk G, Angelo M, Engle EL, Gnjatic S et al (2020) The Society for Immunotherapy in cancer statement on best practices for multiplex immunohistochemistry (IHC) and immunofluorescence (IF) staining and validation. J Immunother Cancer 8(1):e000155
64. Tan WCC, Nerurkar SN, Cai HY, Ng HHM, Wu D et al (2020) Overview of multiplex immunohistochemistry/immunofluorescence techniques in the era of cancer immunotherapy. Cancer Commun 40(4):135–153
65. Maekawa N, Konnai S, Nishimura M, Kagawa Y, Takagi S et al (2021) PD-L1 immunohistochemistry for canine cancers and clinical benefit of anti-PD-L1 antibody in dogs with pulmonary metastatic oral malignant melanoma. NPJ Precis Oncol 5:10
66. Reggeti F, Bienzle D (2011) Flow cytometry in veterinary oncology. Vet Pathol 48(1):223–235
67. Riondato F, Comazzi S (2021) Flow cytometry in the diagnosis of canine B-cell lymphoma. Front Vet Sci 8:600986
68. Bellesi S, Fiorita A, Corina L, D'Agostino G, Maiolo E et al (2023) The role of flow cytometry for the timely diagnosis of lymphoma in the head and neck district. Oral Oncol Rep 6:100045
69. Parys M, Bavcar S, Mellanby RJ, Argyle D, Kitamura T (2023) Use of multi-color flow cytometry for canine immune cell characterization in cancer. PLoS One 18(3):e0279057
70. Bonilla DL, Reinin G, Chua E (2021) Full spectrum flow cytometry as a powerful technology for cancer immunotherapy research. Front Mol Biosci 7:612801
71. Himmel LE, Hackett TA, Moore JL, Adams WR, Thomas G et al (2018) Beyond the H&E: advanced technologies for in situ tissue biomarker imaging. ILAR J 59(1):51–65
72. Maes RK, Langohr IM, Wise AG, Smedley RC, Thaiwong T, Kiupel M (2014) Beyond H&E: integration of nucleic acid–based analyses into diagnostic pathology. Vet Pathol 51(1):238–256
73. Culver S, Ito D, Borst L, Bell JS, Modiano JF, Breen M (2013) Molecular characterization of canine BCR-ABL–positive chronic myelomonocytic leukemia before and after chemotherapy. Vet Clin Pathol 42:314–322
74. Nowakowski GS, Czuczman MS (2015) ABC, GCB, and double-hit diffuse large B-cell lymphoma: does subtype make a difference in therapy selection? Am Soc Clin Oncol Educ Book 35(1):e449–e457
75. Choi WWL, Weisenburger DD, Greiner TC, Piris MA, Banham AH et al (2009) A new immunostain algorithm classifies diffuse large B-cell lymphoma into molecular subtypes with high accuracy. Clin Cancer Res 15(17):5494–5402
76. Lone SN, Nisar S, Masoodi T, Singh M, Rizwan A et al (2022) Liquid biopsy: a step closer to transform diagnosis, prognosis, and future of cancer treatments. Mol Cancer 21:79
77. Clebak KT, Nickolich S, Mendez-Miller M (2022) Multitarget stool DNA testing (Cologuard) for colorectal cancer screening. Am Fam Physician 105(2):198–200
78. Stürzlinger H, Conrads-Frank A, Eisenmann A, Invansits S, Jahn B, Janzic A et al (2023) Stool DNA testing for early detection of colorectal cancer: systematic review using the HTA core model. Ger Med Sci 21:Doc06
79. Liu MC, Oxnard GR, Klein EA, Swanton C et al (2020) Sensitive and specific multi-cancer detection and localization using methylation signatures in cell-free DNA. Ann Oncol 31(6):745–759
80. Beer TM, McDonnell CH, Nadauld L, Liu MC, Klein EA, Reid RL, Marinac C, Chung K, Lopatin M, Fung ET, Schrag D (2021) Interim results of PATHFINDER, a clinical use study using a methylation-based multi-cancer early detection test. J Clin Oncol 39(15):3010–3010
81. Klein EA, Richards D, Cohn A, Tummala M, Lapham R, Cosgrove D et al (2021) Clinical validation of a targeted methylation-based multi-cancer early detection test using an independent validation set. Ann Oncol 32(9):1167–1177
82. Selting KA, Sharp CR, Ringold R, Knouse J (2015) Serum thymidine kinase 1 and C-reactive protein as biomarkers for screening clinically healthy dogs for occult disease. Vet Comp Oncol 13(4):373–384
83. Wilson-Robles HM, Bygott T, Kelly TK, Miller TM, Miller P, Matsushita M et al (2022) Evaluation of plasma nucleosome concentrations in dogs with a variety of common cancers and in healthy dogs. BMC Vet Res 18(1):329

Comparative Radiobiology and Radiation Therapy

Charles A. Maitz and Ravi Patel

1 Introduction

Since the discovery of x-rays by Roentgen in 1895, descriptions of x-rays for medical uses in dogs and other animals have accompanied those describing use in humans. Richard Eberlein, a German physician and veterinarian, described the use of x-rays for diagnosis in 1896 and reported radiation therapy in 1905 [51]. Eberlein published radiographs of several veterinary species, and many credit him as likely the first to use radiation to treat cancer in animals. Alois Pommer, director of the Roentgen Institute, published on the skin tolerance of horses and dogs during the 1940s and 1950s and continued to report on the treatment of carcinomas and sarcomas using protocols that continued in veterinary use until only the last two to three decades [187, 188]. In 1969, Ed Gillette started a program in clinical and experimental radiation therapy at Colorado State University. In 1994, the American College of Veterinary Radiology designated Radiation Oncology as a recognized subspecialty, charging Mark Dewhirst, Pat Gavin, Ed Gillette, and Don Thrall as the organizing committee [75]. The members of the founding committee all played key roles in the development of veterinary radiation oncology, all had strong foundations in radiation biology, and all were committed to a shared vision of comparative radiation oncology. In the three decades since the ACVR-RO was recognized, membership has grown to over 100 board-certified veterinary radiation oncologists spanning several continents.

Much like human radiation oncology, veterinary radiation oncology initially used orthovoltage units to treat superficial tumors in patients, before adopting cobalt-60 units, and then linear accelerators. In 2001, a survey of veterinary radiation therapy facilities was conducted, revealing a total of 42 sites, 17 (40%) of which were academic institutions, and 25 (60%) of which were private practice facilities. At that time, 3 facilities used orthovoltage units, 18 used linear accelerators (three off-site at a human facility), and 22 used cobalt-60 [148]. A similar survey was performed in 2010 and reported that the number of sites had nearly doubled to 76, 24 (32%) of which were academic, and 52 (68%) of which were private practice. At that time, all veterinary radiation therapy facilities were using on-site linear accelerators [55]. Eight years later, it was reported that 37 veterinary facilities (55% of respondents of the survey) provide stereotactic radiation therapy, either with a linear accelerator, helical tomotherapy, or CyberKnife [49]. Historically, most veterinary facilities sourced equipment second-hand, often purchasing equipment previously used in

C. A. Maitz (✉)
College of Veterinary Medicine, University of Missouri, Columbia, MO, USA
e-mail: maitzc@missouri.edu

R. Patel
UPMC Hillman Cancer Center, Pittsburg, PA, USA

M. W. Nolan et al. (eds.), *Comparative Oncology*, https://doi.org/10.1007/978-3-032-04454-9_6

human facilities. Today, there is an increasing number of veterinary facilities purchasing equipment new, capable of providing state-of-the-art care to patients.

The use of modern radiotherapy equipment provides an opportunity for veterinary radiation oncologists to provide the same standard of care to their patients as their physician counterparts. It also provides an environment where the comparative aspects of veterinary radiation oncology and radiobiology can flourish. While finely fractionated protocols have been limited by logistical factors including machine availability and the need for patient anesthesia, stereotactic radiation therapy protocols in veterinary patients can match those used to treat people with cancer. With the same advanced planning techniques and treatment delivery devices used in human clinical trials, novel radiation therapy modalities and protocols can be delivered to veterinary patients. With advanced imaging systems, disease response and progression, pharmacokinetics, and even radiopharmaceutical uptake can be tracked and quantitated. Veterinary radiation oncology has continued to advance rapidly over the last 30 years, and this chapter will describe how comparative radiation oncology and radiobiology have been important to these advances and will continue to contribute to the treatment of cancer in pets and people.

2 Normal Tissue Tolerance to Radiation

In 2010, the Red Journal (International Journal of Radiation Oncology • Biology • Physics) published a special issue on the Quantitative Analyses of Normal Tissue Effects in the Clinic (QUANTEC) which compiled a breadth of data in an effort to relate clinical radiation therapy outcomes with normal tissue delivered doses [136]. Before this special issue, which relied on the effort of a number of investigators across many institutions, clinicians leaned on a hallmark paper by Emami et al., which amassed clinical data on normal tissues complemented by expert opinions of experienced clinicians [53]. However, while the fields of radiation oncology and radiation biology were still in their infancy, translational research was being carried out in a number of different models to evaluate the response of normal tissues to radiation. In 1922, George Whipple and Stafford Warren published a series of papers in the Journal of Experimental Medicine describing "Roentgen Ray Intoxication," in which they report the effects of thoracic and abdominal irradiation on a variety of animals, including dogs [238–241]. Dogs were specifically chosen as a test subject in these studies due to familiarity with canine behavior and digestive physiology. In these studies, Warren and Whipple described the development of diarrhea and observed histologic loss of crypt epithelium as well as bacterial translocation from the gastrointestinal tract into the bloodstream after whole abdomen irradiation [238]. In another study, the investigators demonstrated little sparing effect of daily fractionation of whole abdominal radiation doses, but a significant sparing effect of weekly fractionation, in addition to a significant volume effect of abdominal irradiation [239]. Additional studies evaluated the physical characteristics of radiation effects through animal subjects, evaluating organs affected and zones of transition between irradiated and unirradiated tissues [240] and comparisons between-whole body radiosensitivity of a variety of different species, including dogs, cats, rats, birds, snakes, and frogs [241].

These initial studies in comparative radiobiology provided groundwork toward the use of large animal models of normal tissue radiation side effects. Early studies carefully described radiation dermatitis in pig skin, which has continued to serve as a model of radiation dermatitis and radiation fibrosis. Many of these studies involve semiquantitative numerical skin effect scores based on observations of degrees of side effects such as erythema and desquamation [17, 19, 64]. These normal tissue animal models have been incredibly useful in the development of dose-response relationships in a variety of tissues beyond skin, including intestine, lung, spinal cord, kidney, oral mucosa, and parotid gland [90, 108]. While the use of both small and large animal preclinical animal models has been important in the understanding of radiobiology, radiobiology research utilizing companion animals has provided significant insight into both tumor and normal tissue responses to radiation that can benefit both veterinary and human medicine.

Over the course of his career and the training of numerous veterinary radiation oncologists, Ed Gillette was a pioneer of not only veterinary radiation oncology, but also comparative radiobiology. Gillette's studies in both research-bred dogs as well as companion dogs with spontaneous cancer defined comparative radiation oncology, strengthening both human and veterinary radiobiology. Systematic studies evaluating the response of thoracic radiation in dogs gave insight into early and late effects of the heart, pericardium, and lungs, drawing isoeffect curves and evaluating the effects of fraction size on outcomes such as fibrosis, stroke volume, pulmonary hypertension, and ultimately determining alpha/beta doses for such effects [76, 78, 143, 145, 146, 189]. Fike and others evaluated radiation dose–response relationships after single-dose hemibrain irradiation to doses from 11.5 Gy to 17 Gy. They evaluated toxicities with serial CT scans and calculated an LD_{50} of 14.9 Gy with a steep dose–response curve, while also describing two different processes of late radiation damage: the classic degenerative late effects, and a more rapid onset "delayed acute" reaction, believed to be caused by demyelination [58, 226]. Similarly, researchers, including Gillette, evaluated the histopathologic dose–response relationship of the canine spinal cord. Following these dogs for several years, researchers were able to characterize a number of different lesions in the spinal cord, including white matter necrosis, massive hemorrhage, and segmental parenchymal atrophy with an ED_{50} of 56.9 Gy in 4 Gy fractions, as well as less severe local fiber loss, with an ED_{50} of 49.5 Gy in 4 Gy fractions [191]. These parameters have been used to guide radiation planning in veterinary medicine for decades. Similar systematic studies were performed to evaluate the dose–response relationship and fractionation effects of the trachea in dogs, where dogs received 36–74 Gy in 2, 3, or 4 Gy fractions. Fractionation sparing effects and alpha/beta doses were determined for a variety of endpoints, including decrease in goblet cells (3.5 Gy), surface ulceration (4.7 Gy), decrease in submucosal glands (4.5 Gy), and increase in connective tissue (1.8 Gy) [190]. These data demonstrated the need for finer fractionated protocols to spare tracheal side effects. The pathogenesis of radiation nephropathy was elucidated by studies involving kidney irradiation and serial biopsy to look for pathologic changes, giving insight into radiation-induced kidney failure and normal tissue tolerances [98]. The use of dogs was essential in the understanding of radiation effects on the bone marrow and, in particular, in the development of bone marrow transplantation procedures, ultimately providing hope for a cure in some forms of leukemia [82]. Rainer Storb, considered one of the pioneers in stem cell transplantation techniques, recognized the important roles dogs can play in understanding tolerances of bone marrow ablation and the nuances of the immune system and graft-versus-host disease [13, 83, 218, 233].

In 2001, the Veterinary Radiation Therapy Oncology Group (VRTOG) published a standardized side effect scoring scheme that is used to quantitate radiation-induced side effects in normal tissues [120]. This scheme was developed to be analogous to the RTOG radiation morbidity scoring scheme. In 2023, the VRTOG toxicity grading scheme was updated into a format which provides a framework which complements the updated Veterinary Cooperative Oncology Group-Common Terminology Criteria for Adverse Events (VCOG-CTCAE v2) [127, 186]. These widely adopted standardized scoring schemes improve comparison between studies and provide a more quantitative method of reporting radiation side effects, which could serve to increase the potential of comparative radiobiologic studies in veterinary patients with naturally occurring tumors. Such studies are currently used to evaluate emerging treatment techniques, such as FLASH radiotherapy, discussed later in this chapter. Research into normal tissue tolerances to radiation are now also expanding beyond just the tissue being irradiated, as researchers have acknowledged that radiodermatitis can cause systemic somatosensory sensitization [169]. The interaction between radiotherapy and the immune system has become important as well, with companion dogs representing an important step in the translation of these treatments [42].

3 DNA Damage Response, Repair, and Radiogenomics

Dysregulation of the DNA Damage Response (DDR) is implicated in the development and progression of cancer. Defects in DDR pathways can render cells more susceptible to genomic instability and mutation, potentially contributing to cancer development [34]. Improved understanding of the DDR allows researchers to develop more effective treatments targeting specific components of the DDR, potentially enhancing the sensitivity of cancer cells to radiation and other therapies, while sparing normal tissues [88]. Most DDR studies are performed in well-established xenograft models of human cancer cell lines. These models can be propagated in cell culture, and in vitro DDR studies such as clonogenic survival studies, COMET assays, and quantification of γH2AX foci can be performed as relatively inexpensive screening assays. Then to test in vivo efficacy of DDR agents, these tumor models can be implanted into immunodeficient mice, and tumor response as well as gene expression and DDR assays could be assessed. Xenograft mouse models have been the backbone of translational DDR research due to their ability to study efficacy of novel treatments in models of human cancer in a relatively inexpensive manner. Evaluating the DDR pathways first in vitro and later in mouse xenograft models provides a robust mechanistic understanding that promotes the translation of new therapeutic interventions.

Yet, despite many agents demonstrating efficacy in xenograft models, relatively few new DDR treatment strategies have been successfully translated into the clinical setting. In contrast to most naturally arising cancers in the clinical setting which have heterogeneous tumor biology and variable sensitivity to DDR agents, xenograft models are relatively homogenous. Moreover, there has been greater appreciation of the importance of the DDR-induced immune response for tumor control. Many new treatment strategies are testing DDR agents in combination with cancer immunotherapies which require an intact immune system to model response. To study these treatment paradigms, syngeneic or genetically modified models of murine cancer can be utilized, but they often have much more rapid proliferation and fail to produce tumors with similar biology to spontaneously arising human cancers.

Comparative oncology models can provide some important advantages in the study and ultimate translation of DDR-directed therapies [89, 92]. The molecular similarities between human and dog cancer have been well documented, particularly with regard to the DDR, where, for instance, the homology between dog and human ATM is roughly 90%, which is greater than the homology between human and pig ATM [72]. While there is generally a high degree of conservation of DDR gene expression among mammalian cells, the rates of DNA repair mechanisms, including base excision repair (BER), nucleotide excision repair (NER), homologous recombination (HR), and non-homologous end-joining (NHEJ) in humans were demonstrated to be more similar to those of dogs than rats or mice [176]. In another study which evaluated fluctuations in the levels of p53 protein across species, the oscillations in p53 expression in canine cells did not significantly differ from those in human cells, while both differed significantly from mouse and rat cells [217]. Alteration of DNA mismatch repair (MMR) genes leads to microsatellite instability, and this has been identified in a number of human cancers, including hereditary nonpolyposis colon cancer (HNPCC), endometrial cancer, gastrointestinal cancers, and others [180]. One study surveying a number of canine tumors with immunolabeling of MMR proteins (MSH2, MSH6, and MLH1) identified MMR deficiency in 60% of the canine oral malignant melanoma and 53% of the hepatocellular carcinoma samples evaluated [103]. Canine OMM was also noted to have significant loss or reduction of p16 expression and loss of nuclear p53 in the majority of tumor samples, a translationally relevant change that is often seen in human malignant melanoma [116, 219].

4 Comparative Radiation Oncology

Since its origins, veterinary radiation oncology has built a foundation upon comparative medicine with strong considerations toward the basic tenets of radiobiology [168, 232]. Conventional radiotherapy and multifraction regimens are based upon earlier investigations into the effects of fractionation, which identified that, through fractionation, radiation oncologists can improve the ratio of tumor death to normal tissue effects. The conceptual framework for fractionation is derived from the four Rs of radiobiology: (1) Repair of sublethal damage, (2) Reassortment of cells within the cell cycle, (3) Reoxygenation, and (4) Repopulation describe the potential benefits and limitations of fractionation in radiotherapy [90].

The linear-quadratic (LQ) model was developed to model in vitro cell killing and has been modified to allow for comparison between different dose-fractionation schemata. These correlations, using either Biologically Effective Dose (BED) or Equivalent Dose in 2 Gy Fractions (EQD2) have been widely used to develop radiotherapy protocols in veterinary medicine, where fraction number is often limited due to cost, anesthetic morbidity, and length of treatment. As a result, while many human radiation protocols use a 2 Gy fraction as a standard fraction size, finely fractionated protocols in veterinary medicine can range from 2.5 to 4.0 Gy per fraction [55]. In 2010, The Red Journal (International Journal of Radiation Oncology, Biology, Physics) published an issue featuring a series of articles describing the Quantitative Analyses of Normal Tissue Effects in the Clinic, or QUANTEC, which summarized maximum tolerated doses with expected toxicity rates and endpoints for several tissues, all normalized to the use of 2 Gy fractions. In veterinary radiation oncology, we have only a limited number of known tissue tolerances, many documented as previously described by Ed Gillette and his fellow researchers. Therefore, it is common practice among veterinary radiation oncologists to extrapolate QUANTEC data for normal tissue tolerances in companion animals, performing BED/EQD2 corrections as appropriate. Table 1 is an example of a toxicity table used at the University of Missouri Veterinary Health Center for planning constraints, with QUANTEC tissue tolerances extrapolated based on EQD2 calculations using α/β values determined from Emami et al. [53, 137].

Recently, there has been an increase in the number of publications describing the interplay between localized radiation therapy and systemic effects, particularly with regard to interactions with the immune system. Nevertheless, classical radiobiology relied on models of cell killing and focused on radiotherapy as a localized treatment with local effects. In this regard, fraction size has been a key factor in the development of radiation therapy protocols in veterinary medicine. Total dose delivered is most predictive of tumor control as well as acute, or short-term side effects. The side effects are generally transient and are often treated symptomatically. In general, a small dose per fraction (1.8–3.0 Gy/fx) allows for tolerance to treat to higher total doses while limiting the occurrence of late side effects, which can cause significant morbidity and mortality. Treating with a higher dose per fraction is associated with a higher risk of late side effects. The effects of fraction size can also be affected by the tissue type being irradiated, and tissues are considered either "early responding" or "late responding." In the LQ formalism, these tissue types are associated with a relatively high (~10) or low (~3) α/β dose, respectively.

With the advent of advanced image guidance and precise radiation delivery, large doses per fraction can be more safely administered through stereotactic radiation therapy (SRT) of the head and stereotactic body radiation therapy (SBRT). While growing, SRT is still limited in veterinary medicine, both in practice and in publication. Though there remains variability, the most common SRT protocols used in veterinary medicine are 3 fractions of 8–12 Gy delivered daily or every other day. In veterinary medicine,

Table 1 A normal tissue dose constraint table adjusted for treatment with 3 Gy fractions, common in veterinary radiation oncology

Structure	Volume	Dose/volume (3 Gy fx)	Max dose (3 Gy fx)	Toxicity rate	Toxicity endpoint
Brain			48.2	<3%	Symptomatic necrosis
Brain			57.9	0.05	Symptomatic necrosis
Brain			72.4	0.1	Symptomatic necrosis
Brain stem			43.4	<5%	Neuropathy or necrosis
Brain stem	D1–10 cc	47.4	0.0	<5%	Neuropathy or necrosis
Brain stem			51.5	<5%	Neuropathy or necrosis
Optic nerve/chiasm			45.8	<3%	Optic neuropathy
Optic nerve/chiasm			50.0	>7–20%	Optic neuropathy
Spinal cord			40.9	0.002	Myelopathy
Spinal cord			49.1	0.06	Myelopathy
Spinal cord			56.5	0.5	Myelopathy
Cochlea	Mean	37.5		<30%	Sensory-neural hearing loss
Parotid, bilateral	Mean	20.8		<20%	Long-term salivary function <25%
Parotid, bilateral	Mean	32.5		<50%	Long-term salivary function <25%
Parotid, unilateral	Mean	16.7		<20%	Long-term salivary function <25%
Pharyngeal constrictors	Mean	42.6		<20%	Symptomatic dysphagia and aspiration
Larynx			56.3	<20%	Vocal dysfunction
Larynx	Mean	42.6		<30%	Aspiration
Larynx	Mean	37.5		<20%	Edema
Larynx	0.27	42.6		<20%	Edema
Lung	0.3	17.3		<20%	Symptomatic pneumonitis
Lung	Mean	6.1		0.05	Symptomatic pneumonitis
Lung	Mean	11.2		0.1	Symptomatic pneumonitis
Lung	Mean	17.3		0.2	Symptomatic pneumonitis
Lung	Mean	20.8		0.3	Symptomatic pneumonitis
Lung	Mean	23.4		0.4	Symptomatic pneumonitis
Esophagus	Mean	28.3		5–20%	Grade 3+ esophagitis
Esophagus	0.5	29.2		<30%	Grade 2+ esophagitis
Esophagus	0.4	41.7		<30%	Grade 2+ esophagitis
Esophagus	0.2	58.3		<30%	Grade 2+ esophagitis
Heart (pericardium)	Mean	20.8		<15%	Pericarditis
Heart (pericardium)	0.46	24.0		<15%	Pericarditis
Heart	0.1	20.0		<1%	Long-term cardiac mortality
Liver	Mean	23.3		<5%	RILD (in normal liver function)
Liver	Mean	32.7		<50%	RILD (in normal liver function)
Liver	Mean	21.8		<5%	RILD (in child-Pugh A or HCC)
Liver	Mean	28.0		<50%	RILD (in child-Pugh A or HCC)
Kidney, bilateral	Mean	12.5		<5%	Clinical dysfunction
Kidney, bilateral	Mean	23.3		<50%	Clinical dysfunction
Kidney, bilateral	0.55	10.0		<5%	Clinical dysfunction
Kidney, bilateral	0.32	16.7		<5%	Clinical dysfunction

(continued)

Table 1 (continued)

Structure	Volume	Dose/volume (3 Gy fx)	Max dose (3 Gy fx)	Toxicity rate	Toxicity endpoint
Kidney, bilateral	0.3	19.2		<5%	Clinical dysfunction
Kidney, bilateral	0.2	23.3		<5%	Clinical dysfunction
Stomach	D100	41.1		<7%	Ulceration
Small bowel (individual loops)	<120 cc	13.5		<10%	Grade 3+ toxicity
Small bowel (peritoneal cavity)	<195 cc	40.5		<10%	Grade 3+ toxicity
Rectum	<50%	42.9		<10%	Grade 3+ toxicity
Rectum	<35%	51.4		<10%	Grade 3+ toxicity
Rectum	<25%	55.7		<10%	Grade 3+ toxicity
Rectum	<20%	60.0		<10%	Grade 3+ toxicity
Rectum	<15%	64.3		<10%	Grade 3+ toxicity
Bladder (bladder cancer)			56.3	<6%	Grade 3+ toxicity
Bladder (prostate cancer)	<50%	56.3			Grade 3+ toxicity
Bladder (prostate cancer)	<35%	60.7			Grade 3+ toxicity
Bladder (prostate cancer)	<25%	65.0			Grade 3+ toxicity
Bladder (prostate cancer)	<15%	69.3			Grade 3+ toxicity

Dose constraints are adjusted from QUANTEC data using α/β conversions from Emami et al. [53]

stereotactic radiation has not yet demonstrated clear survival advantages over finely fractionated radiation therapy, but minimization of patient time in hospital and improvement in perceived quality of life should not be understated. The advent of SRT and SBRT in veterinary medicine provides an opportunity for comparative radiation oncology to adopt human radiation therapy protocols, since treatment duration and repeated anesthetic events no longer limit veterinarians' ability to treat to comparable doses. This dose and fraction similarity will only help to further reinforce the role of comparative radiation oncology and radiobiology in the coming years.

4.1 Soft Tissue Sarcoma

Soft tissue sarcomas include several different types of mesenchymal neoplasia (e.g., peripheral nerve sheath tumor, perivascular wall tumor, fibrosarcoma, schwannoma, etc.) and the histology is similar between dogs and humans. While soft tissue sarcomas tend to occur more commonly in companion animals (they account for 8–15% of cutaneous and subcutaneous tumors in dogs) than in humans (comprising less than 1% of all tumors), there is overlapping biology [114, 155]. In both species, tumor grade is strongly associated with clinical outcomes including local recurrence and metastasis. Soft tissue sarcomas are typically considered locally invasive and infrequently metastasize; however, histologic grade and mitotic index are the factors most associated with metastasis and local disease recurrence in both dogs and people. Local treatment modalities form the foundation of soft tissue sarcoma treatment. Surgical excision is generally considered the treatment of choice. If complete excision is not achievable or for high-grade tumors with increased risk of recurrence, then treatment with RT, either in the adjuvant or neoadjuvant setting, should be considered. The treatment of gross soft tissue sarcoma is a challenge in both humans and veterinary patients, and sarcomas in dogs provide an excellent platform for comparative studies of novel and emerging therapies.

In humans, wound complications are more common with preoperative versus postoperative RT, but long-term local tumor control rates are comparable [33, 172]. In veterinary medicine, there have been no head-to-head comparisons of how RT timing impacts oncologic outcomes (e.g., tumor control, overall survival time). In a study evaluating the impacts of RT on cutaneous and mucosal flap complications in dogs, it was found that the severity of complications was decreased when RT was postoperative, but ultimately (and similar to the human experience), 85% of irradiated flaps were successful [205].

When surgery is combined with RT in dogs and cats with soft tissue sarcoma, it has been common to use high radiation doses (42–63 Gy) delivered in 15–21 fractions. This is associated with good local control and prolonged survival (1851–2270 days) [63, 151]. These protocols are comparable to those used in humans, which generally range from 40 to 66 Gy delivered in up to 33 fractions. The advent of improved image guidance technologies on-board modern linear accelerators has invited an increased interest in hypofractionated protocols. Preoperative RT protocols have become more hypofractionated for a number of different types of human cancers, including soft tissue sarcoma. For example, it was recently reported that 35 Gy given in 5 daily fractions 4 to 6 weeks prior to surgery led to excellent rates of local control with wound complications occurring in 25% of patients [15]. Likewise, the safety of similarly short-course hypofractionated, neoadjuvant RT has been evaluated in 34 dogs treated with 25 Gy in 5 fractions via helical TomoTherapy. Surgical complications were noted in 17% of dogs, and there was no association between surgical complications and presence of acute radiation side effects, though there was an association between disease location (trunk) and likelihood of complications [211].

When RT is used alone to treat bulky canine soft tissue sarcomas, long-term tumor control is limited, but there is a clear dosee-response relationship. In dogs randomized to receive 35, 40, 45, or 50 Gy in 10 fractions, the dose to control 50% of tumors at 12 months (TCD_{50}) was 45.3 Gy, and this dose to cause normal tissue necrosis in 50% of animals (ND_{50} at 12 months) was 54 Gy [147]. Protocols delivering lower total doses (3–4 weekly fractions of 8 Gy) have been less successful, with low response rates, short progression-free intervals (155–263 days), and survival times under a year [123, 182]. Stereotactic body RT may provide improved local control in some cases of gross soft tissue sarcoma. In a study of 35 dogs receiving 3 fractions of 9–16 Gy, the progression-free and overall survival times were 521 and 713 days, respectively; 46% of dogs had objective responses and 3/28 evaluable dogs experienced a complete response [68]. Response to SBRT was less favorable in another study of 52 dogs receiving 20–50 Gy in 1–5 fractions; here, the median PFS was 173 days and the median OST was 228 days, though this increased to 475 days for the 30% of dogs that had an objective response to treatment. In this study, dogs with metastasis and large primary tumors were more likely to progress and die, with every 100 cm^3 increase in tumor volume resulting in a 5% increase in risk of progression [225]. In both studies, risk of late skin toxicity was considered to be dose-limiting.

4.2 Head and Neck Tumors

Oral tumors are common in dogs and cats; neck tumors including thyroid tumors, tonsillar squamous cell carcinoma, and carotid body tumors have also been well reported. Canine sinonasal tumors, including adenocarcinoma, carcinoma, chondrosarcoma, fibrosarcoma, osteosarcoma, and others, comprise approximately 1% of all tumors in dogs and are locally aggressive tumors with a relatively low rate of metastasis at diagnosis. In humans with head and neck tumors, HPV status and degree of hypoxia have been associated with prognosis [81, 106]. While papillomavirus has not been associated with canine sinonasal tumors, the correlations of glucose metabolism (FDG), cell proliferation (FLT), and hypoxia (Cu-ATSM) were characterized in 20 dogs with sinonasal tumors [23]. These imaging parameters were also investigated as biomarkers of response and resistance to treatment in dogs receiving external beam radiotherapy; in particular, FLT avidity (a marker of tumor cell proliferation) at mid-treatment was inversely correlated with oncologic outcome [24]. Additionally, human and canine sinonasal carcinoma share a similar pattern of p53 overexpression and receptor tyrosine kinase expression including PDGFR,

EGFR, and VEGFR2 [66, 69, 96]. A prospective, multicenter, VRTOG study evaluated combination toceranib phosphate (Palladia) and radiotherapy in 63 dogs, identifying improved tumor response and rates in dogs receiving combination compared to radiation alone [52]. A number of different RT protocols have been used over the years to treat canine sinonasal tumors, including palliative-intent protocols consisting of 20 Gy total in 5 daily fractions or weekly fractions of 6–8 Gy total for 4 to 6 fractions, definitive-intent protocols that are either conventionally fractionated (i.e., 42–63 Gy in 10–20 fractions) or administered with stereotactic body RT (15–36 Gy total in 1–5 fractions) [3, 29, 65, 73, 74, 101, 124, 141, 170, 214, 221]. Despite these efforts, long-term local control of these tumors remains challenging, with most tumors recurring within the treatment volume [185]. A better understanding of the ability of radiation to activate the immune system, particularly in head and neck tumors, could be an important key to improving tumor control, and comparative radiation oncology research in dogs can help to identify those key relationships [42].

Another translationally relevant and common head and neck neoplasm encountered in the veterinary radiation oncology clinic is feline oral squamous cell carcinoma (FOSCC), which is an extremely aggressive cancer that has been likened to HPV-negative oral squamous cell carcinoma in people due to the fact that it is a clinically aggressive disease most often developing in the absence of a detectable feline papillomavirus infection. Much like in the human disease, epidemiologic studies have identified environmental carcinogens that serve as risk factors for FOSCC [36, 164]. Additionally, the best levels of disease control have been achieved with protocols that incorporate accelerated radiation fractionation and/or radiosensitizing chemotherapy. Despite intensive treatment, oncologic outcomes are generally poor; median survival times range from 3 to 6 months [57, 184]. Treatment of FOSCC remains challenging, and this represents an opportunity for using FOSCC clinical trials to evaluate novel treatment strategies.

4.3 Osteosarcoma

Osteosarcoma (OS) most commonly affects the long bones of large breed dogs; it is locally aggressive, and approximately 85% of dogs have micrometastatic disease present at the time of diagnosis. The gold standard treatment for canine appendicular OS is amputation of the affected limb plus adjunctive cytotoxic platinum chemotherapy. For dogs who do not receive amputation, external beam palliative-intent RT improves OS pain, lameness scores, and quality of life in at least 80% of affected dogs [84, 149, 192]. Additionally, stereotactic body RT given together with platinum-based chemotherapy has been used as a definitive-intent limb-sparing treatment [40, 41, 54, 87, 138]. With definitive RT (either finely fractionated or stereotactic), there is a risk of pathologic fracture, but most dogs experience improved lameness and analgesia, with survival comparable to surgery plus chemotherapy [138, 171]. The majority of comparative studies in OS focus on the treatment of metastatic disease, rather than the improvement of local disease, but radiobiology could still play a very important role in these studies.

Similarities in the biology of human and canine OS can be leveraged to accelerate development of new approaches to combinatorial and/or tumor-targeted therapy. For example, Osteosarcoma Tumor Proteins 1 and 3 (TP1 and TP3, respectively) have been used to develop monoclonal murine antibodies specific to human OS cells. TP3 has also been shown to be expressed on pulmonary metastatic OS lesions in dogs, and an F-18 labeled Fab fragment of TP3 further demonstrated uptake and binding in dogs with naturally occurring OS [142, 175]. More recently, TP1 and TP3 were determined to target the ALPL1 cell receptor, which is overexpressed in bone and pulmonary OS lesions of dogs and humans. This target has been used to develop a chimeric antigen receptor therapy for OS in humans [152]. The safety and feasibility of prophylactic whole lung irradiation, a technique described in human patients with Ewing's sarcoma, was demonstrated in series of 12 dogs with appendicular OS and could invite future studies evaluating combination therapies [25, 163, 197, 242]. Osteosarcoma is a disease that is frequently evaluated using the novel and emerging radiotherapy techniques (e.g., Flash RT, spatially fractionated RT, radiopharmaceuticals) described later in this chapter, where the interplay between human and veterinary radiation oncology can inform one another.

4.4 Malignant Melanoma

Many canine malignant melanoma (CMM) lesions originate in the oral cavity, and while not UV-induced, CMM shares biological behavior and many molecular similarities and alterations in signaling pathways with human mucosal melanoma [8]. Treatment of CMM with cytotoxic chemotherapy has been generally unrewarding, and small-molecule inhibitors targeting key mutations, such as BRAF, are not feasible given the lack of any predominant mutation among canine melanomas [216]. In light of these challenges, there has been a great deal of investigation into immunotherapy, which has played a significant role in the treatment of humans with malignant melanoma [6]. The Oncept melanoma vaccine is a xenogeneic DNA vaccine encoding human tyrosinase, which has been USDA approved to stage II to III canine oral melanoma. This vaccine is generally regarded as safe to administer, though there are some disagreements about its effectiveness in improving patient survival [179]. There are no specific studies evaluating the combination of RT and the Oncept vaccine, though recent studies illuminating the complex interplay between RT and the immune system suggest that a combination may improve outcomes [27, 62, 220]. In a multi-institutional retrospective analysis of 131 dogs with oral melanoma who received multimodal therapy including Oncept vaccine, those who received RT as part of their treatment regimen had a decreased risk of progression. Prospective studies evaluating the combination of RT and immunotherapy in CMM could help to better characterize this relationship. The development of canine-specific immune checkpoint blockade has been slow but may become an important avenue of treatment for CMM patients. Merck Animal Health has recently received FDA approval for the use of a PD1 monoclonal antibody in dogs with melanoma, and a veterinary clinical trial of RT plus an anti-CTLA4 monoclonal antibody is underway. The development of these agents and these veterinary clinical trials represents a scaffold upon which oncology researchers can further investigate the interplay between RT and immune checkpoint inhibition.

While RT is a mainstay of CMM treatment, it has a limited role in the treatment of human melanoma, especially since the advent of immune checkpoint blockers. The TROG 2.01 study did demonstrate that adjuvant nodal radiation therapy of 48 Gy in 20 fractions could reduce risk of nodal relapse; however, current guidelines recommend adjuvant immune checkpoint blockade in these patients [91]. Nevertheless, there is evidence that RT can potentiate the effect of immune checkpoint blockade, and, perhaps, comparative oncology can further enable research into such combination therapies [181].

4.5 Intracranial Neoplasia

Over the past decade, researchers have bolstered the translational role of brain tumors in companion dogs [94, 115, 126]. The most common primary brain tumor types in dogs are meningioma (predominately atypical meningioma), and gliomas including astrocytomas, oligodendrogliomas, glioblastoma, and undifferentiated subtypes. While advanced molecular techniques are used to classify glioma subtypes in humans, these methods are not well described in canine glioma. Nevertheless, the Comparative Brain Tumor Consortium (CBTC) has developed a simplified revised pathologic classification scheme which better matches human glioma characterization [115].

Stereotactic RT has become commonplace in the treatment of canine brain tumors, particularly in cases not amenable to surgery [86]. Survival times with SRT alone vary between 1 and 2 years, with most dogs dying of recurrent local disease

[46, 158, 229, 250]. Several different immunotherapy techniques have been attempted, including gene and vaccine therapy. Tumor vaccination combined with losartan and propranolol resulted in objective tumor response, with a significantly improved survival time in vaccine responders (500 days vs. 218 days) [7, 183]. However, at the time of death, there were no differences in the two groups in lymphocyte or macrophage infiltrates in the tumor. The gross and histologic appearance of tumor types, underlying molecular changes, and advanced imaging and treatment techniques all contribute to improved translatability between treatment of intracranial tumors in dogs and humans [153].

There are important challenges in the development of comparative brain tumor studies in dogs. For example, most canine intracranial neoplasms are irradiated in the gross disease setting, without biopsy for confirmatory diagnosis. Using patient clinical data and evaluating MRI features, sensitivity and specificity of identifying intracranial glioma are fairly high (91% and 94%, respectively), though important alternative diagnoses are certainly possible, and histopathology remains the gold standard for brain tumor diagnosis [16, 244]. This diagnostic accuracy can vary between different institutions and imaging protocols. To improve consistency, the Comparative Brain Tumor Consortium has released consensus recommendations for MRI imaging protocols for multi-institutional studies [174].

In humans with metastatic brain cancer, it is common to treat with SRS or whole-brain RT, and hippocampal sparing has been found to improve cognitive function in patients posttreatment [80]. Metastatic intracranial disease has been observed with moderate frequency in dogs, with the most common histologies being hemangiosarcoma, melanoma, and lymphoma [194, 213]. Most canine patients with metastatic CNS lesions have widespread metastatic disease to other distant organs and further treatment of brain metastases is therefore rarely pursued [213]. Nevertheless, treatment of dogs with metastatic brain lesions could provide useful comparative information on the palliative effects of whole-brain RT.

4.6 Urogenital Carcinoma

Canine genitourinary carcinomas (CGUC) are the most common tumors of the lower urinary tract in dogs and often affect the transitional epithelium of the urinary bladder. These tumors are frequently invasive into the deeper muscularis layers at the time of diagnosis [67]. The vast majority occur in the trigone, making bladder-sparing surgery difficult. Partial cystectomy for apical tumors and total cystectomy for trigonal tumors have been reported, and chemoradiation is becoming commonplace [95]. A recent study evaluating IMRT in combination with NSAIDs and mitoxantrone resulted in a prolonged overall median survival time of 510 days, with 30% of dogs developing urinary incontinence as a side effect. Additionally, roughly half of these dogs developed acute colitis during the course of treatment [37]. There are several reports in the veterinary literature describing different fractionation schemes for both palliative and definitive intent, and these protocols are generally based upon bladder-sparing protocols used in humans [5, 35, 102, 165].

There has been growing enthusiasm for targeted therapies and immunotherapy in the treatment of CGUC. The dual-kinase (EGFR and HER2/NEU) inhibitor lapatinib, when combined with piroxicam in dogs with transitional cell carcinoma of the bladder, demonstrated improved survival and better response to therapy when compared to piroxicam alone [131]. A clinical trial evaluating the use of anti-PD-1 antibody in dogs with bladder carcinoma is also currently underway. Chemoradiation protocols are generally considered front-line therapy for dogs with bladder tumors, and most patients are treated in the gross disease setting. This could be a key advantage to the use of dogs for the development of novel RT techniques and combinations that could ultimately benefit humans with muscle-invasive bladder cancer.

In addition to CGUC of the bladder, dogs can also develop prostate carcinoma, which, as most male pet dogs in North America are neutered, is castration-resistant. Canine prostate carcinoma is both locally and metastatically highly aggressive, and survival times in medically treated patients are less than 3 months [193]. Prostatectomy and prostate embolization have been described, but survival times are regarded as poor due to metastatic spread [215]. Due to the highly metastatic nature of this disease, palliative RT is often considered for prostatic carcinoma, though reports on its efficacy are limited. One multi-institutional retrospective study evaluating definitive intent IMRT (50 Gy in 20 fractions) for 18 canine patients with prostatic carcinoma achieved extended survival times of 563 days [237]. Many of these dogs received additional concurrent therapy including chemotherapy, additional courses of RT, and stent placement. An important consideration is that it can be challenging to distinguish true canine prostate cancers from urothelial carcinomas affecting the prostatic urethra. Prostate-specific membrane antigen (PSMA) cannot reliably distinguish the two entities since it can be expressed by either tumor type [18]. In addition to evaluating treatment outcomes, dogs are an excellent model of RT since humans and dogs share many functional, anatomic, and physiologic features, allowing for comparative radiobiology studies evaluating radiation-induced effects of prostate physiology [166, 199]. Dogs with prostate carcinoma also served as a model for the evaluation of radioactive gold nanoparticles as a novel brachytherapy for prostate cancer, demonstrating minimal toxicity [10].

5 Comparative Radiation Oncology in Novel and Emerging Radiotherapy Techniques

5.1 Intraoperative Radiation Therapy

In the 1980s, the National Cancer Institute (NCI) funded preclinical and clinical research evaluating the safety and efficacy of intraoperative irradiation (IORT) for a number of different disease sites. One key component of these investigations was studies in dogs that generated data which were leveraged to inform rational design of clinical applications in humans [210]. In these studies, 9–15 MeV electrons were delivered at doses ranging from 15 to 80 Gy to a number of different organs of research-bred dogs. These studies were designed to characterize late radiation effects via histopathology. These studies represent a key historic example of the role that clinical investigations in dogs can play to broaden an understanding of radiobiology in the development of treatments ultimately intended for human patients. Studies in the canine bladder concluded that the trigone will tolerate IORT up to 20 Gy, beyond which inflammation and fibrosis resulted in obstructive hydronephrosis, while the bladder mucosa can tolerate doses up to 40 Gy [113]. Evaluation of IORT to the mediastinum of dogs, which, in small volumes, was tolerated up to 20 Gy, helped to guide studies in people with lung cancer [12, 30]. Further studies evaluated the tolerability of vasculature and nerves of the head and neck, abdomen, and retroperitoneum, as well as to surgical anastomoses of the aorta and jejunum [4, 77, 99, 156, 209, 222]. A particular advantage of using dogs was that the accelerated course of their lives and disease progression revealed an increased rate of sarcomas in and around the radiation fields of dogs that received IORT [97, 107].

Beyond normal dog studies, there are reports of IORT used in tumor-bearing dogs. Thirteen dogs with partial surgical excision of bladder tumors (11 TCC, 1 rhabdomyosarcoma, 1 leiomyosarcoma) were prescribed 27 Gy delivered by means of a ^{137}Cs source in a single intraoperative fraction. While 61% of dogs were alive at 1 year, only 23% survived until 2 years, and nearly half of the dogs were pollakiuric and nearly half were incontinent. Additionally, 46% of dogs were found to have either persistent disease or disease recurrence during the study period [236]. Intraoperative extracorporeal irradiation was performed in 13 dogs treated for appendicular osteosarcoma in a limb-sparing technique. In these dogs, the tumor-containing bone segment was removed, irradiated under a linear accelerator to 70 Gy in a single fraction, then replaced in the patient and stabilized with internal fixation. While 10/13 dogs retained good to excellent limb function, complications were common (9/13) and severe, including fracture, infection, and implant failure. Additionally, 3/13 dogs had tumor recur in the irradiated section of bone. The investigators concluded that, while complications may be high, particularly in distal limbs, the procedure could still potentially be considered in more proximal portions of the limbs [130]. The use of dogs to evaluate IORT techniques was incredibly valuable in the understanding of normal tissue tolerances of single, high doses, which would eventually be relevant in the development of SBRT and other hypofractionated protocols.

5.2 Hyperthermia

When combined with RT, hyperthermia can enhance therapeutic efficacy by increasing tumor sensitivity to radiation and perpetuating DNA strand breaks. While preclinical and clinical studies have demonstrated the potential benefits of this combined modality, investigations in canine cancer patients have provided valuable insights due to their similarities in tumor biology, response to treatment, and translational relevance to human cancer therapy.

Hyperthermia enhances the radiosensitivity of tumor cells through a variety of mechanisms. Increased heat-induced blood perfusion can improve oxygenation within the tumor microenvironment, mitigating hypoxic conditions that contribute to radioresistance [85]. Additionally, hyperthermia promotes the disruption of DNA repair mechanisms, leading to the accumulation of unrepaired DNA damage, which synergizes with radiation-induced DNA damage [246]. Hyperthermia can also exert immunomodulatory effects, which may contribute to improved tumor control. Studies have suggested that hyperthermia-induced heat shock proteins (HSPs) can enhance antigen presentation, leading to improved activation of T cells and natural killer (NK) cells [20]. A series of clinical trials investigating the safety and efficacy of hyperthermia in combination with RT in humans with various tumor types have shown promising results [43].

Combining hyperthermia with RT in canine cancer patients provided valuable insights into the potential benefits and underlying mechanisms of this combined treatment modality. Findings from canine studies support the relevance of hyperthermia-radiation combination therapy to human cancer treatment. Combination hyperthermia and external beam RT was used to treat a large mast cell tumor in a dog, noting substantial tumor necrosis, but no evidence of disease recurrence at 1 year posttreatment [128]. The combination was also used to treat oral/nasomaxillary fibrosarcoma, with 9/10 dogs treated experiencing a tumor response, 5/10 disease free at 1 year posttreatment, and an overall mean survival of 398 days; one dog died of fatal septicemia [26]. A randomized phase II study evaluated RT alone vs. RT plus hyperthermia in 64 dogs, identifying a statistically significant duration of control when the combination therapy was delivered, with no difference in metastatic rate [79]. Further studies compared localized vs. whole-body hyperthermia and found, while there was no difference in local control, dogs treated with whole-body hyperthermia had a significantly higher rate of metastasis, suggesting that whole-body hyperthermia might alter the biology of the metastatic process and should not be considered in the treatment of localized soft tissue sarcoma [223]. A study in 122 dogs identified a correlation of thermal dose and duration of heating with local control [224]. This correlation was not present in a similar human study, though it should be noted that the sample size in the human study ($n = 35$) was smaller than in the aforementioned canine study ($n = 122$) [133]. Further research and clinical trials are warranted to optimize treatment protocols, define appropriate patient selection criteria, and determine the long-term outcomes of this combined modality in both dogs and humans. The advent of advanced heating devices and specialized activated nanoparticles broadens the potential applications of clinical hyperthermia. Dogs with spontaneous tumors represent an excellent model to aid in the development of these new technologies in hyperthermia, due to their similar size to human patients, the accessibility of imaging technologies such as MRI, and the amenability of canine tumors to direct sampling for measuring temperature and oxygenation. The scale of mouse models and murine tumors doesn't represent well the geometry and depth of penetration needed to aid in the development of new hyperthermia delivery devices. Additionally, mouse models often lack intact immune systems, and the distribution of vasculature and hypoxia in xenograft tumors can differ substantially from naturally occurring tumors [39, 134, 249].

5.3 Boron Neutron Capture Therapy

Boron neutron capture therapy (BNCT) is a binary form of RT that involves the specific delivery of a boron-10 containing drug to cancer cells, followed by the irradiation of that tissue with thermal (<0.4 eV) neutrons. Individually, the boron agent and the thermal neutron should have little biologic effect, but when combined, the boron-10, which has a high neutron cross section, captures the thermal neutron, resulting in the fissile release of an alpha particle and a lithium nucleus, each of which is a high-LET particle which travels approximately one cell diameter. These high-LET particles cause large amounts of highly potent DNA damage locally. BNCT was first proposed in the 1930s and has undergone several renaissances of avid research. In the 1990s, during one such renaissance, dogs were used to evaluate neutron dosimetry and normal tissue tolerances at the clinical neutron beam developed at Brookhaven National Laboratory [32, 38, 70]. Dogs with spontaneous intracranial tumors were also used to evaluate biodistribution for boron-delivery agents that would be used in these trials [118]. Through these studies, relative biologic effectiveness and compound biologic effectiveness factors could be determined that would be used to help guide and evaluate clinical BNCT in people using these agents [71]. BNCT has also been used to treat a series of three cats with nasal planum squamous cell carcinoma at the Argentina RA-6 nuclear reactor [227]. This study was limited by suboptimal boron-10 delivery and neutron penetration, but the cats treated did demonstrate at least a period of clinical improvement and the treatment was well tolerated. More recently, five dogs with head and neck tumors (two nasal squamous cell carcinoma, one nasal chondrosarcoma, two oral melanoma) were treated with BNCT using L-boronophenylalanine (BPA) as the boron-delivery agent. All of the dogs had been refractory to prior treatment, and all experienced a partial response following treatment with a noted improvement in quality of life, though most responses were relatively short-lived with only one dog surviving beyond 1 year [204]. Currently, the primary limitations to BNCT are due to inadequate specific delivery of boron to target tissues, and companion animal studies can be key to agent selection, as agents that show promise in preclinical mouse models may not translate into other species. As an example, boron-laden liposomes which demonstrate very good boron biodistribution (67 ppm B tumor with 1.88:1 tumor:blood ratio) and efficacy in murine flank tumor models resulted in poor biodistribution in a pilot study in dogs with spontaneous tumors, where the average tumor boron concentration was 7.3 ppm and the tumor:blood ratio was 0.71, with only one dog accumulating more boron in the tumor than in the blood 72 h postinjection [119] (unpublished data). Current BNCT research is being fueled by the advent of accelerator-based neutron sources that can be placed in regional centers, and the recent clinical approval of BPA-based BNCT in refractory head and neck cancer and glioblastoma patients in Japan. While it is unlikely that these accelerators will be housed in veterinary facilities, BNCT is poised for a resurgence, and comparative oncology studies could help guide the development of this treatment modality, as they have in the past. While BNCT may not be readily feasible for widespread use in veterinary patients, if applied to veterinary patients, it could be a very useful tool in the elucidation of high-LET radiobiology studies. Furthermore, BNCT stands as another opportunity for veterinary trials with patients treated in a front-line setting for head and neck tumors or gliomas to be performed in tandem with human clinical trials with tumors more heavily pretreated and refractory to other therapies.

5.4 Radiopharmaceutical Therapy

Another form of targeted therapy that is amid a scientific and clinical revival is radiopharmaceutical therapy. The development of a broad repertoire of tumor targeting mechanisms, quantitative nuclear imaging techniques, and voxel-based radiopharmaceutical dosimetry has led to the enrichment of the field of theranostics, where therapeutic and diagnostic radionuclides are combined to improve the effectiveness of radiopharmaceuticals in the treatment of a variety of diseases, including cancer. As new theranostics are being developed, the need to understand dosimetry and biologic effects of the systemically delivered RT becomes more important, particularly as highly potent radiopharmaceuticals using targeted alpha therapy become clinically utilized, and more realistic models of human cancer are necessary. With these physiologic modeling needs, the role of comparative oncology gains importance in radiopharmaceutical sciences. Furthermore, the scale and geometry of tumors in dogs more closely mimic those in humans than murine tumor models, so radiation physics and dosimetry modeling can be developed more accurately. Key translational challenges in oncology, such as alterations in tumor microenvironment, hypoxia, heterogeneity, and geometry, are also addressed by companion animal models.

In both human and veterinary oncology, the best described example of radiopharmaceutical therapy is [^{131}I]NaI, for thyroid carcinoma. In published retrospective studies describing dogs treated with radioiodine (with or without surgery and chemotherapy), the median survival times range from 564 to 1020 days, with most dogs showing an improvement in clinical signs [105, 228, 245]. In general, the dosing of [^{131}I]NaI has been calculated on a mCi/kg basis. Quantitative imaging of iodine distribution (e.g., via ^{124}I-based positron emission tomography (PET)) may enable voxel-based dosimetry of radioiodine and potentially improve clinical outcomes (Fig. 2) [206, 208]. It should also be noted that hyperthyroidism is not required for a patient to benefit from radioiodine therapy, and the aforementioned studies include patients who are hypothyroid and euthyroid, in addition to those who are hyperthyroid [150].

Bone metastasis is another common target for radiopharmaceutical therapy in people, particularly with the recent FDA approval of Xofigo™ [^{223}Ra]$RaCl_2$, the first FDA-approved alpha emitter. Decades before this agent was on the market, studies in dogs played an important role in the FDA approval of Quadramet™, or [^{153}Sm]Sm-EDTMP, which is also used to treat metastatic bone lesions in people. Manuscripts published in the Journal of Nuclear Medicine by Lattimer et al. in 1990 describe the toxicity of [^{153}Sm]Sm-EDTMP in research-bred dogs, as well as the clinical response and clinicopathologic changes in client-owned dogs with naturally occurring bone tumors [121, 122]. Further studies by others describe the use of [^{153}Sm]Sm-EDTMP in appendicular and skull OS, where the clinical response rates vary from 57% to 78% and 20%, respectively [1, 11, 154, 231]. The bone tumor model has also been used to evaluate the effect of different radionuclides as well as novel targeting techniques such as in vivo tumor pretargeting [28, 135].

Dogs with naturally occurring diseases have also been used in the evaluation of low-dose targeted radionuclide therapy for immunomodulation. A study by Magee et al. examined the feasibility of using the theranostic [^{90}Y]Y-NM600 with EBRT and intratumoral immunocytokines (hu14.18-IL2) in canine patients with advanced-stage cancer. The investigators demonstrated that low-dose immunomodulatory radiation was safely delivered with [^{90}Y]Y-NM600,and post treatment biopsy confirmed immune modulation of the tumor microenvironment [132]. This study also utilized advanced, voxel-based, patient-specific dosimetry of the radiopharmaceutical to evaluate dose response. This veterinary clinical study was developed to complement mechanistic studies carried out in rodent models to determine that the combination of low-dose targeted radionuclide therapy and external beam radiotherapy can promote response to immune checkpoint inhibition for a variety of different tumor types [178]. These studies demonstrate the complementary role that small animal and large animal studies can play in the development of novel treatment techniques and agents and highlight the importance of comparative oncology studies in radiobiology and radiation oncology.

The scale of the canine organs and tumors is important to its comparative role in radiopharmaceuticals in terms of dosimetry, but it is also a key component in the application and development of radioembolization and liquid brachytherapy techniques. The safety of Gum Arabic-coated radioactive gold nanoparticles (GA-^{198}AuNPs) was evaluated in nine dogs with prostatic carcinoma [10]. The investigators identified lower than anticipated levels of radioactivity within the prostate and recommended further refinement of retention and dosimetry prior to Phase 1 trials in men. Researchers have used dogs with prostatic hyperplasia to demonstrate proof of concept of ^{90}Y radioembolization of the prostate using PET and MR imaging to visualize localization and coverage, as well as changes in prostate size [161]. Healthy dogs and dogs with naturally occurring brain tumors were used to demonstrate technical feasibility and safety of ^{90}Y radioembolization of brain tumors with ^{90}Y glass microspheres [177]. ^{90}Y has also been evaluated in radioembolization of liver tumors in dogs, and as an intralesional treatment in both dogs and cats with sarcomas [60]. Intratumoral injection of radioactive ^{166}Ho microspheres has demonstrated local disease responses in a number of different tumor types, including FOSCC, soft tissue sarcomas of dogs, and even a dog with a pituitary tumor [159, 160, 230].

At present, there are only a few veterinary facilities equipped to handle patients treated with longer-lived therapeutic radioisotopes. Such facilities require designated areas for radioactive patients where their waste and the risk of contamination can be well controlled. In general, shielding requirements are as much a limiting factor as are the risks associated with contamination. While therapeutic radiopharmaceuticals may not become commonplace in veterinary medicine, molecular imaging with PET is becoming more commonplace, which could increase comparative research in the development of new molecular diagnostics and allow for new metrics of disease response in the evaluation of novel treatment techniques [61, 135].

5.5 Spatially Fractionated Radiation Therapy

In spatially fractionated radiation therapy (SFRT), only portions of the treatment volume are intentionally irradiated with high doses, while other regions of the tumor are intentionally spared, resulting in a large amount of dose heterogeneity within the irradiated volume. After initial experiments demonstrated normal tissue sparing effects of SFRT, further studies identified a marked advantageous effect of SFRT on the tumor microenvironment, both in terms of immune and vascular effects. Clinical SFRT has been possible for decades in the form of GRID RT, which implements a specialized collimator to deliver the unique radiation dose distribution. Most commonly, GRID therapy is used immediately before beginning a course of conventionally fractionated radiation [157, 212]. The GRID is thought to enable effective tumor debulking, whereas the adjuvant open-field conventional RT enables long-term tumor control. Lattice RT (LRT) is an iteration of SFRT that utilizes modern SBRT technology to deliver high-dose spheres within a low-dose treatment volume. LRT can also be used to deliver a modest dose to an entire treatment volume, while delivering a simultaneous integrated boost to spherical subvolumes within that gross tumor volume. Marked responses to SFRT are often attributed to a number of different mechanisms.

Responses within the low-dose regions are believed to be mediated by the bystander effect, where the killed irradiated tumor cells could trigger a tumoricidal effect on contiguous cells that were unirradiated or received a low dose and responses at distant sites by the abscopal effect [44, 62, 129]. LRT is believed to augment these effects by increasing the presentation of tumor-specific antigens from dying tumor cells in an immunostimulatory context (in situ cancer vaccination), lymphocyte recruitment and activation or loss of immunosuppressive cells such as myeloid-derived suppressor cells (MDSCs) or regulatory T cells (Tregs) [59, 200, 201, 207]. Lattice high-dose irradiation compared to whole tumor volume irradiation of tumors in murine models resulted in robust antitumor IFNγ and Th1 responses, increased T cells, and TRAIL-mediated cell death and distant tumor growth delay, indicating that LRT is superior to whole volume irradiation at activating the immune system [109]. The combination of high and low-dose RT (peaks and valleys) may also augment radiation-induced immune modulation by preserving perfusion of circulating factors essential for antitumor immunity.

While murine models help to identify mechanisms of SFRT, irradiation of murine tumors differs greatly from how human tumors are irradiated, on account of differences of scale. Companion animal models provide tumor volumes similar to those seen in human radiation oncology, and the use of equivalent treatment planning systems and delivery infrastructure makes comparative oncology critical to the development of SFRT treatment protocols. A pilot study in dogs receiving GRID therapy for bulky soft tissue sarcomas demonstrated tolerability, with 3 of 6 dogs experiencing grade 1 skin toxicity (erythema). While no dogs in this study had a measurable disease response using RECIST criteria, the investigators identified a decrease in secretory sphingomyelinase activity 48 hours after 25 Gy GRID, and all patients with measurable tumor necrosis factor α had levels decrease at all time points after treatment (1, 4, 24, and 48 h) [167]. In a separate unpublished study, a form of integrated LRT was administered to dogs with soft tissue sarcomas via a prospective randomized study wherein dogs received either LRT or standard palliative RT. Dogs received either 20 Gy in 5 daily fractions, or LRT consisting of 20 Gy to the total Planned Target Volume (PTV), with a simultaneous integrated boost of 66.7 Gy to 1.2 cm diameter spheres within the treatment volume, delivered in 5 fractions every other day. LRT was well tolerated and resulted in a measurable disease response and palliation in all dogs and resulted in a significantly prolonged time to progression when compared with the standard palliative RT group (Unpublished). This veterinary clinical trial was designed in conjunction with a phase 1 study delivering LRT to human patients with large sarcomas and allowed for the inclusion of serial tumor biopsies and blood analysis, which were not feasible in the human patient population [50, 111]. Currently, there is a clinical trial evaluating LRT in dogs with nasopharyngeal carcinoma as well. These comparative studies demonstrate that LRT can be safely delivered to human-scale tumors and that veterinary patients are an advantageous model for studying its radiobiologic and immunologic effects.

SFRT can also be delivered in smaller fields. Minibeam (on the order of millimeters) and microbeam (500–1000 μm) RT demonstrate similar biologic effects to GRID and LRT, namely improved tumor response, with normal tissue sparing, and similar changes to the tumor microenvironment [202, 247]. Microbeam RT generally requires the use of a synchrotron, making large veterinary trials difficult, though safety and efficacy have been demonstrated in a dog with a presumed glioma, who had marked clinical improvement and 87.4% tumor volume decrease 3 months after a single fraction of conformal microbeam therapy [2]. Minibeam therapy is more readily available, particularly as it can be readily adapted to modern orthovoltage machines [140]. This configuration could make comparative studies in dogs or cats with superficial tumors incredibly valuable in the development of the radiobiology surrounding SFRT.

5.6 Flash Radiation Therapy

The universal goal of research in radiation oncology is to maximize tumor control while minimizing effects to normal tissues. Fractionation, inclusion of radiosensitizers and radioprotectors, radiopharmaceuticals, and SFRT all seek to expand that therapeutic window. In the 2010s, researchers at multiple institutions across France identified a differential response between normal and tumor tissue in mice after irradiation with ultrahigh dose rates, termed FLASH radiation therapy (FLASH-RT) [56]. Since this discovery, radiation chemists, physicists, and biologists have all been fervently investigating the delivery and biochemical nature of this FLASH effect. The FLASH effect is generally seen independent of radiation modality (i.e., electrons, photons, protons) when very high-dose rates (as high as 1500 Gy/s) are administered in small pulses, resulting in average dose rates of more than 40 Gy/s with irradiation times <500 ms. Preclinical studies in mice have demonstrated a preferential sparing of late responding tissues/organs including brain and lung, a more modest sparing of acute responding organs, without any detriment to tumor control [235]. These preclinical studies have shown much promise toward treatment of cancer and efforts to translate this work into the clinic have been very rapid, with the description of a patient with heavily resistant cutaneous lymphoma safely treated using FLASH-RT within 5 years of the initial description of the FLASH effect [22]. Studies in domestic mammals have been a key part to the development of clinical FLASH-RT, and description of tumor and normal tissue effects were described in mini-pigs and in cats with naturally occurring nasal planum SCC. The feline study was a clinical, phase I, single-dose escalation trial from 25 to 41 Gy in 6 cats, 3 of which experienced no acute toxicity, and 3 of which exhibited mild to moderate transient mucositis. The progression-free survival of cats at 16 months was 84%, with 5/6 in complete remission [234]. One of the advantages of veterinary tumor models is the advanced rate of progression, both in terms of disease and side effects. This feature was paramount in a follow-up study that prospectively randomized cats to receive either 10 × 4.8 Gy standard of care (SoC) MV radiotherapy or 1 × 30 Gy FLASH-RT. This study identified an increased rate in the late tissue effect of maxillary bone necrosis 9–15 months after RT, which occurred in 3 of 7 cats receiving FLASH-RT and in none (of 9) of the cats receiving standard of care [196]. This study demonstrates the importance of comparative models in the implementation of new treatment techniques and will help to safely implement FLASH-RT toward clinical studies in humans. Additional studies are evaluating the role of FLASH RT in veterinary patients. FLASH-RT was safely administered in a single fraction ranging from 15 to 35 Gy to 13 dogs with a variety of different tumor locations and histologies. In total, 11/13 tumors experienced either a CR or SD, and adverse effects were mild, with only one patient experiencing a grade 3 skin adverse event (desquamation to the nasal planum), though the duration of follow-up in this study was short (3–6 months) and late effects cannot be fully evaluated at this time point [117]. A clinical trial evaluating FLASH protons in dogs with naturally occurring OS is also currently underway.

5.7 Radioprotectors and Radiosensitizers

The integration of radioprotectors and radiosensitizers into clinical practice has the potential to play a crucial role in enhancing the therapeutic efficacy of RT while reducing its harmful effects on healthy tissues. The translation of these findings from preclinical studies to clinical trials requires reliable animal models that closely mimic human physiology and response to radiation. During the course of drug development, agents are often tested on a rodent and a nonrodent species for evaluation of toxicity. Dogs are frequently selected as the nonrodent species, meaning that there is often existing pharmacokinetic and safety data of such agents in dogs, making clinical evaluation in tumor-bearing dogs a logical step in agent development. A number of additional factors make dogs excellent candidates for testing novel radiation-affecting pharmacologics, including a shared environment with humans, which has led to a similarity in gut anatomy, physiology, and microbiota, similar renal and hepatic metabolism, and a behavioral familiarity [139].

Radioprotectors are agents that help protect healthy tissues from the harmful effects of radiation exposure and are categorized into three different classes of agents: prophylactic agents, mitigating agents, and therapeutic agents. Prophylactic agents are given prior to radiation exposure and most frequently seek to decrease the number of DNA radicals produced, either by scavenging free radicals or restoring DNA radicals prior to strand breakage. WR-2721, more commonly known as amifostine, a phosphorothioate which is reduced into an aminothiol, is such an agent. Mitigating agents are administered after radiation exposure to minimize the effects of radiation and therapeutic agents are administered well after exposure to overcome the outcomes caused by radiation. Companion animal models have played a vital role in identifying and assessing potential radioprotectors, allowing researchers to gauge their safety and efficacy before moving on to human trials. Amifostine, in particular, was investigated in both canine and human studies to mitigate radiation-induced toxicities in healthy tissues during cancer treatment. A multi-institution randomized clinical trial in dogs with soft tissue sarcoma receiving fractionated radiation therapy demonstrated no significant reduction in normal tissue effects and suggested that there may be a slight indication of tumor protection at low doses [144]. This study, while not demonstrating a clear protective effect of amifostine, helped to direct future incorporation of radioprotectors into clinical use. A prospective study in beagles demonstrated that administration of a Smad7-based Tat protein mitigated radiation-induced oral mucositis while reducing inflammation and cell death, and increasing cell growth and DNA repair [21]. This study was performed in research-bred animals, using clinical radiation delivery techniques and doses, and could be easily translated into a clinical, tumor-bearing dog clinical trial.

Radiosensitizers are compounds that enhance the sensitivity of tumor cells to radiation, thus increasing the effectiveness of RT. There are several radiosensitization techniques, including targeting hypoxia, targeting DNA damage repair mechanisms, and targeting cells in more radioresistant phases of the cell cycle. As discussed previously in this chapter, hyperthermia is synergistic with radiation therapy because it achieves all three of these techniques, reducing tumor hypoxia, causing denaturation of DDR proteins, and being most effective in the S phase of the cell cycle, a phase which is typically considered to be radioresistant [45, 90]. The evaluation of radiosensitizers in companion animal models has provided critical insights into their mechanisms of action and potential side effects. The tumor penetration of misonidazole, a hypoxic cell radiosensitizer, was clinically evaluated in six dogs with spontaneous tumors, finding concentrations in nonbrain tumors to be comparable to plasma [243]. Combinations of chemotherapy and RT have been evaluated prospectively in several veterinary studies, including combination of radiotherapy with tyrosine-kinase inhibition and radiosensitizing carboplatin, which were well tolerated [31, 52]. Combination with radiosensitizing gemcitabine was also evaluated and resulted in a higher than expected rate of hematologic and local radiation toxicity [125].

5.8 Treatment of Benign Diseases

RT has long been recognized for its value in treating cancer, and its potential in managing benign diseases is now also growing. Improved understanding of the interactions between radiation and inflammation has broadened the role of radiation into orthopedic pain management, neurogenic tremors, trigeminal neuralgia, and, more recently, arrhythmias [100]. Companion animal models provide a platform for developing and refining treatment protocols using radiation therapy for benign diseases. These models allow researchers to optimize dosage, fractionation, and delivery techniques, ultimately improving treatment outcomes. A report describing 13 dogs with acral lick granuloma treated with coarse fraction radiation resulted in generally good control ranging from 0.5 to 3 years, though none of these lesions were permanently resolved [173]. Low-dose radiation has been used to treat osteoarthritis by reducing inflammation in humans using a variety of different protocols [48]. As it is in humans, osteoarthritis is a very common, often under-treated chronic disease affecting dogs, which has few reports, but growing interest. A single 10 Gy fraction of external beam radiation therapy improved lameness in five Labrador Retrievers with elbow osteoarthritis unresponsive to medical therapy [110]. A larger study of 25 dogs with osteoarthritis in a variety of sites evaluated a course of 3 daily fractions of 2 Gy. Clinical improvement, both in terms of lameness and pain score, was seen in 92% of patients for a median benefit duration of 356 days, without any reported side effects [198]. An intra-articular [^{117m}Sn]Tin colloid has also been approved for use in dogs with elbow osteoarthritis after a prospective study demonstrated improvement in gait and pain management in 23 dogs administered 37–92.5 MBq (1.0–2.5 mCi) without any noted side effects or contamination concerns identified [9, 47].

More recently, low-dose whole-brain irradiation has been investigated as a treatment for Alzheimer's dementia in people. Such techniques can result in altered gene expression of DNA repair, cell cycle, and lipid metabolism pathways, functionally reducing oxidative stress and promoting microglial activation [104, 248]. Early clinical trials in humans with Alzheimer's dementia demonstrated a positive safety profile with most patients either stabilizing or having improved cognition, though sample sizes are low and early clinical trials were closed due to COVID-19-related challenges [112, 195]. At this time, there have been no studies of total brain irradiation to treat Alzheimer's disease in dogs; however, there are data to suggest that Canine Cognitive Dysfunction has several physiological similarities to Alzheimer's dementia, including the deposition of amyloid-β plaques, and could be a valuable model of the neurodegenerative processes at work in Alzheimer's disease [203]. Despite no reports of low-dose radiation for Canine Cognitive Dysfunction, there are reports of whole-brain radiation of dogs for other non-neoplastic etiologies. Meningoencephalitis of Unknown Origin (MUO) is a heterogeneous group of noninfectious inflammatory brain diseases of an unknown etiology which occurs in dogs. MUO has a variety of treatment options, without a defined standard of care. Full-course radiation therapy (40–49.5 Gy in 12–15 fractions) has been described as an effective treatment for MUO [162]. More recently, lower doses of radiation have demonstrated efficacy in the treatment of MUO as well. An abbreviated course of 3 Gy × 10 fractions resulted in 6/6 dogs improving in neurological status, with 4/6 dogs having lesion improvement on MRI at 3 months post-RT [14]. An even shorter course of treatment consisting of 4 Gy × 5 fractions resulted in 10/10 dogs improving during treatment, with 4/10 returning to normal shortly after RT. Ultimately 4/10 dogs had disease progression with a mean time to progression of 691 days. The mean overall survival for all dogs was 723 days, and no radiation-induced side effects were seen [93].

6 Conclusion

Veterinary radiation oncology has a rich history founded in the tenets of radiobiology and comparative medicine. For decades, veterinary radiation oncologists have endeavored in comparative studies using the spontaneous disease that develops in their canine patients as an opportunity to provide state-of-the-art care to their patients, while also furthering discovery in the treatment of humans. Cancer disease states in both human and veterinary patient populations share many similarities with regard to tumorigenesis, tumor microenvironment, and clinical studies in each population individually that have helped advance outcomes in both. However, future studies which could be developed for both populations simultaneously could potentially increase study power and improve efficiency (i.e., co-clinical trials addressing similar problems in parallel, both in dogs and humans). Creating and fostering opportunities for collaboration between both human and veterinary radiation oncologists and scientists are vital to achieve these goals.

Advances in technology have resulted in a treatment landscape where veterinary radiation oncologists can continue to contribute to advances in radiobiology and in novel radiotherapy techniques (Figs. 1, 2, and 3).

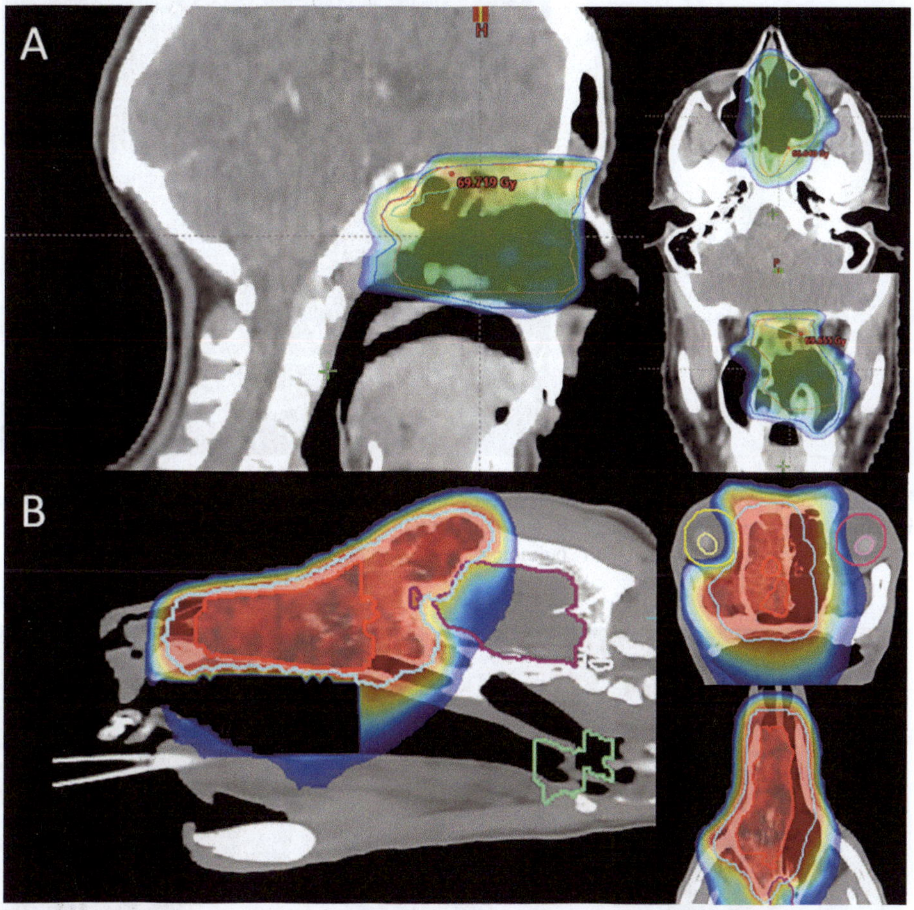

Fig. 1 Sinonasal carcinoma VMAT plans in a human (**a**) and in a dog (**b**). Both plans use intensity modulated photons to maximize dose to tumor (GTV: red, PTV: cyan) while minimizing dose to the surrounding tissues including eyes (left: yellow, right: magenta), brain (purple), and hard palate

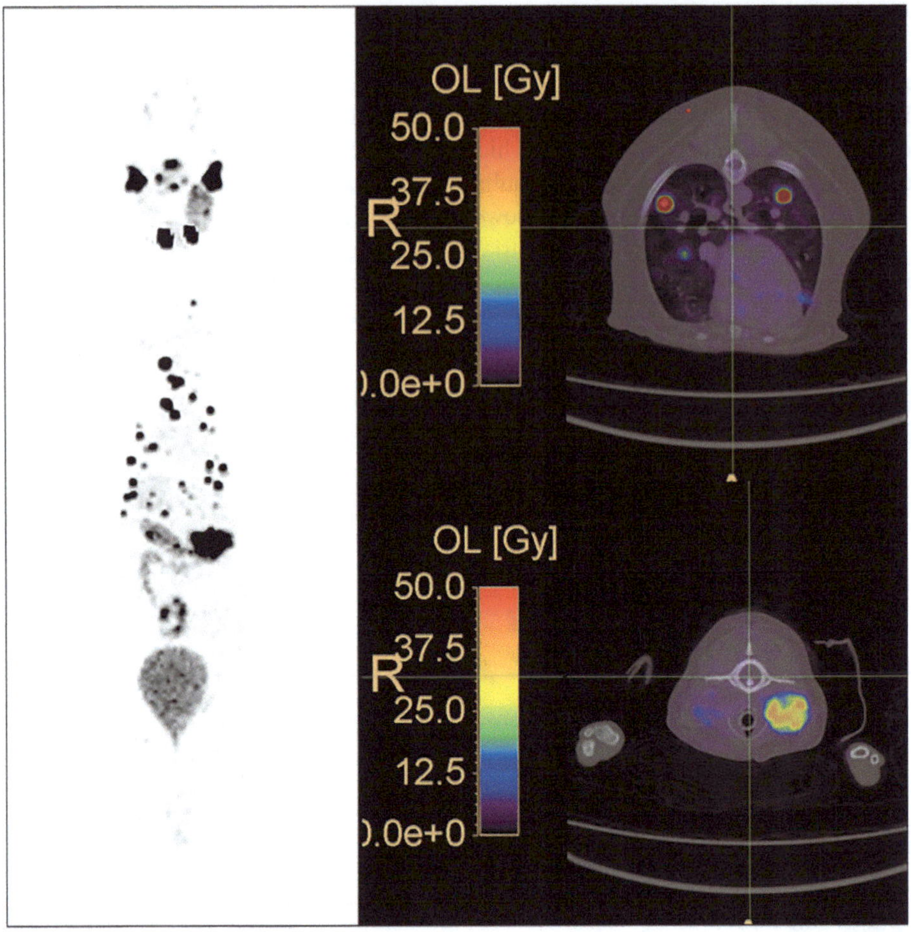

Fig. 2 ^{124}I-based dosimetry for a dog with widespread metastasis from a thyroid carcinoma. Patient progression correlated with dosimetric analysis, with pulmonary metastases with high dose responding to treatment, while recurrence and lymph nodes progressed

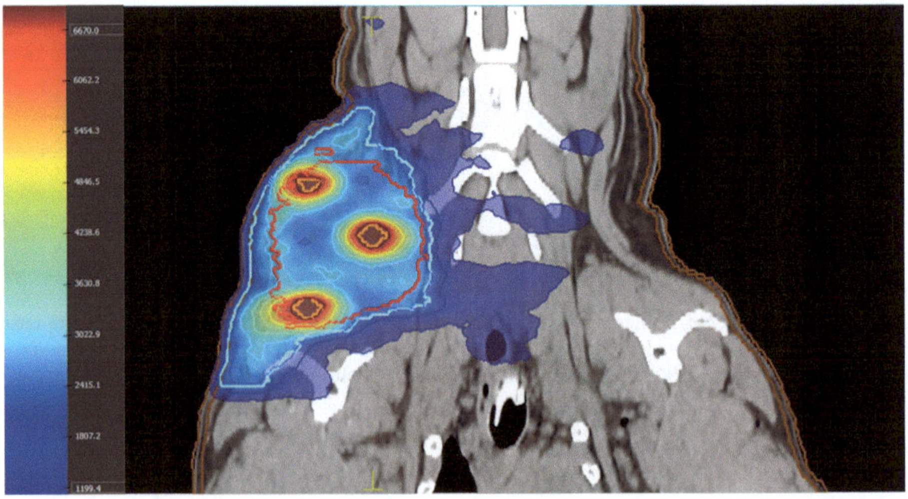

Fig. 3 Dose IsoFill coronal view of a spatially fractionated photon radiation therapy plan in a dog with soft tissue sarcoma. In this case, 20 Gy was delivered to the PTV (cyan) margin, while 66.7 Gy was delivered to latticed subvolumes (orange circles) within the GTV (red). The plan was delivered in five fractions via simultaneous integrated boost

References

1. Aas M, Moe L, Gamlem H, Skretting A, Ottesen N, Bruland OS (1999) Internal radionuclide therapy of primary osteosarcoma in dogs, using 153Sm-ethylene-diamino-tetramethylene-phosphonate (EDTMP). Clin Cancer Res 5:3148s–3152s
2. Adam JF, Balosso J, Bayat S, Berkvens P, Berruyer G, Bräuer-Krisch E, Brochard T, Chamel G, Desagneaux A, Drevon-Gaud R, Eling L, Estève F, Flandin I, Gaudin M, Giraud JY, Giraud L, Gonzalez H, Kefs S, Keshmiri S, Krainik A, Krisch M, Laissue JA, Lemaire G, Mauro A, Nemoz C, Pellicioli P, Renier M, Verry C, Serduc R (2022) Toward neuro-oncologic clinical trials of high-dose-rate synchrotron microbeam radiation therapy: first treatment of a spontaneous canine brain tumor. Int J Radiat Oncol Biol Phys 113:967–973
3. Adams WM, Bjorling DE, McAnulty JE, Green EM, Forrest LJ, Vail DM (2005) Outcome of accelerated radiotherapy alone or accelerated radiotherapy followed by exenteration of the nasal cavity in dogs with intranasal neoplasia: 53 cases (1990–2002). J Am Vet Med Assoc 227:936–941
4. Ahmadu-Suka F, Gillette EL, Withrow SJ, Husted PW, Nelson AW, Whiteman CE (1988) Pathologic response of the pancreas and duodenum to experimental intraoperative irradiation. Int J Radiat Oncol Biol Phys 14:1197–1204
5. Ahrens C, Beatrice L, Meier V, Rohrer Bley C (2024) Radiation toxicity grading after chemoradiotherapy of canine urinary tract carcinomas: comparing VRTOG to VRTOG_v2.0. Vet Comp Oncol 22:255–264
6. Almela RM, Ansón A (2019) A review of immunotherapeutic strategies in canine malignant melanoma. Vet Sci 6:15
7. Ammons DT, Guth A, Rozental AJ, Kurihara J, Marolf AJ, Chow L, Griffin Iv JF, Makii R, MacQuiddy B, Boss M-K (2022) Reprogramming the canine glioma microenvironment with tumor vaccination plus oral losartan and propranolol induces objective responses. Cancer Res Commun 2:1657–1667
8. Atherton MJ, Morris JS, McDermott MR, Lichty BD (2016) Cancer immunology and canine malignant melanoma: a comparative review. Vet Immunol Immunopathol 169:15–26
9. Aulakh KS, Lopez MJ, Hudson C, Gaschen L, Fabiani M, Beale B, Andrews FM, Liu CC, Lattimer J (2021) Prospective clinical evaluation of intra-articular injection of tin-117m ((117m)Sn) radiosynoviorthesis agent for management of naturally occurring elbow osteoarthritis in dogs: a pilot study. Vet Med (Auckl) 12:117–128
10. Axiak-Bechtel SM, Upendran A, Lattimer JC, Kelsey J, Cutler CS, Selting KA, Bryan JN, Henry CJ, Boote E, Tate DJ, Bryan ME, Katti KV, Kannan R (2014) Gum arabic-coated radioactive gold nanoparticles cause no short-term local or systemic toxicity in the clinically relevant canine model of prostate cancer. Int J Nanomedicine 9:5001–5011
11. Barnard S, Zuber R, Moore A (2007) Samarium Sm 153 lexidronam for the palliative treatment of dogs with primary bone tumors: 35 cases (1999–2005). J Am Vet Med Assoc 230:1877–1881
12. Barnes M, Pass H, Deluca A, Tochner Z, Potter D, Terrill R, Sindelar WF, Kinsella TJ (1987) Response of the mediastinal and thoracic viscera of the dog to intraoperative radiation therapy (IORT). Int J Radiat Oncol Biol Phys 13:371–378
13. Baron F, Sandmaier BM, Zellmer E, Sorror M, Storer B, Storb R (2006) Failure of donor lymphocyte infusion to prevent graft rejection in dogs given DLA-identical marrow after 1 Gy of total body irradiation. Biol Blood Marrow Transplant 12:813–817
14. Beckmann K, Carrera I, Steffen F, Golini L, Kircher PR, Schneider U, Bley CR (2015) A newly designed radiation therapy protocol in combination with prednisolone as treatment for meningoencephalitis of unknown origin in dogs: a prospective pilot study introducing magnetic resonance spectroscopy as monitor tool. Acta Vet Scand 57:4
15. Bedi M, Singh R, Charlson JA, Kelly T, Johnstone C, Wooldridge A, Hackbarth DA, Moore N, Neilson JC, King DM (2022) Is 5 the new 25? Long-term oncologic outcomes from a phase II, prospective, 5-fraction preoperative radiation therapy trial in patients with localized soft tissue sarcoma. Adv Radiat Oncol 7:100850
16. Bentley RT, Ober CP, Anderson KL, Feeney DA, Naughton JF, Ohlfest JR, O'Sullivan MG, Miller MA, Constable PD, Pluhar GE (2013) Canine intracranial gliomas: relationship between magnetic resonance imaging criteria and tumor type and grade. Vet J 198:463–471
17. Berry RJ, Wiernik G, Patterson TJ (1974) Skin tolerance to fractionated x-irradiation in the pig—how good a predictor is the NSD formula? Br J Radiol 47:185–190
18. Berry MR, Fadl-Alla BA, Samuelson J, Rosol TJ, Fan TM (2022) Investigating PSMA differential expression in canine uroepithelial carcinomas to aid disease-based stratification and guide therapeutic selection. BMC Vet Res 18:441
19. Bewley DK, Fowler JF, Morgan RL, Silvester JA, Turner BA (2014) VII. Experiments on the skin of pigs with fast neutrons and 8 MV X rays, including some effects of dose fractionation. Br J Radiol 36:107–115
20. Binder RJ (2014) Functions of heat shock proteins in pathways of the innate and adaptive immune system. J Immunol 193:5765–5771
21. Boss M-K, Ke Y, Bian L, Harrison LG, Lee B-I, Prebble A, Martin T, Trageser E, Hall S, Wang DD, Wang S, Chow L, Holwerda B, Raben D, Regan D, Karam SD, Dow S, Young CD, Wang X-J (2022) Therapeutic intervention using a Smad7-based tat

protein to treat radiation-induced oral mucositis. Int J Radiat Oncol Biol Phys 112:759–770
22. Bourhis J, Sozzi WJ, Jorge PG, Gaide O, Bailat C, Duclos F, Patin D, Ozsahin M, Bochud F, Germond JF, Moeckli R, Vozenin MC (2019) Treatment of a first patient with FLASH-radiotherapy. Radiother Oncol 139:18–22
23. Bradshaw TJ, Bowen SR, Jallow N, Forrest LJ, Jeraj R (2013) Heterogeneity in intratumor correlations of 18F-FDG, 18F-FLT, and 61Cu-ATSM PET in canine sinonasal tumors. J Nucl Med 54:1931–1937
24. Bradshaw TJ, Bowen SR, Deveau MA, Kubicek L, White P, Bentzen SM, Chappell RJ, Forrest LJ, Jeraj R (2015) Molecular imaging biomarkers of resistance to radiation therapy for spontaneous nasal tumors in canines. Int J Radiat Oncol Biol Phys 91:787–795
25. Brehm A, Wilson-Robles H, Miller T, Jarvis J, Deveau M (2022) Feasibility and safety of whole lung irradiation in the treatment of canine appendicular osteosarcoma. Vet Comp Oncol 20:20–28
26. Brewer WG Jr, Turrel JM (1982) Radiotherapy and hyperthermia in the treatment of fibrosarcomas in the dog. J Am Vet Med Assoc 181:146–150
27. Bryan JN, Maitz CA (2024) Translational history and Hope of immunotherapy of canine tumors. Clin Cancer Res 30(19):4272–4285
28. Bryan JN, Bommarito D, Kim DY, Berent LM, Bryan ME, Lattimer JC, Henry CJ, Engelbrecht H, Ketring A, Cutler C (2009) Comparison of systemic toxicities of 177Lu-DOTMP and 153Sm-EDTMP administered intravenously at equivalent skeletal doses to normal dogs. J Nucl Med Technol 37:45–52
29. Buchholz J, Hagen R, Leo C, Ebling A, Roos M, Kaser-Hotz B, Bley CR (2009) 3D conformal radiation therapy for palliative treatment of canine nasal tumors. Vet Radiol Ultrasound 50:679–683
30. Calvo FA, Ortiz De Urbina D, Abuchaibe O, Azinovic I, Aristu J, Santos M, Escude L, Herreros J, Llorens R (1990) Intraoperative radiotherapy during lung cancer surgery: technical description and early clinical results. Int J Radiat Oncol Biol Phys 19:103–109
31. Carlsten K, London C, Haney S, Burnett R, Avery A, Thamm D (2012) Multicenter prospective trial of hypofractionated radiation treatment, toceranib, and prednisone for measurable canine mast cell tumors. J Vet Intern Med 26:135–141
32. Chadha M, Capala J, Coderre JA, Elowitz EH, Iwai J, Joel DD, Liu HB, Wielopolski L, Chanana AD (1998) Boron neutron-capture therapy (BNCT) for glioblastoma multiforme (GBM) using the epithermal neutron beam at the Brookhaven National Laboratory. Int J Radiat Oncol Biol Phys 40:1243
33. Cheng EY, Dusenbery KE, Winters MR, Thompson RC (1996) Soft tissue sarcomas: preoperative versus postoperative radiotherapy. J Surg Oncol 61:90–99
34. Choi W, Lee ES (2022) Therapeutic targeting of DNA damage response in cancer. Int J Mol Sci 23:1701
35. Choy K, Fidel J (2016) Tolerability and tumor response of a novel low-dose palliative radiation therapy protocol in dogs with transitional cell carcinoma of the bladder and urethra. Vet Radiol Ultrasound 57:341–351
36. Chu S, Wylie TN, Wylie KM, Johnson GC, Skidmore ZL, Fleer M, Griffith OL, Bryan JN (2020) A virome sequencing approach to feline oral squamous cell carcinoma to evaluate viral causative factors. Vet Microbiol 240:108491
37. Clerc-Renaud B, Gieger TL, Larue SM, Nolan MW (2021) Treatment of genitourinary carcinoma in dogs using nonsteroidal anti-inflammatory drugs, mitoxantrone, and radiation therapy: a retrospective study. J Vet Intern Med 35(2):1052–1061
38. Coderre J, Gavin P, Capala J et al (2000) Tolerance of the normal canine brain to epithermal neutron irradiation in the presence of p-boronophenylalanine. J Neurooncol 48(1):27–40
39. Colombié M, Gouard S, Frindel M, Vidal A, Chérel M, Kraeber-Bodéré F, Rousseau C, Bourgeois M (2015) Focus on the controversial aspects of 64Cu-ATSM in Tumoral hypoxia mapping by PET imaging. Front Med 2:58
40. Coomer A, Farese J, Milner R, Liptak J, Bacon N, Lurie D (2009) Radiation therapy for canine appendicular osteosarcoma. Vet Comp Oncol 7:15–27
41. Covey JL, Farese JP, Bacon NJ, Schallberger SP, Amsellem P, Cavanaugh RP, Milner RJ (2014) Stereotactic radiosurgery and fracture fixation in 6 dogs with appendicular osteosarcoma. Vet Surg 43:174–181
42. Darragh LB, Gadwa J, Pham TT, Van Court B, Neupert B, Olimpo NA, Nguyen K, Nguyen D, Knitz MW, Hoen M, Corbo S, Joshi M, Zhuang Y, Amann M, Wang X-J, Dow S, Kedl RM, Samedi V, Boss M-K, Karam SD (2022) Elective nodal irradiation mitigates local and systemic immunity generated by combination radiation and immunotherapy in head and neck tumors. Nat Commun 13:7015
43. Datta NR, Ordóñez SG, Gaipl US, Paulides MM, Crezee H, Gellermann J, Marder D, Puric E, Bodis S (2015) Local hyperthermia combined with radiotherapy and-/or chemotherapy: recent advances and promises for the future. Cancer Treat Rev 41:742–753
44. Demaria S, Guha C, Schoenfeld J, Morris Z, Monjazeb A, Sikora A, Crittenden M, Shiao S, Khleif S, Gupta S, Formenti SC, Vikram B, Coleman CN, Ahmed MM (2021) Radiation dose and fraction in immunotherapy: one-size regimen does not fit all settings, so how does one choose? J Immunother Cancer 9:e002038
45. Dewhirst MW, Vujaskovic Z, Jones E, Thrall D (2005) Re-setting the biologic rationale for thermal therapy. Int J Hyperth 21:779–790
46. Dolera M, Malfassi L, Bianchi C, Carrara N, Finesso S, Marcarini S, Mazza G, Pavesi S, Sala M, Urso G (2018) Frameless stereotactic radiotherapy alone

and combined with temozolomide for presumed canine gliomas. Vet Comp Oncol 16:90–101
47. Donecker J, Lattimer JC, Gaschen L, Aulakh KS (2021) Safety and clinical response following a repeat Intraarticular injection of tin-117m ((117m) Sn) colloid in dogs with elbow osteoarthritis. Vet Med (Auckl) 12:325–335
48. Dove APH, Cmelak A, Darrow K, McComas KN, Chowdhary M, Beckta J, Kirschner AN (2022) The use of low-dose radiation therapy in osteoarthritis: a review. Int J Radiat Oncol Biol Phys 114:203–220
49. Dunfield EM, Turek MM, Buhr KA, Christensen NI (2018) A survey of stereotactic radiation therapy in veterinary medicine. Vet Radiol Ultrasound 59:786–795
50. Duriseti S, Kavanaugh JA, Szymanski J, Huang Y, Basarabescu F, Chaudhuri A, Henke L, Samson P, Lin A, Robinson C, Spraker MB (2022) LITE SABR M1: a phase I trial of lattice stereotactic body radiotherapy for large tumors. Radiother Oncol 167:317–322
51. Eberlein R (1905) Stand und ziele der röntgenologie in der tierheilkunde. Verhandlungen der Deutschen Röntgen-Gesellschaft 1:70–73
52. Ehling TJ, Klein MK, Smith L, Prescott D, Haney S, Looper J, Ladue T, Brawner W, Fidel J, Shiomitsu K, Green E, Saba C, Turek M, Farrelly J (2022) A prospective, multi-centre, veterinary radiation therapy oncology group study reveals potential efficacy of toceranib phosphate (palladia) as a primary or adjuvant agent in the treatment of canine nasal carcinoma. Vet Comp Oncol 20:293–303
53. Emami B, Lyman J, Brown A, Coia L, Goitein M, Munzenrider J, Shank B, Solin L, Wesson M (1991) Tolerance of normal tissue to therapeutic irradiation. Int J Radiat Oncol Biol Phys 21:109–122
54. Farese JP, Milner R, Thompson MS, Lester N, Cooke K, Fox L, Hester J, Bova FJ (2004) Stereotactic radiosurgery for treatment of osteosarcomas involving the distal portions of the limbs in dogs. J Am Vet Med Assoc 225:1567–1572, 1548
55. Farrelly J, McEntee MC (2014) A survey of veterinary radiation facilities in 2010. Vet Radiol Ultrasound 55:638–643
56. Favaudon V, Caplier L, Monceau V, Pouzoulet F, Sayarath M, Fouillade C, Poupon MF, Brito I, Hupé P, Bourhis J, Hall J, Fontaine JJ, Vozenin MC (2014) Ultrahigh dose-rate FLASH irradiation increases the differential response between normal and tumor tissue in mice. Sci Transl Med 6:245ra93
57. Fidel J, Lyons J, Tripp C, Houston R, Wheeler B, Ruiz A (2011) Treatment of oral squamous cell carcinoma with accelerated radiation therapy and concomitant carboplatin in cats. J Vet Intern Med 25:504–510
58. Fike JR, Cann CE, Turowski K, Higgins RJ, Chan ASL, Phillips TL, Davis RL (1988) Radiation dose response of normal brain. Int J Radiat Oncol Biol Phys 14:63–70
59. Filatenkov A, Baker J, Mueller AM, Kenkel J, Ahn GO, Dutt S, Zhang N, Kohrt H, Jensen K, Dejbakhsh-Jones S, Shizuru JA, Negrin RN, Engleman EG, Strober S (2015) Ablative tumor radiation can change the tumor immune cell microenvironment to induce durable complete remissions. Clin Cancer Res 21:3727–3739
60. Fisher DR, Fidel J, Maitz CA (2019) Direct interstitial treatment of solid tumors using an injectable Yttrium-90-polymer composite. Cancer Biother Radiopharm 35:1
61. Flesner BK, Torres BT, Hutcheson KD, Rindt H, Zalcman AR, Maitz CA (2021) A pilot study of cancer-induced bone pain using validated owner questionnaires, serum N-telopeptide concentration, kinetic analysis, and PET/CT. Front Vet Sci 8:637195
62. Formenti SC, Demaria S (2013) Combining radiotherapy and cancer immunotherapy: a paradigm shift. J Natl Cancer Inst 105:256–265
63. Forrest LJ, Chun R, Adams WM, Cooley AJ, Vail DM (2000) Postoperative radiotherapy for canine soft tissue sarcoma. J Vet Intern Med 14:578–582
64. Fowler JF, Morgan RL, Silvester JA, Bewley DK, Turner BA (1963) Experiments with fractionated x-ray treatment of the skin of pigs. Br J Radiol 36:188–196
65. Fox-Alvarez S, Shiomitsu K, Lejeune AT, Szivek A, Kubicek L (2020) Outcome of intensity-modulated radiation therapy-based stereotactic radiation therapy for treatment of canine nasal carcinomas. Vet Radiol Ultrasound 61:370–378
66. Fu DR, Kadosawa T (2022) Comparison of epidermal growth factor receptor (EGFR) and cyclooxygenase-2 (COX-2) immunohistochemical expression and outcomes in canine nasal carcinomas treated with radiation therapy. J Vet Med Sci 84:1237–1243
67. Fulkerson CM, Knapp DW (2020) Tumors of the urinary system. In: Vail D, Thamm D, Liptak J (eds) Withrow & MacEwen's small animal clinical oncology, 6th edn. Elsevier, St. Louis
68. Gagnon J, Mayer MN, Belosowsky T, Mauldin GN, Waldner CL (2020) Stereotactic body radiation therapy for treatment of soft tissue sarcomas in 35 dogs. J Am Vet Med Assoc 256:102–110
69. Gamblin RM, Sagartz JE, Couto CG (1997) Overexpression of p53 tumor suppressor protein in spontaneously arising neoplasms of dogs. Am J Vet Res 58:857–863
70. Gavin PR, Huiskamp R, Wheeler FJ, Kraft SL, Dehaan CE (1993) Large animal normal tissue tolerance using an epithermal neutron beam and borocaptate sodium. Strahlenther Onkol 169:48–56
71. Gavin PR, Kraft SL, Huiskamp R, Coderre JA (1997) A review: CNS effects and normal tissue tolerance in dogs. J Neuro-Oncol 33:71–80
72. Gentilini F, Turba ME, Forni M, Cinotti S (2009) Complete sequencing of full-length canine ataxia telangiectasia mutated mRNA and characterization

of its putative promoter. Vet Immunol Immunopathol 128:437–440
73. Gieger T, Rassnick K, Siegel S, Proulx D, Bergman P, Anderson C, Ladue T, Smith A, Northrup N, Roberts R (2008) Palliation of clinical signs in 48 dogs with nasal carcinomas treated with coarse-fraction radiation therapy. J Am Anim Hosp Assoc 44:116–123
74. Gieger T, Siegel S, Rosen K, Jackson D, Ware K, Kiselow M, Shiomitsu K (2013) Reirradiation of canine nasal carcinomas treated with coarsely fractionated radiation protocols: 37 cases. J Am Anim Hosp Assoc 49:318
75. Gillette EL (1997) History of veterinary radiation oncology. Vet Clin North Am Small Anim Pract 27:1–6
76. Gillette EL, McChesney SL, Hoopes PJ (1985) Isoeffect curves for radiation-induced cardiomyopathy in the dog. Int J Radiat Oncol Biol Phys 11:2091–2097
77. Gillette EL, Powers BE, McChesney SL, Withrow SJ (1988) Aortic wall injury following intraoperative irradiation. Int J Radiat Oncol Biol Phys 15:1401–1406
78. Gillette SM, Powers BE, Orton EC, Gillette EL (1991) Early radiation response of the canine heart and lung. Radiat Res 125:34–40
79. Gillette SM, Dewhirst MW, Gillette EL, Thrall DE, Page RL, Powers BE, Withrow SJ, Rosner G, Wong C, Sim DA (1992) Response of canine soft tissue sarcomas to radiation or radiation plus hyperthermia: a randomized phase II study. Int J Hyperth 8:309–320
80. Gondi V, Bauman G, Bradfield L, Burri SH, Cabrera AR, Cunningham DA, Eaton BR, Hattangadi-Gluth JA, Kim MM, Kotecha R, Kraemer L, Li J, Nagpal S, Rusthoven CG, Suh JH, Tomé WA, Wang TJC, Zimmer AS, Ziu M, Brown PD (2022) Radiation therapy for brain metastases: an ASTRO clinical practice guideline. Pract Radiat Oncol 12:265–282
81. Göttgens EL, Ostheimer C, Span PN, Bussink J, Hammond EM (2019) HPV, hypoxia and radiation response in head and neck cancer. Br J Radiol 92:20180047
82. Granot N, Storb R (2020) History of hematopoietic cell transplantation: challenges and progress. Haematologica 105:2716–2729
83. Graves SS, Rezvani A, Sale G, Stone D, Parker M, Rosinski S, Spector M, Swearingen B, Kean L, Storb R (2017) A canine model of chronic graft-versus-host disease. Biol Blood Marrow Transplant 23:420–427
84. Green E, Adams W, Forrest L (2002) Four fraction palliative radiotherapy for osteosarcoma in 24 dogs. J Am Anim Hosp Assoc 38:445–451
85. Griffin RJ, Dings RP, Jamshidi-Parsian A, Song CW (2010) Mild temperature hyperthermia and radiation therapy: role of tumour vascular thermotolerance and relevant physiological factors. Int J Hyperth 26:256–263
86. Griffin LR, Nolan MW, Selmic LE, Randall E, Custis J, Larue S (2016) Stereotactic radiation therapy for treatment of canine intracranial meningiomas. Vet Comp Oncol 14:e158–e170
87. Griffin MA, Martin TW, Thamm DH, Worley DR (2023) Partial ulnar ostectomy, stereotactic body radiation therapy, and palliative radiation therapy as local limb sparing treatment modalities for ulnar tumors in dogs. Front Vet Sci 10:1172139
88. Groelly FJ, Fawkes M, Dagg RA, Blackford AN, Tarsounas M (2023) Targeting DNA damage response pathways in cancer. Nat Rev Cancer 23:78–94
89. Grosse N, Van Loon B, Rohrer Bley C (2014) DNA damage response and DNA repair – dog as a model? BMC Cancer 14:203
90. Hall EJ, Giaccia AJ (2018) Radiobiology for the radiologist. Wolters Kluwer Health, Philadelphia
91. Henderson MA, Burmeister BH, Ainslie J, Fisher R, Di Iulio J, Smithers BM, Hong A, Shannon K, Scolyer RA, Carruthers S, Coventry BJ, Babington S, Duprat J, Hoekstra HJ, Thompson JF (2015) Adjuvant lymph-node field radiotherapy versus observation only in patients with melanoma at high risk of further lymph-node field relapse after lymphadenectomy (ANZMTG 01.02/TROG 02.01): 6-year follow-up of a phase 3, randomised controlled trial. Lancet Oncol 16:1049–1060
92. Hernández-Suárez B, Gillespie DA, Pawlak A (2022) DNA damage response proteins in canine cancer as potential research targets in comparative oncology. Vet Comp Oncol 20:347–361
93. Herzig R, Beckmann K, Körner M, Steffen F, Rohrer Bley C (2023) A shortened whole brain radiation therapy protocol for meningoencephalitis of unknown origin in dogs. Front Vet Sci 10:1132736
94. Hicks J, Platt S, Kent M, Haley A (2017) Canine brain tumours: a model for the human disease? Vet Comp Oncol 15:252–272
95. Hildebrandt I, Culp WTN, Griffin MA (2023) A systematic review of canine cystectomy: indications, techniques, and outcomes. Animals (Basel) 13:2896
96. Hocker SE, Higginbotham ML, Schermerhorn T, Henningson J (2017) Receptor tyrosine kinase expression and phosphorylation in canine nasal carcinoma. Res Vet Sci 115:484–489
97. Hoekstra HJ, Sindelar WF, Kinsella TJ, Mehta DM (1989) Intraoperative radiation therapy-induced sarcomas in dogs. Radiat Res 120:508–515
98. Hoopes PJ, Gillette EL, Benjamin SA (1985) The pathogenesis of radiation nephropathy in the dog. Radiat Res 104:406–419
99. Hoopes PJ, Gillette EL, Withrow SJ (1987) Intraoperative irradiation of the canine abdominal aorta and vena cava. Int J Radiat Oncol Biol Phys 13:715–722
100. Howell K, Matuszak M, Maitz CA, Eisaman SH, Padilla L, Brown SL, Joiner MC, Dominello MM, Burmeister J (2020) Three discipline collaborative

radiation therapy (3DCRT) special debate: in the future, at least 20% of NIH funding for radiotherapy research should be allocated to non-oncologic applications. J Appl Clin Med Phys 21:7–13
101. Hunley D, Mauldin G, Shiomitsu K, Mauldin G (2010) Clinical outcome in dogs with nasal tumors treated with intensity-modulated radiation therapy. Can Vet J/La revue vétérinaire canadienne 51:293–300
102. Hwang T-S, An S, Choi M-Y, Huh C, Song J-H, Jung D-I, Lee HC (2022) Piroxicam, mitoxantrone, and hypofractionated radiation therapy with volumetric modulated arc therapy for treating urinary transitional cell carcinoma in a dog: a case report. J Vet Clin 39:16–22
103. Inanaga S, Igase M, Sakai Y, Tanabe M, Shimonohara N, Itamoto K, Nakaichi M, Mizuno T (2021) Mismatch repair deficiency in canine neoplasms. Vet Pathol 58:1058–1063
104. Jebelli J, Hamper MC, Van Quelef D, Caraballo D, Hartmann J, Kumi-Diaka J (2022) The potential therapeutic effects of low-dose ionizing radiation in Alzheimer's disease. Cureus 14:e23461
105. Jegatheeson S, Zuber M, Woodward AP, Cannon CM (2022) Response of canine thyroid carcinomas to radioiodine. Vet Comp Oncol 20:235–245
106. Johnson DE, Burtness B, Leemans CR, Lui VWY, Bauman JE, Grandis JR (2020) Head and neck squamous cell carcinoma. Nat Rev Dis Prim 6:92
107. Johnstone PAS, Laskin WB, Deluca AM, Barnes M, Kinsella TJ, Sindelar WF (1996) Tumors in dogs exposed to experimental intraoperative radiotherapy. Int J Radiat Oncol Biol Phys 34:853–857
108. Joiner M, van der Kogel A (2009) Basic clinical radiobiology. CRC Press, Boca Raton
109. Kanagavelu S, Gupta S, Wu X, Philip S, Wattenberg MM, Hodge JW, Couto MD, Chung KD, Ahmed MM (2014) In vivo effects of lattice radiation therapy on local and distant lung cancer: potential role of immunomodulation. Radiat Res 182:149–162
110. Kapatkin AS, Nordquist B, Garcia TC, Griffin MA, Theon A, Kim S, Hayashi K (2016) Effect of single dose radiation therapy on weight-bearing lameness in dogs with elbow osteoarthritis. Vet Comp Orthop Traumatol 29:338–343
111. Kavanaugh JA, Spraker MB, Duriseti S, Basarabescu F, Price A, Goddu M, Knutson N, Prusator M, Robinson C, Mazur T (2022) LITE SABR M1: planning design and dosimetric endpoints for a phase I trial of lattice SBRT. Radiother Oncol 167:172–178
112. Kim DY, Kim JS, Seo YS, Park WY, Kim BH, Hong EH, Kim JY, Cho SJ, Rhee HY, Kim A, Kim KY, Oh DJ, Chung WK (2023) Evaluation of efficacy and safety using low dose radiation therapy with Alzheimer's disease: a protocol for multicenter phase II clinical trial. J Alzheimer's Dis 95:1263–1272
113. Kinsella TJ, Sindelar WF, Deluca AM, Barnes M, Tochner Z, Mixon A, Glatstein E (1988) Tolerance of the canine bladder to intraoperative radiation therapy: an experimental study. Int J Radiat Oncol Biol Phys 14:939–946
114. Klosowski M, Haines L, Alfino L, McMellen A, Leibowitz M, Regan D (2023) Naturally occurring canine sarcomas: bridging the gap from mouse models to human patients through cross-disciplinary research partnerships. Front Oncol 13:1130215
115. Koehler JW, Miller AD, Miller CR, Porter B, Aldape K, Beck J, Brat D, Cornax I, Corps K, Frank C (2018) A revised diagnostic classification of canine glioma: towards validation of the canine glioma patient as a naturally occurring preclinical model for human glioma. J Neuropathol Exp Neurol 77:1039–1054
116. Koenig A, Bianco SR, Fosmire S, Wojcieszyn J, Modiano JF (2002) Expression and significance of p53, rb, p21/waf-1, p16/ink-4a, and PTEN tumor suppressors in canine melanoma. Vet Pathol 39:458–472
117. Konradsson E, Arendt ML, Bastholm Jensen K, Børresen B, Hansen AE, Bäck S, Kristensen AT, Munck Af Rosenschöld P, Ceberg C, Petersson K (2021) Establishment and initial experience of clinical FLASH radiotherapy in canine cancer patients. Front Oncol 11:658004
118. Kraft S, Gavin P, Dehaan C, Leathers C, Bauer W, Miller D, Dorn R (1992) Borocaptate sodium: a potential boron delivery compound for boron neutron capture therapy evaluated in dogs with spontaneous intracranial tumors. Proc Natl Acad Sci USA 89:11973–11977
119. Kueffer P, Maitz C, Khan A, Schuster S, Shlyakhtina N, Jalisatgi S, Brockman J, Nigg D, Hawthorne M (2013) Boron neutron capture therapy demonstrated in mice bearing EMT6 tumors following selective delivery of boron by rationally designed liposomes. Proc Natl Acad Sci USA 110:E5038
120. Ladue T, Klein MK (2001) Toxicity criteria of the veterinary radiation therapy oncology group. Vet Radiol Ultrasound 42:475–476
121. Lattimer JC, Corwin LA, Stapleton J, Volkert WA, Ehrhardt GJ, Ketring AR, Anderson SK, Simon J, Goeckeler WF (1990a) Clinical and clinicopathologic response of canine bone tumor patients to treatment with Samarium-153-EDTMP. J Nucl Med 31:1316–1325
122. Lattimer JC, Corwin LA, Stapleton J, Volkert WA, Ehrhardt GJ, Ketring AR, Hewett JE, Simon J, Goeckeler WF (1990b) Clinical and clinicopathologic effects of Samarium-153-EDTMP administered intravenously to normal beagle dogs. J Nucl Med 31:586–593
123. Lawrence J, Forrest L, Adams W, Vail D, Thamm D (2008) Four-fraction radiation therapy for macroscopic soft tissue sarcomas in 16 dogs. J Am Anim Hosp Assoc 44:100–108
124. Lawrence JA, Forrest LJ, Turek MM, Miller PE, Mackie TR, Jaradat HA, Vail DM, Dubielzig RR, Chappell R, Mehta MP (2010) Proof of principle of ocular sparing in dogs with sinonasal tumors treated

with intensity-modulated radiation therapy. Vet Radiol Ultrasound 51:561–570
125. LeBlanc AK, Ladue TA, Turrel JM, Klein MK (2004) Unexpected toxicity following use of gemcitabine as a radiosensitizer in head and neck carcinomas: a veterinary radiation therapy oncology group pilot study. Vet Radiol Ultrasound 45:466–470
126. LeBlanc AK, Mazcko C, Brown DE, Koehler JW, Miller AD, Miller CR, Bentley RT, Packer RA, Breen M, Boudreau CE (2016) Creation of an NCI comparative brain tumor consortium: informing the translation of new knowledge from canine to human brain tumor patients. Neuro-Oncology 18:1209–1218
127. LeBlanc AK, Atherton M, Bentley RT, Boudreau CE, Burton JH, Curran KM, Dow S, Giuffrida MA, Kellihan HB, Mason NJ, Oblak M, Selmic LE, Selting KA, Singh A, Tjostheim S, Vail DM, Weishaar KM, Berger EP, Rossmeisl JH, Mazcko C (2021) Veterinary cooperative oncology group-common terminology criteria for adverse events (VCOG-CTCAE v2) following investigational therapy in dogs and cats. Vet Comp Oncol 19:311–352
128. Legorreta RA, Denman DL, Kelley MC, Lewis GC Jr (1988) Use of hyperthermia and radiotherapy in treatment of a large mast cell sarcoma in a dog. J Am Vet Med Assoc 193:1545–1548
129. Lhuillier C, Rudqvist N-P, Elemento O, Formenti SC, Demaria S (2019) Radiation therapy and anti-tumor immunity: exposing immunogenic mutations to the immune system. Genome Med 11:40
130. Liptak JM, Dernell WS, Lascelles BD, Larue SM, Jameson VJ, Powers BE, Huber DJ, Withrow SJ (2004) Intraoperative extracorporeal irradiation for limb sparing in 13 dogs. Vet Surg 33:446–456
131. Maeda S, Sakai K, Kaji K, Iio A, Nakazawa M, Motegi T, Yonezawa T, Momoi Y (2022) Lapatinib as first-line treatment for muscle-invasive urothelial carcinoma in dogs. Sci Rep 12:4
132. Magee K, Marsh IR, Turek MM, Grudzinski J, Aluicio-Sarduy E, Engle JW, Kurzman ID, Zuleger CL, Oseid EA, Jaskowiak C, Albertini MR, Esbona K, Bednarz B, Sondel PM, Weichert JP, Morris ZS, Hernandez R, Vail DM (2021) Safety and feasibility of an in situ vaccination and immunomodulatory targeted radionuclide combination immuno-radiotherapy approach in a comparative (companion dog) setting. PLoS One 16:e0255798
133. Maguire PD, Samulski TV, Prosnitz LR, Jones EL, Rosner GL, Powers B, Layfield LW, Brizel DM, Scully SP, Harrelson JM, Dewhirst MW (2001) A phase II trial testing the thermal dose parameter CEM43 degrees T90 as a predictor of response in soft tissue sarcomas treated with pre-operative thermoradiotherapy. Int J Hyperth 17:283–290
134. Maitz CA, Tate D, Bechtel S, Lunceford J, Henry C, Flesner B, Collins A, Varterasian M, Tung D, Zhang L, Saha S, Bryan JN (2021) Paired 18F-Fluorodeoxyglucose (18F-FDG), and 64Cu-copper(II)-diacetyl-bis(N(4)-methylthiosemicarbazone) (64Cu-ATSM) PET scans in dogs with spontaneous tumors and evaluation for hypoxia-directed therapy. Radiat Res 197:253–260
135. Maitz CA, Delaney S, Cook BE, Genady AR, Hoerres R, Kuchuk M, Makris G, Valliant JF, Sadeghi S, Lewis JS, Hennkens HM, Bryan JN, Zeglis BM (2022) Pretargeted PET of osteodestructive lesions in dogs. Mol Pharm 19:3153–3162
136. Marks LB, Ten Haken RK, Martel MK (2010a) Guest editor's introduction to QUANTEC: a users guide. Int J Radiat Oncol Biol Phys 76:S1–S2
137. Marks LB, Yorke ED, Jackson A, Ten Haken RK, Constine LS, Eisbruch A, Bentzen SM, Nam J, Deasy JO (2010b) Use of normal tissue complication probability models in the clinic. Int J Radiat Oncol Biol Phys 76:S10–S19
138. Martin TW, Griffin L, Custis J, Ryan SD, Lafferty M, Boss MK, Regan D, Rao S, Leary D, Withrow SJ, Larue SM (2021) Outcome and prognosis for canine appendicular osteosarcoma treated with stereotactic body radiation therapy in 123 dogs. Vet Comp Oncol 19:284–294
139. Martinez MN, Mochel JP, Neuhoff S, Pade D (2021) Comparison of canine and human physiological factors: understanding interspecies differences that impact drug pharmacokinetics. AAPS J 23:59
140. Mateus CQ, Grams M, Mashayekhi M (2024) Clinical commissioning of orthovoltage-based mini-beam radiation therapy (MBRT). Int J Radiat Oncol Biol Phys 120:e179
141. Mayer MN, Dewalt JO, Sidhu N, Mauldin GN, Waldner CL (2019) Outcomes and adverse effects associated with stereotactic body radiation therapy in dogs with nasal tumors: 28 cases (2011–2016). J Am Vet Med Assoc 254:602–612
142. Mb KMS (2017) The distribution of pulmonary metastases in dogs with osteosarcoma: Immunohistochemical characterization of TP3 and PCNA; a novel method for studying the distribution of pulmonary micrometastases. Norwegian University of Life Sciences, Ås
143. McChesney Gillette S, Gillette EL, Shida T, Boon J, Miller CW, Powers BE (1992) Late radiation response of canine mediastinal tissues. Radiother Oncol 23:41–52
144. McChesney SL, Gillette EL, Dewhirst MW, Withrow SJ (1986) Influence of wr 2721 on radiation response of canine soft tissue sarcomas. Int J Radiat Oncol Biol Phys 12:1957–1963
145. McChesney SL, Gillette EL, Orton EC (1988) Canine cardiomyopathy after whole heart and partial lung irradiation. Int J Radiat Oncol Biol Phys 14:1169–1174
146. McChesney SL, Gillette EL, Powers BE (1989a) Response of the canine lung to fractionated irradiation: pathologic changes and isoeffect curves. Int J Radiat Oncol Biol Phys 16:125–132
147. McChesney SL, Withrow SJ, Gillette EL, Powers BE, Dewhirst MW (1989b) Radiotherapy of soft

tissue sarcomas in dogs. J Am Vet Med Assoc 194:60–63
148. McEntee MC (2004) A survey of veterinary radiation facilities in the United States during 2001. Vet Radiol Ultrasound 45:476–479
149. McEntee MC, Page RL, Novotney CA, Thrall DE (1993) Palliative radiotherapy for canine appendicular osteosarcoma. Vet Radiol Ultrasound 34:367–370
150. McGuire AR, Maitz CA, Lattimer JC, Flesner BK (2017) What is your diagnosis? J Am Vet Med Assoc 251:273–275
151. McKnight JA, Mauldin GN, McEntee MC, Meleo KA, Patnaik AK (2000) Radiation treatment for incompletely resected soft-tissue sarcomas in dogs. J Am Vet Med Assoc 217:205–210
152. Mensali N, Köksal H, Joaquina S, Wernhoff P, Casey NP, Romecin P, Panisello C, Rodriguez R, Vimeux L, Juzeniene A, Myhre MR, Fåne A, Ramírez CC, Maggadottir SM, Duru AD, Georgoudaki A-M, Grad I, Maturana AD, Gaudernack G, Kvalheim G, Carcaboso AM, De Alava E, Donnadieu E, Bruland ØS, Menendez P, Inderberg EM, Wälchli S (2023) ALPL-1 is a target for chimeric antigen receptor therapy in osteosarcoma. Nat Commun 14:3375
153. Miller AD, Miller CR, Rossmeisl JH (2019) Canine primary intracranial cancer: a clinicopathologic and comparative review of glioma, meningioma, and choroid plexus tumors. Front Oncol 9:1151
154. Milner RJ, Dormehl I, Louw WK, Croft S (1998) Targeted radiotherapy with Sm-153-EDTMP in nine cases of canine primary bone tumours. J S Afr Vet Assoc 69:12–17
155. Milovancev M, Hauck M, Keller C, Stranahan LW, Mansoor A, Malarkey DE (2015) Comparative pathology of canine soft tissue sarcomas: possible models of human non-rhabdomyosarcoma soft tissue sarcomas. J Comp Pathol 152:22–27
156. Mittal BB, Pelzer H, Tsao C-S, Ward WF, Johnson P, Friedman C, Sisson GA Sr, Kies M (1990) Intraoperative radiation of canine carotid artery, internal jugular vein, and vagus nerve: therapeutic applications in the management of advanced head and neck cancers. Arch Otolaryngol Head Neck Surg 116:1425–1430
157. Mohiuddin M, Fujita M, Regine WF, Megooni AS, Ibbott GS, Ahmed MM (1999) High-dose spatially-fractionated radiation (GRID): a new paradigm in the management of advanced cancers. Int J Radiat Oncol Biol Phys 45:721–727
158. Moirano SJ, Dewey CW, Haney S, Yang J (2020) Efficacy of frameless stereotactic radiotherapy for the treatment of presumptive canine intracranial gliomas: a retrospective analysis (2014–2017). Vet Comp Oncol 18:528–537
159. Morsink NC, Klaassen NJM, Meij BP, Kirpensteijn J, Grinwis GCM, Schaafsma IA, Hesselink JW, Nijsen JFW, van Nimwegen SA (2021) Case report: radioactive holmium-166 microspheres for the intratumoral treatment of a canine pituitary tumor. Front Vet Sci 8:748247
160. Morsink NC, Nijsen JFW, Grinwis GCM, Hesselink JW, Kirpensteijn J, van Nimwegen SA (2022) Intratumoral injection of holmium-166 microspheres as neoadjuvant therapy of soft tissue sarcomas in dogs. Front Vet Sci 9:1015248
161. Mouli SK, Raiter S, Harris K, Mylarapu A, Burks M, Li W, Gordon AC, Khan A, Matsumoto M, Bailey KL, Pasciak AS, Manupipatpong S, Weiss CR, Casalino D, Miller FH, Gates VL, Hohlastos E, Lewandowski RJ, Kim DH, Dreher MR, Salem R (2021) Yttrium-90 radioembolization to the prostate gland: proof of concept in a canine model and clinical translation. J Vasc Interv Radiol 32:1103–1112.e12
162. Muñana KR, Luttgen PJ (1998) Prognostic factors for dogs with granulomatous meningoencephalomyelitis: 42 cases (1982–1996). J Am Vet Med Assoc 212:1902–1906
163. Nesbit ME Jr, Gehan EA, Burgert EO Jr, Vietti TJ, Cangir A, Tefft M, Evans R, Thomas P, Askin FB, Kissane JM et al (1990) Multimodal therapy for the management of primary, nonmetastatic Ewing's sarcoma of bone: a long-term follow-up of the First Intergroup study. J Clin Oncol 8:1664–1674
164. Noall L, Lee S, Burton JH, Marquardt TM, Cermak J, Thombs LA, Rogic AM, Bryan JN, Chu S (2023) A multi-institutional epidemiologic study evaluating environmental risk factors for feline oral squamous cell carcinoma. Vet Comp Oncol 21(3):509–519
165. Nolan M, Kogan L, Griffin L, Custis J, Harmon J, Biller B, Larue S (2012) Intensity-modulated and image-guided radiation therapy for treatment of genitourinary carcinomas in dogs. J Vet Intern Med 26:987–995
166. Nolan MW, Marolf AJ, Ehrhart EJ, Rao S, Kraft SL, Engel S, Yoshikawa H, Golden AE, Wasserman TH, Larue SM (2015) Pudendal nerve and internal pudendal artery damage may contribute to radiation-induced erectile dysfunction. Int J Radiat Oncol Biol Phys 91:796–806
167. Nolan MW, Gieger TL, Karakashian AA, Nikolova-Karakashian MN, Posner LP, Roback DM, Rivera JN, Chang S (2017) Outcomes of spatially fractionated radiotherapy (GRID) for bulky soft tissue sarcomas in a large animal model. Technol Cancer Res Treat 16:357–365
168. Nolan MW, Kent MS, Boss MK (2019) Emerging translational opportunities in comparative oncology with companion canine cancers: radiation oncology. Front Oncol 9:1291
169. Nolan MW, Kelsey KL, Enomoto M, Ru H, Gieger TL, Lascelles BDX (2020) Pet dogs with subclinical acute radiodermatitis experience widespread somatosensory sensitization. Radiat Res 193:241–248
170. Nolan MW, Berman AR, Watson-Skaggs ML, Quinn CN, Marcus KL, Russell K, Yoshikawa H, Olby NJ, Gieger TL (2022) Stereotactic radiotherapy (10 Gy X 3) for canine nonlymphomatous intranasal tumors is associated with prolonged survival and minimal

risk of severe radiotoxicity. J Am Vet Med Assoc 260:1496–1506
171. Norquest CJ, Maitz CA, Keys DA, Moore M, Bryan JN, Ehling TJ, Lattimer JC, Flesner BK (2022) Fracture rate and time to fracture in dogs with appendicular osteosarcoma receiving finely fractionated compared to coarsely fractionated radiation therapy: A single institution study. Vet Med Sci 8:1013–1024
172. O'Sullivan B, Davis AM, Turcotte R, Bell R, Catton C, Chabot P, Wunder J, Kandel R, Goddard K, Sadura A, Pater J, Zee B (2002) Preoperative versus postoperative radiotherapy in soft-tissue sarcoma of the limbs: a randomised trial. Lancet 359:2235–2241
173. Owen LN (1989) Canine lick granuloma treated with radiotherapy. J Small Anim Pract 30:454
174. Packer RA, Rossmeisl JH, Kent MS, Griffin Iv JF, Mazcko C, LeBlanc AK (2018) Consensus recommendations on standardized magnetic resonance imaging protocols for multicenter canine brain tumor clinical trials. Vet Radiol Ultrasound 59:261–271
175. Page RL, Garg PK, Garg S, Archer GE, Bruland OS, Zalutsky MR (1994) PET imaging of osteosarcoma in dogs using a fluorine-18-labeled monoclonal antibody fab fragment. J Nucl Med 35:1506–1513
176. Park S-H, Kang H-J, Kim H-S, Kim M-J, Heo J-I, Kim J-H, Kho Y-J, Kim SC, Kim J, Park J-B, Lee J-Y (2011) Higher DNA repair activity is related with longer replicative life span in mammalian embryonic fibroblast cells. Biogerontology 12:565–579
177. Pasciak AS, Manupipatpong S, Hui FK, Gainsburg L, Krimins R, Zink MC, Brayton CF, Morris M, Sage J, Donahue DR, Dreher MR, Kraitchman DL, Weiss CR (2020) Yttrium-90 radioembolization as a possible new treatment for brain cancer: proof of concept and safety analysis in a canine model. EJNMMI Res 10:96
178. Patel RB, Hernandez R, Carlson P, Grudzinski J, Bates AM, Jagodinsky JC, Erbe A, Marsh IR, Arthur I, Aluicio-Sarduy E, Sriramaneni RN, Jin WJ, Massey C, Rakhmilevich AL, Vail D, Engle JW, Le T, Kim K, Bednarz B, Sondel PM, Weichert J, Morris ZS (2021) Low-dose targeted radionuclide therapy renders immunologically cold tumors responsive to immune checkpoint blockade. Sci Transl Med 13:eabb3631
179. Pellin MA (2022) The use of oncept melanoma vaccine in veterinary patients: a review of the literature. Vet Sci 9:597
180. Peltomäki P (1997) DNA mismatch repair gene mutations in human cancer. Environ Health Perspect 105(Suppl 4):775–780
181. Pilones KA, Vanpouille-Box C, Demaria S (2015) Combination of radiotherapy and immune checkpoint inhibitors. Semin Radiat Oncol 25:28–33
182. Plavec T, Kessler M, Kandel B, Schwietzer A, Roleff S (2006) Palliative radiotherapy as treatment for non-resectable soft tissue sarcomas in the dog – a report of 15 cases. Vet Comp Oncol 4:98–103
183. Pluhar GE, Grogan PT, Seiler C, Goulart M, Santacruz KS, Carlson C, Chen W, Olin MR, Lowenstein PR, Castro MG (2010) Anti-tumor immune response correlates with neurological symptoms in a dog with spontaneous astrocytoma treated by gene and vaccine therapy. Vaccine 28:3371–3378
184. Poirier VJ, Kaser-Hotz B, Vail DM, Straw RC (2013) Efficacy and toxicity of an accelerated hypofractionated radiation therapy protocol in cats with oral squamous cell carcinoma. Vet Radiol Ultrasound 54:81–88
185. Poirier VJ, Koh ESY, Darko J, Fleck A, Pinard C, Vail DM (2021) Patterns of local residual disease and local failure after intensity modulated/image guided radiation therapy for sinonasal tumors in dogs. J Vet Intern Med 35:1062–1072
186. Poirier VJ, Keyerleber M, Gordon IK, Turek MM, Kent MS, Bentley E, Lawrence J (2023) ACVR and ECVDI consensus statement: reporting elements for toxicity criteria of the veterinary radiation therapy oncology group v2.0. Vet Radiol Ultrasound 64:789–797
187. Pommer A (1947) Influence of the X-ray quality and intensity as well as the radiation method on the tolerance dose of the skin in horses. Wien Tierarztl Monatsschr 34:676–699
188. Pommer A (1958) X-ray therapy in veterinary medicine. Adv Vet Sci Comp Med 4:97–131
189. Poulson JM, Vujaskovic Z, Gillette SM, Chaney EL, Gillette EL (2000) Volume and dose-response effects for severe symptomatic pneumonitis after fractionated irradiation of canine lung. Int J Radiat Biol 463–468:463
190. Powers BE, McChesney SL, Gillette EL (1987) Late radiation response of the canine trachea with change in dose per fraction. Int J Radiat Oncol Biol Phys 13:1673–1680
191. Powers BE, Beck ER, Gillette EL, Gould DH, Lecouter RA (1992) Pathology of radiation injury to the canine spinal cord. Int J Radiat Oncol Biol Phys 23:539–549
192. Ramirez O 3rd, Dodge RK, Page RL, Price GS, Hauck ML, Ladue TA, Nutter F, Thrall DE (1999) Palliative radiotherapy of appendicular osteosarcoma in 95 dogs. Vet Radiol Ultrasound 40:517–522
193. Ravicini S, Baines SJ, Taylor A, Amores-Fuster I, Mason SL, Treggiari E (2018) Outcome and prognostic factors in medically treated canine prostatic carcinomas: a multi-institutional study. Vet Comp Oncol 16:450–458
194. Razmara AM, Wittenburg LA, Al-Nadaf S, Toedebusch RG, Meyers FJ, Toedebusch CM (2022) Prevalence and clinicopathologic features of canine metastatic melanoma involving the central nervous system: a retrospective analysis and comparative review. Front Oncol 12:868004
195. Rogers CL, Lageman SK, Fontanesi J, Wilson GD, Boling PA, Bansal S, Karis JP, Sabbagh M, Mehta MP, Harris TJ (2023) Low-dose whole brain radiation therapy for Alzheimer's dementia: results from a pilot trial in humans. Int J Radiat Oncol Biol Phys 117:87–95

196. Rohrer Bley C, Wolf F, Gonçalves Jorge P, Grilj V, Petridis I, Petit B, Böhlen TT, Moeckli R, Limoli C, Bourhis J, Meier V, Vozenin M-C (2022) Dose- and volume-limiting late toxicity of FLASH radiotherapy in cats with squamous cell carcinoma of the nasal planum and in mini pigs. Clin Cancer Res 28:3814–3823
197. Ronchi L, Buwenge M, Cortesi A, Ammendolia I, Frakulli R, Abate ME, Arcelli A, Donati CM, Macchia G, Morganti AG, Cammelli S (2018) Whole lung irradiation in patients with osteosarcoma and Ewing sarcoma. Anticancer Res 38:4977–4985
198. Rossi F, Cancedda S, Leone VF, Rohrer Bley C, Laganga P (2018) Megavoltage radiotherapy for the treatment of degenerative joint disease in dogs: results of a preliminary experience in an Italian radiotherapy centre. Front Vet Sci 5:74
199. Ryman-Tubb T, Lothion-Roy JH, Metzler VM, Harris AE, Robinson BD, Rizvanov AA, Jeyapalan JN, James VH, England G, Rutland CS, Persson JL, Kenner L, Rubin MA, Mongan NP, De Brot S (2022) Comparative pathology of dog and human prostate cancer. Vet Med Sci 8:110–120
200. Sathishkumar S, Dey S, Meigooni AS, Regine WF, Kudrimoti MS, Ahmed MM, Mohiuddin M (2002) The impact of TNF-alpha induction on therapeutic efficacy following high dose spatially fractionated (GRID) radiation. Technol Cancer Res Treat 1:141–147
201. Sathishkumar S, Boyanovsky B, Karakashian AA, Rozenova K, Giltiay NV, Kudrimoti M, Mohiuddin M, Ahmed MM, Nikolova-Karakashian M (2005) Elevated sphingomyelinase activity and ceramide concentration in serum of patients undergoing high dose spatially fractionated radiation treatment: implications for endothelial apoptosis. Cancer Biol Ther 4:979–986
202. Schültke E, Balosso J, Breslin T, Cavaletti G, Djonov V, Esteve F, Grotzer M, Hildebrandt G, Valdman A, Laissue J (2017) Microbeam radiation therapy – grid therapy and beyond: a clinical perspective. Br J Radiol 90:20170073
203. Schütt T, Helboe L, Pedersen LØ, Waldemar G, Berendt M, Pedersen JT (2016) Dogs with cognitive dysfunction as a spontaneous model for early Alzheimer's disease: a translational study of neuropathological and inflammatory markers. J Alzheimer's Dis 52:433–449
204. Schwint AE, Monti Hughes A, Garabalino MA, Santa Cruz GA, González SJ, Longhino J, Provenzano L, Oña P, Rao M, Cantarelli M, Leiras A, Olivera MS, Trivillin VA, Alessandrini P, Brollo F, Boggio E, Costa H, Ventimiglia R, Binia S, Pozzi ECC, Nievas SI, Santa Cruz IS (2020) Clinical veterinary boron neutron capture therapy (BNCT) studies in dogs with head and neck cancer: bridging the gap between translational and clinical studies. Biology (Basel) 9:327
205. Séguin B, McDonald DE, Kent MS, Walsh PJ, Théon AP (2005) Tolerance of cutaneous or mucosal flaps placed into a radiation therapy field in dogs. Vet Surg 34:214–222
206. Sgouros G, Hobbs RF, Atkins FB, Van Nostrand D, Ladenson PW, Wahl RL (2011) Three-dimensional radiobiological dosimetry (3D-RD) with 124I PET for 131I therapy of thyroid cancer. Eur J Nucl Med Mol Imaging 38:41–47
207. Shareef MM, Cui N, Burikhanov R, Gupta S, Satishkumar S, Shajahan S, Mohiuddin M, Rangnekar VM, Ahmed MM (2007) Role of tumor necrosis factor-alpha and TRAIL in high-dose radiation-induced bystander signaling in lung adenocarcinoma. Cancer Res 67:11811–11820
208. Shumway KL, Bryan JN, Donnelly LL, Flesner BK, Lattimer JC, McCleary-Wheeler AL, Lunceford JM, Maitz CA (2022) Biodistribution and image characteristics of (124) I-positron emission tomography in dogs with neuroendocrine neoplasia. Vet Radiol Ultrasound 63:298–305
209. Sindelar WF, Tepper J, Travis EL, Terrill R (1982) Tolerance of retroperitoneal structures to intraoperative radiation. Ann Surg 196:601–608
210. Sindelar WF, Johnstone PAS, Hoekstra HJ, Kinsella TJ (1999) Normal tissue tolerance to intraoperative irradiation. In: Gunderson LL, Willet CG, Harrison LB, Calvo FA (eds) Intraoperative irradiation: techniques and results. Humana Press, Totowa
211. Smith-Oskrochi L, Wustefeld-Janssens BG, Hollenbeck D, Stocks C, Deveau M (2023) Safety and feasibility of short course pre-operative radiation therapy followed by surgical excision for canine solid tumours. Vet Comp Oncol 21:82–90
212. Snider JW, Molitoris J, Shyu S, Diwanji T, Rice S, Kowalski E, Decesaris C, Remick JS, Yi B, Zhang B, Hall A, Hanna N, Ng VY, Regine WF (2020) Spatially fractionated radiotherapy (GRID) prior to standard neoadjuvant conventionally fractionated radiotherapy for bulky, high-risk soft tissue and osteosarcomas: feasibility, safety, and promising pathologic response rates. Radiat Res 194:707–714
213. Snyder JM, Lipitz L, Skorupski KA, Shofer FS, Van Winkle TJ (2008) Secondary intracranial neoplasia in the dog: 177 cases (1986–2003). J Vet Intern Med 22:172–177
214. Sones E, Smith A, Schleis S, Brawner W, Almond G, Taylor K, Haney S, Wypij J, Keyerleber M, Arthur J, Hamilton T, Lawrence J, Gieger T, Sellon R, Wright Z (2012) Survival times for canine intranasal sarcomas treated with radiation therapy: 86 cases (1996–2011). Vet Radiol Ultrasound 54:194–201
215. Stans J (2020) Prostatectomy as a treatment for canine prostate cancer: a literature review. Open Vet J 10:317–322
216. Stevenson VB, Klahn S, Leroith T, Huckle WR (2023) Canine melanoma: a review of diagnostics and comparative mechanisms of disease and immu-

notolerance in the era of the immunotherapies. Front Vet Sci 9:1046636
217. Stewart-Ornstein J, Cheng HWJ, Lahav G (2017) Conservation and divergence of p53 oscillation dynamics across species. Cell Syst 5:410–417.e4
218. Storb R, Yu C, Zaucha JM, Deeg HJ, Georges G, Kiem H-P, Nash RA, McSweeney PA, Wagner JL (1999) Stable mixed hematopoietic Chimerism in dogs given donor antigen, CTLA4Ig, and 100 cGy total body irradiation before and pharmacologic immunosuppression after marrow transplant. Blood 94:2523–2529
219. Straume O, Sviland L, Akslen LA (2000) Loss of nuclear p16 protein expression correlates with increased tumor cell proliferation (Ki-67) and poor prognosis in patients with vertical growth phase melanoma. Clin Cancer Res 6:1845–1853
220. Tagliaferri L, Lancellotta V, Fionda B, Mangoni M, Casà C, Di Stefani A, Pagliara MM, D'aviero A, Schinzari G, Chiesa S, Mazzarella C, Manfrida S, Colloca GF, Marazzi F, Morganti AG, Blasi MA, Peris K, Tortora G, Valentini V (2022) Immunotherapy and radiotherapy in melanoma: a multidisciplinary comprehensive review. Hum Vaccin Immunother 18:1903827
221. Tan-Coleman B, Lyons J, Lewis C, Rosenberg M, Ruiz A (2013) Prospective evaluation of A 5 × 4 Gy prescription for palliation of canine nasal tumors. Vet Radiol Ultrasound 54:89–92
222. Tepper JE, Sindelar W, Travis EL, Terrill R, Padikal T (1983) Tolerance of canine anastomoses to intra-operative radiation therapy. Int J Radiat Oncol Biol Phys 9:987–992
223. Thrall DE, Prescott DM, Samulski TV, Rosner GL, Denman DL, Legorreta RL, Dodge RK, Page RL, Cline JM, Lee J, Case BC, Evans SM, Oleson JR, Dewhirst MW (1996) Radiation plus local hyperthermia versus radiation plus the combination of local and whole-body hyperthermia in canine sarcomas. Int J Radiat Oncol Biol Phys 34:1087–1096
224. Thrall DE, Larue SM, Yu D, Samulski T, Sanders L, Case B, Rosner G, Azuma C, Poulson J, Pruitt AF, Stanley W, Hauck ML, Williams L, Hess P, Dewhirst MW (2005) Thermal dose is related to duration of local control in canine sarcomas treated with thermoradiotherapy. Clin Cancer Res 11:5206–5214
225. Tierce R, Martin T, Hughes KL, Harrison L, Swancutt KL, Rao S, Leary D, Larue SM, Boss M-K (2021) Response of canine soft tissue sarcoma to stereotactic body radiotherapy. Radiat Res 196:587–601, 15
226. Tiller-Borcich JK, Fike JR, Phillips TL, Davis RL (1987) Pathology of delayed radiation brain damage: an experimental canine model. Radiat Res 110:161–172
227. Trivillin V, Heber E, Rao M, Cantarelli M, Itoiz M, Nigg D, Calzetta O, Blaumann H, Longhino J, Schwint A (2008) Boron neutron capture therapy (BNCT) for the treatment of spontaneous nasal planum squamous cell carcinoma in felines. Radiat Environ Biophys 47:147–155
228. Turrel J, McEntee M, Burke B, Page R (2006) Sodium iodide I 131 treatment of dogs with nonresectable thyroid tumors: 39 cases (1990-2003). J Am Vet Med Assoc 229:542–548
229. Van Asselt N, Christensen N, Meier V, Rohrer Bley C, Laliberte S, Poirier VJ, Desai N, Chen Y, Turek M (2020) Definitive-intent intensity-modulated radiation therapy provides similar outcomes to those previously published for definitive-intent three-dimensional conformal radiation therapy in dogs with primary brain tumors: a multi-institutional retrospective study. Vet Radiol Ultrasound 61:481–489
230. van Nimwegen SA, Bakker RC, Kirpensteijn J, Van Es RJJ, Koole R, Lam M, Hesselink JW, Nijsen JFW (2018) Intratumoral injection of radioactive holmium ((166) Ho) microspheres for treatment of oral squamous cell carcinoma in cats. Vet Comp Oncol 16:114–124
231. Vancil J, Henry C, Milner R, McCoig A, Lattimer J, Villamil J, McCaw D, Bryan J (2012) Use of samarium Sm 153 lexidronam for the treatment of dogs with primary tumors of the skull: 20 cases (1986–2006). J Am Vet Med Assoc 240:1310–1315
232. Vanhaezebrouck IF, Scarpelli ML (2023) Companion animals as a key to success for translating radiation therapy research into the clinic. Cancers (Basel) 15:3377
233. Venkataraman GM, Geraghty D, Fox J, Graves SS, Zellmer E, Storer BE, Torok-Storb BJ, Storb R (2013) Canine DLA-79 gene: an improved typing method, identification of new alleles and its role in graft rejection and graft-versus-host disease. Tissue Antigens 81:204
234. Vozenin MC, De Fornel P, Petersson K, Favaudon V, Jaccard M, Germond JF, Petit B, Burki M, Ferrand G, Patin D, Bouchaab H, Ozsahin M, Bochud F, Bailat C, Devauchelle P, Bourhis J (2018) The advantage of FLASH radiotherapy confirmed in mini-pig and cat-cancer patients. Clin Cancer Res 25:35
235. Vozenin M-C, Bourhis J, Durante M (2022) Towards clinical translation of FLASH radiotherapy. Nat Rev Clin Oncol 19:791–803
236. Walker M, Breider M (1987) Intraoperative radiotherapy of canine bladder cancer. Vet Radiol 28:200–204
237. Walz JZ, Desai N, Van Asselt N, Poirier VJ, Hansen K, Selmic L (2020) Definitive-intent intensity-modulated radiation therapy for treatment of canine prostatic carcinoma: a multi-institutional retrospective study. Vet Comp Oncol 18:381–388
238. Warren SL, Whipple GH (1923a) Roentgen ray intoxication: I. Bacterial invasion of the blood stream as influenced by X-ray destruction of the mucosal epithelium of the small intestine. J Exp Med 38:713–723
239. Warren SL, Whipple GH (1923b) Roentgen ray intoxication: II. The cumulative effect or summation of X-ray exposures given at varying intervals. J Exp Med 38:725–730

240. Warren SL, Whipple GH (1923c) Roentgen ray intoxication: III. The path of a beam of hard rays in the living organism. J Exp Med 38:731–739
241. Warren SL, Whipple GH (1923d) Roentgen ray intoxication: IV. Intestinal lesions and acute intoxication produced by radiation in a variety of animals. J Exp Med 38:741–752
242. Whelan JS, Burcombe RJ, Janinis J, Baldelli AM, Cassoni AM (2002) A systematic review of the role of pulmonary irradiation in the management of primary bone tumours. Ann Oncol 13:23–30
243. White RA, Workman P, Owen LN, Bleehen NM (1979) The penetration of misonidazole into spontaneous canine tumours. Br J Cancer 40:284–294
244. Wolff CA, Holmes SP, Young BD, Chen AV, Kent M, Platt SR, Savage MY, Schatzberg SJ, Fosgate GT, Levine JM (2012) Magnetic resonance imaging for the differentiation of neoplastic, inflammatory, and cerebrovascular brain disease in dogs. J Vet Intern Med 26:589–597
245. Worth AJ, Zuber RM, Hocking M (2005) Radioiodide (131I) therapy for the treatment of canine thyroid carcinoma. Aust Vet J 83:208–214
246. Wust P, Hildebrandt B, Sreenivasa G, Rau B, Gellermann J, Riess H, Felix R, Schlag PM (2002) Hyperthermia in combined treatment of cancer. Lancet Oncol 3:487–497
247. Yan W, Khan MK, Wu X, Simone CB 2nd, Fan J, Gressen E, Zhang X, Limoli CL, Bahig H, Tubin S, Mourad WF (2020) Spatially fractionated radiation therapy: history, present and the future. Clin Transl Radiat Oncol 20:30–38
248. Yin E, Nelson DO, Coleman MA, Peterson LE, Wyrobek AJ (2003) Gene expression changes in mouse brain after exposure to low-dose ionizing radiation. Int J Radiat Biol 79:759–775
249. Yuan H, Schroeder T, Bowsher JE, Hedlund LW, Wong T, Dewhirst MW (2006) Intertumoral differences in hypoxia selectivity of the PET imaging agent 64Cu(II)-diacetyl-bis(N4-methylthiosemicarbazone). J Nucl Med 47:989–998
250. Zwingenberger AL, Pollard RE, Taylor SL, Chen RX, Nunley J, Kent MS (2016) Perfusion and volume response of canine brain tumors to stereotactic radiosurgery and radiotherapy. J Vet Intern Med 30:827–835

Comparative Aspects of Chemotherapy and Targeted Therapy: How Different Species Process Drugs

Luke A. Wittenburg and Ai-Ming Yu

An understanding of the fate of a drug throughout the body and how that drug is acted upon or processed by the body, termed pharmacokinetics, is essential in building and optimizing treatment plans involving that drug. Particularly for drugs with a narrow therapeutic window, such as traditional cytotoxic antineoplastic compounds, safe and effective use is ideally based on knowledge of key pharmacokinetic parameters such as the maximum systemic concentration, distribution within the body, systemic clearance, area under the drug concentration time curve (AUC) and half-life. Linking one or more of these parameters with measures of outcome, be it efficacy or toxicity, has the potential to provide a mechanism to "fine tune" or personalize the therapeutic regimen. To date, much of the knowledge of the processing of chemotherapy drugs has come from studies performed in human cancer patients, and in some cases, this information has been applied to veterinary cancer therapy, although a complete validation of equivalence between species may be lacking. Even within a species, a high degree of variability in pharmacokinetic parameters is often seen following standardized doses, making it difficult to predict how an individual patient might respond. Dosing many of cytotoxic chemotherapy drugs in humans and animals is generally based on body surface area (mg/m^2) instead of patient weight (mg/kg). This was originally instituted as a means of normalizing the maximum tolerated dose of drug between species and was based on the idea that physiologic processes that influence drug movement and activity in the body, such as glomerular filtration rate and cardiac output, correlate better with body surface area than weight. The commonly used formula for converting weight to body surface area in veterinary patients is:

$$\text{Surface Area} = \frac{\text{Body Weight}^{0.67} \times \text{K}}{10^4}$$

where surface area is given in square meters, and K is a species constant with a value of 10.1 for dogs and 10.0 for cats. Numerous variations exist for calculating body surface area in humans, with the most common being the Du Bois and Du Bois formula [33] which incorporates height as well as body weight:

$$\text{Surface Area} = 0.00718 \times \left(\text{Height}\,(\text{cm})^{0.725}\right) \times \left(\text{Weight}\,(\text{kg})^{0.425}\right)$$

L. A. Wittenburg (✉)
Department of Surgical and Radiological Sciences, Center for Companion Animal Health, School of Veterinary Medicine, University of California, Davis, Davis, CA, USA
e-mail: lwittenburg@ucdavis.edu

A.-M. Yu
Department of Biochemistry and Molecular Medicine, School of Medicine, University of California, Davis, Sacramento, CA, USA
e-mail: aimyu@ucdavis.edu

M. W. Nolan et al. (eds.), *Comparative Oncology*, https://doi.org/10.1007/978-3-032-04454-9_7

However, exceptions to BSA-based dosing exist in both veterinary and human cancer therapy, particularly in the case of smaller dogs and cats where weight-based dosing is often used to prevent excessive toxicity due to the relatively higher dose that BSA-based dosing would provide [109, 114]. In contrast to many of the cytotoxic compounds, dosing of targeted therapies generally utilizes weight-based dosing in veterinary patients and/or a fixed dose administered per day in humans.

Differences in some pharmacokinetic parameters of anticancer agents measured between human and veterinary patients undoubtedly result, in part, from differences in distribution, metabolism and excretion pathways but also from a fundamental difference in the goals of treatment; the greater focus on quality of life over obtaining a cure in veterinary medicine often results in lower relative doses (sometimes as much as 50% less) and selection of more convenient dosing regimens. In addition, many combination dosing regimens in human oncology involve administration of multiple drugs at once, while drug combinations are administered to veterinary patients as a single drug at a time almost exclusively.

For some drugs, differences in disposition between human and veterinary patients might be anticipated based on known mechanisms of metabolism or transport protein specificity and species differences in expression or activity of metabolizing enzymes and drug transporters. Drugs that are primarily eliminated through glucuronidation may be anticipated to cause unacceptable levels of toxicity in cats due to the presence of a pseudogene for UDP-glucuronyltransferase (UGT) 1A6 in the cat genome, demonstrated by their increased sensitivity to phenolic drugs such as acetaminophen [128]. In addition, metabolism by conjugation reactions other than glucuronidation (sulfation, glycination) also tends to occur slower in cats [24]. An absence of N-acetyltransferase (NAT) genes in dogs leads to an inability to acetylate and metabolize arylamine and hydrazine compounds [139]. While not completely unable to acetylate substrate drugs, cats also have a relative deficiency in acetylation compared to humans due to the presence of only a single NAT gene [140].

1 Specific Classes of Chemotherapeutic Drugs

1.1 Antitumor Antibiotics

The most frequently used chemotherapeutic agent in veterinary medicine, doxorubicin, belongs to the anthracycline class of antitumor antibiotics. Daunorubicin, another anthracycline antibiotic sometimes used in human oncology, is not commonly used in veterinary medicine and pharmacokinetic comparisons of daunorubicin in veterinary and human cancer patients have not been made. The anthracenedione mitoxantrone has been used in both human and veterinary oncology, but fewer studies investigating pharmacokinetics have been performed in animals, and there is a paucity of PK information in cancer-bearing animals.

1.1.1 Doxorubicin

The pharmacokinetics of doxorubicin have been well described in human and canine cancer patients. Comparative metabolism studies have identified that doxorubicin undergoes carbonyl reduction and glycosidic cleavage in both species to form doxorubicinol and 7-hydroxy aglycone, respectively [91]. Elimination of doxorubicin occurs through metabolism and elimination of parent drug via renal and biliary routes. Comparative in vitro metabolism studies evaluating aldo-keto reductase activity suggest a greater affinity for doxorubicin in dogs based on calculated Michaelis-Menten parameters (i.e., lower K_m and a higher V_{max}). Pharmacokinetic profiles in dogs and humans are best fit by a three-compartment model with rapid clearance from plasma, deposition in tissues and slow excretion. Half-lives of each phase of doxorubicin disposition are strikingly similar between species, with α half-lives of 10 min vs. 3 min, β half-lives of 1 h vs. 30 min and λ half-lives of 30 h vs. 20 h in humans and dogs, respectively. The terminal phase represents the majority of the total exposure to doxorubicin in both species. Tissue distribution and binding have been correlated with DNA and cardiolipin content, and physiologic models that incorporate DNA and cardiolipin binding have accurately predicted blood and tissue pharmacokinetics in mice, dogs and humans [59]. Tissue to plasma doxorubicin ratios have been measured to range from 10:1 to 500:1 due to the high affinity of doxorubicin for DNA. A single pharmacokinetic study in cats has evaluated the impact of infusion rate on doxorubicin PK parameters. In this study, the data were best fit by a two-compartment model; however, concentrations were only evaluated out to 3 h post infusion, which likely limited the ability to identify a prolonged terminal elimination phase [60].

In veterinary medicine, the impact of drug transporters on the pharmacokinetic and toxicity profiles of doxorubicin, particularly in dogs, is frequently considered as some breeds of dog are known to harbor inactivating deletion mutations of the ABCB1/MDR1 gene encoding the P-glycoprotein efflux pump [99, 100]. Simulated pharmacokinetic modeling of dogs homozygous for the MDR1 mutation predicts that gastrointestinal exposure to doxorubicin in this population would likely require dose reductions to levels that may be subtherapeutic, although this has not been investigated in clinical patients [58]. Polymorphisms of P-glycoprotein have also been identified in human populations and are suggested to play a role in pharmacokinetic variability, but inactivating mutations analogous to those seen in dogs have not been identified [95]. In human and canine cancer patients, a direct correlation between doxorubicin activity, measured as either antitumor activity or toxicity, and area-under-the-curve has been identified, while maximum plasma concentration appears to correlate with the incidence of hypersensitivity reactions and acute cardiac toxicity during infusion [112, 145].

In both human and canine patients, doxorubicin-induced cardiotoxicity can potentially lead to congestive heart failure (CHF). In both species, this toxicity appears to be mainly cumulative, although there are reports of individual patients developing CHF following a single dose. Cumulative doses greater than 450–500 mg/m^2 in humans and 240 mg/m^2 in dogs significantly increase the risk of developing noninflammatory cardiomyopathy and congestive heart failure [32, 97], leading to lifetime limits on doxorubicin exposure. In dogs, the limit is often set at 150 mg/m^2, allowing for approximately five doses of doxorubicin. Histopathologic changes seen in doxorubicin-induced cardiomyopathy are similar in humans and dogs, with evidence of myocardiocytolysis, degeneration and myocardial fibrillar vacuolation [16, 97]. The underlying mechanism of doxorubicin-induced cardiomyopathy is thought to be the same in humans and dogs, in part due to the doxorubicin semiquinone generating oxygen free radicals, triggering damage to the sarcoplasmic reticulum, with iron playing an important role in catalyzing the formation of these free radicals [48]. Importantly, the addition of dexrazoxane, an iron chelating agent, has been shown to reduce the risk of cardiotoxicity from doxorubicin in human and canine cancer patients [35], demonstrating the comparative potential of doxorubicin-induced cardiomyopathy in dogs to investigate novel preventive or therapeutic interventions for this toxicity in human cancer patients.

Doxorubicin has a very broad spectrum of antitumor activity and, in veterinary medicine, is used as a single agent and as a component of combination protocols for canine and feline lymphoma, osteosarcoma and most tumors of mesenchymal (sarcoma) or epithelial (carcinoma) origin. Similarly, doxorubicin is used against a wide variety of human cancers including hematopoietic tumors, many carcinomas, sarcomas of bone and soft tissue and many pediatric malignancies.

Resistance to doxorubicin has been well studied, and multiple mechanisms in canine and human cancer cell lines have been identified in vitro. Reduced intracellular drug accumulation is probably the best-known mechanism of doxorubicin resistance and has been associated with upregulation of a number of ATP-binding cassette (ABC) drug transport proteins, of which ABCB1 (MDR1/P-glycoprotein) is frequently identified as a cause of reduced sensitivity [26, 104, 108]. Additional transporters associated with resistance to doxorubicin include the ABCC (MRP proteins) and ABCG (BCRP proteins) subfamilies of transporters. While in vitro studies have demonstrated a clear link between increased expression of ABCB1, ABCG2 and ABCC proteins with reduced doxorubicin sensitivity, the precise extent to which overexpression of each of these proteins accounts for clinical resistance is less clear. Furthermore, pharmacologic inhibitors of transporter activity, particularly P-glycoprotein, have not proven to be useful doxorubicin-sensitizing agents, often due to the development of unacceptable toxicity. The expression of a major doxorubicin target, topoisomerase IIa (TOP2A) has also been associated with drug sensitivity. Reduced expression of TOP2A has been associated with anthracycline resistance in vitro and in vivo in some human cancers [68, 113]. One in vitro study in which doxorubicin-resistant canine prostate and bladder cancer cells were generated did not identify alterations in TOP2A associated with the resistant state [104], while a study evaluating TOP2A expression in canine B- and T cell lymphoma demonstrated higher expression in B cell lymphomas which tend to be relatively more sensitive to doxorubicin [75]. However, the impact of increased or reduced TOP2A expression on clinical resistance to doxorubicin in veterinary medicine remains unknown.

1.1.2 Mitoxantrone

Mitoxantrone has a narrower spectrum of antitumor activity than doxorubicin, but also carries a reduced risk of cardiotoxicity due to its reduced ability to undergo one-electron reduction and generate free radicals [44]. Thus, in veterinary medicine, mitoxantrone may be chosen as a doxorubicin alternative in patients with increased risk of cardiac disease or in patients that have already received their maximum dose of doxorubicin, discussed in the previous section. Mitoxantrone is also sometimes used for treatment of transitional cell carcinoma of the urinary bladder. In human cancer patients, mitoxantrone is not frequently chosen as an alternative to doxorubicin, but is approved for use in acute nonlymphocytic leukemia and as a palliative treatment in some prostate cancers. Additionally, mitoxantrone has been shown to have some efficacy in breast cancers, non-Hodgkin's lymphoma and palliation in advanced hepatic and ovarian cancers [41].

The available information on the disposition of mitoxantrone in humans and veterinary patients suggests that the drug is processed in a very similar manner, being somewhat independent of species. In humans, dogs and cats, mitoxantrone serum concentration profiles are best fit by a three-compartment model, and kinetics are defined by rapid initial loss of drug due to accumulation within formed components of the blood, followed by wide distribution to tissues in a blood-flow-dependent manner and a prolonged and variable terminal elimination phase [13, 76]. The terminal half-life in humans is reported to be quite variable, with values ranging from 3 to 298 h. The reported half-life in cats is much shorter and ranges from 15 to 90 min; however, a short sampling period (200 min) may have resulted in underestimation of the true terminal elimination phase [76]. Elimination of mitoxantrone in humans and dogs is primarily through biliary excretion of parent drug and two inactive metabolites, with only a small percentage of drug lost via renal excretion [13].

Resistance to mitoxantrone, similar to doxorubicin, can be in part mediated via drug efflux by P-glycoprotein (MDR1) as well as the breast cancer resistance protein (BCRP) [40], as cytotoxicity is dependent on intracellular drug concentration and duration of exposure. Furthermore, cross-resistance to mitoxantrone and doxorubicin associated with reduced levels of TOP2A, in the absence of increased P-glycoprotein, has been demonstrated in vitro in human leukemia cells [63]. Resistance to mitoxantrone may also develop from a reduced ability of cells to undergo apoptosis in response to DNA damage, as seen in lymphoma cells with mutations in both p53 and ataxia-telangiectasia mutated (ATM), while cells with mutations in only one DNA damage response gene retained mitoxantrone sensitivity [42].

1.2 Alkylating Agents

The alkylating agents are a frequently used class of drugs in veterinary and human cancer therapy. This class includes the nitrogen mustards (cyclophosphamide, ifosfamide, mechlorethamine, melphalan and chlorambucil), ethyleneimines (altretamine, thiotepa), alkyl sulfonates (busulfan), nitrosoureas (lomustine, carmustine) and methylating agents (dacarbazine, procarbazine). The ethyleneimines and alkyl sulfonates are rarely used in veterinary medicine and comparative aspects will not be discussed here.

1.2.1 Cyclophosphamide

The most widely used nitrogen mustard in veterinary medicine is cyclophosphamide, and it is considered one of the most versatile of the nitrogen mustards in human oncology. Extensive use of cyclophosphamide is seen in veterinary and human oncology, most commonly as a component of multiagent treatment protocols. In human oncology, cyclophosphamide is used in the treatment of numerous solid tumors including breast cancer, rhabdomyosarcoma, Ewing sarcoma and neuroblastoma as well as serving a key role in the management of hematologic cancers such as chronic lymphocytic leukemia, non-Hodgkin's lymphoma and rarely multiple myeloma [65]. In veterinary medicine, the use of cyclophosphamide is primarily in the treatment of hematologic cancers, with some limited use in combination with doxorubicin for canine mammary carcinoma. Myeloablative conditioning prior to allogeneic or autologous stem cell transplantation is another area where high-dose cyclophosphamide has been used in human oncology. Similarly, immunosuppressive doses of cyclophosphamide have been used in dogs with high-grade B cell lymphoma prior to hematopoietic stem cell transplantation [51].

Cyclophosphamide requires hepatic transformation by the mixed function oxidase system to form the intermediate compound 4-hydroxycyclophosphamide (4-OHCP), which then undergoes spontaneous degradation to form active phosphoramide mustard. The formation of 4-OHCP in humans is mediated by the CYP2B6 enzyme, and some reports suggest polymorphisms of CYP2B6 or CYP2C19 contribute to the large interindividual differences in observed ratios of 4-OHCP to parent drug [105, 137], while other studies have not identified these same relationships [37]. The canine CYP2B11 enzyme is the ortholog to human CYP2B6, and a CYP2B11 haplotype that results in reduced metabolic activity of this enzyme has been identified in the Greyhound breed [94]; an effect on biotransformation of cyclophosphamide has not been evaluated. In vitro studies of cyclophosphamide biotransformation suggest that there are species differences in the enzymes most responsible for CP metabolism, with CYP2B inhibition decreasing metabolism only in cat microsomes, while CYP2C inhibition reduced metabolism in mouse, cat, human and dog microsomes. Pharmacokinetic studies in dog and human cancer patients have identified that cyclophosphamide is well absorbed, and that exposure to the 4-OHCP metabolite is equivalent between oral and intravenous dosing of the parent drug in both species [134, 143]. Furthermore, a pharmacokinetic study performed in cats has also identified equivalent exposures to 4-OHCP when administered via intravenous, oral and intraperitoneal routes [133]. Comparisons between dog, cat and human CP pharmacokinetics demonstrate an increased total exposure and longer half-life of parent drug and 4-OHCP in humans, with dog and cat values being similar, although dogs do have a slightly lower exposure and shorter half-life relative to cats [115]. The species differences in PK can be explained by the differences in microsomal CP metabolism; dog microsomes appear to be 55-fold more efficient than human microsomes and 2.8-fold more efficient than cat microsomes in the bioactivation of CP [115]. In human patients administered high-dose CP in a 3- to 5-day fractionated protocol, an auto-induction of CP metabolism has been identified that leads to increased formation of 4-OHCP when compared to bolus dosing [18]. This increase in exposure to the metabolite was not identified during fractionated oral dosing in dogs administered a standard dose of 200–250 mg/m^2 [142], and thus, the impact of fractionated dosing with regard to antitumor activity in dogs is likely of little clinical relevance.

In both human and veterinary cancer patients, the use of cyclophosphamide has been associated with the development of sterile hemorrhagic cystitis (SHC) which can occur acutely or may develop weeks to months after therapy. In the acute form, exposure to acrolein, a CP metabolite, has been identified as causative, and forced diuresis and administration of MESNA may prevent acute SHC by reducing acrolein contact time with the bladder wall and forming nontoxic adducts, respectively [23, 25, 39]. The risk of developing SHC increases with increasing dose as well as with chronic low-dose, or metronomic, treatments in canines and humans [96, 132]. The development of late-onset SHC in humans has been reported to have a viral etiology in many cases, usually secondary to the ubiquitous BK polyoma virus that infects humans during childhood and resides permanently in the urinary tract, becoming reactivated during periods of impaired immunity [8, 14]. A viral etiology has not been reported in dogs experiencing late-onset SHC. Discontinuation of CP is typically the first step in the management of SHC. Further management strategies reported in humans and canines include administration of anticholinergic bladder medications such as oxybutynin and/or pentosan polysulfate. More severe or persistent cases of SHC have been managed similarly in dogs and humans, with intravesicular instillations of anti-inflammatory and/or hemostatic compounds such as DMSO, alum, aminocaproic acid, silver nitrate and, in the most severe or refractory cases, formalin [82, 90].

1.2.2 Ifosfamide

An analog of cyclophosphamide also requiring hepatic activation, ifosfamide has a reduced rate of initial metabolism compared to cyclophosphamide, and the presence of a secondary metabolic pathway that generates chloroacetaldehyde results in the requirement of larger doses when compared to cyclophosphamide; this is reflected in the doses that produce clinical toxicity. For example, the MTD values for ifosfamide and CP in the cat are 900 mg/m^2 and 200 mg/m^2, respectively, while dogs have a smaller difference in the MTD between ifosfamide and CP (350–375 mg/^{2} vs. 250 mg/m^2, respectively). No studies have been performed to identify the difference in doses tolerated by dogs and cats, although it is likely to involve differences in metabolism and exposure levels to active and/or toxic metabolites. In humans, the reported half-life for the parent drug (approximately 1.5 h) is shorter than that reported for CP (ranges from 5 to 12 h) and a large degree of variability in ifosfamide pharmacokinetics is present. Very few pharmacokinetic studies have been performed with ifosfamide in veterinary cancer patients. In cats, following a 30-min infusion of 900 mg/m^2, an average maximum plasma concentration of 122.8 μg/mL was identified with a half-life of approximately 3 h [116]. Similar to the administration protocols for humans, cats are administered saline diuresis prior to and following ifosfamide administration, and are administered multiple doses of MESNA to prevent urothelial toxicity (SHC). The doses that are tolerated in cats and in dogs are substantially lower than those used in humans, where doses range from 1.8 to 3 g/m^2/day for 2 to 5 days [19]. Auto-induction of ifosfamide metabolism with increased amounts of metabolite formation following fractionation of dosing has been reported in humans [71, 81] and may partly explain the higher response rates in soft tissue sarcomas that were reported with doses administered over 3 days versus 24 h [70]. This effect has not been evaluated in veterinary cancer patients.

Use of ifosfamide in veterinary oncology has primarily been for the treatment of sarcomas. In cats, ifosfamide has demonstrated some activity against vaccine-associated sarcomas [117] and has been used in combination with doxorubicin in canine soft tissue sarcomas. Similarly, doxorubicin and ifosfamide appear to be the most effective single agents for the treatment of soft tissue sarcomas in human oncology [118].

1.2.3 Chlorambucil

Chlorambucil, another nitrogen mustard alkylating agent, is used in veterinary oncology primarily in the treatment of feline small cell (low grade) gastrointestinal lymphoma and was a standard treatment for most human patients with indolent (low-grade) non-Hodgkin's lymphoma until the 1990s [65]. Metronomic chemotherapy using chlorambucil for a variety of cancers in dogs is also reported [85]. Although chlorambucil use has been largely replaced by other agents in human oncology, studies performed in humans and in cats demonstrate strikingly similar pharmacokinetic properties of the orally administered formulation. In both species, there is rapid and nearly complete oral absorption and a biphasic elimination profile. The distribution and elimination half-life of chlorambucil in humans and cats have been reported as 0.49 h vs. 0.32 h and 1.3–1.5 h vs. 1.7 h, respectively [4, 64, 98]. One published study evaluating pharmacokinetics of metronomic, or low dose, chlorambucil in dogs demonstrates a similar profile to that seen in cats and humans, with a rapidly achieved T_{max} (0.7 hrs) and a terminal elimination half-life of 1.7 h [120]. No studies in dogs or cats have been performed to compare the concentrations of the primary metabolite, phenylacetic acid mustard, with those seen in human cancer patients following oral dosing.

1.2.4 Lomustine

The nitrosourea alkylating agent lomustine (CCNU) is another orally administered chemotherapeutic that has been evaluated in veterinary and human cancer patients. In dogs, CCNU is primarily used in the treatment of histiocytic sarcoma, mast cell tumors, relapsed lymphomas and/or cancers of the brain and neurologic system. In humans, lomustine is FDA approved and routinely used for patients with brain tumors following surgery and/or radiation therapy [146]. In cats, lomustine has also been used as part of combination therapy protocols for treatment-naïve and relapsed high-grade lymphomas [119].

The pharmacokinetics of lomustine have been reported in dogs and humans, and in neither species is the parent drug found in plasma following oral administration; this is because first pass through the gastrointestinal tract and liver produces two monohydroxylated metabolites which presumably provide the antitumor activity as well as systemic toxicity seen following administration [86]. In both species, the trans-4-hydroxy and cis-4-hydroxy metabolites are found, with the first being found in the highest concentrations. Peak metabolite concentrations in humans occur 2–4 h after dosing, while they are found to peak at 1 h in dogs. In humans, half-lives of the two metabolites are similar within an individual but vary up to two-fold between individuals, from 1.3 to 2.9 h. In dogs, a similar pattern is seen, although the half-lives are shorter, ranging from 30 min to 1.9 h.

For nearly all of the alkylating agents, increased detoxification via increased levels of sulfhydryl molecules or related enzymes and enhanced DNA repair have been identified as mechanisms contributing to resistance. Conjugation of some alkylating agents to the abundant intracellular thiol, glutathione, results in the removal of the reactive chlorine atoms and thus limits cytotoxicity, and increased glutathione levels have been commonly identified in resistant cell lines. Evidence in cell lines and some human tumor tissues has also demonstrated that increased expression of the glutathione S-transferase enzymes may accelerate conjugation of alkylating agents to glutathione and lead to treatment resistance [61]. In the case of cyclophosphamide, increased expression of aldehyde dehydrogenase (ALDH) in tumor cells can lead to resistance through increased conversion of activated cyclophosphamide to the inactive carboxyphosphamide metabolite [138]. An additional major mechanism of resistance to alkylating agents is the enhanced repair of DNA alkylation lesions, mediated by multiple DNA repair systems. One of the most studied is the direct removal of alkyl groups from the O^6-position of guanine by the alkylguanine-O^6-alkyl transferase enzyme which is encoded by the MGMT gene. Increased activity or expression of MGMT has been linked to reduced response to alkylating agent treatment of brain tumors in human patients [83]. In canine oncology, one study has reported increased MGMT expression in localized GI lymphoma tumors from dogs with shorter survival times, although that study was retrospective in nature and no consistent chemotherapy protocol was used [148]. In vitro, canine lymphoma cell lines resistant to lomustine were found to have elevated expression of MGMT [73], but a clear association between clinical response to alkylating agents and MGMT expression or activity is yet to be identified in veterinary oncology.

1.3 Platinum Compounds

Platinum compounds, including cisplatin, carboplatin, oxaliplatin and others, are often a mainstay of therapy for human germ cell tumors, head and neck tumors, bladder cancer, small cell and nonsmall cell lung cancers, colorectal cancers as well as osteosarcoma, and it is estimated that nearly half of all human patients receiving chemotherapy will receive some form of platinum-based drug [50]. In veterinary medicine, the platinum drugs, primarily cisplatin and carboplatin, have also been evaluated for treatment of germinal cell tumors, osteosarcoma, bladder cancer (TCC), squamous cell carcinoma and mesothelioma as well as intracavitary therapy of carcinomatosis [12]. The utility of cisplatin in some human tumor types (head and neck and cervical cancers) is also due, in part, to its role as a radiation sensitizer. Use of platinum drugs in combination with radiation therapy has also been evaluated for a number of canine cancers [45, 84, 136], but inclusion of cisplatin or carboplatin in radiotherapy for the purpose of sensitization is not currently a common practice in veterinary oncology.

Carboplatin is the most widely used platinum compound in veterinary medicine, although direct comparisons of antitumor activity have not been performed to demonstrate equivalence with cisplatin for many tumor types. Carboplatin is often chosen over cisplatin because of the significant time commitment involved with aggressive fluid therapy required to prevent nephrotoxicity with cisplatin administration. Cisplatin and carboplatin both demonstrate extensive binding to plasma and tissue proteins, although the degree may be less with carboplatin than with cisplatin. Early pharmacokinetic studies in humans and dogs demonstrated similar elimination half-lives of carboplatin at 131 min vs. 155 min, respectively. Additionally, a large percentage of the drug is recovered in the urine shortly after administration; approximately 30–50% of the dose within 4 h in dogs and approximately 70% of the dose within 24 h in human patients [77, 110]. There is a significant correlation between renal function and carboplatin exposure (AUC) reported in humans as well as in cats, and dosing strategies that incorporate a target exposure have been reported for both species [10, 11, 36]. The maximum tolerated AUC in cats is suggested to be less than 3 min*mg/mL while the target AUC in humans associated with greater efficacy is generally more than 5 min*mg/mL. With regard to membrane transporters that may play a role in the pharmacokinetics, efficacy and adverse reactions to carboplatin, species differences have been identified through in vitro studies. The canine ATP-binding cassette transporter, breast cancer resistance protein (BCRP/ABCG2), was identified to confer resistance to carboplatin, while the feline protein was not, nor has carboplatin been reported to be a substrate for human BCRP [89]. A clinical impact of this species difference in substrate specificity for carboplatin is not known.

Cisplatin is not commonly used in canine cancer therapy and is not used in cats due to the development of fatal pulmonary edema following cisplatin therapy in this species. In dogs, the requirement for lengthy saline diuresis prior to (3–4 h) and post (1–2 h) cisplatin administration to reduce nephrotoxicity combined with the substantially higher emetogenic potential of cisplatin often leads to the choice of alternative agents such as carboplatin. Although cisplatin has been considered a model, renally cleared anticancer agent, the pharmacokinetics in both humans and dogs demonstrate that total body clearance is over two-fold higher than renal clearance [2]. In addition, human studies suggest a poor correlation between glomerular filtration and renal cisplatin clearance. Thus, dose determination using glomerular filtration rate is not performed with cisplatin as can be done with carboplatin. In dogs, however, renal clearance of cisplatin displays a closer relationship with GFR, although renal clearance values are less than GFR indicating some renal tubular reabsorption [2]. While some data in humans suggests that the pharmacokinetic profile of cisplatin is best fit by a three-compartment model, available data in dogs is best fit by a two-compartment model. Regardless, the half-life of the terminal elimination phase is similar in both at approximately 24 h in humans and 13–30 h in dogs. One study available in birds (sulfur-crested cockatoos) also shows bi-phasic elimination of cisplatin with a prolonged terminal half-life of 70 h [43].

As with the classic alkylating agents, the main mechanism of antitumor effect for the platinum agents is the induction of DNA damage. Platinum-DNA adduct formation measured in tumor tissues and in circulating blood cells has been positively correlated with assessments of tumor response. Platinum-DNA adducts can be repaired via the nucleotide excision repair (NER) pathway, and expression levels of the critical NER gene ERCC excision repair 1 (ERCC1) in tumors directly correlate with platinum therapy response in human ovarian, gastric, colorectal and lung cancers [28, 102, 107, 127]. Direct relationships between NER proteins such as ERCC1 and response to platinum therapy have not yet been identified in veterinary cancer.

1.4 Antimetabolites

1.4.1 Cytidine Analogs

Cytosine arabinoside (ara-C) is a cytidine analog that is metabolized to the active triphosphate ara-CTP through the activity of intracellular kinases. The disposition of ara-C is characterized by a rapid disappearance from plasma due to deamination of drug in plasma forming ara-U, which then becomes the predominant form of drug found in the plasma within minutes. The presence of the metabolizing enzyme, cytidine deaminase, is found in high levels in the gastrointestinal tract, preventing oral administration of ara-C, although a lipophilic prodrug of ara-C (cytarabine ocfosfate) has demonstrated an ability to achieve potentially effective systemic levels of ara-C following oral dosing [152]. In humans and dogs, subcutaneous dosing protocols can produce similar systemic exposures to intravenous dosing, and the pharmacokinetics of ara-C are linear over a wide dose range, until concentrations that saturate cytidine deaminase are achieved. Peak plasma concentrations in dogs administered a 50 mg/m^2 subcutaneous dose or a 25 mg/m^2 CRI for 8 h are similar at approximately 5 μM, while peak plasma concentrations in humans following a 100 mg/m^2 dose are reported to be approximately 10 μM [22, 27]. The elimination half-life of ara-C when given by intravenous infusion or subcutaneous injection in dogs is approximately 1.5 h, similar to the 30–150 min measured in humans [27, 69, 88]. Although very water-soluble, ara-C has the ability to cross the blood-brain-barrier in both dogs and humans, with CSF to plasma ratios of approximately 0.6 [126]. The use of cytarabine in veterinary oncology is primarily in the setting of relapsed or refractory lymphoma as a component of rescue protocols in combination with melphalan and vincristine [34], carboplatin [54] or dexamethasone, melphalan and actinomycin-D [111, 129]. Cytarabine is also commonly used in veterinary medicine for the treatment of granulomatous meningoencephalitis of unknown origin (GME). Cytarabine use in human oncology is primarily for treatment of myeloid and lymphoid leukemias and lymphomas as a mainstay of induction and rescue protocols [3, 17, 56].

Gemcitabine is another cytidine analog antimetabolite that has similar metabolism to its triphosphate form (dFdCTP) and similar effects on DNA, yet differences in kinetics of inhibition as well as additional sites of activity result in a wider clinical spectrum of activity than ara-C. While there are a limited number of studies in veterinary oncology suggesting a therapeutic benefit of gemcitabine, primarily in solid tumors [53, 78, 93], the importance of dosing regimen on therapeutic efficacy that has been identified in human oncology suggests that further studies of proper scheduling and dosing in veterinary medicine are warranted. While numerous dose regimens have been evaluated in veterinary medicine, including 350–400 mg/m^2 weekly for 5 weeks, 800 mg/m^2 given over 60 min every 7 days, 625 mg/m^2 biweekly, and 2 mg/kg on days 1 and

8 of a 21 day cycle, there have been very few studies that have evaluated the impact of using a fixed-dose-rate, which has been found in humans to provide superior efficacy, albeit with slightly greater toxicity, to bolus or short infusion dosing. Pharmacokinetic studies in dogs have evaluated bolus dosing and infusions of gemcitabine and have demonstrated linear pharmacokinetics of gemcitabine, but not the metabolite dFdU, with increasing doses. With both bolus dosing and a 30-min CRI, the time to maximum dFdU plasma concentration is approximately 2 h, and following CRI the half-life of dFdU is approximately 14 h [46, 47] which is the same as that found in human patients. The half-life of gemcitabine in plasma of dogs is approximately 1.8–3 h following bolus and CRI dosing which is substantially longer than what has been measured in human patients at 8–17 min [22, 46]. In both humans and dogs, gemcitabine has a relatively large volume of distribution suggesting there is extensive tissue distribution. In human oncology, a relationship between plasma gemcitabine concentration and maximum accumulation of intracellular dFdCTP has been identified, and thus, a fixed-dose rate of 10 mg/m^2/min over prolonged periods is commonly used to maintain plasma gemcitabine concentrations of 15–20 μM [57]. In cats, a fixed-dose-rate between 2.5 and 5 mg/m^2/min given over a period of >1 h may achieve similar plasma concentrations, although accumulation of dFdCTP has not been evaluated in this situation [52]. A potential reason for reaching a target plasma concentrations at a lower dose rate in cats may have to do with a slower inactivation of gemcitabine to dFdU in cat blood than is seen in dogs or humans [106]. Indications for gemcitabine in human oncology are also primarily in the treatment of solid tumors where it has been a first-line therapy for pancreatic, bladder and non-small cell lung cancers [124, 125, 131].

Several mechanisms have been proposed that lead to reduced sensitivity to the cytidine analogs, and they tend to correlate with alterations in the rate limiting enzyme required to either activate the parent drug (deoxycytidine kinase; CdR) or in the activity of the enzyme responsible for metabolism (cytidine deaminase). In the case of gemcitabine, increased expression of ribonucleotide reductase is also identified to reduce sensitivity of tumor cells [30], and as compounds that require active transport into tumor cells it is not then surprising that reduced or absent expression of the equilibrative nucleoside transporter 1 on tumor cells is associated with reduced survival in pancreatic cancer patients treated with gemcitabine [55].

1.5 Microtubule Targeting Agents

The most commonly used microtubule targeting drugs in veterinary medicine are the vinca alkaloids, with vincristine and vinblastine being the most common. The taxanes have found limited use in veterinary medicine; although a micellar formulation of paclitaxel that did not contain the solvent cremophor, to which dogs are particularly sensitive, was previously available in veterinary medicine through conditional approval, this medication is no longer available.

The vinca alkaloids are a class of microtubule poisons that inhibit microtubule dynamics and tubulin polymerization. In humans and dogs, the drivers of distribution and elimination of vincristine and vinblastine are tubulin binding within the cell, a high degree of plasma protein binding to alpha 1-acid glycoprotein, transport by ABCB1/P-glycoprotein and cytochrome P450-mediated metabolism with elimination through glomerular filtration and biliary excretion. Pharmacokinetic profiles are characterized by a large volume of distribution and triphasic elimination with an early rapid systemic clearance followed by prolonged half-lives [121]. In dogs and humans, vincristine and vinblastine bind extensively to formed blood elements, particularly platelets due to tubulin concentrations. In vitro and in vivo, plasma concentrations reduce by nearly 50% within minutes as the vinca alkaloids distribute to blood elements and extensively into tissues, with the spleen accumulating drug at the greatest extent [20]. In dogs and humans, a prolonged clearance from tissues is demonstrated by terminal elimination half-lives of vinblastine that are approximately 24 h [121, 144]. The vast majority of elimination of the vinca alkaloids results from hepatic metabolism and elimination of metabolites via biliary excretion, with only small amounts of parent drug and metabolites eliminated in urine. Reaction phenotyping in the dog has identified the primary vinblastine metabolizing enzyme to be Cyp3A12, the ortholog to human Cyp3A4 which metabolizes vinblastine in that species [1]. The importance of CYP3A-mediated metabolism in humans is exemplified by increased clearance of vinca alkaloids when coadministered with CYP3A-inducing drugs and increased toxicity when administered with CYP3A inhibitors. The desacetyl metabolites of vinblastine in particular, products of CYP3A-mediated metabolism, have been identified in dogs and humans following treatment. The importance of drug transporters, particularly ABCB1/P-glycoprotein, in drug distribution is evident for the vinca alkaloids in dogs as the presence of the truncating mutation can predict those dogs in which severe hematologic toxicity, specifically neutropenia and thrombocytopenia, will occur [101]. Furthermore, brain exposure to vinblastine has been shown to be 13-fold higher in mice that are homozygous null for Mdr1a/b, demonstrating the importance of this transporter in preventing CNS exposure to vinca alkaloids [144].

Vincristine use in veterinary medicine has predominantly been as a component of multidrug protocols for dogs and cats with high-grade lymphoma, specifically as part of CHOP (cyclophosphamide, doxorubicin, vincristine, prednisolone) therapy. Similarly, vincristine has use in the treatment of human lymphoma in the related R-CHOP protocol, which differs by the addition of a monoclonal antibody (Rituximab) targeting human CD20. In dogs, vincristine can be curative as a single agent in the treatment of canine transmissible venereal tumor [5], and while it has been evaluated in treatment of mast cell tumors, vinblastine is more commonly chosen to treat this disease. Vinblastine is most often utilized in the treatment of canine mast cell tumors but is also sometimes used as a component of rescue protocols for lymphoma. Vinblastine is also used in the treatment of canine transitional cell carcinoma (TCC) of the bladder. In veterinary oncology, vinblastine has also been utilized in place of vincristine in some cases as it is reported to be associated with reduced gastrointestinal adverse effects compared to vincristine [80]. Similarly, gastrointestinal autonomic dysfunction in human patients is reported to occur most commonly with vincristine than with other vinca alkaloids when given at standard doses.

As discussed with the antitumor antibiotics, resistance to vinca alkaloids can also be mediated through the increased expression of ATP binding cassette transport proteins, particularly MDR1 and MRP1. A second mechanism of resistance to vinca alkaloids is related to expression of various isotypes of α and β-tubulin, the cellular targets of vinca alkaloids, with structural alterations that influence microtubule dynamics [49, 62]. Interestingly, the presence of tubulin subunits that confer resistance to vinca alkaloids, generally through hyperstabilization of microtubules, results in collateral sensitivity to taxanes. A study in dogs has identified increased expression of one isotype of β-tubulin in cell lines resistant to taxanes, but the reciprocal sensitivity to vinca alkaloids in these cells was not evaluated [9].

2 Targeted Therapies

2.1 Small-Molecule Inhibitors

In veterinary medicine, only one small-molecule inhibitor is fully approved for use in cancer patients: the tyrosine kinase inhibitor (TKI) toceranib, which is structurally and functionally quite similar to the human-approved drug sunitinib. In dogs, toceranib is characterized by a very large volume of distribution, moderate systemic clearance and a prolonged half-life [149]. The maximum plasma concentration of toceranib following oral dosing occurs approximately 8 h post dose. Oral bioavailability is nearly 80% in dogs, with no differences in fed or fasted states, and the volume of distribution >20 L/kg suggests extensive tissue distribution. While distribution occurs to numerous tissues, the greatest accumulation of toceranib is seen in the liver and bile, demonstrating the importance of hepatobiliary elimination. Metabolism studies have identified only a single N-oxide metabolite of toceranib which has been identified in both microsomal fractions and isolated hepatocytes [150]. The activity of this metabolite is not known in dogs, although the efficacy of N-oxide metabolites in general is often reduced compared to the parent drug. The half-life of toceranib in dogs is approximately 30 h, supporting every-other-day dosing of this drug. With regard to comparisons, sunitinib is the drug that is most closely related to toceranib, and some similarities are seen in how these drugs are processed between species. Maximum plasma concentrations following oral dosing also occur at approximately 8 h in humans, and the majority of sunitinib is eliminated via hepatobiliary routes. While oral bioavailability of sunitinib has not been determined in humans, food does not affect its systemic exposure [15]. Additionally, terminal half-lives of sunitinib are approximately 50 h, and moderate systemic clearance is evident [130]. In contrast to dogs where a single N-oxide metabolite has been identified, numerous sunitinib metabolites have been identified, with the major metabolite being an active N-desethyl metabolite or norsunitinib primarily produced by CYP3A4 [66, 130] which exhibits high plasma binding (90%) as sunitinib itself (95%).

Including sunitinib, many small-molecule TKIs have been approved for the treatment of various types of human cancers [31, 67, 123]. Almost all TKIs are orally bioavailable while showing some variations (e.g., high: imatinib 98%; medium: gefitinib 57%; low: nilotinib 30%) and thus can be administered orally as tablets or capsules. Likewise, the rates of absorption of TKIs vary from rapid to slow, leading to relatively shorter (e.g., imatinib 2–4 h) to longer (sunitinib 6–12 h) time to reach the C_{max}. With a few exceptions (e.g., gefitinib 79%), nearly all TKIs have high plasma protein binding (over 90%). The plasma half-lives of many TKIs (e.g., sunitinib, erlotinib, gefitinib and pazopanib) are fairly long, ranging from 30 to 50 h that enables once daily dosing therapy. By contrast, some TKIs exhibit relatively shorter half-lives (3–17 h) demanding twice daily dosing (e.g., dasatinib and nilotinib) or a once daily, high dose (lapatinib, 1.25 g). Phase 1 metabolism of TKIs is mainly mediated by CYP3A4, although other CYPs (e.g., CYP2D6 and CYP2C8) may be involved in the process for specific TKIs (e.g., gefitinib and nilotinib, respectively). The metabolites norimatinib and norsunitinib, generated from imatinib and sunitinib, respectively, are pharmacologically active, exhibiting comparable plasma protein binding, whereas half-lives are about twice as long as their respective parent drugs which is known to contribute to overall antitumor effects. Depending upon the impact of food intake on its oral bioavailability, a TKI may be taken with (e.g., imatinib and bosutinib) or without (e.g., sorafenib, nilotinib, lapatinib and pazopanib) food, or either way (dasatinib, gefitinib, ponatinib and sunitinib). In addition, the solubility of some TKIs may be significantly affected by gastric acidity, or pH, leading to changes in their pharmacokinetics [141]. For example, dasatinib exposure (Cmax and AUC) is reduced by about 60% in humans who take the H(2)-receptor antagonist famotidine 10 h before dasatinib [38]. Similarly, dasatinib exposure is about 55% lower when the antacid Maalox is coadministered in humans [38]. The risk of such unwanted drug-drug interactions [141] warrants precaution to concomitantly use these TKIs with H(2)-receptor antagonists, proton pump inhibitors or other drugs that sharply alter gastric pH.

While most TKIs have not been approved for the treatment of veterinary cancer patients, understanding the species difference and consistency in TKI pharmacokinetics could help rational, off-label use in veterinary medicine. Orally administered nilotinib is rapidly absorbed in dogs with a short Tmax (2 h) [147] which is similar to that (3 h) in humans. The apparent plasma half-life of nilotinib in dogs is approximately 5 h, in comparison to an average of 16 h in humans. The oral bioavailability of nilotinib in dogs is 27%, similar to that (30%) in humans. Indeed, good correlations in pharmacokinetic parameters (e.g., CL and Vss) have been disclosed for both nilotinib and imatinib from rodents to dogs by using allometric scaling [7], supporting the utility of this approach to predict or explain interspecies pharmacokinetics between animal and human patients. There has been recent interest and increased utilization of TKIs labeled for human use in the treatment of a variety of canine cancers, and pharmacokinetic studies are now being published allowing for better design of rational dosing strategies. The dual EGFR and HER2 inhibitor lapatinib, approved for treatment of HER2-positive breast cancer in humans, has also demonstrated activity in HER2-positive canine mammary carcinoma cell lines [87] as well as canine transitional cell and prostatic carcinoma cell lines [72, 122]. Clinically, lapatinib has demonstrated some encouraging activity in treatment-naïve canine bladder cancer that demonstrated a role for HER2 overexpression associated with response [92]. A pharmacokinetic study in dogs and cats was also performed, demonstrating that maximum plasma concentrations following administration of the clinically used dose (25 mg/kg) in dogs approximated concentrations achieved in humans, while cats experienced maximum plasma concentrations 3.5 times lower, suggesting a potential need for alternate dosing strategies in this species [151]. There has also been recent interest in targeting MEK in canine cancers utilizing the TKI trametinib, which has shown in vitro activity against a variety of canine tumor types including histiocytic sarcoma, melanoma and transitional cell carcinomas, among others [29]. Population pharmacokinetics of trametinib in dogs with cancer has also identified that dogs may reach steady-state concentrations of trametinib associated with clinical efficacy in humans within 2 weeks of daily dosing [135]. Clinical trials are currently ongoing in veterinary oncology evaluating the clinical effects of trametinib in canine histiocytic sarcoma, oral squamous cell carcinoma and when used in combination with a PI3K/mTOR inhibitor for numerous tumor types (veterinaryclinicaltrials.org). The potential for precision medicine in veterinary oncology has also brought about the advent of opportunities that attempt to match tumor mutations in dogs with drugs that have demonstrated activity in tumors with similar mutations in human oncology. Veterinarians now have the opportunity to submit tumor tissues for sequencing to identify the mutational landscape of a specific tumor and obtain a list of human-approved drugs that target those mutations. Further comparative studies into target engagement in tumors, in vitro activity, pharmacokinetics of the FDA-approved drugs as well as compounded formulations, commonly utilized in this setting, will be required to fully appreciate the potential benefit of these platforms.

2.2 Monoclonal Antibodies

Currently, there are no fully approved monoclonal antibodies (mAbs) for use in veterinary oncology, while bedinvetmab is the first canine mAb approved by the FDA for the control of pain associated with osteoarthritis in dogs. The Tmax of serum bedinvetmab is approximately 7 days after subcutaneous injection, and the elimination half-life is about 8–10 days [79, 103] which enables monthly injections for the treatment of dog patients. A conditional license from the USDA Center for Veterinary Biologics has been granted for the first canine immune checkpoint inhibitor mAb, Gilvetmab, which targets canine programmed death receptor-1 (PD1). Published pharmacokinetic data specific to gilvetmab are not available, but unpublished data suggest a prolonged half-life similar to bedinvetmab. Indeed, different from small-molecule drugs in physicochemical properties such as molecular size and hydrophilicity as well as gastrointestinal stability, therapeutic mAbs and proteins commonly exhibit distinct pharmacokinetic properties characterized by slow absorption and tissue distribution, low elimination rate, long elimination half-life (e.g., 6–27 days) and lack of oral bioavailability in human and animal subjects. As such, therapeutic mAbs, including TKIs [74] and the more recent immune checkpoint inhibitors (ICIs), are usually administered parenterally (e.g., intravenously, intramuscularly and subcutaneously) and much less frequently (e.g., weekly to monthly) than most small-molecule medications.

All ICI mAbs are given to human cancer patients via intravenous infusion, and their pharmacokinetic profiles can be described by a two-compartment model with linear elimination, with the exception of durvalumab which shows both linear and nonlinear elimination [21]. Upon entering the central circulating system, the sizes of therapeutic mAbs often limit their distribution from the blood to peripheral tissues, leading to their presence mainly in plasma or extracellular fluids. Rather, binding of mAbs to their target antigens or neonatal Fc receptor (FcRn) may largely affect their pharmacokinetic properties, such as fraction unbound, volume of distribution and half-life. Unlike small-molecule drugs, all mAbs are extensively metabolized by various circulating or peripheral peptidases or hydrolases to peptides and amino acids that can be reused for peptide or protein synthesis within the body or eliminated via renal excretion. Furthermore, nonlinear pharmacokinetics is often observed for mAb drugs and may be explained by target-mediated drug disposition (TMDD) when high-affinity binding of a drug to a therapeutic target determines its clearance, which can be viewed as a scenario of "pharmacodynamics affecting pharmacokinetics" [6]. In addition, the clearance of some therapeutic mAbs may also vary over time after treatment starts, which is partially attributable to the generation of antibodies against the mAbs, or antidrug antibodies (ADAs) [21].

References

1. Achanta S, Maxwell LK (2016) Reaction phenotyping of vinblastine metabolism in dogs. Vet Comp Oncol 14:161–169
2. Achanta S, Sewell A, Ritchey JW, Broaddus K, Bourne DW, Clarke CR, Maxwell LK (2016) Anatomical and physiological basis for the allometric scaling of cisplatin clearance in dogs. J Vet Pharmacol Ther 39:224–236
3. Aldoss IT, Weisenburger DD, Fu K, Chan WC, Vose JM, Bierman PJ, Bociek RG, Armitage JO (2008) Adult Burkitt lymphoma: advances in diagnosis and treatment. Oncology (Williston Park) 22:1508–1517
4. Al-Nadaf S, Wittenburg LA, Skorupski KA, Burton JH (2022) Population pharmacokinetics identifies rapid gastrointestinal absorption and plasma clearance of oral chlorambucil administered to cats with indolent lymphoproliferative malignancies. Am J Vet Res 83:1–9
5. Amber EI, Henderson RA, Adeyanju JB, Gyang EO (1990) Single-drug chemotherapy of canine transmissible venereal tumor with cyclophosphamide, methotrexate, or vincristine. J Vet Intern Med 4:144–147
6. An G (2020) Concept of pharmacologic target-mediated drug disposition in large-molecule and small-molecule compounds. J Clin Pharmacol 60:149–163
7. Ananthula HK, Parker S, Touchette E, Buller RM, Patel G, Kalman D, Salzer JS, Gallardo-Romero N, Olson V, Damon IK, Moir-Savitz T, Sallans L, Werner MH, Sherwin CM, Desai PB (2018) Preclinical pharmacokinetic evaluation to facilitate repurposing of tyrosine kinase inhibitors nilotinib and imatinib as antiviral agents. BMC Pharmacol Toxicol 19:80
8. Apperley JF, Rice SJ, Bishop JA, Chia YC, Krausz T, Gardner SD, Goldman JM (1987) Late-onset hemorrhagic cystitis associated with urinary excretion of polyomaviruses after bone marrow transplantation. Transplantation 43:108–112
9. Arai K, Maruo K, Ara KY, Uehara K, Matsuda H (2001) Characterization of isotype-specific regions of five classes of canine beta-tubulin and their expression in several tissues and cell culture. J Vet Med Sci 63:1297–1302
10. Bailey DB, Rassnick KM, Erb HN, Dykes NL, Hoopes PJ, Page RL (2004) Effect of glomerular filtration rate on clearance and myelotoxicity of carboplatin in cats with tumors. Am J Vet Res 65:1502–1507
11. Bailey DB, Rassnick KM, Dykes NL, Pendyala L (2009) Phase I evaluation of carboplatin by use of a dosing strategy based on a targeted area under the platinum concentration-versus-time curve and individual glomerular filtration rate in cats with tumors. Am J Vet Res 70:770–776
12. Barabas K, Milner R, Lurie D, Adin C (2008) Cisplatin: a review of toxicities and therapeutic applications. Vet Comp Oncol 6:1–18
13. Batra VK, Morrison JA, Woodward DL, Siverd NS, Yacobi A (1986) Pharmacokinetics of mitoxantrone in man and laboratory animals. Drug Metab Rev 17:311–329
14. Bedi A, Miller CB, Hanson JL, Goodman S, Ambinder RF, Charache P, Arthur RR, Jones RJ (1995) Association of BK virus with failure of prophylaxis against hemorrhagic cystitis following bone marrow transplantation. J Clin Oncol 13:1103–1109
15. Bello CL, Sherman L, Zhou J, Verkh L, Smeraglia J, Mount J, Klamerus KJ (2006) Effect of food on the pharmacokinetics of sunitinib malate (SU11248), a multi-targeted receptor tyrosine kinase inhibitor: results from a phase I study in healthy subjects. Anti-Cancer Drugs 17:353–358

16. Billingham ME, Mason JW, Bristow MR, Daniels JR (1978) Anthracycline cardiomyopathy monitored by morphologic changes. Cancer Treat Rep 62:865–872
17. Burnett A, Wetzler M, Lowenberg B (2011) Therapeutic advances in acute myeloid leukemia. J Clin Oncol 29:487–494
18. Busse D, Busch FW, Schweizer E, Bohnenstengel F, Eichelbaum M, Fischer P, Schumacher K, Aulitzky WE, Kroemer HK (1999) Fractionated administration of high-dose cyclophosphamide: influence on dose-dependent changes in pharmacokinetics and metabolism. Cancer Chemother Pharmacol 43:263–268
19. Carli M, Passone E, Perilongo G, Bisogno G (2003) Ifosfamide in pediatric solid tumors. Oncology 65(Suppl 2):99–104
20. Castle MC, Margileth DA, Oliverio VT (1976) Distribution and excretion of (3H)vincristine in the rat and the dog. Cancer Res 36:3684–3689
21. Centanni M, Moes D, Troconiz IF, Ciccolini J, Van Hasselt JGC (2019) Clinical pharmacokinetics and pharmacodynamics of immune checkpoint inhibitors. Clin Pharmacokinet 58:835–857
22. Chabner BA, Glass J (2011) Cytidine analogues. In: Chabner BA, Longo DL (eds) Cancer chemotherapy and biotherapy: principles and practice, 5th edn. Lippincott Williams & Wilkins, Philadelphia
23. Chan CM, Frimberger AE, Moore AS (2016) Incidence of sterile hemorrhagic cystitis in tumor-bearing dogs concurrently treated with oral metronomic cyclophosphamide chemotherapy and furosemide: 55 cases (2009–2015). J Am Vet Med Assoc 249:1408–1414
24. Court MH (2013) Feline drug metabolism and disposition: pharmacokinetic evidence for species differences and molecular mechanisms. Vet Clin North Am Small Anim Pract 43:1039–1054
25. Cox PJ (1979) Cyclophosphamide cystitis—identification of acrolein as the causative agent. Biochem Pharmacol 28:2045–2049
26. Cox J, Weinman S (2016) Mechanisms of doxorubicin resistance in hepatocellular carcinoma. Hepat Oncol 3:57–59
27. Crook KI, Early PJ, Messenger KM, Munana KR, Gallagher R, Papich MG (2013) The pharmacokinetics of cytarabine in dogs when administered via subcutaneous and continuous intravenous infusion routes. J Vet Pharmacol Ther 36:408–411
28. Dabholkar M, Bostick-Bruton F, Weber C, Bohr VA, Egwuagu C, Reed E (1992) ERCC1 and ERCC2 expression in malignant tissues from ovarian cancer patients. J Natl Cancer Inst 84:1512–1517
29. Das S, Idate R, Cronise KE, Gustafson DL, Duval DL (2019) Identifying candidate druggable targets in canine cancer cell lines using whole-exome sequencing. Mol Cancer Ther 18:1460–1471
30. Davidson JD, Ma L, Flagella M, Geeganage S, Gelbert LM, Slapak CA (2004) An increase in the expression of ribonucleotide reductase large subunit 1 is associated with gemcitabine resistance in non-small cell lung cancer cell lines. Cancer Res 64:3761–3766
31. Di Gion P, Kanefendt F, Lindauer A, Scheffler M, Doroshyenko O, Fuhr U, Wolf J, Jaehde U (2011) Clinical pharmacokinetics of tyrosine kinase inhibitors: focus on pyrimidines, pyridines and pyrroles. Clin Pharmacokinet 50:551–603
32. Doroshow JH (2011) Topoisomerase II inhibitors: anthracyclines. In: Chabner B, Longo DL (eds) Cancer chemotherapy and biotherapy: principles and practice, 5th edn. Lippincott Williams & Wilkins, Philadelphia
33. Du Bois D, Du Bois EF (1989) A formula to estimate the approximate surface area if height and weight be known. 1916. Nutrition 5:303–311; discussion 312–3
34. Duckett ME, Curran KM, Bracha S, Leeper HJ (2024) Retrospective evaluation of melphalan, vincristine, and cytarabine chemotherapy for the treatment of relapsed canine lymphoma. J Am Anim Hosp Assoc 60:7–14
35. Ducroq J, Moha Ou Maati H, Guilbot S, Dilly S, Laemmel E, Pons-Himbert C, Faivre JF, Bois P, Stucker O, Le Grand M (2010) Dexrazoxane protects the heart from acute doxorubicin-induced QT prolongation: a key role for I(Ks). Br J Pharmacol 159:93–101
36. Duffull SB, Robinson BA (1997) Clinical pharmacokinetics and dose optimisation of carboplatin. Clin Pharmacokinet 33:161–183
37. Ekhart C, Doodeman VD, Rodenhuis S, Smits PH, Beijnen JH, Huitema AD (2008) Influence of polymorphisms of drug metabolizing enzymes (CYP2B6, CYP2C9, CYP2C19, CYP3A4, CYP3A5, GSTA1, GSTP1, ALDH1A1 and ALDH3A1) on the pharmacokinetics of cyclophosphamide and 4-hydroxycyclophosphamide. Pharmacogenet Genomics 18:515–523
38. Eley T, Luo FR, Agrawal S, Sanil A, Manning J, Li T, Blackwood-Chirchir A, Bertz R (2009) Phase I study of the effect of gastric acid pH modulators on the bioavailability of oral dasatinib in healthy subjects. J Clin Pharmacol 49:700–709
39. Emadi A, Jones RJ, Brodsky RA (2009) Cyclophosphamide and cancer: golden anniversary. Nat Rev Clin Oncol 6:638–647
40. Evison BJ, Sleebs BE, Watson KG, Phillips DR, Cutts SM (2016) Mitoxantrone, more than just another topoisomerase II poison. Med Res Rev 36:248–299
41. Faulds D, Balfour JA, Chrisp P, Langtry HD (1991) Mitoxantrone. A review of its pharmacodynamic and pharmacokinetic properties, and therapeutic potential in the chemotherapy of cancer. Drugs 41:400–449
42. Ferrer A, Marce S, Bellosillo B, Villamor N, Bosch F, Lopez-Guillermo A, Espinet B, Sole F, Montserrat E, Campo E, Colomer D (2004) Activation of mitochondrial apoptotic pathway in mantle cell lymphoma: high sensitivity to mitoxantrone in cases

with functional DNA-damage response genes. Oncogene 23:8941–8949
43. Filippich LJ, Bucher AM, Charles BG (2000) Platinum pharmacokinetics in Sulphur-crested cockatoos (Cacatua galerita) following single-dose cisplatin infusion. Aust Vet J 78:406–411
44. Fisher GR, Patterson LH (1992) Lack of involvement of reactive oxygen in the cytotoxicity of mitoxantrone, CI941 and ametantrone in MCF-7 cells: comparison with doxorubicin. Cancer Chemother Pharmacol 30:451–458
45. Freeman KP, Hahn KA, Harris FD, King GK (2003) Treatment of dogs with oral melanoma by hypofractionated radiation therapy and platinum-based chemotherapy (1987–1997). J Vet Intern Med 17:96–101
46. Freise KJ, Martin-Jimenez T (2006a) Pharmacokinetics of gemcitabine and its primary metabolite in dogs after intravenous bolus dosing and its in vitro pharmacodynamics. J Vet Pharmacol Ther 29:137–145
47. Freise KJ, Martin-Jimenez T (2006b) Pharmacokinetics of gemcitabine and its primary metabolite in dogs after intravenous infusion. J Vet Pharmacol Ther 29:147–152
48. Gammella E, Maccarinelli F, Buratti P, Recalcati S, Cairo G (2014) The role of iron in anthracycline cardiotoxicity. Front Pharmacol 5:25
49. Gan PP, Kavallaris M (2008) Tubulin-targeted drug action: functional significance of class ii and class IVb beta-tubulin in vinca alkaloid sensitivity. Cancer Res 68:9817–9824
50. Gandin V, Hoeschele JD, Margiotta N (2023) Special issue "Cisplatin in cancer therapy: molecular mechanisms of action 3.0". Int J Mol Sci 24:7917
51. Gareau A, Sekiguchi T, Warry E, Ripoll AZ, Sullivan E, Westfall T, Chretin J, Fulton LM, Harkey M, Storb R, Suter SE (2022) Allogeneic peripheral blood haematopoietic stem cell transplantation for the treatment of dogs with high-grade B-cell lymphoma. Vet Comp Oncol 20:862–870
52. Garnett CL, Guerrero TA, Rodriguez CO Jr (2016) Fixed-dose-rate administration of gemcitabine in cancer-bearing cats: A pilot study. Can Vet J 57:1149–1155
53. Ghisoni G, Foglia A, Sabattini S, Agnoli C, Dondi F, Perfetti S, Marconato L (2023) A retrospective clinico-pathologic study of 35 dogs with urethral transitional cell carcinoma undergoing treatment. Animals (Basel) 13:2395
54. Gillem J, Giuffrida M, Krick E (2017) Efficacy and toxicity of carboplatin and cytarabine chemotherapy for dogs with relapsed or refractory lymphoma (2000–2013). Vet Comp Oncol 15:400–410
55. Giovannetti E, Del Tacca M, Mey V, Funel N, Nannizzi S, Ricci S, Orlandini C, Boggi U, Campani D, Del Chiaro M, Iannopollo M, Bevilacqua G, Mosca F, Danesi R (2006) Transcription analysis of human equilibrative nucleoside transporter-1 predicts survival in pancreas cancer patients treated with gemcitabine. Cancer Res 66:3928–3935
56. Gokbuget N, Hoelzer D (2009) Treatment of adult acute lymphoblastic leukemia. Semin Hematol 46:64–75
57. Grunewald R, Kantarjian H, Keating MJ, Abbruzzese J, Tarassoff P, Plunkett W (1990) Pharmacologically directed design of the dose rate and schedule of 2′,2′-difluorodeoxycytidine (gemcitabine) administration in leukemia. Cancer Res 50:6823–6826
58. Gustafson DL, Thamm DH (2010) Pharmacokinetic modeling of doxorubicin pharmacokinetics in dogs deficient in ABCB1 drug transporters. J Vet Intern Med 24:579–586
59. Gustafson DL, Rastatter JC, Colombo T, Long ME (2002) Doxorubicin pharmacokinetics: macromolecule binding, metabolism, and excretion in the context of a physiologic model. J Pharm Sci 91:1488–1501
60. Hahn KA, Frazier DL, Cox SK, Legendre AM (1997) Effect of infusion regime on doxorubicin pharmacokinetics in the cat. J Am Anim Hosp Assoc 33:427–433
61. Hall AG, Tilby MJ (1992) Mechanisms of action of, and modes of resistance to, alkylating agents used in the treatment of haematological malignancies. Blood Rev 6:163–173
62. Hari M, Wang Y, Veeraraghavan S, Cabral F (2003) Mutations in alpha- and beta-tubulin that stabilize microtubules and confer resistance to colcemid and vinblastine. Mol Cancer Ther 2:597–605
63. Harker WG, Slade DL, Dalton WS, Meltzer PS, Trent JM (1989) Multidrug resistance in mitoxantrone-selected HL-60 leukemia cells in the absence of P-glycoprotein overexpression. Cancer Res 49:4542–4549
64. Hartvig P, Simonsson B, Oberg G, Wallin I, Ehrsson H (1988) Inter- and intraindividual differences in oral chlorambucil pharmacokinetics. Eur J Clin Pharmacol 35:551–554
65. Highley MS, Landuyt B, Prenen H, Harper PG, De Bruijn EA (2022) The nitrogen mustards. Pharmacol Rev 74:552–599
66. Houk BE, Bello CL, Kang D, Amantea M (2009) A population pharmacokinetic meta-analysis of sunitinib malate (SU11248) and its primary metabolite (SU12662) in healthy volunteers and oncology patients. Clin Cancer Res 15:2497–2506
67. Huang L, Jiang S, Shi Y (2020) Tyrosine kinase inhibitors for solid tumors in the past 20 years (2001–2020). J Hematol Oncol 13:143
68. Jarvinen TA, Tanner M, Rantanen V, Barlund M, Borg A, Grenman S, Isola J (2000) Amplification and deletion of topoisomerase IIalpha associate with ErbB-2 amplification and affect sensitivity to topoisomerase II inhibitor doxorubicin in breast cancer. Am J Pathol 156:839–847
69. Jones A, McGrath S, Gustafson DL (2019) The pharmacokinetics of cytarabine administered at three

distinct subcutaneous dosing protocols in dogs with meningoencephalomyelitis of unknown origin. J Vet Pharmacol Ther 42:588–592
70. Judson I, Verweij J, Gelderblom H, Hartmann JT, Schoffski P, Blay JY, Kerst JM, Sufliarsky J, Whelan J, Hohenberger P, Krarup-Hansen A, Alcindor T, Marreaud S, Litiere S, Hermans C, Fisher C, Hogendoorn PC, Dei Tos AP, Van Der Graaf WT, European Organisation and Treatment of Cancer Soft Tissue and Bone Sarcoma Group (2014) Doxorubicin alone versus intensified doxorubicin plus ifosfamide for first-line treatment of advanced or metastatic soft-tissue sarcoma: a randomised controlled phase 3 trial. Lancet Oncol 15:415–423
71. Kaijser GP, Beijnen JH, Bult A, Underberg WJ (1994) Ifosfamide metabolism and pharmacokinetics (review). Anticancer Res 14:517–531
72. Kaji K, Motegi T, Yonezawa T, Momoi Y, Maeda S (2024) Anti-tumour effects of lapatinib on HER2-positive canine prostatic carcinoma cell lines. Open Vet J 14:1259–1268
73. Kambayashi S, Minami K, Ogawa Y, Hamaji T, Hwang CC, Igase M, Hiraoka H, Miyama TS, Noguchi S, Baba K, Mizuno T, Okuda M (2015) Expression of O(6)-methylguanine-DNA methyltransferase causes lomustine resistance in canine lymphoma cells. Can J Vet Res 79:201–209
74. Keizer RJ, Huitema AD, Schellens JH, Beijnen JH (2010) Clinical pharmacokinetics of therapeutic monoclonal antibodies. Clin Pharmacokinet 49:493–507
75. Klimiuk P, Lopuszynski W, Bulak K, Smiech A, Brzana A (2020) Study of DNA topoisomerase IIa expression in canine lymphomas and its potential role as a marker of sensitivity to anthracycline-based chemotherapy in dogs. Folia Histochem Cytobiol 58:46–53
76. Kochevar DT, Middendorf DL, Mealey KL, Meyers RO, Rogers KS, Barton CL, Habron L, Alberts DS, Polzer JP (1995) Pharmacokinetics and haematological effects of a single intravenous dose of mitoxantrone in cats. J Vet Pharmacol Ther 18:471–475
77. Koeller JM, Trump DL, Tutsch KD, Earhart RH, Davis TE, Tormey DC (1986) Phase I clinical trial and pharmacokinetics of carboplatin (NSC 241240) by single monthly 30-minute infusion. Cancer 57:222–225
78. Kosarek CE, Kisseberth WC, Gallant SL, Couto CG (2005) Clinical evaluation of gemcitabine in dogs with spontaneously occurring malignancies. J Vet Intern Med 19:81–86
79. Krautmann M, Walters R, Cole P, Tena J, Bergeron LM, Messamore J, Mwangi D, Rai S, Dominowski P, Saad K, Zhu Y, Guillot M, Chouinard L (2021) Laboratory safety evaluation of bedinvetmab, a canine anti-nerve growth factor monoclonal antibody, in dogs. Vet J 276:105733
80. Krick EL, Cohen RB, Gregor TP, Salah PC, Sorenmo KU (2013) Prospective clinical trial to compare vincristine and vinblastine in a COP-based protocol for lymphoma in cats. J Vet Intern Med 27:134–140
81. Kurowski V, Cerny T, Kupfer A, Wagner T (1991) Metabolism and pharmacokinetics of oral and intravenous ifosfamide. J Cancer Res Clin Oncol 117(Suppl 4):S148–S153
82. Laing EJ, Miller CW, Cochrane SM (1988) Treatment of cyclophosphamide-induced hemorrhagic cystitis in five dogs. J Am Vet Med Assoc 193:233–236
83. Lalezari S, Chou AP, Tran A, Solis OE, Khanlou N, Chen W, Li S, Carrillo JA, Chowdhury R, Selfridge J, Sanchez DE, Wilson RW, Zurayk M, Lalezari J, Lou JJ, Ormiston L, Ancheta K, Hanna R, Miller P, Piccioni D, Ellingson BM, Buchanan C, Mischel PS, Nghiemphu PL, Green R, Wang HJ, Pope WB, Liau LM, Elashoff RM, Cloughesy TF, Yong WH, Lai A (2013) Combined analysis of O6-methylguanine-DNA methyltransferase protein expression and promoter methylation provides optimized prognostication of glioblastoma outcome. Neuro-Oncology 15:370–381
84. Lana SE, Dernell WS, Lafferty MH, Withrow SJ, Larue SM (2004) Use of radiation and a slow-release cisplatin formulation for treatment of canine nasal tumors. Vet Radiol Ultrasound 45:577–581
85. Leach TN, Childress MO, Greene SN, Mohamed AS, Moore GE, Schrempp DR, Lahrman SR, Knapp DW (2012) Prospective trial of metronomic chlorambucil chemotherapy in dogs with naturally occurring cancer. Vet Comp Oncol 10:102–112
86. Lee FY, Workman P, Roberts JT, Bleehen NM (1985) Clinical pharmacokinetics of oral CCNU (lomustine). Cancer Chemother Pharmacol 14:125–131
87. Leis-Filho AF, De Faria Lainetti P, Emiko Kobayashi P, Fonseca-Alves CE, Laufer-Amorim R (2021) Effects of lapatinib on HER2-positive and HER2-negative canine mammary carcinoma cells cultured in vitro. Pharmaceutics 13:897
88. Levitin HA, Foss KD, Li Z, Reinhart JM, Hague DW, Fan TM (2021) Pharmacokinetics of a cytosine arabinoside subcutaneous protocol in dogs with meningoencephalomyelitis of unknown aetiology. J Vet Pharmacol Ther 44:696–704
89. Lewis RS, Fidel J, Dassanayake S, Court MH, Burke NS, Mealey KL (2017) Comparison of chemotherapeutic drug resistance in cells transfected with canine ABCG2 or feline ABCG2. Vet Comp Oncol 15:411–420
90. Li KD, Jones CP, Hakam N, Erickson BA, Vanni AJ, Chancellor MB, Breyer BN (2023) Haemorrhagic cystitis: a review of management strategies and emerging treatments. BJU Int 132:631–637
91. Loveless H, Arena E, Felsted RL, Bachur NR (1978) Comparative mammalian metabolism of adriamycin and daunorubicin. Cancer Res 38:593–598
92. Maeda S, Sakai K, Kaji K, Iio A, Nakazawa M, Motegi T, Yonezawa T, Momoi Y (2022) Lapatinib as first-line treatment for muscle-invasive urothelial carcinoma in dogs. Sci Rep 12:4
93. Marconato L, Finotello R, Bonfanti U, Dacasto M, Beatrice L, Pizzoni S, Leone VF, Balestra G, Furlanello T, Rohrer Bley C, Aresu L (2015) An

open-label phase 1 dose-escalation clinical trial of a single intravenous administration of gemcitabine in dogs with advanced solid tumors. J Vet Intern Med 29:620–625
94. Martinez SE, Andresen MC, Zhu Z, Papageorgiou I, Court MH (2020) Pharmacogenomics of poor drug metabolism in greyhounds: cytochrome P450 (CYP) 2B11 genetic variation, breed distribution, and functional characterization. Sci Rep 10:69
95. Marzolini C, Paus E, Buclin T, Kim RB (2004) Polymorphisms in human MDR1 (P-glycoprotein): recent advances and clinical relevance. Clin Pharmacol Ther 75:13–33
96. Matsuyama A, Woods JP, Mutsaers AJ (2017) Evaluation of toxicity of a chronic alternate day metronomic cyclophosphamide chemotherapy protocol in dogs with naturally occurring cancer. Can Vet J 58:51–55
97. Mauldin GE, Fox PR, Patnaik AK, Bond BR, Mooney SC, Matus RE (1992) Doxorubicin-induced cardiotoxicosis. Clinical features in 32 dogs. J Vet Intern Med 6:82–88
98. McLean A, Woods RL, Catovsky D, Farmer P (1979) Pharmacokinetics and metabolism of chlorambucil in patients with malignant disease. Cancer Treat Rev 6(Suppl):33–42
99. Mealey KL, Meurs KM (2008) Breed distribution of the ABCB1-1Delta (multidrug sensitivity) polymorphism among dogs undergoing ABCB1 genotyping. J Am Vet Med Assoc 233:921–924
100. Mealey KL, Bentjen SA, Gay JM, Cantor GH (2001) Ivermectin sensitivity in collies is associated with a deletion mutation of the mdr1 gene. Pharmacogenetics 11:727–733
101. Mealey KL, Fidel J, Gay JM, Impellizeri JA, Clifford CA, Bergman PJ (2008) ABCB1-1Delta polymorphism can predict hematologic toxicity in dogs treated with vincristine. J Vet Intern Med 22:996–1000
102. Metzger R, Leichman CG, Danenberg KD, Danenberg PV, Lenz HJ, Hayashi K, Groshen S, Salonga D, Cohen H, Laine L, Crookes P, Silberman H, Baranda J, Konda B, Leichman L (1998) ERCC1 mRNA levels complement thymidylate synthase mRNA levels in predicting response and survival for gastric cancer patients receiving combination cisplatin and fluorouracil chemotherapy. J Clin Oncol 16:309–316
103. Michels GM, Honsberger NA, Walters RR, Kira STJ, Cleaver DM (2023) A prospective, randomized, double-blind, placebo-controlled multisite, parallel-group field study in dogs with osteoarthritis conducted in The United States of America evaluating bedinvetmab, a canine anti-nerve growth factor monoclonal antibody. Vet Anaesth Analg 50:446–458
104. Morita A, Aoshima K, Gulay KCM, Onishi S, Shibata Y, Yasui H, Kobayashi A, Kimura T (2019) High drug efflux pump capacity and low DNA damage response induce doxorubicin resistance in canine hemangiosarcoma cell lines. Res Vet Sci 127:1–10
105. Nakajima M, Komagata S, Fujiki Y, Kanada Y, Ebi H, Itoh K, Mukai H, Yokoi T, Minami H (2007) Genetic polymorphisms of CYP2B6 affect the pharmacokinetics/pharmacodynamics of cyclophosphamide in Japanese cancer patients. Pharmacogenet Genomics 17:431–445
106. O'Brien D, Ta G, Frazier S, Rebhun R, Skorupski K, Rodrigues C (2012) Gemcitabine degradation in whole blood from humans, dogs, cats, and horses. J Vet Sci Technol 3:119
107. Olaussen KA, Dunant A, Fouret P, Brambilla E, Andre F, Haddad V, Taranchon E, Filipits M, Pirker R, Popper HH, Stahel R, Sabatier L, Pignon JP, Tursz T, Le Chevalier T, Soria JC, Investigators IB (2006) DNA repair by ERCC1 in non-small-cell lung cancer and cisplatin-based adjuvant chemotherapy. N Engl J Med 355:983–991
108. Packeiser EM, Engels L, Nolte I, Goericke-Pesch S, Murua Escobar H (2023) MDR1 inhibition reverses doxorubicin-resistance in six doxorubicin-resistant canine prostate and bladder cancer cell lines. Int J Mol Sci 24:8136
109. Page RL, Macy DW, Thrall DE, Dewhirst MW, Allen SL, Heidner GL, Sim DA, McGee ML, Gillette EL (1988) Unexpected toxicity associated with use of body surface area for dosing melphalan in the dog. Cancer Res 48:288–290
110. Page RL, McEntee MC, George SL, Williams PL, Heidner GL, Novotney CA, Riviere JE, Dewhirst MW, Thrall DE (1993) Pharmacokinetic and phase I evaluation of carboplatin in dogs. J Vet Intern Med 7:235–240
111. Parsons-Doherty M, Poirier VJ, Monteith G (2014) The efficacy and adverse event profile of dexamethasone, melphalan, actinomycin D, and cytosine arabinoside (DMAC) chemotherapy in relapsed canine lymphoma. Can Vet J 55:175–180
112. Piscitelli SC, Rodvold KA, Rushing DA, Tewksbury DA (1993) Pharmacokinetics and pharmacodynamics of doxorubicin in patients with small cell lung cancer. Clin Pharmacol Ther 53:555–561
113. Press MF, Sauter G, Buyse M, Bernstein L, Guzman R, Santiago A, Villalobos IE, Eiermann W, Pienkowski T, Martin M, Robert N, Crown J, Bee V, Taupin H, Flom KJ, Tabah-Fisch I, Pauletti G, Lindsay MA, Riva A, Slamon DJ (2011) Alteration of topoisomerase II-alpha gene in human breast cancer: association with responsiveness to anthracycline-based chemotherapy. J Clin Oncol 29:859–867
114. Price GS, Frazier DL (1998) Use of body surface area (BSA)-based dosages to calculate chemotherapeutic drug dose in dogs: I. Potential problems with current BSA formulae. J Vet Intern Med 12:267–271
115. Ramirez DA, Collins KP, Aradi AE, Conger KA, Gustafson DL (2019) Kinetics of cyclophosphamide metabolism in humans, dogs, cats, and mice and relationship to cytotoxic activity and pharmacokinetics. Drug Metab Dispos 47:257–268

116. Rassnick KM, Moore AS, Northrup NC, Kristal O, Beaulieu BB, Lewis LD, Page RL (2006a) Phase I trial and pharmacokinetic analysis of ifosfamide in cats with sarcomas. Am J Vet Res 67:510–516
117. Rassnick KM, Rodriguez CO, Khanna C, Rosenberg MP, Kristal O, Chaffin K, Page RL (2006b) Results of a phase II clinical trial on the use of ifosfamide for treatment of cats with vaccine-associated sarcomas. Am J Vet Res 67:517–523
118. Ratan R, Patel SR (2016) Chemotherapy for soft tissue sarcoma. Cancer 122:2952–2960
119. Rau SE, Burgess KE (2017) A retrospective evaluation of lomustine (CeeNU) in 32 treatment naive cats with intermediate to large cell gastrointestinal lymphoma (2006-2013). Vet Comp Oncol 15:1019–1028
120. Reese MJ, Knapp DW, Anderson KM, Mund JA, Case J, Jones DR, Packer RA (2018) In vitro effect of chlorambucil on human glioma cell lines (SF767 and U87-MG), and human microvascular endothelial cell (HMVEC) and endothelial progenitor cells (ECFCs), in the context of plasma chlorambucil concentrations in tumor-bearing dogs. PloS One 13:e0203517
121. Rowinsky EK, Donehower RC (1991) The clinical pharmacology and use of antimicrotubule agents in cancer chemotherapeutics. Pharmacol Ther 52:35–84
122. Sakai K, Maeda S, Saeki K, Nakagawa T, Murakami M, Endo Y, Yonezawa T, Kadosawa T, Mori T, Nishimura R, Matsuki N (2018) Anti-tumour effect of lapatinib in canine transitional cell carcinoma cell lines. Vet Comp Oncol 16:642–649
123. Scheffler M, Di Gion P, Doroshyenko O, Wolf J, Fuhr U (2011) Clinical pharmacokinetics of tyrosine kinase inhibitors: focus on 4-anilinoquinazolines. Clin Pharmacokinet 50:371–403
124. Schiller JH, Harrington D, Belani CP, Langer C, Sandler A, Krook J, Zhu J, Johnson DH, Eastern Cooperative Oncology Group (2002) Comparison of four chemotherapy regimens for advanced non-small-cell lung cancer. N Engl J Med 346:92–98
125. Schlack K, Boegemann M, Steinestel J, Schrader AJ, Krabbe LM (2016) The safety and efficacy of gemcitabine for the treatment of bladder cancer. Expert Rev Anticancer Ther 16:255–271
126. Scott-Moncrieff JC, Chan TC, Samuels ML, Cook JR, Coppoc GL, Denicola DB, Richardson RC (1991) Plasma and cerebrospinal fluid pharmacokinetics of cytosine arabinoside in dogs. Cancer Chemother Pharmacol 29:13–18
127. Shirota Y, Stoehlmacher J, Brabender J, Xiong YP, Uetake H, Danenberg KD, Groshen S, Tsao-Wei DD, Danenberg PV, Lenz HJ (2001) ERCC1 and thymidylate synthase mRNA levels predict survival for colorectal cancer patients receiving combination oxaliplatin and fluorouracil chemotherapy. J Clin Oncol 19:4298–4304
128. Shrestha B, Reed JM, Starks PT, Kaufman GE, Goldstone JV, Roelke ME, O'Brien SJ, Koepfli KP, Frank LG, Court MH (2011) Evolution of a major drug metabolizing enzyme defect in the domestic cat and other felidae: phylogenetic timing and the role of hypercarnivory. PLoS One 6:e18046
129. Smallwood K, Tanis JB, Grant IA, Blackwood L, Killick DR, Amores-Fuster I, Elliott J, Mas A, Harper A, Marrington M, Finotello R (2019) Evaluation of a multi-agent chemotherapy protocol combining dexamethasone, melphalan, actinomycin D, and cytarabine for the treatment of resistant canine non-Hodgkin high-grade lymphomas: a single centre's experience. Vet Comp Oncol 17:165–173
130. Speed B, Bu HZ, Pool WF, Peng GW, Wu EY, Patyna S, Bello C, Kang P (2012) Pharmacokinetics, distribution, and metabolism of [14C]sunitinib in rats, monkeys, and humans. Drug Metab Dispos 40:539–555
131. Springfeld C, Jager D, Buchler MW, Strobel O, Hackert T, Palmer DH, Neoptolemos JP (2019) Chemotherapy for pancreatic cancer. Presse Med 48:e159–e174
132. Stillwell TJ, Benson RC Jr, Deremee RA, McDonald TJ, Weiland LH (1988) Cyclophosphamide-induced bladder toxicity in Wegener's granulomatosis. Arthritis Rheum 31:465–470
133. Stroda KA, Murphy JD, Hansen RJ, Brownlee L, Atencio EA, Gustafson DL, Lana SE (2017) Pharmacokinetics of cyclophosphamide and 4-hydroxycyclophosphamide in cats after oral, intravenous, and intraperitoneal administration of cyclophosphamide. Am J Vet Res 78:862–866
134. Struck RF, Alberts DS, Horne K, Phillips JG, Peng YM, Roe DJ (1987) Plasma pharmacokinetics of cyclophosphamide and its cytotoxic metabolites after intravenous versus oral administration in a randomized, crossover trial. Cancer Res 47:2723–2726
135. Takada M, Kitagawa K, Zhang Y, Bulitta JB, Moirano S, Jones A, Borgen J, Onsager A, Thaiwong T, Vail DM (2024) Population pharmacokinetics, pharmacodynamics and safety properties of trametinib in dogs with cancer: a phase I dose escalating clinical trial. Vet Comp Oncol 22:410–421
136. Theon AP, Madewell BR, Ryu J, Castro J (1994) Concurrent irradiation and intratumoral chemotherapy with cisplatin: a pilot study in dogs with spontaneous tumors. Int J Radiat Oncol Biol Phys 29:1027–1034
137. Timm R, Kaiser R, Lotsch J, Heider U, Sezer O, Weisz K, Montemurro M, Roots I, Cascorbi I (2005) Association of cyclophosphamide pharmacokinetics to polymorphic cytochrome P450 2C19. Pharmacogenomics J 5:365–373
138. Tomita H, Tanaka K, Tanaka T, Hara A (2016) Aldehyde dehydrogenase 1A1 in stem cells and cancer. Oncotarget 7:11018–11032
139. Trepanier LA, Ray K, Winand NJ, Spielberg SP, Cribb AE (1997) Cytosolic arylamine N-acetyltransferase (NAT) deficiency in the dog and other canids due to an absence of NAT genes. Biochem Pharmacol 54:73–80

140. Trepanier LA, Cribb AE, Spielberg SP, Ray K (1998) Deficiency of cytosolic arylamine N-acetylation in the domestic cat and wild felids caused by the presence of a single NAT1-like gene. Pharmacogenetics 8:169–179
141. Van Leeuwen RW, Van Gelder T, Mathijssen RH, Jansman FG (2014) Drug-drug interactions with tyrosine-kinase inhibitors: a clinical perspective. Lancet Oncol 15:e315–e326
142. Veluvolu S, Willcox JL, Skorupski KA, Al-Nadaf S, Rebhun R, Wittenburg L (2023) Fractionated oral dosing and its effect on cyclophosphamide pharmacokinetics in dogs with high-grade multicentric lymphoma. Vet Comp Oncol 21:20–27
143. Warry E, Hansen RJ, Gustafson DL, Lana SE (2011) Pharmacokinetics of cyclophosphamide after oral and intravenous administration to dogs with lymphoma. J Vet Intern Med 25:903–908
144. Witta S, Collins KP, Ramirez DA, Mannheimer JD, Wittenburg LA, Gustafson DL (2023) Vinblastine pharmacokinetics in mouse, dog, and human in the context of a physiologically based model incorporating tissue-specific drug binding, transport, and metabolism. Pharmacol Res Perspect 11:e01052
145. Wittenburg LA, Weishaar K, Ramirez D, Gustafson DL (2019) Doxorubicin area under the curve is an important predictor of neutropenia in dogs with naturally occurring cancers. Vet Comp Oncol 17:147–154
146. Wu W, Klockow JL, Zhang M, Lafortune F, Chang E, Jin L, Wu Y, Daldrup-Link HE (2021) Glioblastoma multiforme (GBM): an overview of current therapies and mechanisms of resistance. Pharmacol Res 171:105780
147. Xia B, Heimbach T, He H, Lin TH (2012) Nilotinib preclinical pharmacokinetics and practical application toward clinical projections of oral absorption and systemic availability. Biopharm Drug Dispos 33:536–549
148. Yamazaki H, Sasai H, Tanaka M, Tanaka T, Nishida H, Noguchi S, Kuwamura M, Akiyoshi H (2021) Assessment of biomarkers influencing treatment success on small intestinal lymphoma in dogs. Vet Comp Oncol 19:123–131
149. Yancey MF, Merritt DA, Lesman SP, Boucher JF, Michels GM (2010a) Pharmacokinetic properties of toceranib phosphate (Palladia, SU11654), a novel tyrosine kinase inhibitor, in laboratory dogs and dogs with mast cell tumors. J Vet Pharmacol Ther 33:162–171
150. Yancey MF, Merritt DA, White JA, Marsh SA, Locuson CW (2010b) Distribution, metabolism, and excretion of toceranib phosphate (Palladia, SU11654), a novel tyrosine kinase inhibitor, in dogs. J Vet Pharmacol Ther 33:154–161
151. Yu TW, Yamamoto H, Morita S, Fukushima R, Elbadawy M, Usui T, Sasaki K (2024) Comparative pharmacokinetics of tyrosine kinase inhibitor, lapatinib, in dogs and cats following single oral administration. J Vet Med Sci 86:317–321
152. Zwueste DM, Vernau KM, Vernau W, Pypendop BH, Knych HK, Rodrigues CA, Kol A, Questa M, Dickinson PJ (2023) Oral cytarabine ocfosfate pharmacokinetics and assessment of leukocyte biomarkers in normal dogs. J Vet Intern Med 37:2429

Intraoperative Image Guidance in Human and Veterinary Surgical Oncology

Joanne Tuohy, William C. Eward, and John Rossmeisl

1 Introduction

As cancer treatments evolve and progress over time in efforts to optimize treatment outcomes and maximize survival prognoses, the contributions of surgical oncologists also evolve accordingly to embrace treatment advances. An important area of development in surgical oncology is in image-guided surgical planning and surgery. The general principles of tumor staging and surgical planning in human and veterinary surgical oncology have remained relatively constant in the face of technological advances. Establishing disease stage allows for informed decisions regarding surgical dose. Advances in imaging technologies have allowed for increasingly sophisticated tumor staging, surgical planning, and intraoperative image-guided surgery. Due to the closer proximity in body size between dogs and humans compared to mice and humans, emerging imaging modalities can be evaluated and refined using dogs with spontaneously occurring tumors for increased translatability to human cancer patients. This chapter will highlight the techniques for image-guided surgical planning and surgery in two illustrative areas: sarcoma and brain tumors in veterinary and human cancer patients.

J. Tuohy (✉) · J. Rossmeisl
Virginia-Maryland College of Veterinary Medicine, Virginia Polytechnic Institute and State University, Blacksburg, VA, USA
e-mail: jltuohy@vt.edu

W. C. Eward
Department of Orthopaedic Surgery, Duke University Medical Center, Durham, NC, USA

2 Techniques for Image-Guided Surgery for Sarcoma: The Perspective in Veterinary Patients

In veterinary oncology, sarcomas represent a heterogeneous group of tumors that broadly include bone and soft tissue sarcomas. Osteosarcoma is the most common primary bone tumor in dogs [1]. Soft tissue sarcoma is a heterogeneous group of tumors that arise from mesenchymal tissues, comprising multiple histological subtypes [2]. Imaging techniques for tumor staging have seen advances in recent years, with the increasing availability of computerized tomography (CT) and positron-emission tomography (PET) CT scanning. Technologies for surgical planning and intraoperative image-guided surgery have also advanced substantially.

2.1 Imaging as a Staging Diagnostic in Veterinary Bone and Soft Tissue Sarcomas

As CT imaging has become increasingly available and affordable for pet owners, CT scans

M. W. Nolan et al. (eds.), *Comparative Oncology*, https://doi.org/10.1007/978-3-032-04454-9_8

have seen increased use for staging canine bone and soft tissue sarcoma patients. The use of whole-body CT scans for staging in canine osteosarcoma allows for thorough evaluation for possible metastatic lesions, especially with the advent of PET-CT scans for veterinary use. Fluorine-18-fluorodeoxyglucose PET-CT has been shown to be effective as a staging diagnostic in canine osteosarcoma with increased detection of bone and soft tissue lesions [3], and with potential prognostic value [4]. A study reported by Brody et al. suggested that fluorine-18-fluorodeoxyglucose PET-CT improved detection of metastatic and concurrent neoplastic lesions in dogs with appendicular osteosarcoma [5], and a report by Slinkard et al. indicated the potential utility of PET-CT for metastatic lymph node identification in canine osteosarcoma [6]. Whole-body CT scans with or without PET imaging are also utilized in staging for human osteosarcoma [7]. Even though MRI imaging is a common diagnostic modality in human osteosarcoma patients, the use of MRI in canine osteosarcoma remains currently limited, potentially due to cost and availability limitations. The need for general anesthesia to perform an MRI compared to the option of performing a CT under sedation in veterinary patients may also contribute to the limited use of MRI. As the imaging modalities for staging cancer increase in their sophistication, it is important to bear in mind the potential implications of stage migration on comparison of scientific reports, on prognostication, and on patient care decisions.

2.2 Preoperative Imaging and Surgical Planning for Canine Sarcomas

Surgical options for resection of the primary appendicular osteosarcoma tumor include full limb amputation +/− hemipelvectomy or limb-salvage surgery [1]. Cross-sectional imaging is especially needed for accurate surgical planning of limb-salvage procedures, with its ability to accurately determine the gross extent of osteosarcoma tumors. In canine osteosarcoma, there are few reports documenting evaluations of imaging modalities to predict tumor extent. In general, both CT and MRI imaging appear to be appropriate for estimating tumor extent, but the comparative accuracy of both techniques remains to be definitively determined [8–10]. As efforts to advance limb-salvage procedures continue, the need for high-quality cross-sectional imaging becomes even more apparent. For example, customized, personalized 3D-printed limb-salvage implants have been investigated for dogs with appendicular osteosarcoma, and CT imaging serves as the template for designing the custom implants and cutting guides [11, 12]. Custom-fabricated limb-salvage implants and cutting guides have potential to decrease surgery time and risk of implant failure for both dogs and people. MRI has been used to provide muscular morphometric data in efforts to design custom limb-salvage implants for the canine proximal humerus [13].

2.3 Fabricated Personalized 3D Surgical Planning Models

3D printing technology such as desktop vat polymerization has increased the accessibility of smaller-scale 3D printing, and together with the rising prevalence of cross-sectional imaging in veterinary clinics, the possibility of utilizing 3D-printed models for surgical planning is becoming increasingly adopted in veterinary medicine. 3D-printed models fabricated from cross-sectional imaging from a patient allow for more thorough evaluations of the spatial relationships between anatomic structures, thereby translating into improved presurgical planning and the possibility of presurgical rehearsal. Such presurgical planning is especially useful in oncologic surgery, where each patient's tumor is unique, and thus requires individualized preparation for resection. This increased presurgical preparation leads to advantages such as a reduction of surgical time and surgical errors. Utilizing 3D-printed models in advanced oral and maxillofacial surgeries has been reported to improve surgical preparation and reduce surgical time by at least

15 minutes [14]. The use of 3D-printed models in veterinary surgery is reported in a recent review [15], and 3D-printed models were used to enhance planning in canine maxillofacial surgeries in another report that included resection of a maxillary osteosarcoma [16]. The potential benefits of 3D-printed models also need to be weighed against considerations such as the quality control needed to ensure that the 3D fabrication process produces models with sufficient accuracy to facilitate surgical planning and rehearsal [15]. Increased use of 3D-printed models can continue to enhance presurgical planning to improve patient outcomes in human and veterinary oncologic surgery. Its use, together with custom-fabricated surgical instrumentation, will be further discussed in the section of the chapter on the human perspective in sarcoma surgical planning.

2.4 Intraoperative Imaging

A primary goal of canine sarcoma resection is achieving a negative or complete margin, and this goal has to be balanced with potential functional morbidity caused by surgery. Current surgical practice involves resecting a wide margin of grossly normal tissue in three dimensions around the tumor to maximize chances of obtaining negative margins, with 3 cm lateral tissue margins and a fascial tissue plane deep representing typical gross surgical margins for canine sarcomas [17, 18]. However, wide surgical margins could negatively impact patient function and mobility after surgery, especially as these wide lateral margins are not relative to the size of the dog and may not be needed in some cases to achieve histologically tumor-free margins. Thus, techniques to provide real-time intraoperative information to guide the surgeon on the precise gross surgical margin needed to eliminate all microscopic residual tumor cells are crucial for reducing excessive tissue resection. The need for accurate intraoperative data to guide tumor resection is especially highlighted by the insufficiency in current techniques in human oncologic surgery, where unacceptably high rates of positive tumor margins have been reported [19]. Intraoperative frozen histopathological sections can aid a surgeon in evaluating tumor resection site margins. However, limitations such as the time needed for processing and evaluation of samples by a pathologist, thus increasing patient time under anesthesia, sampling technique biases and errors, cost and resource limitations—which are especially pronounced in veterinary medicine—pose substantial challenges to widespread implementation of intraoperative frozen section assessment. Additionally, bone and soft tissue sarcomas present unique challenges for frozen section histopathological evaluation such as tissue limitations, as not all sarcoma samples are amenable to accurate frozen section processing [20]. Although intraoperative imaging techniques to assess surgical margins in sarcoma resections are not currently available in standard clinical practice, they represent exciting progress made toward advancing real-time image-guided veterinary surgery. The following section highlights examples of intraoperative imaging for margin evaluation that have been reported in veterinary studies of canine sarcoma.

2.4.1 Fluorescence Imaging

Near-infrared (NIR) imaging is one modality being explored for intraoperative tumor imaging in veterinary medicine. The technique utilizes locally or systemically administered fluorescent agents that preferentially target tumor tissue and requires a compatible intraoperative imaging system. These fluorescent agents, depending on their mechanism of action, can target specific tumors (tumor-targeting) or can non-specifically target tumor tissue. A novel system utilizing tumor-targeting NIR fluorescent probes to detect residual disease in the tumor bed after canine soft tissue sarcoma resection has been reported [21, 22]. This particular NIR probe used is optically activated after cleavage by cathepsin proteases, which are overexpressed in tumors such as soft tissue sarcomas [22]. Preclinical studies using a murine tumor model demonstrated that the detection of residual fluorescence correlated with local tumor recurrence [23]. The canine studies reported minimal adverse reactions to intravenous injection of the NIR probe and successful detection of residual disease with fluorescence imaging; however, limitations such as the incidence of false positives and negatives were noted [21, 22]. Additionally, the small number of cases where there was positive identification of residual tumor foci potentially due to the wide tumor resections limited the investigators' ability to determine the sensitivity of the system [21, 22]. The utility of this system using NIR probes needs to be further explored in larger canine studies and across different tumor types. This early work with the NIR probes did lead to a phase 1 human clinical trial [24], which is referenced in the portion of this chapter focusing on human intraoperative imaging.

Another reported tumor-targeting NIR fluorescent agent capable of targeting soft tissue sarcomas is a peptide bound to indocyanine green that binds Annexin A2, which is overexpressed in many tumors [25, 26]. There was a discordance between NIR imaging and histopathological evaluation in one dog with a soft tissue sarcoma, where the absence of fluorescence in the surgical resection site did not correlate with the positive margins determined by histopathological tumor evaluation. The small number of dogs in this study with specific tumor types precluded evaluation of the sensitivity of the fluorescent agent to identify microscopic residual disease within the tumor resection bed [25].

A novel tumor-targeting NIR fluorescent agent that targets the integrin $\alpha_v\beta_3$ expressed in various tumors. A canine study involving multiple tumor types reported accumulation of fluorescence in tumors such as mammary tumors, mast cell tumors and sarcomas. In the one osteosarcoma and one soft tissue sarcoma evaluated in this study, there was false positive fluorescence in the resection bed, as supported by negative histopathological margins [27].

Indocyanine green (ICG) is a small water-soluble molecule (MW 744), non-specific fluorescent agent that has been used for intraoperative tumor imaging. ICG uptake in tumors depends on the increased permeability of neoangiogenic tumor vasculature and decreased tumor lymphatic drainage, hence its non-specificity and potential application to various tumor types. A study reported evaluation of ICG intraoperatively to detect residual disease after canine (n = 15) and human (n = 2) sarcoma resection [28]. In total, 14 out of 15 canine sarcomas in this study fluoresced positively with ICG, 5 surgical resection sites exhibited positive ICG fluorescence indicating microscopic residual disease, and 4 of these 5 sites were confirmed via biopsy to contain residual tumor. The surgical site of the two human subjects did not exhibit ICG fluorescence, and histopathological evaluation of the resected tumors confirmed complete resections with negative margins [28]. ICG has its limitations, including a low signal in poorly vascularized tumors and a low specificity that inhibits discrimination between tumor tissue and peritumoral inflammation, which have similarly permeable vasculature [29]. Further discussion on indocyanine green is presented in the section on intraoperative imaging from the human patient perspective.

A novel non-targeted lipid nanoparticle fluorescence agent has been reported for intraoperative imaging in nine dogs with mesenchymal tumors [30]. In the six dogs that underwent tumor resection with wide surgical margins, the fluorescence intensity of the surgical site was high in one dog, whose tumor subsequently was confirmed to have positive margins on histopathological evaluation. In the three dogs that underwent limb amputation, the fluorescence intensity in the regional lymph nodes identified two out of three histologically confirmed metastatic lymph nodes [30].

2.4.2 Optical Coherence Tomography

Optical coherence tomography (OCT) is a rapidly emerging tool that has been recently explored for intraoperative surgical margin imaging in veterinary oncology patients. This technology utilizes the backscatter of light to visualize tissue microstructures and has the potential to differentiate between tumor and non-tumorous tissues. OCT has been reported to differentiate between soft tissue sarcoma, muscle and adipose tissue using sarcoma samples from 17 dogs and 2 cats [31]. This group of investigators then went on to establish that OCT can further differentiate between tumor and normal tissue at the surgical margin after soft tissue sarcoma resection in dogs, supporting the use of OCT to intraoperatively identify positive surgical margins [32]. OCT images are generated and reviewed in real-time, and the large volume of images takes time for human observers to process. In order to facilitate the practicality of rapid intraoperative margin assessment, machine learning has been investigated for its accuracy in detecting canine soft tissue sarcomas and found to be accurate and precise for interpreting OCT surgical margin imaging in a study using 25 canine soft tissue sarcomas [33]. OCT has thus far exhibited high potential for intraoperative margin assessment in canine soft tissue sarcomas, offering the advantage over traditional histopathological evaluation of real-time assessment of possibly the entire tumor resection bed.

3 Techniques for Image-Guided Surgery for Sarcoma: The Perspective in Human Patients

In the spectrum of solid tumor malignancy, few resections are as challenging and multifaceted as resecting sarcomas. While soft tissue sarcomas and sarcomas of bone represent two fundamentally different diseases, they are united by their mesenchymal origin and similarly morbid impact upon patients. These large, rare, and complex malignancies have devastating effects on patients such that even those individuals that are cured often have permanently altered levels of function. When a surgeon resects a sarcoma, the necessary operation is a wide excision such that a margin of normal tissue surrounds the tumor [34]. However, it is unknown what size of a margin is sufficient for any given tumor, and any dictum about a specific size is based on dogma rather than data [34]. What is clear, however, is that having a negative, or clean, margin has a positive impact on local recurrence-free and disease-free survival. This assessment of the surgical margin is performed grossly first by the surgeon and then microscopically by a pathologist using the gold standard of tumor either contacting (a positive margin) or not contacting (a negative margin) ink placed on the specimen shortly after removal. The problem with this method is twofold: First, it is an indirect answer to the question, “Did we completely resect this tumor?” A negative margin is only an inference to the answer to this question based on evaluating *what was removed* from the patient. A direct answer would require an evaluation of the *tissue that remains* in the patient. Second, the report on surgical margin status from the pathologist typically takes one to two weeks, by which time the surgery is long completed, and any action taken to correct a positive margin requires revision surgery. Therefore, the ideal solution for this problem would be an intraoperative imaging system which can deliver information about the presence or absence of residual cancer in the patient in such a way that this information is available to the surgeon in real time. At present, such a technology does not exist in an effective form. However, great progress has been made. In the process of attempting to assess completion of tumor resection, many advances have been made in areas of computer navigation and intraoperative imaging that—at the very least—make sarcoma resections safer, technically easier, and more precise. In this section, we will discuss advancements in human medicine toward real-time, image-guided resection of sarcomas.

3.1 Soft Tissue Sarcoma

For soft tissue sarcomas, there is great latitude with regard to where definitive resection cuts are made. After all, a surgical margin may be taken as wide as it need be, and involved structures must be sacrificed as required. For this reason, intraoperative imaging modalities are primarily about one ultimate goal: ensuring a negative margin and the total resection of all known disease. Unfortunately, the attainment of this goal has lagged behind the available technologies. It is one thing to apply various technologies to the pursuit of intraoperative margin assessment. It is another matter altogether to demonstrate that this can be done in a way that matches or exceeds the standard of histopathology. The following section will review those technologies regularly employed.

3.1.1 Conventional Imaging Modalities Such as Ultrasound and MRI

Intraoperative imaging has undergone significant advancements in recent years, facilitating several improvements in the surgical management of soft tissue sarcomas. The primary paradigm shift has been to utilize modalities such as ultrasound, MR imaging, and CT scans to guide biopsy needle placement. This allows a core needle biopsy to be planned in line with the desired resection path while ascertaining that the tip of the biopsy needle is in the desired location [35]. However, while these modalities have been translated to the operating room, their utilization has not been widespread in the treatment of soft tissue sarcoma for a variety of reasons—from cost to limitations of resolution to perceived difficulty in application. Intraoperative ultrasound (IOUS) offers—in principle—real-time imaging during surgery, allowing surgeons to precisely assess tumor extent, identify adjacent vital structures, and guide tumor resection with enhanced accuracy. In reality, surgeons have found it difficult to make confident inferences about the extent of tumor, thus relegating its presence in the literature largely to case reports about very specific niche applications (such as delimiting margins in the rare, infiltrative sarcoma known as dermatofibrosarcoma protuberans) [36]. Intraoperative magnetic resonance imaging (iMRI) offers superior soft tissue resolution, which is typically more familiar to surgeons and may offer a complementary imaging tool for real-time assessment of tumor volume and margins during the surgical procedure [37]. This has been predominantly described in the neurosurgical literature. Mesko et al. described the approach taken to adopt this to a soft tissue sarcoma patient [37]. It is possible that the effort required to make such an adaptation has been a deterrent to its expanded use. At the author's own institution, we have successfully accessed an operative suite with intraoperative MRI only to be met by an unexpected opponent: insurance companies often do not approve the additional expense, citing a lack of data. Intraoperative CT offers a more accessible and cost-effective means of obtaining intraoperative images, and this modality is more relevant in resection of sarcomas of bone (given the limitations of soft tissue imaging with CT). Interestingly, the challenges and limitations of utilizing conventional imaging modalities in the operating room coincided with the explosion of custom, 3D-printed implants. While such implants are generally not necessary in soft tissue sarcoma surgery, 3D-printed models have proven useful in visualizing soft tissue sarcomas, the surrounding anatomy, and the steps in the surgical plan. This concept—that a 3D-printed model can be studied and brought into the operating room—has been explored in urological surgery [38], colorectal surgery [39], thoracic surgery [40], and orthopedic trauma surgery [41]. Li et al. created 3D-printed models of two patients' soft tissue sarcomas [42]. They subsequently asked groups of junior, intermediate, and senior surgeons, as well as a group of interns, to evaluate the models and to utilize them in making preoperative plans. They also evaluated the operations themselves regarding utilization of the models. Through this work, they demonstrated that 3D-printed models of complex sarcoma cases can provide great value for preoperative planning, intraoperative navigation, and medical education.

3.1.2 Tumor-Selective Intraoperative Fluorescence Imaging

Although there are limitations of conventional intraoperative imaging modalities, one area of great interest in soft tissue sarcoma resection has been the ability to use fluorescence imaging to assess surgical margins in real time. Intraoperative frozen sections are subject to sampling bias and error—and, in the case of large soft tissue sarcomas—are impractical due to the large amounts of tissue required to be processed [34]. A group from Duke University has demonstrated the efficacy of protease-activated, tumor-selective probes to detect microscopic residual disease in the tumor bed in real time [22, 23]. The early canine studies have been referenced in the veterinary sarcoma section. A phase I clinical trial of one of these probes—LUM015—was published in 2016 [24], but phase II and phase III trials have been relegated to breast cancer resection rather than sarcoma because of the relatively smaller number of human sarcoma patients. An interesting limitation of this technology was identified: the fluorescence imaging system can detect cancer cells within the tumor bed at the single-cell level, but this level of detection is more sensitive than what the surgeon's eyes and hands can address technically [24]. In other words, even if the surgeon is alerted to the presence of microscopic residual disease in the body, they may lack the technical ability to remove single cells and can only resect gross amounts of tissue in response. This led to the development of an attached laser ablation system so that the precision of the detection system can have a similarly precise ablative response, but this remains in the preclinical stage [43]. It is the view of this author that the ideal solution will involve tumor-selective imaging modalities and an ablation system with a level of precision that exceeds the limits of the human eye and hands. Multiple systems are currently underway, from different activation enzymes attached to specific fluorophores to antibody-fluorophore conjugates with targets such as EGFR and VEGF-A. Whichever system prevails, the basic workflow for fluorescence imaging involves some version of the following (adapted from Keereweer et al. [44] and described by Visgauss et al. [45]):

1. *A light source emits light at a specific wavelength known to excite the chosen fluorophore.*
2. *The fluorophore may be endogenous to tissues (autofluorescence) or administered to the patient at a given time prior to the procedure (fluorescent probe).*
3. *This light wavelength (photon) travels into the tissue and is absorbed by the fluorophore. It is subjected to reflection, refraction, and scattering as it penetrates the tissues.*
4. *The fluorophore enters a state of excitation for a fraction of a second (depending on the lifetime of the fluorophore).*
5. *When the fluorophore returns to its ground state, it emits the photon at another given wavelength of light.*
6. *This light wavelength travels out of the tissue (again subjected to reflection, refraction, and scattering) and is captured and recorded by the camera system.*
7. *An ablative system targets the cells emitting the specific light wavelength.*

3.1.3 Autofluorescence

There are specific techniques under development which utilize autofluorescence to guide surgical resections. Such techniques exploit differences in the inherent optical properties that have known variance between normal and pathological tissues, resulting in alterations in light refraction [45]. Wilke et al. capitalize on the fact that tumor tissue has a different level of expression in β-carotene and hemoglobin from adjacent normal tissue [46]. The authors described a detection of positive margins at a rate of 79% when compared to the gold standard histopathology. While this is impressive, it would certainly require significant improvement to become widely used. False negative errors were the result of cancer cells located beyond the penetration depth of this technique (2 mm). False positive errors were attributed to tissue changes that accompany resection.

3.1.4 Indocyanine Green Fluorescence Imaging

Indocyanine green (ICG) fluorescence imaging deserves its own section as it has, despite its lack of specificity, offered a great deal of promise in resecting sarcomas and a variety of other solid tumor malignancies [47]. ICG is a well-studied and historically safe fluorophore that has a successful track record for guiding intraoperative margin assessment in breast [48], gastrointestinal [49], and thoracic cancers [50]. Gong et al. are currently exploring the utility of ICG fluorescence imaging to assess margin status during resection of soft tissue sarcomas [47]. Using a threshold of 77% of the maximum intensity in the resected tumor, they report 56% concordance with histopathology in their series of 18 sarcoma patients. While many users continue to explore ICG for margin interrogation, a new role for ICG fluorescence imaging has opened in soft tissue sarcoma surgery: assessment of wound healing potential. Lazarides et al. [51] attempted to address the problem of increased rates of wound dehiscence in soft tissue sarcoma patients who receive neoadjuvant radiation therapy followed by surgery. They performed ICG fluorescence imaging of the tumor bed at different time points following resection of soft tissue sarcomas. Based on inflow into the skin flaps, surgeons blinded to the ultimate wound healing outcomes were able to predict wound complications in 75% of cases. By experimenting with different fluorescence parameters, the authors were able to demonstrate that flow during the peak phase could predict wound complications with a sensitivity of 88.9% and a specificity of 100% [51]. It is possible that this technology may be used to make real-time surgical decisions not about surgical margins but, rather, about whether or not a wound should be closed (as opposed to treated with a flap, a skin graft, or a wound V.A.C.).

3.2 Sarcoma of Bone

For the various sarcomas of bone, a different set of intraoperative imaging needs presents itself to the surgeon. Indeed, the need for a negative margin remains paramount. However, cutting the bone in the right anatomic location must also consider the safe positioning of osteotomes or other cutting instruments relative to the adjacent soft tissues as well as making cuts which are shaped to accommodate reconstructive prosthetic implants. For these latter two reasons, intraoperative imaging modalities differ in both type and application from those used in soft tissue sarcoma resection. Whereas intraoperative imaging for margin assessment in soft tissue sarcoma surgery may be useful in any anatomic location, intraoperative imaging is primarily used to assist bone tumor resection in the pelvis and sacrum, where three-dimensional anatomy is complex and adjacent soft tissue structures are vitally important. The following section will review available technologies and their applications.

3.2.1 Computer Navigation

Computer navigation has been utilized in a variety of orthopedic subspecialties (for example, arthroplasty [52], traumatology [53], and spine surgery [54] to increase the level of surgical precision with which osteotomies are made. The earliest mainstream publications about using computer navigation to improve the quality of bone tumor resection appeared in 2012 and 2013 [55, 56]. A variety of companies provide computer navigation systems suitable for resecting bone tumors, and all share a common workflow:

1. *Place a tracking array securely into a fixed location within the skeleton (ideally in a different bone from the one being resected).*
2. *Obtain an intraoperative CT scan to register the tracking array within the patient's current operative anatomy.*
3. *Position the navigational robot so that it can "see" the tracking array and verify the accuracy of the system with reference points of either known bony landmarks or small fiducials* (e.g., *mini-frag screws) placed into the skeleton prior to the scan.*
4. *Attach tracking arrays to instruments such as osteotomes, routers, or saws so that cuts can be visualized in real time on the display screen.*

Staats et al. evaluated the learning curve of the above workflow in 24 patients in whom computer navigation was utilized [56]. They found the mean registration error to be 0.9 mm. While this is certainly a reasonable amount of error to accept, at our institution we typically utilize an error of 0.2 mm, and we repeat registration/calibration until such a level of procedure can be obtained. There were no intraoperative complications. Except for one patient in whom a marginal resection was planned, there were negative margins in 23 cases. One patient experienced local recurrence, and one patient died of distant metastasis. Jeys et al. from the Birmingham orthopedic oncology group reviewed 23 consecutive patients with bone tumors treated with an oncology-specific navigation system (Stryker

OrthoMap 3D Navigation System II; Kalamazoo, MI) [57]. In these 23 patients, negative bony margins were attained in all 23, while negative soft tissue margins were attained in 21, and the rate of local recurrence was 13%. Notably, these were significant decreases from the 27% negative margins and 29% local recurrence from the 539 primary bone tumor resections previously published from the same institution but using conventional techniques.

3.2.2 Imaging-Informed Patient-Specific Cutting Instrumentation

It may seem counterintuitive to discuss instrumentation such as cutting guides in a chapter about surgical imaging techniques. However, the two concepts are definitively linked. Ultimately, computer navigation allows the surgeon to make cuts precisely and safely. The cost of this is increased operative time and increased radiation to both the patient and the operative team. In the era of readily available, patient-specific 3D printing, surgeons asked a simple question: Can we use preoperative imaging, obtained near the time of the planned resection, to design and fabricate cutting guides that allow the hands and instruments to be positioned as they would be during a navigated resection? The answer has been a resounding "yes." Benady et al. described a typical workflow which also illustrates the close association between imaging and patient-specific instruments (PSIs) such that it becomes clear how such instruments translate advanced imaging into the live operative setting [58]. In Benady's work, a biomedical engineer is first provided with CT scans and MRI scans of the patient. 2D images are inputted into an imaging processing software system approved by the FDA (Mimics®, Materialise, N.V. Leuven, Belgium, or Intellispace Portal V9 and V11, Philips Healthcare, Best, Netherlands). Images are merged and segmented such that a 3D model of the bony anatomy is created, and planned tumor margins are then digitally superimposed. Based on this work, cutting planes for resection are chosen and refined by the surgeon. A cutting PSI is then designed with specific bony footprints selected for attachment adjacent to the tumor, and this PSI is printed and processed. In a cohort of 11 patients with complex pelvic sarcomas treated with the above workflow, the authors reported negative margins in 10 of the 11 patients, with a remarkable operative time of 3:38 ± 0.05 hours [58]. It is this last statistic—operative time—which illustrates the advantage of the PSI as an extension of live, intraoperative imaging and navigation. With classical computer navigation, every step of the process, from placement of tracking arrays, to obtaining an intraoperative CT scan (a resource not readily available) to checking registration and tracking instruments, is happening with the patient under general anesthesia and with an open surgical wound. With a PSI, the imaging is admittedly obtained in the near-preoperative period, but this allows a simulated plan to be exacted before the patient is under anesthesia and before an incision has been made. The linchpin in this process is the availability of 3D (additive) printing materials. With the availability of rapid fabrication of the PSIs, the time-consuming part of intraoperative imaging can be separated from the operation, and the simulation can be used to obtain the end result—accurate positioning of hands and instruments for cutting—in the form of a printed implement that replaces the need for actual navigation in real time.

3.2.3 Haptic and Other Feedback Systems

The natural progression from reliable computer navigation systems or PSIs would be systems which provide corrective feedback. Such systems do exist, and they provide feedback through either haptic or visual means. Mustahsan et al. note that both navigation modalities and customized 3D-printed cutting guides based on simulated surgical fields can have clinically meaningful errors in technique for a variety of reasons [59]. They have developed an inexpensive optical feedback system (OFS) that compares intraoperative camera images to the preoperative plan. This feedback system provides visual feedback on the surgeon's placement of a PSI into the body. In their study, they simulated wide resections on a total of 24 femurs using 3 types of cutting guides with a second study in a total of 20 sawbones, with and without the surgeon using the OFS to adjust the guide position before cutting. The OFS increased the accuracy of cuts about the sagittal and transverse planes by a remarkable 33% and 53%, respectively [59]. The same group has also described a novel intraoperative method to project osteotomy lines onto bone [60]. Their so-called projector method literally projects visible light onto the bones so that preoperatively planned osteotomies can be visualized in the live operative setting. In controlled experiments using both cadavers and sawbones, the authors were able to reduce the corner deviation from 2.53 mm to 0.35 mm, the angular deviation from 2.10° to 0.31°, and the point deviation from 4.66 mm to 0.48 mm ($p < 0.001$) when compared to traditional, manual methods [60].

Robotic and haptic feedback systems have been used in orthopedic surgery since the first system—the ROBODOC—was introduced in 1992 and used to improve accuracy in total hip arthroplasty [61]. Since the ROBODOC, there are now a multitude of robotic or haptic feedback systems. The MAKO RIO (Mako Surgical, USA) is a haptic feedback system which guides the surgeon's hands when making cuts during knee arthroplasty. The robotic system, TiRobot (Tinavi, China), has been used in a variety of minimally invasive and open surgical tasks. These tasks can be divided into semi-active and fully active robotic paradigms [61]. The former uses haptic inputs that allow the surgeon to retain control of instrument placement, while the latter allows the robot to perform a task independently, with the surgeon taking on a task-setting and supervisory role [61]. At present, these systems are useful for the reconstructive aspects of orthopedic oncology—from accurate placement of arthroplasty implants, safe screw placement, and even guiding intramedullary nail stabilization of long bones. However, there has been almost no utilization of these systems for guidance of the resection.

4 Techniques for Image-Guided Brain Tumor Surgery: The Perspectives in Human and Veterinary Patients

While preoperative neuroimaging techniques, such as MRI and CT, have greatly facilitated the surgical management of central nervous system cancers by providing excellent macroscopic localization of lesions identified for biopsy or resection, veterinary surgeons are still faced with a lack of practical and economical, real-time, image-based intraoperative feedback that can guide successful completion of procedures [62]. Neurosurgeons have traditionally employed subjective and experientially biased criteria, such as visual or textural differences to discriminate neoplastic from normal tissues, which can result in undesirable outcomes such as subtotal tumor resection or unintentional removal of normal brain tissue [62, 63]. In addition, the neurosurgeon is continually and further challenged by the dynamic visual appearances, tactile features, and locations of brain structures due to loss of cerebrospinal fluid, presence of edema, and removal of abnormal tissue, which can all contribute to brain shift that occurs during the course of an operation.

In human neuro-oncology, numerous techniques to improve the safety and accuracy of brain biopsy procedures and to optimize brain tumor resection have been developed including neuronavigation systems (NNS), intraoperative MRI (iMRI), intraoperative ultrasound (iUS), intraoperative Raman spectroscopy (RS), and fluorescent imaging (FLI) [64]. Several of these methods have been evaluated in dogs and cats with brain tumors. However, as no studies in veterinary medicine have systematically or objectively (i.e., based on early postoperative imaging assessments) reported on the incidence of residual tumor following conventional brain tumor resection nor on the influence of the extent of resection (EOR) on the prognosis of any type or grade of brain tumor, it is difficult to currently define the utility or roles of these techniques in veterinary neuro-oncology [65]. However, given the frequency with which brain tumor recurrences are identified within the operative field, it is clear that there is a need for techniques that can facilitate complete brain tumor resections in dogs and cats [62, 65]. As has been emerging with more widespread use in humans, these modalities may eventually be shown to improve veterinary patient outcomes through more complete initial tumor resections, reducing surgical complications, and streamlining operating room workflows and efficiency [64].

4.1 Neuronavigation Systems (NNS)

NNS refer to a group of computer-assisted technologies that incorporate traditional principles of stereotactic neurosurgery to integrate preoperative imaging (usually MRI or CT) data to generate patient-specific 3D neuroanatomic imaging atlases (image space) [66, 67]. Through the use of fiducials incorporated into preoperative images and surgical instrumentation and an intraoperative optical or electromagnetic tracking system, NNS create a translatable virtual map between image space, the actual spatial position of the patient's head in the operating theater (anatomic space) and any registered calibrated surgical instrumentation, thus allowing real-time viewing of coregistered and fused imaging, patient anatomic, and instrument positional data in any plane [67]. NNS allow the neurosurgeon to precisely identify surgical targets, plan, and monitor surgical approaches and manipulations. NNS platforms can also integrate advanced imaging datasets such as diffusion tensor imaging, fiber tracking, and MR-spectroscopy and be used with other technologies such as intraoperative microscopy, FLI, or tissue resection devices that assist the neurosurgeon [68].

Detailed workflows for the use of both framed and frameless NNS in veterinary neurosurgery have been described elsewhere [67–70]. NNS are being utilized in veterinary neuro-oncology practice for both diagnostic and therapeutic procedures, and the positional accuracies of NNS for brain biopsy in dogs are reported to range from 0.5 to 3 mm, which are on par with frame-based stereotactic systems [67–71]. Major challenges associated with the use of NNS for tumor resection are their reliance on preoperative imaging for registration and thus navigational accuracy. Intraoperative brain shift that inevitably occurs during tumor resection or brain parenchymal manipulations significantly reduces the navigational accuracy of NNS, and thus, NNS cannot be solely relied upon to guide tumor resection [68]. Additional postoperative imaging is also required to evaluate the EOR, or other objective measure of surgical success, following the use of NNS.

4.2 Intraoperative MRI (iMRI)

Given the negative impact that brain shift introduces into NNS or other procedures that rely on preoperative image sets to guide surgery, use of iMRI has been incorporated into the workflow of some neurosurgical indications in humans [72]. Operative theaters that utilize iMRI can be configured with scanners contained within the operating theater, or in a specialized imaging room adjacent to the surgical suite. Use of iMRI allows near real-time assessment of the extent of tumor resection and evaluation of surgical manipulations on neighboring critical structures, allowing modifications to treatment to be easily and readily incorporated into the operation. In humans, utilization of iMRI has demonstrated significant improvements in EOR, quality of life, and survival in glioma patients [72]. Despite advantages of iMRI being demonstrated for some indications in human neuro-oncology, this technology is associated with several notable disadvantages that will likely limit its incorporation into veterinary clinical practice in the immediate future. The physical plant, equipment, and personnel requirements necessary to operate and maintain integrated iMRI operating theaters are substantially higher than standalone imaging or surgical suites, as are initial hardware installation costs. In humans, neurosurgical procedures utilizing iMRI guidance have also been shown to take significantly longer than conventional or NNS procedures, which translates into higher procedural fees.

4.3 Intraoperative Ultrasound (iUS)

iUS offers the distinct advantages of not exposing the patient or surgical team to ionizing radiation and compared to other intraoperative imaging techniques, is relatively economical and readily available. When applied during open intracranial procedures, iUS performed with 5 to 8 MHz transducers has been used to identify the appearance, position, and margination of brain tumors relative to the craniectomy defect and surrounding normal tissues, and to subsequently aid in determining the extent of resection (Fig. 1) [73]. iUS imaging data is acquired rapidly and in real time, can be repeated as necessary without significantly impeding operative workflows, and images can be readily visualized in 2D or 3D depending on system capabilities [73]. The iUS imaging characteristics of tissues are heavily dependent on the frequency and incident angle of the ultrasound waves, and challenges can be encountered acquiring and interpreting iUS images, especially at the limits of craniectomy defects due to beam attenuation and shadowing, as well as comparing iUS images to preoperative MRI or CT scans. The use of 3D iUS can assist in the interpretation of multi-modality imaging by generating a volumetric image that is viewable in any plane, which facilitates registration with MRI or CT images. It is also possible to integrate iUS into neuronavigational platforms such that iUS images can be visualized contemporaneously with corresponding preoperative MRI or CT datasets [74]. Disadvantages of iUS include heavily operator-dependent image quality and low-image resolution which can restrict iUS utility for deep intraparenchymal tumors.

4.4 Raman Spectroscopy (RS)

Raman spectroscopy is an optical-based technology that provides information about the molecular characteristics of tissues by applying incident light and assessing changes in vibrational frequencies in chemical bonds resulting from the inelastic scattering of that light [14]. Each tissue has a vibrational spectral signature due to the concentrations of nucleic acids, lipids, and proteins it contains, and different vibrational signatures can be detected and compared to distinguish different types of tissues (i.e., white vs. gray matter or normal vs. neoplastic brain tissue) [14]. Intra-operative Raman detection systems consist of handheld transducers, similar in size to ultrasound probes, which contain a miniaturized fiber-coupled Raman spectrometer and operate in real time [14, 15]. Raman spectroscopy is also advantageous in that it is capable of providing real-time

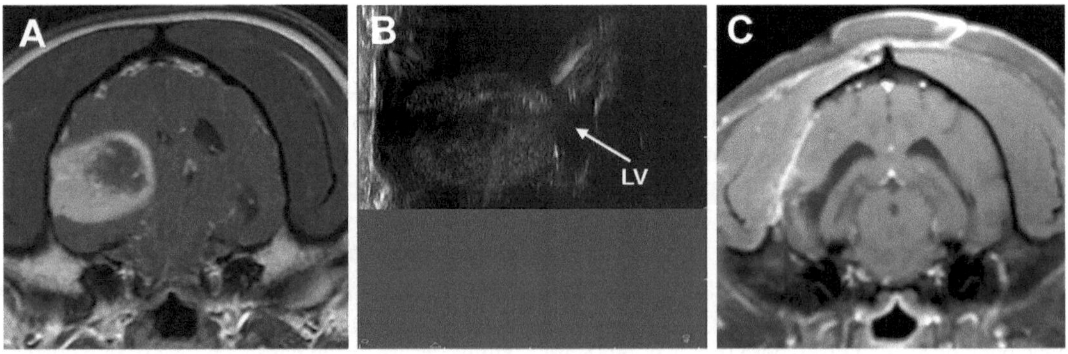

Fig. 1 Intraoperative ultrasound-guided resection of canine cerebral convexity meningioma encroaching the lateral ventricle (LV). (**a**) Preoperative T1W post-contrast MRI with heterogeneously contrast-enhancing tumor in the temporal lobe attenuating the LV. (**b**) Intraoperative ultrasound delineating hyperechoic, ovoid tumor, and temporal horn of the LV (arrow) deep to the mass. (**c**) Postoperative T1W post-contrast MRI illustrating complete tumor resection

imaging without exposing operating room staff to ionizing radiation. Intraoperative RS has been shown to be feasible in dogs with brain tumors, with an 85% sensitivity and 90% specificity for differentiating neoplastic from normal brain tissue [15]. In humans, RS has been used to successfully detect diffusely invasive brain cancer cells in patients with high-grade gliomas [16]. However, given the tissue heterogeneities present within and between brain tumors, as well as in adjacent tissues with microscopic tumor invasion, discrimination between cancerous and noncancerous tissue based on small differences in spectral shifts may ultimately require the use of machine-learning models [14, 16].

4.5 Fluorescent Imaging (FLI)

Although in vivo fluorescent imaging was first used in human brain tumors in 1948, it was not until the early part of the next century that intraoperative FLI techniques were further explored, developed, and widely utilized [75]. Intraoperative FLI using the near-infrared (NIR) fluorescent spectra has subsequently reemerged as a powerful tool that provides surgeons with real-time information about the location and margination of tumors, thus facilitating tumor resection. Advantages of NIR-FLI that have been demonstrated in human neuro-oncologic indications include a high sensitivity, lower cost, and relative ease of incorporation of detection instrumentation into existing surgical technological platforms and workflows compared to other intraoperative imaging modalities [76]. However, all FLI approaches currently used in the clinic share important limitations with respect to resolution, quantification, depth of penetration, and tumor specificity.

All FLI approaches that are routinely utilized in human neurosurgery involve the systemic administration of exogenous agents that are either fluorescent in the visible or NIR electromagnetic spectra (fluorescein [FS] and indocyanine green [ICG]), or pro-drugs that are metabolized into fluorophores within neoplastic tissue (5-aminolevulinic acid; 5-ALA). These biochemical agents can be visualized in the operative field using white light, modified surgical microscopes with special filters or fluorescent excitation/detection channels, in vivo fluorescence microscopy, or handheld spectrophotometric instruments [77]. In neuro-oncology, FS, ICG, and 5-ALA have been investigated the most extensively, and each of these agents is FDA-approved for use in humans.

Fluorescein Sodium FS is a small organic salt with a molecular weight of 376 that has been used extensively for retinal angiography as well as for FLI-guided resection of gliomas, meningiomas, and brain metastases in humans and dogs [77, 78]. FS accumulates within tumors in regions of blood-brain barrier (BBB) disruption, is excited at 460–500 nm, and emits a yellow-green fluorescent emission at 540–690 nm wavelength. Intraoperative visualization of FS within tumors is similar to contrast-enhancing areas of tumors evident in preoperative gadolinium-enhanced T1W MR images (Fig. 2) [78]. While FS can be visualized under white light (Fig. 2), the use of an operating microscope with a dedicated filter can intensify regions of fluorescence with lower systemic SF doses. Although the optimal timing and dose of FS to administer to maximize tumor fluorescence is not known, it is typically administered IV 30–90 minutes before the planned tumor resection at doses ranging from 1 to 20 mg/kg (Table 1) [77, 78]. The FS-guided resection technique is advantageous because it is safe, easy to perform, and can be utilized in an operating room with no need for extra surgical equipment. Disadvantages of FS include lack of specificity for tumors, with areas of the brain lacking BBB (dura, choroid plexus) also demonstrating intense fluorescence.

Indocyanine Green Indocyanine green (ICG), described in prior sections of this chapter, has been used extensively in medicine for liver and cardiac functional studies, as well as in neurosurgical procedures requiring blood flow monitoring, such as resection of arteriovenous malformations and aneurysm treatment. As ICG

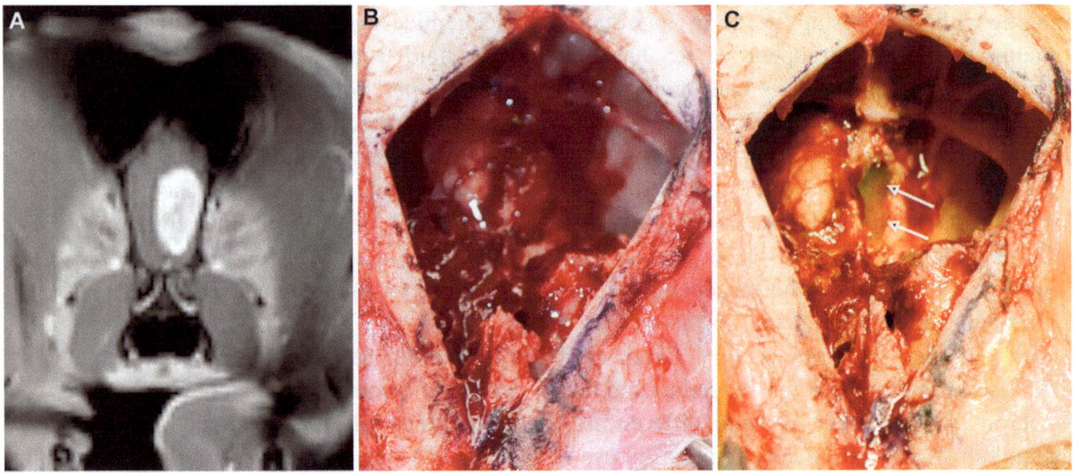

Fig. 2 Fluorescein sodium (FS)-guided resection of canine olfactory meningioma. (**a**) Preoperative T1W post-contrast MRI with homogenously contrast-enhancing tumor in the olfactory region. (**b**) Intraoperative view of the tumor exposed via a transfrontal craniotomy prior to administration of FS. (**c**) Following the administration of FS, the tumor demonstrates yellow-green fluorescence under white light (arrows), with fluorescence correlating with gadolinium enhancement observed on MRI

Table 1 Summary of fluorophores used for FLI-guided brain tumor surgery

Agent	Administration route	Dose (mg/kg)	$T_{1/2}$ (mins)	Time to tumor visualization	Excitation (nm)	Emission (nm)	Duration of fluorescence in target tissue
Fluorescein sodium	IV	1–20	25	30 min–4 h	460–500	540–690	2–4 h
Indocyanine green	IV	0.2–5	3–5	< 1 min	780	700–850	5–10 min
Second window ICG	IV	2–5		24 h			72 h
5-ALA	PO	20	60–180	2–8 h	375–440	640–710	20–24 h

Data derived from humans

is highly protein bound and remains confined within the vasculature following administrations, it is also a passive tumor-targeting agent that accumulates within brain tumors in regions of BBB breakdown [76, 77]. ICG is a NIR fluorophore (Table 1), which affords the advantages of higher resolution imaging with increasing tissue penetration depths and an excellent signal-to-noise ratio (SNR) [77].

ICG has a short half-life (3–5 minutes) and is rapidly cleared from the bloodstream. For intraoperative use in humans, it is delivered at doses of <0.5 mg/kg as an IV bolus immediately prior to the period in which the neurosurgeon requires NIR imaging as tumor fluorescence is only visible for 5–10 minutes using this technique, which limits its intraoperative utility. A second window ICG (SWICG) technique, in which the higher doses of ICG are injected (2–5 mg/kg) and intraoperative NIR imaging employed 24 hours after ICG administration, has been described to overcome this limitation [79]. In humans with gliomas, the SWICG signal correlates with the degree of gadolinium enhancement on MRI and also provides practical and sensitive means of intraoperative delineation of tumors [77, 79]. Currently, there are no reports of the use of ICG in veterinary neuro-oncology.

5-Aminolevulinic Acid 5-ALA is a naturally occurring precursor metabolized in the heme biosynthetic pathway, which is present in all mammalian cells, to protoporphyrin (PpIX). It is typical that neoplastic cells produce more PpIX, and significantly higher PpIX has been found in human and rodent models of brain tumors compared to normal brain tissues [76, 77]. Administration of exogenous 5-ALA to patients with brain tumors leverages this difference in tissue PpIX production, resulting in high intratumoral concentrations of PpIX that are detectable using intraoperative fluorescent microscopy. PpIX absorbs light between 375 and 440 nm and emits a violet-red fluorescence at 640–710 nm (Table 1) [77].

A randomized controlled multicenter phase III trial showed that humans with high-grade gliomas who underwent surgery using 5-ALA guidance had significantly improved tumor resections and 6-month progression-free survival rates than patients who underwent conventional surgery under white light conditions [76]. Due to the success of 5-ALA as a tumor margin demarcation tool in neurosurgical resection of human gliomas, a large body of research on ALA-induced PpIX fluorescence of brain tumors currently exists, and 5-ALA is currently the only FLI agent approved by the FDA specifically for the resection of brain tumors [76, 77].

The human experience has identified limitations of using 5-ALA for brain tumor resections, some of which have been observed in pilot studies in dogs [76, 77]. A substantial percentage of low-grade (>90%) gliomas will not demonstrate fluorescence after standard dosing of 5-ALA, and delineation of tumor margins can be complicated by non-specific and vague peritumoral fluorescence, which can occur in edematous or necrotic tissues. There are also practical considerations which may limit the utility of 5-ALA in companion animals, including the expense and availability of the agent, the requirement for relatively large volume oral dosing in close proximity to anesthetic induction time (and subsequent risk of aspiration), and the potential for phototoxicity in patients. To date, the use of 5-ALA in veterinary neurosurgery has not been rigorously studied.

5 Conclusion

Continued advances in imaging and image-guided surgery will improve the diagnosis, staging, and treatment of veterinary and human cancer patients. The phenotypic similarities of cancers such as sarcomas and brain tumors shared by dogs and humans, together with the physical size of the dog, provide opportunities to utilize the pet dog with spontaneously occurring cancers to advance the development of cancer imaging and image-guided surgery for animals and humans.

References

1. Fenger JM, London CA, Kisseberth WC (2014) Canine osteosarcoma: a naturally occurring disease to inform pediatric oncology. ILAR J 55:69–85
2. Bray JP (2016) Soft tissue sarcoma in the dog - part 1: a current review. J Small Anim Pract 57:510–519
3. Crooks C, Randall E, Griffin L (2021) The use of fluorine-18-fluorodeoxyglucose-positron emission tomography/computed tomography as an effective method for staging in dogs with primary appendicular osteosarcoma. Vet Radiol Ultrasound 62:350–359
4. Griffin LR, Thamm DH, Brody A, Selmic LE (2019) Prognostic value of fluorine(18) flourodeoxyglucose positron emission tomography/computed tomography in dogs with appendicular osteosarcoma. J Vet Intern Med 33:820–826
5. Brody A, Crooks JC, French JM et al (2022) Staging canine patients with appendicular osteosarcoma utilizing fluorine-18 fluorodeoxyglucose positron emission tomography/computed tomography compared to whole body computed tomography. Vet Comp Oncol 20:541–550
6. Slinkard PT, Randall EK, Griffin LR (2021) Retrospective analysis of use of fluorine-18 fluorodeoxyglucose-positron emission tomography/computed tomography ((18)F-FDG PET/CT) for detection of metastatic lymph nodes in dogs diagnosed with appendicular osteosarcoma. Can J Vet Res 85:131–136
7. Oh C, Bishop MW, Cho SY et al (2023) (18)F-FDG PET/CT in the Management of Osteosarcoma. J Nucl Med 64:842–851
8. Davis GJ, Kapatkin AS, Craig LE et al (2002) Comparison of radiography, computed tomography,

and magnetic resonance imaging for evaluation of appendicular osteosarcoma in dogs. J Am Vet Med Assoc 220:1171–1176
9. Karnik KS, Samii VF, Weisbrode SE et al (2012) Accuracy of computed tomography in determining lesion size in canine appendicular osteosarcoma. Vet Radiol Ultrasound 53:273–279
10. Wallack ST, Wisner ER, Werner JA et al (2002) Accuracy of magnetic resonance imaging for estimating intramedullary osteosarcoma extent in preoperative planning of canine limb-salvage procedures. Vet Radiol Ultrasound 43:432–441
11. Seguin B, Pinard C, Lussier B et al (2020) Limb-sparing in dogs using patient-specific, three-dimensional-printed endoprosthesis for distal radial osteosarcoma: a pilot study. Vet Comp Oncol 18:92–104
12. Timercan A, Brailovski V, Petit Y et al (2019) Personalized 3D-printed endoprostheses for limb sparing in dogs: modeling and in vitro testing. Med Eng Phys 71:17–29
13. Llido M, Le Bras LA, Brailovski V et al (2023) Muscular morphometric study of the canine shoulder for the design of 3D-printed endoprostheses in dogs with osteosarcoma of the proximal humerus: a pilot cadaveric study by MRI. Am J Vet Res 84
14. Winer JN, Verstraete FJM, Cissell DD et al (2017) The application of 3-dimensional printing for preoperative planning in oral and maxillofacial surgery in dogs and cats. Vet Surg 46:942–951
15. Altwal J, Wilson CH, Griffon DJ (2022) Applications of 3-dimensional printing in small-animal surgery: a review of current practices. Vet Surg 51:34–51
16. Huang YH, Lee B, Chuy JA, Goldschmidt SL (2022) 3D printing for surgical planning of canine oral and maxillofacial surgeries. 3D Print Med 8:17
17. Bray JP (2017) Soft tissue sarcoma in the dog - part 2: surgical margins, controversies and a comparative review. J Small Anim Pract 58:63–72
18. Culp WCEN (2022) Principles of surgical oncology. In: Seguin BKS (ed) Veterinary surgical oncology, 2nd edn. Wiley, pp 1–16
19. Orosco RK, Tapia VJ, Califano JA et al (2018) Positive surgical margins in the 10 Most common solid cancers. Sci Rep 8:5686
20. Bui MM, Smith P, Agresta SV et al (2008) Practical issues of intraoperative frozen section diagnosis of bone and soft tissue lesions. Cancer Control 15:7–12
21. Bartholf DeWitt S, Eward WC, Eward CA et al (2016) A novel imaging system distinguishes neoplastic from Normal tissue during resection of soft tissue sarcomas and mast cell tumors in dogs. Vet Surg 45:715–722
22. Eward WC, Mito JK, Eward CA et al (2013) A novel imaging system permits real-time in vivo tumor bed assessment after resection of naturally occurring sarcomas in dogs. Clin Orthop Relat Res 471:834–842
23. Mito JK, Ferrer JM, Brigman BE et al (2012) Intraoperative detection and removal of microscopic residual sarcoma using wide-field imaging. Cancer 118:5320–5330
24. Whitley MJ, Cardona DM, Lazarides AL et al (2016) A mouse-human phase 1 co-clinical trial of a protease-activated fluorescent probe for imaging cancer. Sci Transl Med 8:320ra324
25. Fidel J, Kennedy KC, Dernell WS et al (2015) Preclinical validation of the utility of BLZ-100 in providing fluorescence contrast for imaging spontaneous solid tumors. Cancer Res 75:4283–4291
26. Huang Y, Jia M, Yang X et al (2022) Annexin A2: the diversity of pathological effects in tumorigenesis and immune response. Int J Cancer 151:497–509
27. Favril S, Brioschi C, Vanderperren K et al (2020) Preliminary safety and imaging efficacy of the near-infrared fluorescent contrast agent DA364 during fluorescence-guided surgery in dogs with spontaneous superficial tumors. Oncotarget 11:2310–2326
28. Holt D, Parthasarathy AB, Okusanya O et al (2015) Intraoperative near-infrared fluorescence imaging and spectroscopy identifies residual tumor cells in wounds. J Biomed Opt 20:76002
29. Holt D, Okusanya O, Judy R et al (2014) Intraoperative near-infrared imaging can distinguish cancer from normal tissue but not inflammation. PLoS One 9:e103342
30. Cabon Q, Sayag D, Texier I et al (2016) Evaluation of intraoperative fluorescence imaging-guided surgery in cancer-bearing dogs: a prospective proof-of-concept phase II study in 9 cases. Transl Res 170:73–88
31. Mesa KJ, Selmic LE, Pande P et al (2017) Intraoperative optical coherence tomography for soft tissue sarcoma differentiation and margin identification. Lasers Surg Med 49:240–248
32. Selmic LE, Samuelson J, Reagan JK et al (2019) Intra-operative imaging of surgical margins of canine soft tissue sarcoma using optical coherence tomography. Vet Comp Oncol 17:80–88
33. Ye Y, Sun WW, Xu RX et al (2021) Intraoperative assessment of canine soft tissue sarcoma by deep learning enhanced optical coherence tomography. Vet Comp Oncol 19:624–631
34. Cendan JC, Coco D, Copeland EM 3rd. (2005) Accuracy of intraoperative frozen-section analysis of breast cancer lumpectomy-bed margins. J Am Coll Surg 201:194–198
35. Wong H, Tarr GP, Anand R et al (2023) Diagnostic yield and concordance of image-guided biopsy in musculoskeletal lesions. Skeletal Radiol 53:75
36. Sanchez-Diaz M, Martinez-Lopez A, Montero-Vilchez T, Arias-Santiago S (2022) Ultrasonography as a novel technique for intraoperative delimitation of dermatofibrosarcoma protuberans. Dermatologic Surg 48:575–577
37. Mesko NW, Joyce DM, Ilaslan H, Joyce MJ (2016) Creating an intraoperative MRI suite for the musculoskeletal tumor center. Clin Orthop Relat Res 474:1516–1522
38. Cacciamani GE, Okhunov Z, Meneses AD et al (2019) Impact of three-dimensional printing in urology: state of the art and future perspectives. A systematic review by ESUT-YAUWP group. Eur Urol 76:209–221

39. Emile SH, Wexner SD (2019) Systematic review of the applications of three-dimensional printing in colorectal surgery. Color Dis 21:261–269
40. Xu J, Tian Y, Yin J et al (2019) Utility of three-dimensional printing in preoperative planning for children with anomalous pulmonary venous connection: a single center experience. Quant Imaging Med Surg 9:1804–1814
41. Yang L, Grottkau B, He Z, Ye C (2017) Three dimensional printing technology and materials for treatment of elbow fractures. Int Orthop 41:2381–2387
42. Li L, Zhang K, Wang R et al (2021) A study of three-dimensional reconstruction and printing models in two cases of soft tissue sarcoma of the thigh. Int J Comput Assist Radiol Surg 16:1627–1636
43. Lazarides AL, Whitley MJ, Strasfeld DB et al (2016) A fluorescence-guided laser ablation system for removal of residual cancer in a mouse model of soft tissue sarcoma. Theranostics 6:155–166
44. Keereweer S, Van Driel PB, Snoeks TJ et al (2013) Optical image-guided cancer surgery: challenges and limitations. Clin Cancer Res 19:3745–3754
45. Visgauss JD, Eward WC, Brigman BE (2016) Innovations in intraoperative tumor visualization. Orthop Clin North Am 47:253–264
46. Wilke LG, Brown JQ, Bydlon TM et al (2009) Rapid noninvasive optical imaging of tissue composition in breast tumor margins. Am J Surg 198:566–574
47. Gong MF, Li WT, Bhogal S et al (2023) Intraoperative evaluation of soft tissue sarcoma surgical margins with Indocyanine green fluorescence imaging. Cancers (Basel) 15:15
48. Liu J, Guo W, Tong M (2016) Intraoperative indocyanine green fluorescence guidance for excision of nonpalpable breast cancer. World J Surg Oncol 14:266
49. Alander JT, Kaartinen I, Laakso A et al (2012) A review of indocyanine green fluorescent imaging in surgery. Int J Biomed Imag 2012:940585
50. Okusanya OT, Holt D, Heitjan D et al (2014) Intraoperative near-infrared imaging can identify pulmonary nodules. Ann Thorac Surg 98:1223–1230
51. Lazarides AL, Saltzman EB, Visgauss JD et al (2022) Intraoperative angiography imaging correlates with wound complications following soft tissue sarcoma resection. J Orthop Res 40:2382–2390
52. Anderson KC, Buehler KC, Markel DC (2005) Computer assisted navigation in total knee arthroplasty: comparison with conventional methods. J Arthroplast 20:132–138
53. Grutzner PA, Suhm N (2004) Computer aided long bone fracture treatment. Injury 35(Suppl 1):S-A57-64
54. Amiot LP, Lang K, Putzier M et al (1976) Comparative results between conventional and computer-assisted pedicle screw installation in the thoracic, lumbar, and sacral spine. Spine (Phila Pa) 2000(25):606–614
55. Cho HS, Oh JH, Han I, Kim HS (2012) The outcomes of navigation-assisted bone tumour surgery: minimum three-year follow-up. J Bone Joint Surg Br 94:1414–1420
56. Staats K, Panotopoulos J, Tiefenboeck TM et al (2017) Computer navigation-assisted surgery for musculoskeletal tumors: a closer look into the learning curve. Eur J Orthop Surg Traumatol 27:851–858
57. Jeys L, Matharu GS, Nandra RS, Grimer RJ (2013) Can computer navigation-assisted surgery reduce the risk of an intralesional margin and reduce the rate of local recurrence in patients with a tumour of the pelvis or sacrum? Bone Joint J 95-B:1417–1424
58. Benady A, Gortzak Y, Sofer S et al (2022) Internal Hemipelvectomy for primary bone sarcomas using intraoperative patient specific instruments- the next step in limb salvage concept. BMC Musculoskelet Disord 23:1012
59. Mustahsan VM, He G, Helguero CG et al (2023) Novel positioning feedback system as a guidance in bone tumor resection. Surg Innov 30:126–129
60. He G, Dai AZ, Mustahsan VM et al (2022) A novel intraoperative method to project osteotomy lines for accurate resection of primary bone sarcomas. J Orthop 32:60–67
61. Fan X, Zhu Q, Tu P et al (2023) A review of advances in image-guided orthopedic surgery. Phys Med Biol 68:02TR01
62. Miller AD, Miller CR, Rossmeisl JH (2019) Canine primary intracranial cancer: a Clinicopathologic and comparative review of glioma, meningioma, and choroid plexus tumors. Front Oncol 9:1151
63. Rosenthal EL, Warram JM, Bland KI, Zinn KR (2015) The status of contemporary image-guided modalities in oncologic surgery. Ann Surg 261:46–55
64. Schipmann-Miletic S, Stummer W (2020) Image-guided brain surgery. Recent Results Cancer Res 216:813–841
65. Rossmeisl JH Jr, Garcia PA, Daniel GB et al (2014) Invited review–neuroimaging response assessment criteria for brain tumors in veterinary patients. Vet Radiol Ultrasound 55:115–132
66. Rossmeisl JH (2014) New treatment modalities for brain tumors in dogs and cats. Vet Clin North Am Small Anim Pract 44:1013–1038
67. Wininger F (2014) Neuronavigation in small animals: development, techniques, and applications. Vet Clin North Am Small Anim Pract 44:1235–1248
68. Packer RA, McGrath S (2020) Onscreen-guided resection of extra-axial and intra-axial forebrain masses through registration of a variable-suction tissue resection device with a neuronavigation system. Vet Surg 49:676–684
69. Chen AV, Wininger FA, Frey S et al (2012) Description and validation of a magnetic resonance imaging-guided stereotactic brain biopsy device in the dog. Vet Radiol Ultrasound 53:150–156
70. Gutmann S, Tastensen C, Bottcher IC et al (2022) Clinical use of a new frameless optical neuronavigation system for brain biopsies: 10 cases (2013-2020). J Small Anim Pract 63:468–481
71. Rossmeisl JH, Andriani RT, Cecere TE et al (2015) Frame-based stereotactic biopsy of canine brain

masses: technique and clinical results in 26 cases. Front Vet Sci 2:20
72. Hlavac M, Wirtz CR, Halatsch ME (2017) Intraoperative magnetic resonance imaging. HNO 65:25–29
73. Shores A, Lee AM, Kornberg ST et al (2021) Intraoperative ultrasound applications in intracranial surgery. Front Vet Sci 8:725867
74. Prada F, Del Bene M, Mattei L et al (2015) Preoperative magnetic resonance and intraoperative ultrasound fusion imaging for real-time neuronavigation in brain tumor surgery. Ultraschall Med 36:174–186
75. Moore GE, Peyton WT et al (1948) The clinical use of fluorescein in neurosurgery; the localization of brain tumors. J Neurosurg 5:392–398
76. Jenkinson MD, Barone DG, Bryant A et al (2018) Intraoperative imaging technology to maximise extent of resection for glioma. Cochrane Database Syst Rev 1:CD012788
77. Nagaya T, Nakamura YA, Choyke PL, Kobayashi H (2017) Fluorescence-guided surgery. *Front.* Oncologia 7:314
78. Nakano Y, Nakata K, Shibata S et al (2018) Fluorescein sodium-guided resection of intracranial lesions in 22 dogs. Vet Surg 47:302–309
79. Zeh R, Sheiksh S, Xia L et al (2017) The second window ICG technique demonstrates a broad plateau period for near infrared fluorescence tumor contrast in glioblastoma. PLoS One 12:e0182034

Comparative Oncology by Tumor Type

Osteosarcoma

Camille A. McAloney, Timothy M. Fan, and Ryan D. Roberts

1 Human Disease

Osteosarcoma is a malignant tumor that arises from multipotent mesenchymal cells with osteoblastic differentiation; these cells produce mineralized bone and/or osteoid [1–3]. Cartilage, cartilage matrix, and fibrous tissue may also be produced by the neoplastic cells [1]. Based on the predominant matrix observed on histology, tumors are subdivided into chondroblastic, fibroblastic, osteoblastic, and telangiectatic types [3]. Tumors can be further subdivided into low-, intermediate-, and high-grade types, with higher grades generally indicating greater risk of metastasis [3].

Osteosarcoma is the most common primary tumor of bone, but is relatively rare, with approximately 1,000 new cases reported each year in the United States [4–7]. This incidence is similar to rates seen in Europe and Asia; however, some countries in South America and Africa have reported higher incidence [8–10]. Despite its rarity, because osteosarcoma predominantly affects children and adolescents, it is linked to many lost years of life and productivity [11]. It has a bimodal incidence, with the first peak in incidence occurring in adolescents and young adults, and the second, smaller peak occurring in individuals over 60 years of age [8, 12].

In adolescents and young adults, the most common site of primary tumor occurrence is the distal femur, followed by the proximal tibia and the proximal humerus, although osteosarcoma may arise in any bone [7, 13]. Most tumors occur within or near growth plates during or shortly after periods of rapid growth, suggesting a link between the mechanisms of bone growth and malignant transformation [13]. Height is also a known risk factor for osteosarcoma [14]. Indeed, female patients have an earlier average age of osteosarcoma diagnosis than males, which is consistent with earlier onset of puberty and growth typically seen in young women [8, 13]. Approximately 18–28% of all patients with osteosarcoma have germline mutations predisposing to cancer development, and these mutations are more common in younger patients [15, 16]. In older patients, bone dysplasias such as Paget's disease of bone and radiation exposure are among the risk factors associated with osteosarcoma development [3, 8, 12, 17]. Tumors occur more commonly in the axial skeleton and

C. A. McAloney (✉)
Charles River Laboratories, Mattawan, MI, USA

T. M. Fan
Department of Veterinary Clinical Medicine, Cancer Center at Illinois, University of Illinois at Urbana-Champaign, Urbana, IL, USA

R. D. Roberts
Abigail Wexner Research Institute, Nationwide Children's Hospital and The James Comprehensive Cancer Institute, The Ohio State University, Columbus, OH, USA

M. W. Nolan et al. (eds.), *Comparative Oncology*, https://doi.org/10.1007/978-3-032-04454-9_9

craniofacial bones in older patients than in adolescents [18].

On a cellular level, the ubiquity of TP53 inactivations and/or MDM2/4 amplifications in osteosarcoma tumors suggests that these are likely oncogenic drivers [19, 20]. The functional silencing of TP53 may enable chromothripsis and other massive chromosomal abnormalities, ultimately resulting in the chaotic genome for which osteosarcoma is known [19, 21]. These catastrophic genetic changes are thought by some to occur within a single cell cycle; however, this remains an area of active discussion and investigation [20, 22]. As a consequence of its marked structural variation, osteosarcoma is known for alterations in the somatic copy numbers of genes [23]. Genes that are frequently amplified include MYC, VEGFA, and CCNE1, while PTEN and CDKN2A/B are frequently deleted [3, 23]. These copy number alterations are thought to be the primary drivers of osteosarcoma; only moderate numbers of point mutations (most often in TP53 and RB1 genes) have been found in large-scale sequencing efforts [23–27].

Osteosarcoma metastasizes almost exclusively to the lungs, with a minority of metastases occurring in bone or local sites [7]. Despite this tropism, once disseminated tumor cells reach the lungs, only a small fraction survive. Indeed, lung colonization is the most inefficient and narrowest point of the metastatic bottleneck [28, 29]. Furthermore, clonal selection occurs when osteosarcoma cells colonize the lung, implying that some cells are fundamentally better suited to metastasis and pulmonary survival than others and/or some cells become more rapidly proliferative once in the lung [30]. Interestingly, despite the selection of the metastatic bottleneck, experimental models have shown that the degree of transcriptional heterogeneity is comparable between primary and metastatic tumors, and perhaps metastatic fitness could be more likely influenced by differences in clonal mRNA translational efficiency [30, 31]. Metastatic disease can behave differently from primary tumors even within the same patient, such as exhibiting resistance to traditional chemotherapeutics and expressing more antiapoptotic proteins [7, 32].

Patients who present with localized disease have a 5-year survival rate of approximately 70% [19, 33–36]. Treatment involves surgical resection of the primary tumor, with efforts made to preserve limb function while achieving complete resection [37]. Prostheses, bone grafts, and expandable implants may all be used to this end [38, 39]. Amputation is still performed when necessary to achieve complete tumor resection or when the functional outcomes of limb-sparing surgery and amputation are predicted to be similar, and the risks of limb-sparing surgery are high [3]. Chemotherapy is given neoadjuvantly and consists of high-dose *m*ethotrexate with leukovorin rescue, doxorubicin (*A*driamycin), and cis*p*latin (“MAP” chemotherapy) [13, 19, 40–42]. Ifosfamide is sometimes added to this combination [7, 13, 19, 40, 42]. When surgical resection of the primary tumor is not possible or would lead to unacceptable morbidity (as in tumors of the pelvis or cranio-facial bones), radiation may be considered for local control [3]. Long-term local control of inoperable osteosarcoma of the pelvis and trunk with ionizing radiation has been shown to be 62% and 67%, respectively [43, 44].

When patients present with disseminated disease, long-term survival is approximately 20% [7, 45]. When possible, the first-line treatment for recurrent or metastatic osteosarcoma is surgical resection, as this is associated with improved outcomes [7, 13, 45–49]. When metastases are few in number and able to be completely excised, patients typically fare better [50]. Response rates of 20–50% may be seen in patients with recurrent disease when treated with high-dose ifosfamide (or fractionated cyclophosphamide) with or without etoposide, or gemcitabine and docetaxel, but unresected metastases almost always regrow. Indeed, in the setting of macroscopic disease, none of these therapies have been shown to improve long-term survival [51–56].

The presence or absence of disseminated disease is by far the most impactful prognostic indicator for patients with osteosarcoma [13, 19, 42, 45]. Indeed, it is the only metric by which patients with high-grade lesions are staged [42, 45]. Other prognostic indicators may include tumor size, elevated serum ALP (alkaline phosphatase), location (appendicular vs. axial vs. craniofacial), surgical margins, age of onset, sex, tumor histologic subtype, and other factors [37, 57–59]. A histologic finding of >90% necrosis of the primary tumor at the time of removal has clearly been associated with better prognosis [13]. However, intensifying chemotherapy regimens to induce greater tumor necrosis in patients with poor tumor necrosis to neoadjuvant MAP therapy has not improved outcomes [13, 37, 42, 60–62].

Numerous therapies have been trialed in vitro, in vivo, and in clinical trials. The drug gefitinib has recently been shown to reduce osteosarcoma invasion and metastasis in vitro and in murine models by inhibiting macrophage receptor interacting protein kinase 2 (RIPK2) in macrophages [63, 64]. The drug trabectedin, which is a transcription regulator that also preferentially kills monocytes and macrophages, has shown some promise in preclinical models of osteosarcoma [65–68]. A number of other immunotherapeutics have been investigated, including PD-1/PD-L1 checkpoint inhibitors, chimeric antigen receptor (CAR) T cells, monoclonal antibodies against tumor antigens, targeting or administering cytokines, and others [69–71]. Attempts at targeting tyrosine kinase receptors have seen limited success, with the most promise seen in drugs that affect multiple RTKs [3, 7, 13, 69, 72]. Ultimately, thus far, no experimental treatments have substantively improved long-term outcomes—especially for patients with high-risk disease. However, these studies have provided insight into disease mechanisms and laid groundwork for future trials. As of this writing approximately 200 osteosarcoma clinical trials are ongoing in the United States, and numerous other treatments are undergoing preclinical evaluation [3, 13, 69, 73].

2 Canine Disease

Much like its human counterpart, the cell of origin for osteosarcoma has yet to be definitively determined, but diagnosis of the canine disease also hinges primarily on the production of osteoid, suggesting that it arises in cells with bone-forming potential [74–78]. These cells may also produce fibrous tissue, cartilage, and cartilage matrix. Histologically, tumors can be classified as osteoblastic, chondroblastic, fibroblastic, telangiectatic, giant cell-rich, and poorly differentiated [75–77, 79].

Also as in humans, osteosarcoma is the most common primary tumor of bone in dogs, comprising approximately 80% of all primary bone tumors. It is relatively common, with roughly 10,000 cases of canine osteosarcoma seen in the United States each year [4, 80]. Indeed, this number is likely an underestimation, given that not all cases are reported and there is an absence of an analogous Surveillance, Epidemiology, and End Results Program (SEER) for reporting canine cancer currently [4, 81]. Unlike their human counterparts, the disease arises predominantly in older dogs, with a median age of 7 years, although a small uptick in cases is seen in dogs aged 18–24 months [82].

Large and giant breed dogs as a whole are at greater risk for developing osteosarcoma [80, 82]. These dogs typically present with tumors within or near appendicular growth plates; the most common sites of primary tumor occurrence are the distal radius and proximal humerus [81–83]. Smaller (less than 15 kg) dogs develop osteosarcoma infrequently, but may develop axial osteosarcoma more often; however, tumors may ultimately occur in any bone in any size dog [84]. Different breeds of dogs also carry varying risks of developing osteosarcoma, even when they are of relatively similar size [80, 85]. This overall genetic diversity contained within well-defined breeds has facilitated research into characterizing the genetic susceptibility to osteosarcomagenesis. Leveraging breed genetics, researchers utilized genome-wide analysis to identify 33 genetic loci that contribute to heritable osteosarcoma in Greyhounds, Rottweilers, and Irish Wolfhounds [86]. Additional loci have been identified in Scottish Deerhounds, Leonbergers, and other breeds [87–90]. Recent studies have found that a driving factor of osteosarcoma development in Scottish Deerhounds is likely a heritable trait with dominant expression [89, 90]. Indeed, while dogs are substantially more outbred than laboratory mice, studies have shown that dog breeds can be considered "distinct genetic units" with unique characteristics that incline them toward specific phenotypes, behaviors, and diseases, including osteosarcoma [91, 92]. Despite these breed differences, osteosarcoma tumors frequently show inactivations of TP53 and RB1 [93]. Some studies showed copy number loss of PTEN in 30–42% of tumors evaluated [94, 95]. Copy number loss and gain are common in canine osteosarcoma; it is characterized by a complex genetic landscape with markedly aneuploid karyotypes [93]. This chaotic genome may be enabled by disruption of the TP53 pathway [93, 96].

Canine companion animals that present with localized disease are offered treatment with either definitive or palliative therapies. For definitive treatment, affected dogs typically are treated with surgical resection and chemotherapy, similar to humans. In appendicular osteosarcoma, surgical resection most often consists of amputation of the affected limb [74]. Limb-sparing surgery can be performed; however, this is uncommon given the expense of endoprosthetics and the requirement for an advanced surgical skill set [74]. Chemotherapy is generally administered after surgical resection, and typically consists of — four to six doses of carboplatin, yielding a median survival time of approximately 321 days [74, 97, 98]. Additional chemotherapies used in dogs adjuvantly include classical MAP agents such as doxorubicin and cisplatin. When surgical resection is performed without chemotherapy, the median survival time is approximately 133 days, supporting the notion that systemic chemotherapy can slow the natural course of metastatic progression [99, 100]. In the palliative setting, when tumors are unresectable or a patient has comorbidities such as osteoarthritis or neurologic deficits precluding functional recovery following amputation, radiation therapy may be performed [74]. Several studies support the achievement of non-inferior outcomes in dogs treated palliatively with radiation therapy and systemic therapies compared to conventional definitive treatments with surgical amputation and chemotherapy [101, 102]. Radiation therapy alone or in combination with bisphosphonates may also be used palliatively to reduce cancer bone pain [103, 104].

As in humans, canine osteosarcoma most frequently metastasizes to the lungs, although bone, skin, and visceral organ metastases can occur, but local lymph node involvement has been rarely reported [74, 76]. When patients present with metastatic disease or experience relapse, mean survival time ranges from approximately 49–79 days [74, 105]. Preliminary studies suggest that dogs may benefit from surgical removal of metastases, and this thoracic surgical intervention so commonly practiced in pediatric patients remains an area of active research for affected dogs [105]. Some veterinarians are pioneering thoracoscopy techniques that might allow for metastases to be surgically removed from canine patients with minimal impairment on quality of life [106].

The most impactful prognostic factor in canine osteosarcoma is the presence or absence of metastasis [74, 96]. Other prognostic factors include serum ALP, tumor size, tumor location (axial vs. appendicular, proximal humeral location), postoperative limb-sparing infection, and administration of chemotherapy [74, 75, 96]. Histologic findings such as mitotic index, cellular pleomorphism, and degree of tumor necrosis have been studied as prognostic factors with mixed results [75, 79, 107–111].

Some experimental treatments have resulted in prolonged survival times in canine patients; however, none have accrued sufficient evidence to be used as mainstays of treatment. The earliest of these trials involved the drug mifamurtide (liposome-encapsulated muramyl tripeptide phosphatidylethanolamine; L-MTP-PE), which is thought to work by shifting the patient's monocytes and macrophages to an antitumor state [7]. In canine patients that received amputation and chemotherapy followed by treatment with mifamurtide or empty liposomes, the mifamurtide group had a 47% greater median survival time [112–114]. Along the lines of myeloid targeting to slow metastatic progression, another trial evaluated co-treatment with losartan and toceranib; this combination of drugs was administered to block monocyte recruitment to metastases. Dogs had clinically detectable metastases at the time of enrollment, and treatment in the higher dose group resulted in reduction of metastasis size or clinically meaningful stable disease in 8/16 dogs [115]. As of 2023 researchers are investigating the efficacy of adding defactinib to losartan and toceranib treatment in dogs with metastatic osteosarcoma [116]. Finally, a *Listeria*-based tumor immunotherapy targeting HER2, ADXS31-164 (also known as OST-HER2), received provisional USDA approval in 2022, and studies remain ongoing [117]. In the initial study, the 18 canine patients that received ADXS31-164 had an overall survival of 956 days, more than double the overall survival of historical HER2+ controls (423 days) [118]. A definitive trial in 80 dogs evaluating ADXS31-164 in pet dogs has been completed. Using a similar technology with a lyophilized formulation called canine osteosarcoma vaccine, live Listeria vector (COV-LLV), some dogs treated with this biotherapy strategy have cultured positive for *Listeria* after receiving this treatment, raising safety concerns [119, 120].

3 Comparative Oncology of Osteosarcoma

One of the difficulties facing human osteosarcoma research is the tumor's rarity. It can take years for enough patients to enroll in a study to provide meaningful data: exemplifying this real-world limitation has been the EURAMOS-1 study, which took 6 years to enroll 2,260 patients across 17 countries [42]. This same study calculated that at least 756 patients would be required in order to detect an absolute improvement in event-free survival of 10% (from 45% to 55%) at 80% power—essentially the same number of new osteosarcoma patients in the entire United States per year [4–7, 42, 121].

In contrast, conservative estimates identify canine osteosarcoma occurring at a rate approximately ten times that of human disease, with roughly 10,000 cases of canine osteosarcoma seen in the United States each year [4, 80]. Additionally, because the disease progresses more often and more quickly in dogs, canine clinical trials can be completed on shorter timelines—recent surveys suggest an average of 18 months [4, 42]. These logistical advantages, the fact that canine osteosarcoma shares many genetic, transcriptional, and pathological qualities with human osteosarcoma, and the reduced number of regulatory hurdles associated with canine clinical trials make integrative approaches to drug development in osteosarcoma extremely attractive (Fig. 1) [4, 81, 86, 93, 96, 122–125].

Further advantages of canine osteosarcoma include the fact that it develops and evolves naturally, in the setting of an intact immune system, and undergoes selective pressures similar to human osteosarcoma [2, 126]. Canine osteosarcoma develops in similar locations and follows a similar disease course to human osteosarcoma [2, 75, 93, 96, 126]. Dogs also have high hepatic enzyme homology with humans and have tumor burden and laws of diffusion comparable to humans, both of which are critical when evaluating drug pharmacokinetics/pharmacodynamics and safety [2, 127].

Dogs also offer unique opportunities for engagement with the stewards of their various breeds: dog fanciers and their clubs. Importantly, scientific advancements have been supported through directed philanthropic support toward osteosarcoma research fostered by different organizations, most notably the Morris Animal Foundation and the American Kennel Club Canine Health Foundation. Notably, the Morris Animal Foundation has provided funding support to conduct one of the largest prospective clinical trials seeking to determine if mTOR inhibition can improve the control of metastatic progression, as well as supporting the definitive evaluation of ADXS31-164 in pet dogs with osteosarcoma [128]. In tandem, the American Kennel Club Canine Health Foundation has raised millions of dollars to research a variety of canine diseases—including osteosarcoma—that have resulted in nearly one thousand peer-reviewed publications [129]. Many of the grants provided by this organization are funded through clubs specializing in breeds predisposed to osteosarcoma, such as Greyhounds and Irish

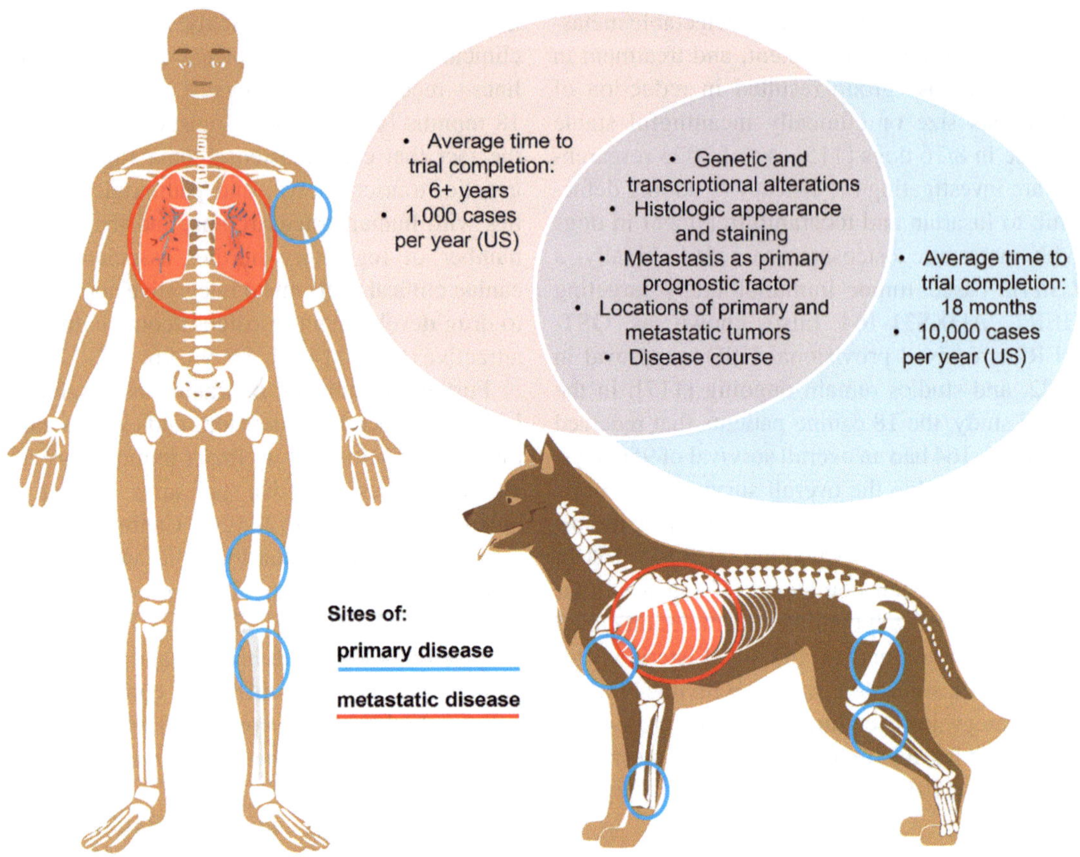

Fig. 1 Similarities and differences of human and canine osteosarcoma. Many traits are shared between human and canine osteosarcoma. The tumors develop in similar anatomic regions, follow a similar disease course, have a similar histologic appearance, exhibit many of the same molecular alterations, and are generally treated using similar approaches. However, the incidence and mortality of the disease are much higher in canines

Wolfhounds. Indeed, breed clubs are often filled with "citizen scientists" eager to contribute, financially or otherwise. The research identifying osteosarcoma heritability in Irish Wolfhounds and Scottish Deerhounds succeeded in part thanks to extensive pedigree and health documentation that was provided to researchers by breeders and other club members [89, 90, 130, 131]. Many breed clubs maintain a database of genetic material from registered dogs, both for the purposes of confirming breed identity and research into specific diseases [132–134]. Club newsletters may include information about available clinical trials, and club websites may have both grants and study results listed [135–137]. Dog fanciers and the clubs they belong to are a unique, enthusiastic source of support for osteosarcoma research.

Clinical findings from clinical studies performed using companion animals diagnosed with osteosarcoma have long shaped approaches in humans (Table 1). For instance, dogs played a critical role in developing limb-sparing surgeries now regularly utilized in human patients [138, 139]. The canine clinical trial utilizing losartan and toceranib in patients with metastatic disease led to a phase 1/1b human clinical trial in 2019 to investigate co-treatment of osteosarcoma patients with losartan and sunitinib, a human-approved sister compound of toceranib [140]. This trial is ongoing as of this writing. Similarly, the results of the canine trial of ADXS31-164 (also known

Table 1 Therapies developed using an integrative/comparative approach

Therapy	Outcome in dogs	Outcome in humans
Limb-sparing surgeries	Key for development and refinement of the procedures	Regularly utilized
Mifamurtide/L--MTP-PE	47% greater median survival time when administered after chemotherapy	Insufficient evidence of benefit to gain FDA approval when administered concurrently with chemotherapy
Losartan and RTK inhibitor (sunitinib or toceranib)	Reduction of metastasis or clinically stable disease in half of dogs enrolled	Phase I/Ib trial ongoing as of 2025
Listeria-based tumor immunotherapy targeting HER2 (ADXS31-164/ OST-HER2)	Double overall survival vs. historical controls Provisional FDA approval as of 2025	Phase IIb trial ongoing as of 2025

as OST-HER2) garnered provisional USDA approval for use in dogs, and in 2022 a phase IIb human trial began that remains ongoing [117].

Finally, the previously described canine trials of mifamurtide were significant enough to warrant human trials. Unfortunately, results in human trials were less significant than those seen in dogs, and insufficient to accrue FDA approval in the United States, although mifamurtide is approved for use in Europe and may be used in the United States under compassionate use [141, 142]. Trial design limited the ability to evaluate efficacy, and the co-administration of chemotherapy and mifamurtide (as opposed to chemotherapy followed by mifamurtide, as was successful in dogs) may have played a role in its lackluster results [7, 142]. While chemotherapy was not shown to impair mifamurtide activation of human-derived monocytes in vitro, studies have not ruled out the effects of chemotherapy-induced leukopenia on hindering the drug's efficacy [143]. Thus, it is difficult to determine if the suboptimal results in humans were due to species differences or study design. Additional human studies of mifamurtide in metastatic disease and in combination with other chemotherapeutics are ongoing, although to date none have studied chemotherapy followed by mifamurtide [69, 142, 144, 145]. Nonetheless, this trial was key in establishing that canine clinical trials can inform human trials, while also highlighting opportunities and challenges inherent in the process.

Veterinarians ethically can, and often do, deviate from "gold standard" therapies for a variety of legitimate reasons. This means that if chemotherapy does not fall within the treatment goals and/or financial abilities of a dog's owner, pet dogs can feasibly and ethically be enrolled in a trial testing a novel drug in patients who have not received chemotherapy. Additionally, the standard approach to treating primary canine tumors is resection followed by chemotherapy. Thus, the tumors of many canine tumors (primary and metastatic) are treatment naïve. This allows researchers the opportunity to evaluate these untreated "controls" against the effects of drugs and drug combinations on primary (and metastatic) tumors from treated individuals. Treatments that could be hindered by traditional chemotherapy—such as immunomodulatory drugs—can be studied ethically and effectively prior to treatment with chemotherapy in dogs. By studying the effects of these drugs on treatment-naïve tumors (and immune systems), their mechanisms of action can be more fully illuminated and refined, and their therapeutic potential more fully evaluated. Furthermore, efforts are being made to find means of removing metastatic tumors from dogs with minimal impacts on quality of life. Beyond potentially prolonging the life of canine patients with metastatic disease, surgical removal of metastases from living canine patients will facilitate the study of metastatic tumors' response to study interventions in detail and facilitate the collection of paired and serial tumor samples collected over the course of treatment. This allows for evaluation of response to treatment, drug resistances and vulnerabilities, and more.

4 Gaps in Human and Veterinary Oncology

Compared to human medicine, veterinary medicine is far less specialized and relies heavily on general practitioners. In 2020, approximately 83% of physicians were certified by the American Board of Medical Specialties or American Osteopathic Association specialty board [146]. In contrast, in 2021, approximately 12% of veterinarians were certified by an American Board of Veterinary Specialties. Only 3% of board-certified veterinarians—and 0.4% of all active veterinarians—are oncologists, and even a smaller subset of veterinary oncologists are engaged in scientific discovery and conduct of investigational clinical trials [147, 148]. As such, the number of veterinarians capable of providing the advanced oncology care necessary for osteosarcoma clinical trials is limited. The small number of specialist practitioners in turn reduces the number of patients that can be seen at each practice. Lack of veterinary oncologists also limits the number of specialty practices that can exist. Indeed, as of 2022 there are only 33 accredited veterinary teaching hospitals in the United States, and BluePearl Specialty and Emergency Pet Hospital—one of the largest veterinary specialist companies—boasts merely "over 100" locations in the United States [149, 150]. Furthermore, not every specialist veterinary clinic maintains an oncology service. Compare this to human medicine, where as of 2022, there are 1,602 oncology-specific practices in the United States, in addition to oncology services within larger practices [151]. The small number of veterinary study sites also geographically limits and pre-selects the patient population: a client may be willing to enroll their dog, but be unable to travel to the clinic regularly. The limited number of study sites can also greatly reduce the likelihood of follow-up should the client and their pet move. Because of these and other factors, clients often return to their referring veterinarian for end-of-life care and euthanasia for their pet. Additionally, an increasing number of clients are choosing at-home euthanasia [152]. Euthanasia away from the study site can limit or eliminate the possibility of sample collection immediately pre- and postmortem.

Unlike people, dogs do not understand that adverse events from treatments are endured in the hopes of improved and prolonged quality of life-long term [124]. Many owners and veterinarians therefore reasonably prioritize patient quality over quantity of life. This can mean reducing or eliminating treatments to minimize side effects, even at the cost of treatment efficacy. Indeed, only 10% of dogs receiving any kind of chemotherapy experience adverse side effects requiring veterinary intervention, and life-threatening adverse events occur in only approximately 1% of dogs [124]. Compare this to humans, where adverse events occur in nearly all patients undergoing chemotherapy for osteosarcoma, and severe adverse events occur in approximately 86% of patients [42, 153]. The reason for these differences in side effects is obvious when comparing canine and human osteosarcoma treatments. Dogs with osteosarcoma are typically given —four to five doses of carboplatin after amputation over the course of weeks, compared to the —five to six cycle methotrexate/doxorubicin/cisplatin (MAP) regimen given to human patients, which can last up to a year [154]. Additionally, in dogs the development of metastasis often signals the end stage of the disease and thereafter only palliative care is generally pursued. In humans, metastases are surgically removed, and patients often receive ifosfamide treatment and other therapies [155–159]. These differences in treatment and the lower threshold for acceptable side effects in dogs may result in otherwise promising therapies appearing less effective when tested in canine populations.

The opposite may also hold true in some cases, with drugs that appear promising in dogs having little effect in humans. The institution of significantly less intensive therapies in dogs can bias investigational therapies to be perceived as effective, yet when transplanted on top of a highly intensive treatment regimen in people, derived therapeutic benefit is dramatically diluted and potentially undetectable. Furthermore, generally human patients must receive standard of care therapy in clinical trials to maximize potential benefits and minimize potential risks [160]. In certain cases, this may confound study results in humans for a drug that showed promise in dogs. For example, if a novel immune-modulating drug is required by study design to be given at the same time as chemotherapy in humans, the chemotherapy may kill immune cells before they can be acted on by the trial drug, yielding lackluster results.

Despite these challenges, dogs remain an important model for osteosarcoma. Indeed, the partnerships between physicians, researchers, and veterinarians studying osteosarcoma have led the way in integrative trials and comparative oncology. As interest in dogs as a spontaneous model of osteosarcoma continues to grow, expanded training for veterinary researchers and oncologists, as well as the expansion of existing comparative oncology centers and the creation of new ones, is necessary to keep pace. Programs to streamline coordination across participating oncology centers to maximize patient enrollment and disseminate data, such as the National Institutes of Health's Comparative Oncology Program, are likewise critical to future success.

5 Conclusions

Continued funding, allocation of resources, and improved awareness will allow comparative research and medicine to flourish. Studying osteosarcoma in dogs offers a unique opportunity to study spontaneous tumors in animals with an intact immune system that share the same environments as their human counterparts. Importantly, canine disease offers an opportunity to study the metastatic process rapidly and in detail. Among other opportunities, the ability to obtain paired primary and metastatic canine tumor samples from patients with and without treatment will aid in elucidating metastatic dependencies. Canine clinical trials likewise offer the chance to rapidly and effectively contribute to pharmacokinetic, pharmacodynamic, and initial efficacy data of promising treatments. Osteosarcoma research, in particular, has led the way in efforts that contribute to both human and canine health. The continued inclusion of pet dogs with osteosarcoma into discovery efforts and drug development pathways affords unique opportunities to provide pet owners and their dogs with therapies that would not otherwise be available for potentially improving the quality and quantity of life. These innovative, comparatively rapid trials offer hope for improved outcomes in people as well.

References

1. Klein MJ, Siegal GP (2006) Osteosarcoma: anatomic and histologic variants. Am J Clin Pathol 125(4):555–581. https://doi.org/10.1309/UC6KQHLD9LV2KENN
2. Fan TM, Roberts RD, Lizardo MM (2020) Understanding and modeling metastasis biology to improve therapeutic strategies for combating osteosarcoma progression. Front Oncol 10:13. https://doi.org/10.3389/fonc.2020.00013
3. Beird HC, Bielack SS, Flanagan AM et al (2022) Osteosarcoma. Nat Rev Dis Primers 8(1):77. https://doi.org/10.1038/s41572-022-00409-y
4. Rowell JL, McCarthy DO, Alvarez CE (2011) Dog models of naturally occurring cancer. Trends Mol Med 17(7):380–388. https://doi.org/10.1016/j.molmed.2011.02.004
5. Key Statistics for Osteosarcoma. Accessed 23 Nov 2022. https://www.cancer.org/cancer/osteosarcoma/about/key-statistics.html
6. Damron TA, Ward WG, Stewart A (2007) Osteosarcoma, chondrosarcoma, and Ewing's sarcoma: national cancer data base report. Clin Orthop Relat Res 459:40–47. https://doi.org/10.1097/BLO.0b013e318059b8c9
7. Meazza C, Bastoni S, Scanagatta P (2020) What is the best clinical approach to recurrent/refractory osteosarcoma? Expert Rev Anticancer Ther 20(5):415–428. https://doi.org/10.1080/14737140.2020.1760848
8. Mirabello L, Troisi RJ, Savage SA (2009) International osteosarcoma incidence patterns in children and adolescents, middle ages and elderly persons. Int J Cancer 125(1):229–234. https://doi.org/10.1002/ijc.24320
9. Parkin DM, Stiller CA, Draper GJ, Bieber CA (1988) The international incidence of childhood cancer. Int J Cancer 42(4):511–520. https://doi.org/10.1002/ijc.2910420408
10. Nie Z, Peng H (2018) Osteosarcoma in patients below 25-years of age: an observational study of incidence, metastasis, treatment and outcomes. Oncol Lett. https://doi.org/10.3892/ol.2018.9453. Published online 18 Sept 2018

11. Force LM, Abdollahpour I, Advani SM et al (2019) The global burden of childhood and adolescent cancer in 2017: an analysis of the global burden of disease study 2017. Lancet Oncol 20(9):1211–1225. https://doi.org/10.1016/S1470-2045(19)30339-0
12. Mirabello L, Troisi RJ, Savage SA (2009) Osteosarcoma incidence and survival rates from 1973 to 2004: data from the surveillance, epidemiology, and end results program. Cancer 115(7):1531–1543. https://doi.org/10.1002/cncr.24121
13. Harrison DJ, Geller DS, Gill JD, Lewis VO, Gorlick R (2018) Current and future therapeutic approaches for osteosarcoma. Expert Rev Anticancer Ther 18(1):39–50. https://doi.org/10.1080/14737140.2018.1413939
14. Mirabello L, Pfeiffer R, Murphy G et al (2011) Height at diagnosis and birth-weight as risk factors for osteosarcoma. Cancer Causes Control 22(6):899–908. https://doi.org/10.1007/s10552-011-9763-2
15. Mirabello L, Zhu B, Koster R et al (2020) Frequency of pathogenic germline variants in cancer-susceptibility genes in patients with osteosarcoma. JAMA Oncol 6(5):724–734. https://doi.org/10.1001/jamaoncol.2020.0197
16. Zhang J, Walsh MF, Wu G et al (2015) Germline mutations in predisposition genes in pediatric cancer. N Engl J Med 373(24):2336–2346. https://doi.org/10.1056/NEJMoa1508054
17. Huvos AG (1986) Osteogenic sarcoma of bones and soft tissues in older persons. A clinicopathologic analysis of 117 patients older than 60 years. Cancer 57(7):1442–1449. https://doi.org/10.1002/1097-0142(19860401)57:7<1442::aid-cncr2820570734>3.0.co;2-3
18. Sadykova LR, Ntekim AI, Muyangwa-Semenova M et al (2020) Epidemiology and risk factors of osteosarcoma. Cancer Investig 38(5):259–269. https://doi.org/10.1080/07357907.2020.1768401
19. Luetke A, Meyers PA, Lewis I, Juergens H (2014) Osteosarcoma treatment – where do we stand? A state of the art review. Cancer Treat Rev 40(4):523–532. https://doi.org/10.1016/j.ctrv.2013.11.006
20. Roberts RD, Lizardo MM, Reed DR et al (2019) Provocative questions in osteosarcoma basic and translational biology: a report from the children's oncology group. Cancer 125(20):3514–3525. https://doi.org/10.1002/cncr.32351
21. Botter SM, Neri D, Fuchs B (2014) Recent advances in osteosarcoma. Curr Opin Pharmacol 16(1):15–23. https://doi.org/10.1016/j.coph.2014.02.002
22. Ma X, Liu Y, Liu Y et al (2018) Pan-cancer genome and transcriptome analyses of 1,699 paediatric leukaemias and solid tumours. Nature 555(7696):371–376. https://doi.org/10.1038/nature25795
23. Sayles LC, Breese MR, Koehne AL et al (2019) Genome-informed targeted therapy for osteosarcoma. Cancer Discov 9(1):46–63. https://doi.org/10.1158/2159-8290.CD-17-1152
24. Perry JA, Kiezun A, Tonzi P et al (2014) Complementary genomic approaches highlight the PI3K/mTOR pathway as a common vulnerability in osteosarcoma. Proc Natl Acad Sci USA 111(51):E5564–E5573. https://doi.org/10.1073/pnas.1419260111
25. Behjati S, Tarpey PS, Haase K et al (2017) Recurrent mutation of IGF signalling genes and distinct patterns of genomic rearrangement in osteosarcoma. Nat Commun 8:15936. https://doi.org/10.1038/ncomms15936
26. Chen X, Bahrami A, Pappo A et al (2014) Recurrent somatic structural variations contribute to tumorigenesis in pediatric osteosarcoma. Cell Rep 7(1):104–112. https://doi.org/10.1016/j.celrep.2014.03.003
27. Wu CC, Beird HC, Andrew Livingston J et al (2020) Immuno-genomic landscape of osteosarcoma. Nat Commun 11(1):1008. https://doi.org/10.1038/s41467-020-14646-w
28. Fidler IJ (1970) Metastasis: quantitative analysis of distribution and fate of tumor emboli labeled with ^{125}I-5-iodo-2′-deoxyuridine. J Natl Cancer Inst 45(4):773–782
29. Cameron MD, Schmidt EE, Kerkvliet N et al (2000) Temporal progression of metastasis in lung: cell survival, dormancy, and location dependence of metastatic inefficiency. Cancer Res 60(9):2541–2546
30. Rajan S, Franz E, McAloney CA et al Osteosarcoma tumors maintain intra-tumoral transcriptional heterogeneity during bone and lung colonization. Published online December 13, 2022:2020.11.03.367342. https://doi.org/10.1101/2020.11.03.367342
31. Morrow JJ, Mendoza A, Koyen A et al (2016) mTOR inhibition mitigates enhanced mRNA translation associated with the metastatic phenotype of osteosarcoma cells in vivo. Clin Cancer Res 22(24):6129–6141. https://doi.org/10.1158/1078-0432.CCR-16-0326
32. McAloney CA, Makkawi R, Budhathoki Y et al (2024) Host-derived growth factors drive ERK phosphorylation and MCL1 expression to promote osteosarcoma cell survival during metastatic lung colonization. Cell Oncol. https://doi.org/10.1007/s13402-023-00867-w. Published online 7 Sept 2023
33. Jaffe N, Puri A, Gelderblom H (2013) Osteosarcoma: evolution of treatment paradigms. Sarcoma 2013:203531. https://doi.org/10.1155/2013/203531
34. Jaffe N (1972) Recent advances in the chemotherapy of metastatic osteogenic sarcoma. Cancer 30(6):1627–1631. https://doi.org/10.1002/1097-0142(197212)30:6<1627::aid-cncr2820300631>3.0.co;2-h
35. Ettinger LJ, Douglass HO, Mindell ER et al (1986) Adjuvant adriamycin and cisplatin in newly diagnosed, nonmetastatic osteosarcoma of the extremity. J Clin Oncol 4(3):353–362. https://doi.org/10.1200/JCO.1986.4.3.353
36. Link MP, Goorin AM, Miser AW et al (1986) The effect of adjuvant chemotherapy on relapse-free

survival in patients with osteosarcoma of the extremity. N Engl J Med 314(25):1600–1606. https://doi.org/10.1056/NEJM198606193142502
37. Bacci G, Longhi A, Versari M, Mercuri M, Briccoli A, Picci P (2006) Prognostic factors for osteosarcoma of the extremity treated with neoadjuvant chemotherapy: 15-year experience in 789 patients treated at a single institution. Cancer 106(5):1154–1161. https://doi.org/10.1002/cncr.21724
38. Tate R, Gerrand C, Hale J (2015) Tibial turn-up procedure as an alternative to rotationplasty in a 4-year-old with osteosarcoma of the distal femur. J Pediatr Orthop B 24(1):50–55. https://doi.org/10.1097/BPB.0000000000000110
39. Hebert JS, Rehani M, Stiegelmar R (2017) Osseointegration for lower-limb amputation: a systematic review of clinical outcomes. JBJS Rev 5(10):e10. https://doi.org/10.2106/JBJS.RVW.17.00037
40. Anninga JK, Gelderblom H, Fiocco M et al (2011) Chemotherapeutic adjuvant treatment for osteosarcoma: where do we stand? Eur J Cancer 47(16):2431–2445. https://doi.org/10.1016/j.ejca.2011.05.030
41. Meyers PA (2015) Systemic therapy for osteosarcoma and Ewing sarcoma. Am Soc Clin Oncol Educ Book 35:e644–e647. https://doi.org/10.14694/EdBook_AM.2015.35.e644
42. Marina NM, Smeland S, Bielack SS et al (2016) Comparison of MAPIE versus MAP in patients with a poor response to preoperative chemotherapy for newly diagnosed high-grade osteosarcoma (EURAMOS-1): an open-label, international, randomised controlled trial. Lancet Oncol 17(10):1396–1408. https://doi.org/10.1016/S1470-2045(16)30214-5
43. Ciernik IF, Niemierko A, Harmon DC et al (2011) Proton-based radiotherapy for unresectable or incompletely resected osteosarcoma. Cancer 117(19):4522–4530. https://doi.org/10.1002/cncr.26037
44. Matsunobu A, Imai R, Kamada T et al (2012) Impact of carbon ion radiotherapy for unresectable osteosarcoma of the trunk. Cancer 118(18):4555–4563. https://doi.org/10.1002/cncr.27451
45. Roberts RD, Wedekind MF, Setty BA (2015) Malignant pediatric bone tumors – treatment & management. Springer
46. Jaffe N (2014) Historical perspective on the introduction and use of chemotherapy for the treatment of osteosarcoma. In: Kleinerman MD, Eugenie S (eds) Current advances in osteosarcoma. Springer, pp 1–30. https://doi.org/10.1007/978-3-319-04843-7_1
47. Briccoli A, Rocca M, Salone M et al (2005) Resection of recurrent pulmonary metastases in patients with osteosarcoma. Cancer 104(8):1721–1725. https://doi.org/10.1002/cncr.21369
48. Harting MT, Blakely ML, Jaffe N et al (2006) Long-term survival after aggressive resection of pulmonary metastases among children and adolescents with osteosarcoma. J Pediatr Surg 41(1):194–199. https://doi.org/10.1016/j.jpedsurg.2005.10.089
49. Kempf-Bielack B, Bielack SS, Jürgens H et al (2005) Osteosarcoma relapse after combined modality therapy: an analysis of unselected patients in the cooperative osteosarcoma study group (COSS). J Clin Oncol 23(3):559–568. https://doi.org/10.1200/JCO.2005.04.063
50. Kager L, Zoubek A, Pötschger U et al (2003) Primary metastatic osteosarcoma: presentation and outcome of patients treated on neoadjuvant cooperative osteosarcoma study group protocols. J Clin Oncol 21(10):2011–2018. https://doi.org/10.1200/JCO.2003.08.132
51. Treatment by Cancer Type. NCCN. Accessed 5 Jan 2023. https://www.nccn.org/guidelines/category_1
52. Strauss SJ, Frezza AM, Abecassis N et al (2021) Bone sarcomas: ESMO-EURACAN-GENTURIS-ERN PaedCan clinical practice guideline for diagnosis, treatment and follow-up. Ann Oncol 32(12):1520–1536. https://doi.org/10.1016/j.annonc.2021.08.1995
53. Gentet JC, Brunat-Mentigny M, Demaille MC et al (1997) Ifosfamide and etoposide in childhood osteosarcoma. A phase II study of the French society of paediatric oncology. Eur J Cancer 33(2):232–237. https://doi.org/10.1016/s0959-8049(96)00439-x
54. Lee JA, Jeon DG, Cho WH et al (2016) Higher gemcitabine dose was associated with better outcome of osteosarcoma patients receiving gemcitabine-docetaxel chemotherapy. Pediatr Blood Cancer 63(9):1552–1556. https://doi.org/10.1002/pbc.26058
55. Miser JS, Kinsella TJ, Triche TJ et al (1987) Ifosfamide with mesna uroprotection and etoposide: an effective regimen in the treatment of recurrent sarcomas and other tumors of children and young adults. J Clin Oncol 5(8):1191–1198. https://doi.org/10.1200/JCO.1987.5.8.1191
56. Rodríguez-Galindo C, Daw NC, Kaste SC et al (2002) Treatment of refractory osteosarcoma with fractionated cyclophosphamide and etoposide. J Pediatr Hematol Oncol 24(4):250–255. https://doi.org/10.1097/00043426-200205000-00006
57. Vasquez L, Tarrillo F, Oscanoa M et al (2016) Analysis of prognostic factors in high-grade osteosarcoma of the extremities in children: a 15-year single-institution experience. Front Oncol 6:22. https://doi.org/10.3389/fonc.2016.00022
58. Bramer JAM, van Linge JH, Grimer RJ, Scholten RJPM (2009) Prognostic factors in localized extremity osteosarcoma: a systematic review. Eur J Surg Oncol 35(10):1030–1036. https://doi.org/10.1016/j.ejso.2009.01.011
59. Prabowo Y, Kamal AF, Kodrat E, Prasetyo M, Maruanaya S, Efar TS (2020) Parosteal osteosarcoma: a benign-looking tumour, amenable to a variety of surgical reconstruction.

Int J Surg Oncol 2020:4807612. https://doi.org/10.1155/2020/4807612
60. Sami SH, Rafati AH, Hodjat P (2008) Tissue necrosis after chemotherapy in osteosarcoma as the important prognostic factor. Saudi Med J 29(8):1124–1129
61. Kim MS, Lee SY, Cho WH et al (2008) Tumor necrosis rate adjusted by tumor volume change is a better predictor of survival of localized osteosarcoma patients. Ann Surg Oncol 15(3):906–914. https://doi.org/10.1245/s10434-007-9779-8
62. Jawad MU, Cheung MC, Clarke J, Koniaris LG, Scully SP (2011) Osteosarcoma: improvement in survival limited to high-grade patients only. J Cancer Res Clin Oncol 137(4):597–607. https://doi.org/10.1007/s00432-010-0923-7
63. Maloney C, Kallis M, Edelman M et al (2020) Gefitinib inhibits invasion and metastasis of osteosarcoma via inhibition of macrophage receptor interacting serine/threonine kinase 2. Am Assoc Cancer Res. https://doi.org/10.1158/1535-7163.MCT-19-0903. Published online 2020
64. Kallis MP, Maloney C, Blank B, Soffer SZ, Symons M, Steinberg BM (2020) Pharmacological prevention of surgery-accelerated metastasis in an animal model of osteosarcoma. J Transl Med 18(1):183. https://doi.org/10.1186/s12967-020-02348-2
65. Ratti C, Botti L, Cancila V et al (2017) Trabectedin overrides osteosarcoma differentiative block and reprograms the tumor immune environment enabling effective combination with immune checkpoint inhibitors. Clin Cancer Res 23(17):5149–5161. https://doi.org/10.1158/1078-0432.CCR-16-3186
66. Igarashi K, Murakami T, Kawaguchi K et al (2017) A patient-derived orthotopic xenograft (PDOX) mouse model of a cisplatinum-resistant osteosarcoma lung metastasis that was sensitive to temozolomide and trabectedin: implications for precision oncology. Oncotarget 8(37):62111–62119. https://doi.org/10.18632/oncotarget.19095
67. Pignochino Y, Capozzi F, D'Ambrosio L et al (2017) PARP1 expression drives the synergistic antitumor activity of trabectedin and PARP1 inhibitors in sarcoma preclinical models. Mol Cancer 16(1):86. https://doi.org/10.1186/s12943-017-0652-5
68. Germano G, Frapolli R, Belgiovine C et al (2013) Role of macrophage targeting in the antitumor activity of trabectedin. Cancer Cell 23(2):249–262. https://doi.org/10.1016/j.ccr.2013.01.008
69. Hattinger CM, Patrizio MP, Magagnoli F, Luppi S, Serra M (2019) An update on emerging drugs in osteosarcoma: towards tailored therapies? Expert Opin Emerg Drugs 24(3):153–171. https://doi.org/10.1080/14728214.2019.1654455
70. Chen C, Xie L, Ren T, Huang Y, Xu J, Guo W (2021) Immunotherapy for osteosarcoma: fundamental mechanism, rationale, and recent breakthroughs. Cancer Lett 500:1–10. https://doi.org/10.1016/j.canlet.2020.12.024
71. Gross AC, Cam H, Phelps DA et al IL6 and CXCL8 mediate osteosarcoma-lung interactions critical to metastasis
72. Greenfield EM, Collier CD, Getty PJ (2020) Receptor tyrosine kinases in osteosarcoma: 2019 update. Adv Exp Med Biol 1258:141–155. https://doi.org/10.1007/978-3-030-43085-6_9
73. Search of: recruiting, active, not recruiting studies | "osteosarcoma" – list results – ClinicalTrials.gov. Accessed 5 Jan 2023. https://clinicaltrials.gov/ct2/results?cond=%22Osteosarcoma%22&Search=Apply&recrs=a&recrs=d&age_v=&gndr=&type=&rslt=
74. Vail DM, Thamm DH, Liptak JM (eds) (2020) Withrow & MacEwen's small animal clinical oncology, 6th edn. Elsevier
75. Beck J, Ren L, Huang S et al (2022) Canine and murine models of osteosarcoma. Vet Pathol 59(3):399–414. https://doi.org/10.1177/03009858221083038
76. Meuten D (2020) Tumors in domestic animals. Wiley
77. Craig L, Dittmer K, Thompson K (2015) Bones and joints. In: Maxie G (ed) Jubb, Kennedy & Palmer's pathology of domestic animals, 6th edn. W.B Saunders
78. Olson EJ, Dykstra JA, Armstrong AR, Carlson CS (2022) Bones, joints, tendons, and ligaments. In: Zachary JF (ed) Pathologic basis of veterinary disease, 7th edn. Elsevier
79. Nagamine E, Hirayama K, Matsuda K et al (2015) Diversity of histologic patterns and expression of cytoskeletal proteins in Canine skeletal osteosarcoma. Vet Pathol 52(5):977–984. https://doi.org/10.1177/0300985815574006
80. Anfinsen KP, Grotmol T, Bruland OS, Jonasdottir TJ (2011) Breed-specific incidence rates of canine primary bone tumors – a population based survey of dogs in Norway. Can J Vet Res 75(3):209–215
81. Mueller F, Fuchs B, Kaser-Hotz B (2007) Comparative biology of human and canine osteosarcoma. Anticancer Res 27(1A):155–164
82. Misdorp W, Hart AA (1979) Some prognostic and epidemiologic factors in canine osteosarcoma. J Natl Cancer Inst 62(3):537–545
83. Trost ME, Kommers GD, Brown CC et al (2012) Primary bone neoplasms in dogs: 90 cases. Pesq Vet Bras 32(12):1329–1335. https://doi.org/10.1590/S0100-736X2012001200018
84. Cooley DM, Waters DJ (1997) Skeletal neoplasms of small dogs: a retrospective study and literature review. J Am Anim Hosp Assoc 33(1):11–23. https://doi.org/10.5326/15473317-33-1-11
85. Dobson JM (2013) Breed-predispositions to cancer in pedigree dogs. ISRN Vet Sci 2013:1–23. https://doi.org/10.1155/2013/941275
86. Karlsson EK, Sigurdsson S, Ivansson E et al (2013) Genome-wide analyses implicate 33 loci in heritable dog osteosarcoma, including regulatory variants near

CDKN2A/B. Genome Biol 14(12):R132. https://doi.org/10.1186/gb-2013-14-12-r132

87. Phillips JC, Lembcke L, Chamberlin T (2010) A novel locus for canine osteosarcoma (OSA1) maps to CFA34, the canine orthologue of human 3q26. Genomics 96(4):220–227. https://doi.org/10.1016/j.ygeno.2010.07.002
88. Letko A, Minor KM, Norton EM et al (2021) Genome-wide analyses for osteosarcoma in Leonberger dogs reveal the CDKN2A/B gene locus as a major risk locus. Genes 12(12):1964. https://doi.org/10.3390/genes12121964
89. Dillberger JE, McAtee SA (2017) Osteosarcoma inheritance in two families of Scottish deerhounds. Canine Genet Epidemiol 4:3. https://doi.org/10.1186/s40575-017-0042-8
90. Phillips JC, Stephenson B, Hauck M, Dillberger J (2007) Heritability and segregation analysis of osteosarcoma in the Scottish deerhound. Genomics 90(3):354–363. https://doi.org/10.1016/j.ygeno.2007.05.001
91. Parker HG, Kim LV, Sutter NB et al (2004) Genetic structure of the purebred domestic dog. Science 304(5674):1160–1164. https://doi.org/10.1126/science.1097406
92. McAloney CA, Silverstein KAT, Modiano JF, Bagchi A (2014) Polymorphisms within the telomerase reverse transcriptase gene (TERT) in four breeds of dogs selected for difference in lifespan and cancer susceptibility. BMC Vet Res 10(1):20. https://doi.org/10.1186/1746-6148-10-20
93. Fan TM, Khanna C (2015) Comparative aspects of osteosarcoma pathogenesis in humans and dogs. Vet Sci 2(3):210–230. https://doi.org/10.3390/vetsci2030210
94. Thomas R, Wang HJ, Tsai PC et al (2009) Influence of genetic background on tumor karyotypes: evidence for breed-associated cytogenetic aberrations in canine appendicular osteosarcoma. Chromosom Res 17(3):365–377. https://doi.org/10.1007/s10577-009-9028-z
95. Angstadt AY, Motsinger-Reif A, Thomas R et al (2011) Characterization of canine osteosarcoma by array comparative genomic hybridization and RT-qPCR: signatures of genomic imbalance in canine osteosarcoma parallel the human counterpart. Genes Chromosomes Cancer 50(11):859–874. https://doi.org/10.1002/gcc.20908
96. Fenger JM, London CA, Kisseberth WC (2014) Canine osteosarcoma: a naturally occurring disease to inform pediatric oncology. ILAR J 55(1):69–85. https://doi.org/10.1093/ilar/ilu009
97. Skorupski KA, Uhl JM, Szivek A, Allstadt Frazier SD, Rebhun RB, Rodriguez CO (2016) Carboplatin versus alternating carboplatin and doxorubicin for the adjuvant treatment of canine appendicular osteosarcoma: a randomized, phase III trial. Vet Comp Oncol 14(1):81–87. https://doi.org/10.1111/vco.12069
98. Selmic LE, Burton JH, Thamm DH, Withrow SJ, Lana SE (2014) Comparison of carboplatin and doxorubicin-based chemotherapy protocols in 470 dogs after amputation for treatment of appendicular osteosarcoma. J Vet Intern Med 28(2):554–563. https://doi.org/10.1111/jvim.12313
99. Brodey RS, Riser WH, Canine osteosarcoma. (1969) A clinicopathologic study of 194 cases. Clin Orthop Relat Res 62:54–64
100. Spodnick GJ, Berg J, Rand WM et al (1992) Prognosis for dogs with appendicular osteosarcoma treated by amputation alone: 162 cases (1978-1988). J Am Vet Med Assoc 200(7):995–999
101. Martin TW, Griffin L, Custis J et al (2021) Outcome and prognosis for canine appendicular osteosarcoma treated with stereotactic body radiation therapy in 123 dogs. Vet Comp Oncol 19(2):284–294. https://doi.org/10.1111/vco.12674
102. Nolan MW, Green NA, DiVito EM, Lascelles BDX, Haney SM (2020) Impact of radiation dose and pretreatment pain levels on survival in dogs undergoing radiotherapy with or without chemotherapy for presumed extremity osteosarcoma. Vet Comp Oncol 18(4):538–547. https://doi.org/10.1111/vco.12576
103. Ramirez O, Dodge RK, Page RL et al (1999) Palliative radiotherapy of appendicular osteosarcoma in 95 dogs. Vet Radiol Ultrasound 40(5):517–522. https://doi.org/10.1111/j.1740-8261.1999.tb00385.x
104. Fan TM, Charney SC, de Lorimier LP et al (2009) Double-blind placebo-controlled trial of adjuvant pamidronate with palliative radiotherapy and intravenous doxorubicin for canine appendicular osteosarcoma bone pain. J Vet Intern Med 23(1):152–160. https://doi.org/10.1111/j.1939-1676.2008.0221.x
105. Turner H, Séguin B, Worley DR et al (2017) Prognosis for dogs with stage III osteosarcoma following treatment with amputation and chemotherapy with and without metastasectomy. J Am Vet Med Assoc 251(11):1293–1305. https://doi.org/10.2460/javma.251.11.1293
106. Minimally Invasive Metastasectomy in Canines (MIMIC). Ethos veterinary health. Accessed 23 Nov 2022. https://www.ethosvet.com/clinical-study/minimally-invasive-metastasectomy-in-canines-mimic/
107. Al-Khan AA, Nimmo JS, Day MJ et al (2020) Fibroblastic subtype has a favourable prognosis in appendicular osteosarcoma of dogs. J Comp Pathol 176:133–144. https://doi.org/10.1016/j.jcpa.2020.02.011
108. Boerman I, Selvarajah GT, Nielen M, Kirpensteijn J (2012) Prognostic factors in canine appendicular osteosarcoma – a meta-analysis. BMC Vet Res 8:56. https://doi.org/10.1186/1746-6148-8-56
109. Kirpensteijn J, Kik M, Rutteman GR, Teske E (2002) Prognostic significance of a new histologic grading system for canine osteosarcoma. Vet Pathol 39(2):240–246. https://doi.org/10.1354/vp.39-2-240
110. Kruse MA, Holmes ES, Balko JA, Fernandez S, Brown DC, Goldschmidt MH (2013) Evaluation of

clinical and histopathologic prognostic factors for survival in canine osteosarcoma of the extracranial flat and irregular bones. Vet Pathol 50(4):704–708. https://doi.org/10.1177/0300985812471542
111. Schott CR, Tatiersky LJ, Foster RA, Wood GA (2018) Histologic grade does not predict outcome in dogs with appendicular osteosarcoma receiving the standard of care. Vet Pathol 55(2):202–211. https://doi.org/10.1177/0300985817747329
112. MacEwen EG, Kurzman ID, Rosenthal RC et al (1989) Therapy for osteosarcoma in dogs with intravenous injection of liposome-encapsulated muramyl tripeptide. J Natl Cancer Inst 81(12):935–938. https://doi.org/10.1093/jnci/81.12.935
113. Kurzman ID, Macewen EG, Rosenthal RC et al (1995) Adjuvant therapy for osteosarcoma in dogs: results of randomized clinical trials using combined liposome-encapsulated Muramyl tripeptide and cisplatin. Clin Cancer Res 1(12):1595–1601
114. MacEwen EG, Kurzman ID (1996) Canine osteosarcoma: amputation and chemoimmunotherapy. Vet Clin North Am Small Anim Pract 26(1):123–133. https://doi.org/10.1016/s0195-5616(96)50011-2
115. Regan DP, Chow L, Das S et al (2022) Losartan blocks osteosarcoma-elicited monocyte recruitment, and combined with the kinase inhibitor Toceranib, exerts significant clinical benefit in Canine metastatic osteosarcoma. Clin Cancer Res 28(4):662–676. https://doi.org/10.1158/1078-0432.CCR-21-2105
116. Klosowski M, Haines L, Alfino L, McMellen A, Leibowitz M, Regan D (2023) Naturally occurring canine sarcomas: bridging the gap from mouse models to human patients through cross-disciplinary research partnerships. Front Oncol 13:1130215. https://doi.org/10.3389/fonc.2023.1130215
117. Therapies OS OS Therapies announces nationwide open enrollment of remaining 36 to 42 patients in phase IIb trial of OST-HER2 (Listeria monocytogenes) in recurred, resected osteosarcoma. Accessed 30 Dec 2022. https://www.prnewswire.com/news-releases/os-therapies-announces-nationwide-open-enrollment-of-remaining-36-to-42-patients-in-phase-iib-trial-of-ost-her2-listeria-monocytogenes-in-recurred-resected-osteosarcoma-301469427.html
118. Mason NJ, Gnanandarajah JS, Engiles JB et al (2016) Immunotherapy with a HER2-targeting listeria induces HER2-specific immunity and demonstrates potential therapeutic effects in a phase I trial in Canine osteosarcoma. Clin Cancer Res 22(17):4380–4390. https://doi.org/10.1158/1078-0432.CCR-16-0088
119. Musser ML, Berger EP, Tripp CD, Clifford CA, Bergman PJ, Johannes CM (2021) Safety evaluation of the canine osteosarcoma vaccine, live listeria vector. Vet Comp Oncol 19(1):92–98. https://doi.org/10.1111/vco.12642
120. Musser ML, Berger EP, Parsons C, Kathariou S, Johannes CM (2019) Vaccine strain listeria monocytogenes abscess in a dog: a case report. BMC Vet Res 15(1):467. https://doi.org/10.1186/s12917-019-2216-y
121. George SL, Desu MM (1974) Planning the size and duration of a clinical trial studying the time to some critical event. J Chronic Dis 27(1):15–24. https://doi.org/10.1016/0021-9681(74)90004-6
122. Gardner HL, Sivaprakasam K, Briones N et al (2019) Canine osteosarcoma genome sequencing identifies recurrent mutations in DMD and the histone methyltransferase gene SETD2. Commun Biol 2(1):1–13. https://doi.org/10.1038/s42003-019-0487-2
123. Paoloni M, Davis S, Lana S et al (2009) Canine tumor cross-species genomics uncovers targets linked to osteosarcoma progression. BMC Genomics 10:625. https://doi.org/10.1186/1471-2164-10-625
124. Paoloni M, Khanna C (2008) Translation of new cancer treatments from pet dogs to humans. Nat Rev Cancer 8(2):147–156. https://doi.org/10.1038/nrc2273
125. Selvarajah GT, Kirpensteijn J, van Wolferen ME, Rao NA, Fieten H, Mol JA (2009) Gene expression profiling of canine osteosarcoma reveals genes associated with short and long survival times. Mol Cancer 8(1):72. https://doi.org/10.1186/1476-4598-8-72
126. Gardner HL, Fenger JM, London CA (2016) Dogs as a model for cancer. Annu Rev Anim Biosci 4:199–222. https://doi.org/10.1146/annurev-animal-022114-110911
127. Pinho SS, Carvalho S, Cabral J, Reis CA, Gärtner F (2012) Canine tumors: a spontaneous animal model of human carcinogenesis. Transl Res 159(3):165–172. https://doi.org/10.1016/j.trsl.2011.11.005
128. LeBlanc AK, Mazcko CN, Cherukuri A et al (2021) Adjuvant Sirolimus does not improve outcome in pet dogs receiving standard-of-care therapy for appendicular osteosarcoma: a prospective, randomized trial of 324 dogs. Clin Cancer Res 27(11):3005–3016. https://doi.org/10.1158/1078-0432.CCR-21-0315
129. AKC Canine Health Foundation | Our Impact. Accessed 2 Dec 2022. https://www.akcchf.org/research/our-impact/
130. Momen M, Kohler NL, Binversie EE, Dentino M, Sample SJ (2021) Heritability and genetic variance estimation of osteosarcoma (OSA) in Irish wolfhound, using deep pedigree information. Canine Med Genet 8(1):9. https://doi.org/10.1186/s40575-021-00109-y
131. The Irish Wolfhound Database IWDB. Accessed 7 Dec 2022. https://iwdb.org/
132. Samples Needed! Deerhound Health. Published 19 Sept 2013. Accessed 2 Dec 2022. https://deerhound-health.org/samples-needed/
133. AKC Canine Health Foundation | Canine Health Information Center (CHIC). Accessed 7 Dec 2022. https://www.akcchf.org/about-us/alliances/canine-health-information.html
134. CHIC Program. OFA. Accessed 7 Dec 2022. https://ofa.org/chic-programs/

135. Studies—The Irish Wolfhound Foundation. Accessed 2 Dec 2022. https://www.iwfoundation.org/studies
136. Wilson J. Health information. Irish Setter Club of America, Inc. Accessed 7 Dec 2022. https://irishsetterclub.org/health/health-information/
137. CANINE CANCER – Mastiff Club of America. Published 13 November 2019. Accessed 7 Dec 2022. https://www.mastiff.org/canine-cancer/
138. Straw RC, Powers BE, Withrow SJ, Cooper MF, Turner AS (1992) The effect of intramedullary polymethylmethacrylate on healing of intercalary cortical allografts in a canine model. J Orthop Res 10(3):434–439. https://doi.org/10.1002/jor.1100100316
139. Mason NJ (2020) Comparative immunology and immunotherapy of Canine osteosarcoma. In: Kleinerman ES, Gorlick R (eds) Current advances in the science of osteosarcoma: research perspectives: tumor biology, organ microenvironment, potential new therapeutic targets, and Canine models, Advances in experimental medicine and biology, pp 199–221. https://doi.org/10.1007/978-3-030-43085-6_14
140. University of Colorado, Denver (2022) A phase I/Ib study of Losartan in combination with Sunitinib in the treatment of pediatric and adult patients with relapsed or refractory osteosarcoma. clinicaltrials.gov. Accessed 4 Jan 2023. https://clinicaltrials.gov/ct2/show/NCT03900793
141. Carlson B (2007) Approvals, FDA actions, clinical trials. Biotechnol Healthc 4(5):14–15
142. Gill J, Gorlick R (2021) Advancing therapy for osteosarcoma. Nat Rev Clin Oncol 18(10):609–624. https://doi.org/10.1038/s41571-021-00519-8
143. Kleinerman ES, Snyder JS, Jaffe N (1991) Influence of chemotherapy administration on monocyte activation by liposomal muramyl tripeptide phosphatidylethanolamine in children with osteosarcoma. J Clin Oncol 9(2):259–267. https://doi.org/10.1200/JCO.1991.9.2.259
144. Heymann MF, Lézot F, Heymann D (2019) The contribution of immune infiltrates and the local microenvironment in the pathogenesis of osteosarcoma. Cell Immunol 343:103711. https://doi.org/10.1016/j.cellimm.2017.10.011
145. Brard C, Piperno-Neumann S, Delaye J et al (2019) Sarcome-13/OS2016 trial protocol: a multicentre, randomised, open-label, phase II trial of mifamurtide combined with postoperative chemotherapy for patients with newly diagnosed high-risk osteosarcoma. BMJ Open 9(5):e025877. https://doi.org/10.1136/bmjopen-2018-025877
146. Young A, Chaudhry HJ, Pei X, Arnhart K, Dugan M, Simons KB (2020) FSMB census of licensed physicians in the United States. Published online 2021:8
147. U.S. veterinarians 2021. American Veterinary Medical Association. Accessed 23 Nov 2022. https://www.avma.org/resources-tools/reports-statistics/market-research-statistics-us-veterinarians
148. Veterinary specialists 2021. American Veterinary Medical Association. Accessed 23 Nov 2022. https://www.avma.org/resources-tools/reports-statistics/veterinary-specialists-2021
149. Accredited veterinary colleges. American Veterinary Medical Association. Accessed 23 Nov 2022. https://www.avma.org/education/center-for-veterinary-accreditation/accredited-veterinary-colleges
150. Job Locations | BluePearl Specialty & Emergency Pet Hospital. Accessed 23 Nov 2022. https://careers.bluepearlvet.com/locations/
151. (2022) 2022 Snapshot: State of the Oncology Workforce in America. JCO Oncol Pract 18(5):396. https://doi.org/10.1200/OP.22.00168
152. Cooney K (2020) Historical perspective of euthanasia in veterinary medicine. Vet Clin Small Anim Pract 50(3):489–502. https://doi.org/10.1016/j.cvsm.2019.12.001
153. Yu D, Zhang S, Feng A et al (2019) Methotrexate, doxorubicin, and cisplatinum regimen is still the preferred option for osteosarcoma chemotherapy: a meta-analysis and clinical observation. Medicine 98(19):e15582. https://doi.org/10.1097/MD.0000000000015582
154. Withrow SJ, Wilkins RM (2010) Cross talk from pets to people: translational osteosarcoma treatments. ILAR J 51(3):208–213. https://doi.org/10.1093/ilar.51.3.208
155. Marti C, Kroner T, Remagen W, Berchtold W, Cserhati M, Varini M (1985) High-dose ifosfamide in advanced osteosarcoma. Cancer Treat Rep 69(1):115–117
156. Berrak SG, Pearson M, Berberoğlu S, Ilhan IE, Jaffe N (2005) High-dose ifosfamide in relapsed pediatric osteosarcoma: therapeutic effects and renal toxicity. Pediatr Blood Cancer 44(3):215–219. https://doi.org/10.1002/pbc.20228
157. Chou AJ, Merola PR, Wexler LH et al (2005) Treatment of osteosarcoma at first recurrence after contemporary therapy: the Memorial Sloan-Kettering Cancer Center experience. Cancer 104(10):2214–2221. https://doi.org/10.1002/cncr.21417
158. Harris MB, Cantor AB, Goorin AM et al (1995) Treatment of osteosarcoma with ifosfamide: comparison of response in pediatric patients with recurrent disease versus patients previously untreated: a pediatric oncology group study. Med Pediatr Oncol 24(2):87–92. https://doi.org/10.1002/mpo.2950240205
159. Harris MB, Gieser P, Goorin AM et al (1998) Treatment of metastatic osteosarcoma at diagnosis: a pediatric oncology group study. J Clin Oncol 16(11):3641–3648. https://doi.org/10.1200/JCO.1998.16.11.3641
160. Kim WO (2012) Institutional review board (IRB) and ethical issues in clinical research. Korean J Anesthesiol 62(1):3–12. https://doi.org/10.4097/kjae.2012.62.1.3

Lymphoma

William C. Kisseberth, Walter Hanel,
and Davis M. Seelig

1 Overview of Hodgkin's and Non-Hodgkin's Lymphoma

1.1 Introduction

Lymphoma consists of a heterogeneous group of hematopoietic malignancies that is comprised of many different histologically and molecularly defined types and subtypes. Many of the non-Hodgkin's lymphoma types defined in humans have histopathologically equivalent diseases occurring in dogs, thus providing an opportunity to study and conduct clinical trials in pet dogs with lymphoma to investigate new therapies, diagnostics, and devices to improve lymphoma patient outcomes. In humans, the diagnosis of lymphoma encompasses over 30 distinct disease entities as currently defined by the fifth edition of the World Health Organization Classification of Hematolymphoid Tumors (WHO-HAEM5) [1]. Hodgkin's lymphoma (HL) is a relatively rare cancer, accounting for about 15% of all lymphomas, and mostly affects young patients, with a second peak occurring in patients above 60 years of age [2, 3]. HL is clinically and morphologically distinct from other lymphomas, i.e., the non-Hodgkin's lymphomas (NHL). Within WHO-HAEMS, the different lymphomas are hierarchically classified based on category, family/class, entity/type, and subtype, with disease entities classified as aggressive or indolent based on typical rate of disease progression, and by immunophenotype/cell of origin, represented by B-cell, T-cell, and NK/null subtypes. Although many of the histological entities/types of lymphoma recognized in humans are also found in spontaneous canine cancers, their frequency of occurrence varies between the species (Fig. 1) [4]. Further, there are lymphoma types and subtypes without a clear equivalent in the other species (e.g., canine T-zone lymphoma) [5]. Human and canine lymphomas overlap in their molecular and genetic basis, with different types and subtypes sharing varying degrees of common gene mutations and common dysregulation of signaling pathways. As such, spontaneous lym-

W. C. Kisseberth (✉)
Department of Veterinary Clinical Sciences, College of Veterinary Medicine, The Ohio State University, Columbus, OH, USA

Division of Hematology, Department of Medicine, The Ohio State University Wexner Medical Center, Columbus, OH, USA
e-mail: kisseberth.2@osu.edu

W. Hanel
Division of Hematology, Department of Medicine, The Ohio State University Wexner Medical Center, Columbus, OH, USA

D. M. Seelig
Department of Veterinary Clinical Sciences, College of Veterinary Medicine, University of Minnesota, St. Paul, MN, USA

M. W. Nolan et al. (eds.), *Comparative Oncology*, https://doi.org/10.1007/978-3-032-04454-9_10

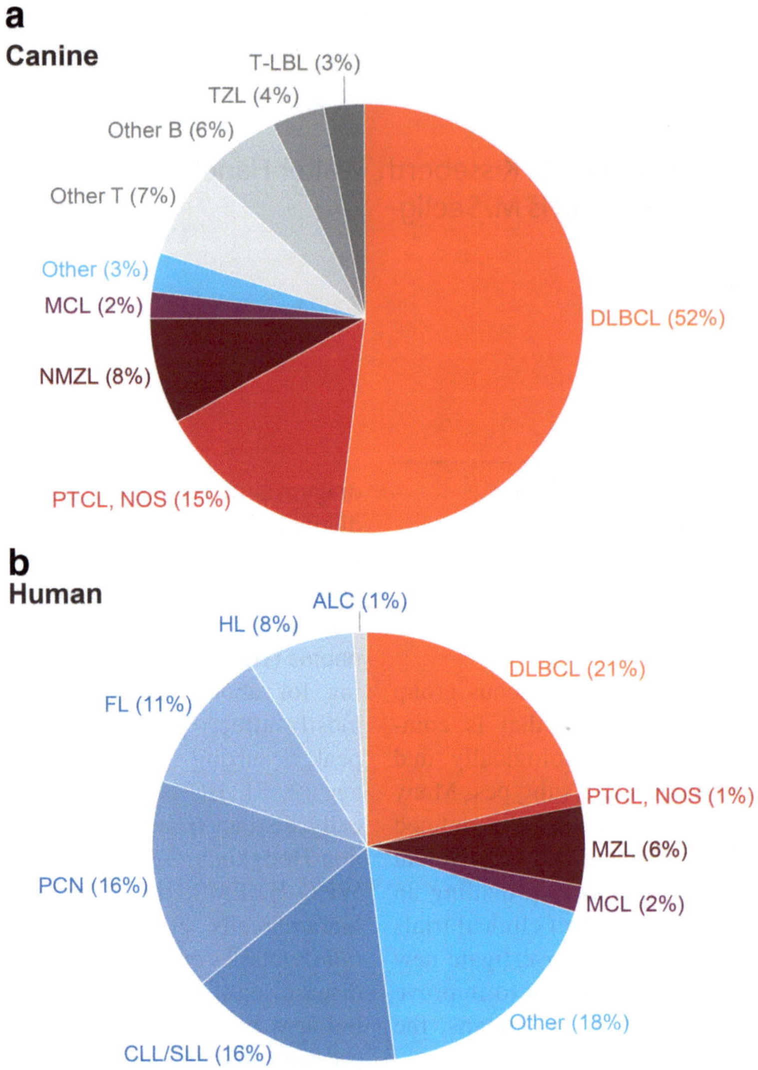

Fig. 1 Incidence of canine (**a**) and human (**b**) lymphoma. Canine data reflect summary data from three publications, whereas human data originates from one. *DLBCL* diffuse large B-cell lymphoma, *PTCL, NOS* peripheral T-cell lymphoma, not otherwise specified, *NMZL* nodal marginal zone lymphoma, *TZL* T-zone lymphoma, *T-LBL* T-cell lymphoblastic lymphoma, *MCL* mantle cell lymphoma, *CLL/SLL* chronic lymphocytic leukemia/small lymphocytic lymphoma, *PCN* plasma cell neoplasia, *FL* follicular lymphoma, *HL* Hodgkin's lymphoma, ALC anaplastic large cell lymphoma. (Modified from Seelig DM, Avery AC, Ehrhart EJ, Linden MA. Vet Sci. 2016 Jun;3(2):11. doi: 10.3390/vetsci3020011. Epub 2016 Jun 9. PMID: 28435836; PMCID: PMC5397114. [4]

phoma in pet dogs is increasingly being used in the preclinical development of new lymphoma treatments, and published translational trials are briefly reviewed here. Here, we will focus primarily on lymphoma types that occur with sufficient frequency in dogs that they can be used as large animal models for human cancers, or are of other comparative interest.

1.2 Clinical Epidemiology and Risk Factors for Lymphoma

1.2.1 Human Lymphoma

In humans, lymphoma represents the most common hematopoietic cancer and is the seventh most common cancer overall in men and the fifth most common in women. There were an estimated 8830 new cases of HL and 80,550 new cases of NHL diagnosed in the United States in 2023. Increasing age is a strong risk factor for lymphoma overall but varies with lymphoma type with the median age at diagnosis being 68 years for NHL and 39 years for HL [6]. Lymphoma risk is higher in men than women and is greater in white populations than in African American or Asian populations in the United States [7]. The pathogenesis of most lymphomas is unknown; however, the underlying genetic basis and environmental factors contributing to lymphomagenesis are areas of intense interest and research. Environmental exposures to certain chemicals (e.g., benzene, trichloroethylene), drugs, including some chemotherapy drugs, drugs to treat rheumatoid arthritis (e.g., methotrexate, TNF inhibitors), and radiation exposure have been epidemiologically associated with greater lymphoma risk, although not in all studies [8–13]. People with a weakened immune system (e.g., HIV infection [14, 15], organ transplant recipients [16, 17], genetic syndromes such as ataxia-telangiectasia and Wiskott-Aldrich syndrome [18] and autoimmune diseases (rheumatoid arthritis, systemic lupus erythematosus, Sjögren disease), celiac disease, and others are at increased risk for NHL [19, 20]. Infection/inflammation associated with a variety of infectious agents may contribute to the development of lymphoma, including specific lymphoma types such as extranodal marginal zone lymphomas (EMZL) [21]. Infectious causes may contribute to lymphoma development by direct lymphocyte transformation, viral-mediated T-cell immunosuppression leading to immune escape of lymphoma cells, and chronic immune stimulation of lymphocytes resulting in transformation [22, 23]. Associated infectious agents include: Epstein-Barr virus (EBV) (HL, Burkitt lymphoma (BL), T-cell lymphoma), HIV (BL, diffuse large B-cell lymphoma (DLBCL), primary CNS lymphoma), hepatitis C virus (HCV) (DLBCL, splenic marginal zone lymphoma (SMZL), nodal marginal zone lymphoma (NMZL)), human T-lymphotropic virus 1 (HTLV-1) (T-cell lymphoma), human herpes virus 8 (HHV-8) (primary effusion lymphoma), *Helicobacter pylori* (gastric mucosa-associated lymphoid tissue MALT) lymphoma, *Campylobacter jejuni* (small intestine MALT), *Chlamydia psittaci* (ocular adnexa malt), *Borrelia afzelii* (cutaneous MALT), and *Plasmodium falciparum* (BL) [24].

1.2.2 Canine Lymphoma

Similarly, in dogs, lymphoma is the most common hematopoietic cancer and is one of the most common cancers overall. Accurate and representative canine cancer incidence data are limited; however, canine lymphoma incidence is reported to be between 13 and 114 per 100,000 dogs at risk, and like humans, risk increases with age with a median age at diagnosis of 7.7 years [25–29]. Similar to humans, genetic and environmental factors influence lymphomagenesis although data on specific environmental exposures and risk factors are more limited. Epidemiological studies showed increased lymphoma risk in boxer dogs living in counties exceeding EPA ozone limits and having higher exposure risk estimates for airborne 1,3-butadiene and formaldehyde [30]. As in humans, herbicide and pesticide exposure and owner chemical use [31] have been associated with increased lymphoma risk in dogs [32–35] and residence in industrial areas [31]. A significant association between distributions of canine lymphoma and waste incinerators, polluted sites, and radioactive waste has been reported [36]. Unlike humans and cats, no transforming or immunosuppressive viral agents have been implicated in canine lymphoma pathogenesis. Although endogenous retroviruses can be found in normal tissue and tumor canine genomes, including lymphoma [37, 38], and other viral sequences detected in a variety of canine cancers, no reliable integration sites were identified [39]. However, high antibody titers to EBV or an EBV-like virus in dogs with spontaneous B-cell lymphoma and EBV-related viral components within malignant lymph nodes are reported [40]. The stomachs of dogs and cats can be colonized by several *Helicobacter* species; however, no association with gastric or other lymphomas has been established [41].

1.3 Diagnosis and Workup

1.3.1 Human Lymphoma

Pathologic diagnosis of lymphoma begins with histopathological assessment of a tumor biopsy, preferably an excisional biopsy, for nodal disease. Morphologic features assessed include cell size, characteristics of nucleus and cytoplasm, and the overall lymph node architecture. Lymphomas are classified using the most current edition of the World Health Classification of Tumors of the Hematopoietic and Lymphoid Tumors [42]. Fine-needle aspiration and cytology alone generally are not suitable for diagnosis. The precise diagnosis of lymphoma requires incorporating clinical information, along with the morphologic features of biopsy specimens. Ancillary studies including immunophenotype characterization immunohistochemistry (IHC) and flow cytometry (FC), conventional cytogenetics and fluorescence in situ hybridization (FISH), clonality studies, and gene mutation analysis significantly complement standard H&E staining and greatly aid in arriving at a final diagnosis. [43].

IHC and FC are critical for determining cell lineage and establishing specific lymphoma diagnoses. Diagnostic IHC and FC antibody panels used vary, and detailed guidelines are provided by the National Comprehensive Cancer Network (NCCN); however, for IHC, this generally includes CD3, CD20, Ki-67, CD10, Bcl-6, MUM-1, Bcl-2, c-myc, EBV ISH for DLBCL; CD3, CD20, CD5, Ki-67, Bcl-2, and CD10 for small/low-grade B-cell lymphoma; CD3, CD20, Ki-67, CD30, CD56, and EBV ISH for T/NK cell lymphomas; CD3, CD20, CD79a, CD10, Ki-67, TdT, and CD99 for precursor lymphomas; and CD3, CD20, Ki-67, CD30, CD15, PAX5, and EBV ISH for Hodgkin's lymphomas [44] [45]. Similarly, FC panels vary [46] [47] [48]; however, efforts are being made toward standardization, including the EuroFlow B-CLPD panel (CD3, CD4, CD5, CD8, CD10, CD11c, CD19, CD20, CD22, CD23, CD27, CD31, CD38, CD39, CD43, CD45, CD49d, CD56, CD62L, CD79b, CD81, CD95, CD103, CD185, CD200, CD305, HLA-DR, IgM, Igλ/Igκ, TCRγδ-1) [49] [50]. Under certain circumstances, and in particular to define specific lymphoma subtypes, other diagnostic tests may be required including molecular analyses to detect gene rearrangements (karyotype, FISH, PCR), next-generation sequencing panels, additional IHC panels, and EBV-encoded RNA in situ hybridization (EBVER-ISH) [1].

In addition to diagnostic assessments of the tumor, clinical stage, prognostic factors, and assessment of comorbidities play an important role in determining a final treatment plan. Standard clinical workup varies with different specific lymphoma diagnoses; however, in general, physical exam, performance status, CBC, comprehensive metabolic panel, LDH, hepatitis and HIV testing, imaging with positron emission tomography/computed tomography (PET/CT) or chest/abdomen/pelvis CT scans, and bone marrow biopsy/aspirate are performed. Additional tests, including immunoglobulin levels and gene mutation testing, may be required with certain lymphoma types as well.

1.3.2 Canine Lymphoma

The diagnosis, staging, and treatment of dogs with lymphoma are poorly standardized and vary between veterinary oncologists and institutions [51, 52]. Only a few consensus documents have been published by different organizations [53, 54]. As the recommended common therapies for canine lymphomas are dictated primarily by whether the tumor is considered aggressive or indolent and to a certain extent by immunophenotype, i.e., B cell or T cell, and not as much by the specific WHO diagnosis, many dogs are diagnosed and treated for lymphoma based solely on fine-needle aspiration and cytology of an affected lymph node and clinical findings. Up to 80% of canine lymphomas are aggressive; thus cytologic diagnosis is often straightforward. When it is not, additional supportive diagnostic tests, including FC of a fine-needle aspirate, or clonality testing (e.g., PCR for antigen receptor rearrangement, PARR), may be performed. As in people, excisional biopsy of a lymph node or, alternatively, multiple needle biopsies, is required to make a specific WHO diagnosis. Canine lymphomas can be classified

Table 1 Canine and human non-Hodgkin lymphomas according to the 2008 WHO guidelines

B-Cell neoplasms	T-Cell neoplasms
B-lymphoblastic leukemia/lymphoma	**T-lymphoblastic leukemia/lymphoma**
Chronic lymphocytic leukemia/small lymphocytic lymphoma	T-cell prolymphocytic leukemia
B-cell prolymphocytic leukemia	**T-cell large granular lymphocytic leukemia**
Splenic marginal zone lymphoma	Chronic lymphoproliferative disorder of NK cells
Hairy cell leukemia	Aggressive NK-cell leukemia
Splenic lymphoma/leukemia, unclassifiable	EBV-positive T-cell disease of childhood
Lymphoplasmacytic lymphoma	Hydroa vacciniforme-like lymphoma
Heavy chain diseases	Adult T-cell leukemia/lymphoma
Plasma cell myeloma	Extranodal NK/T-cell lymphoma, nasal type
Solitary plasmacytoma of bone	**Enteropathy-associated T-cell lymphoma**[a]
Extraosseous plasmacytoma	**Hepatosplenic T-cell lymphoma**
MALT lymphoma	Subcutaneous panniculitis-like T-cell lymphoma
Nodal marginal zone lymphoma	**Mycosis fungoides**
Follicular lymphoma	**Sézary syndrome**
Primary cutaneous follicle center lymphoma	Cutaneous $CD30^+$ T-cell disorders
Mantle cell lymphoma	**Peripheral T-cell lymphoma, NOS**
Diffuse large B-cell lymphoma	**T-zone lymphoma**[b]
Lymphomatoid granulomatosis	Angioimmunoblastic T-cell lymphoma
Primary mediastinal large B-cell lymphoma	Anaplastic large cell lymphoma, ALK-positive
Intravascular large B-cell lymphoma	Anaplastic large cell lymphoma, ALK-negative
ALK-positive large B-cell lymphoma	
Plasmablastic lymphoma	
Large B-cell lymphoma in Castleman disease	
Primary effusion lymphoma	
Burkitt lymphoma	
B-cell lymphoma, unclassifiable	

Non-bolded entities represent malignancies in humans only whereas bolded entities reflect malignancies reported in both humans and canines.

[a] A neoplasm with an EATL-like morphology has been described in dogs, but an association with celiac disease has not been documented.

[b] In humans, TZL is considered a morphologic variant of PTCL, NOS. Modified from Seelig DM, Avery AC, Ehrhart EJ, Linden MA. Vet Sci. 2016 Jun;3(2):11. doi: 10.3390/vetsci3020011. Epub 2016 Jun 9. PMID: 28435836; PMCID: PMC5397114. [4]

using a modified WHO classification (Table 1) [55]. Determination of B-cell or T-cell lineage is made either by IHC of tumor biopsies or FC of fine-needle aspirates, with the latter providing more extensive characterization of lineage and phenotype. PARR may also be used in selected cases.

Diagnosis and Staging of Canine Lymphoma

Although histopathology is the gold standard for lymphoma diagnosis in the dog, cytologic diagnosis is much more common for a variety of reasons. First, the majority of canine lymphomas are high-grade and thus differentiating lymphoma from other disease entities is generally clearer for high-grade, aggressive lymphomas compared to low-grade, indolent lymphomas. Also, fine needle aspiration cytology is minimally invasive, rapid, accessible, and inexpensive. Finally, compared to lymphoma in people, treatment options for canine lymphomas are more limited and are much less dictated by the specific histologically determined type, i.e., a less precise lymphoma type diagnosis is needed in order to guide treatment. For all of these reasons, in many cases a specific lymphoma histologic type is often not obtained.

When a histologic diagnosis is made, excisional lymph node biopsy, or wedge biopsy including capsule, is preferred. Alternatively, needle core biopsies can be taken, in which case it is important that multiple cores be obtained so that there is sufficient tissue available for histologic examination and for IHC. In one small study, comparing the diagnostic utility of needle core biopsies to excisional biopsy, needle core biopsies accurately confirmed the presence of lymphoma in 12/14 (86%) of cases [56]. However, needle core biopsies have not been sufficiently evaluated for their utility in accurately determining WHO-type diagnosis. Compared to histologic diagnosis, the cytologic diagnostic accuracy for lymphoma versus other diagnoses in dogs and cats was reported to be 92.3% (24/26) in one study [57]. In another report, six evaluators reviewed fine needle aspirate samples from 161 lymph nodes (146 lymphoma, 15 other pathologies) [58]. Lymphoma classification accuracy ranged from 82.9% to 93.2%, with an overall sensitivity of 92.6%.

Immunophenotyping for lymphoma involves using antibody-based detection methods to identify proteins specific to different lymphocyte lineages or subsets. Immunophenotyping is necessary for WHO lymphoma classification. Immunophenotype cannot be determined reliably based on histologic or cytologic morphologic criteria [59]. Most commonly, immunophenotyping is done either using IHC on histologic specimens or FC on needle aspirates. The main advantage of IHC is that it allows concurrent evaluation of both histomorphology and immunophenotype. Unfortunately, fixation and processing of paraffin-embedded tissue can alter the conformation of protein epitopes, especially for cell surface proteins, thus limiting the number of antibodies detectable by IHC. Antibodies commonly used for IHC-based lymphoma diagnosis and immunophenotyping include CD3, CD79a, CD20, and Pax-5.

FC is typically performed on live cells collected by fine needle aspiration; thus, it complements cytologic diagnosis well. As antigenic degradation due to fixation is less of an issue with FC compared to IHC, a broader array of antigens can be detected and a greater number of immunophenotypes determined. Diagnostic FC, like IHC, lacks standardization of reagents, instrumentation, techniques, and reporting [60]. FC panels and protocols are not standardized and vary; however, commonly used markers in veterinary clinical flow cytometry include CD3, CD4, CD5, CD8, CD11b, CD14, CD18, CD20, CD21, CD22, CD25, CD34, CD45, CD61, CD79a, CD117, IgG/IgM, Ki67, and MHC II, but vary with laboratory [60–65]. Representative scatterplots of common canine lymphoma diagnoses are shown (Fig. 2) [66]. Furthermore, FC can detect aberrant antigen expression, such as loss of CD45, or co-expression of antigens normally restricted to a single lineage, e.g., CD3+/CD21+, CD4+/CD8+ [67–70]. Besides its role in WHO classification, i.e., determining B- and T-cell lineage, some immunophenotypes are highly correlated with specific morphologic types and prognostic profiles. Notably, TZL, which typically is CD45-, CD21+, CD3+, CD5+, CD4+/−, CD8+/−, and MHCII^{hi} can be diagnosed with a combination of FC and cytopathology [5, 71]. Additionally, FC can identify immunophenotypes within WHO-defined types that have prognostic significance. For example, as in humans, PTCL is a heterogeneous disease in dogs. The most common immunophenotype in dogs is CD3^{+}/CD4^{+}/MHC II^{-}; however, CD4^{-}/CD8^{+}, CD4^{+}/CD8^{+}, CD4^{-}/CD8^{-} immunophenotypes, and MHC II^{hi} immunophenotypes occur too, although the prognostic significance of different immunophenotypes and potential impact on response to treatment have not been established [72–74].

Assessment of clonality in canine lymphoid malignancies is most commonly done using PCR-based methods to evaluate the immunoglobulin (Ig) receptor and T-cell receptor (TCR) genes. PCR primers target the DNA sequences encoding the third complementarity determining region (CDR3). PCR-based amplification of this region yields a uniquely sized amplicon from each lymphocyte and its clonal progeny within the sampled population. Assessment of clonality can be used to support a diagnosis of lymphoma in morphologically or immunophenotypically ambiguous cases, where a monoclonal population of lymphocytes is supportive of (although not specific to) a diagnosis of lymphoma, whereas a polyclonal population is inconsistent with lym-

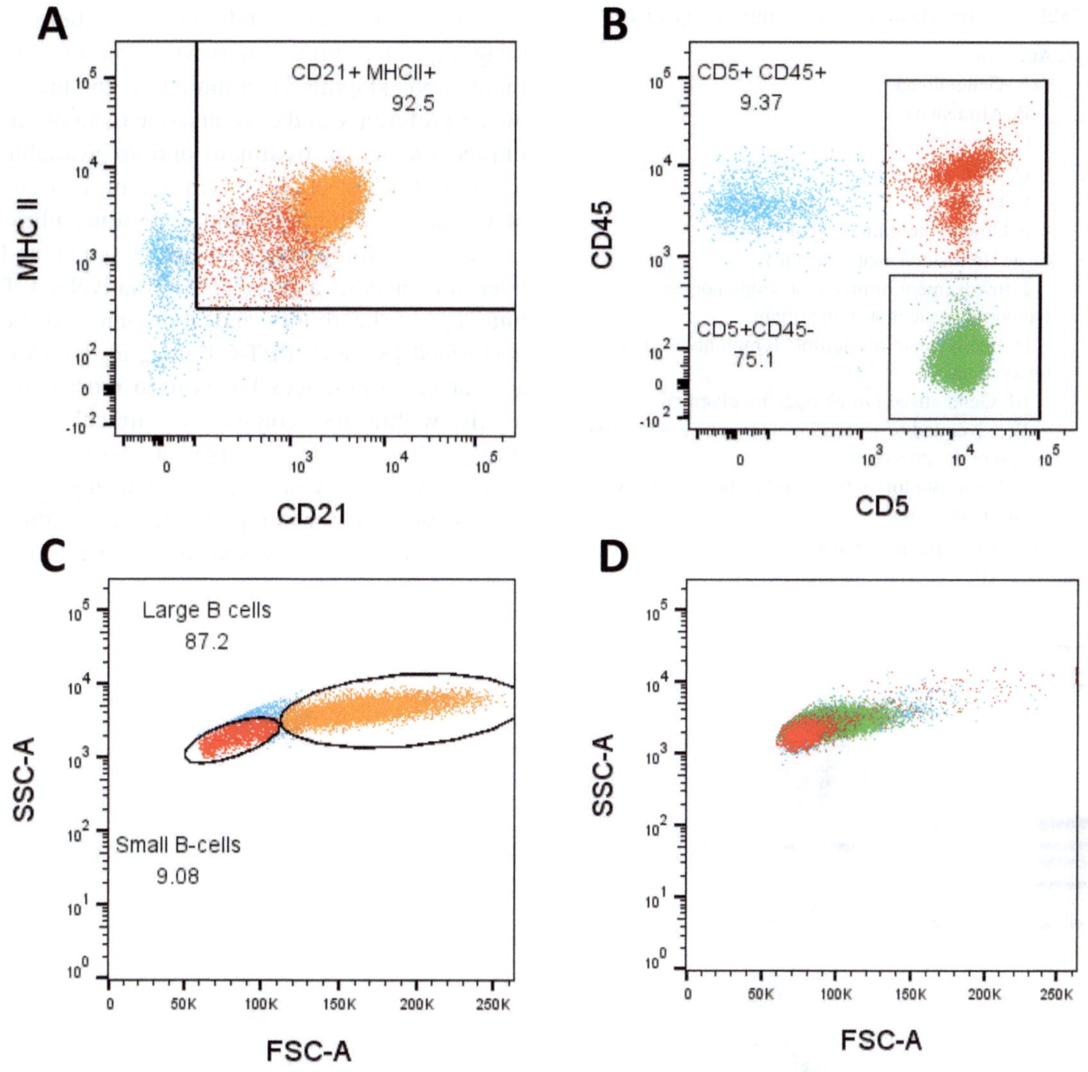

Fig. 2 Representative scatterplots from common canine lymphomas. Panels **a**, **c** = Large B-cell lymphoma. In panel **a**, note the near monotypic population of CD21+ MHCII+ B-cells (orange) that, in panel **c**, demonstrate increased forward and side scattered as compared to this patients non-neoplastic B-cells (red). Panels **b**, **d** = T-Zone lymphoma. In panel **b**, note the dominant population of phenotypically aberrant T-cells that express the pan-T cell antigen CD5, but lack appropriate expression of the pan-leukocyte antigen CD45 (green). These cells are medium sized as demonstrated by their slightly higher forward scatter as compared to this patient's phenotypically normal T-cells (green, panel **d**)

phoma [75]. It can also be used to establish B- or T-cell lineage where immunophenotyping is otherwise not available. Finally, clonality assays can be used to assess molecular disease status in lymph node/tumor aspirates, bone marrow, or peripheral blood, for molecular disease staging, or for detection of minimal residual disease (MRD) during the course of therapy [76–79].

TNM classification and staging of canine lymphomas was defined by the WHO but has not been updated (Table 2) [80]. Complete staging of a canine patient with a new diagnosis of lymphoma typically includes physical exam, caliper measurements of peripheral lymph nodes, a minimum database of a complete blood cell count (CBC), serum biochemi-

Table 2 WHO classification of canine lymphoma

1. Anatomic type
A. Generalized
B. Alimentary
C. Thymic
D. Skin
E. Leukemia
F. Others (including solitary renal)
2. Stage (to include anatomic site)
I. Involvement limited to a single node or lymphoid tissue in a single organ
II. Involvement of multiple lymph nodes in a regional area
III. Generalized lymph node involvement
IV. Liver and/or spleen involvement (± generalized lymph node involvement)
V. Manifestation in the blood or bone marrow ± other organ system

Substage (a) without systemic signs
Substage (b) with systemic signs

cal profile, urinalysis, abdominal and thoracic imaging, and bone marrow aspirate/core. Incomplete staging is common, both due to owner preference and cost, and due to an often-limited impact on treatment options available or offered. Most commonly, imaging consists of thoracic radiography and abdominal ultrasound +/− cytologic assessment of spleen and liver fine needle aspirates. Alternatively, CT imaging of the thorax and abdomen may be performed [81–84]. PET-CT imaging is available at some practices but is used most commonly within the context of clinical trials (Fig. 3) [85, 86]. Bone marrow assessment, by aspiration cytology or core biopsy histopathology, is required for complete clinical staging; however, due to its invasive nature it is often

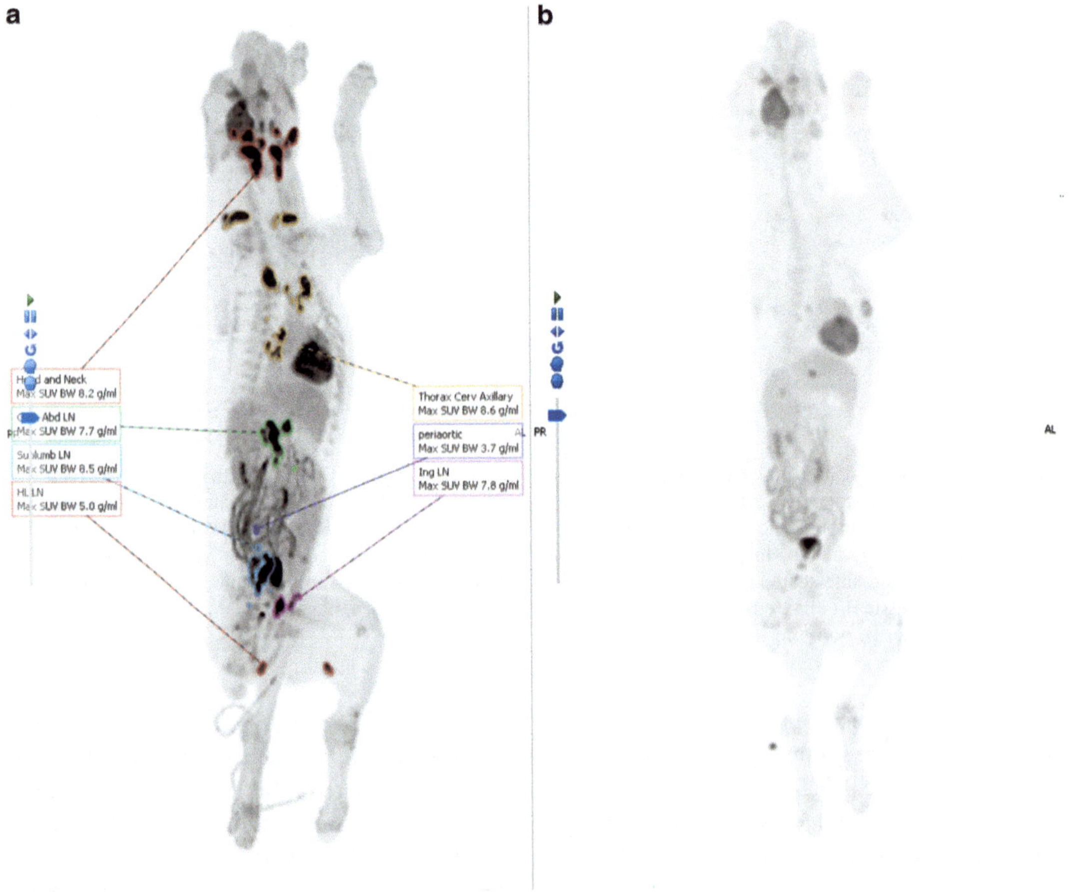

Fig. 3 18F-FDG uptake in a canine patient with multicentric lymphoma. 18F-fluoro-2-deoxy-D-glucose (18F-FDG) positron emission tomography/computed tomography (PET/CT), obliqued dorsal/lateral image. Increased FDG uptake in the lymphocenters of the head, neck, thorax, abdomen, and hind limb pretreatment (**a**) with diminished uptake post-CHOP chemotherapy treatment (**b**). (Courtesy of © Lynn Griffin)

omitted. As imaging techniques have improved and more sensitive tests have been developed to assess for the presence of disease, i.e., minimal residual disease (MRD), as in people, "stage migration" has become evident [87]. Based on these staging tests, dogs with lymphoma can be assigned a WHO clinical stage and substage which have prognostic significance [88].

1.4 Lymphoma Types

Classification of human lymphomas is updated periodically, with the most recent consensus documents being the fifth edition of the World Health Organization (WHO) classification and the international consensus of mature lymphoid neoplasms (ICC2022) [1, 61]. The 2008 REAL-WHO guidelines have been adapted for the dog and diagnostic applicability assessed by a panel of 18 international veterinary pathologists. Using this canine-adapted system, 300 cases of canine lymphoma were diagnosed with an overall accuracy of 83% and an inter-observer variability of 65% [54, 89, 90].

1.4.1 Human and Canine Diffuse Large B-Cell Lymphoma

Diffuse large B-cell lymphoma (DLBCL) is the most common aggressive B-cell lymphoma in people representing about a third of NHL diagnoses, but its incidence ranges between 20% and 50% by country. Incidence is generally higher in males, and in the United States, it is highest among non-Hispanic whites. The median age at diagnosis is 66 years and incidence increases with age [8].

Pathology

Although DLBCL, NOS (not otherwise specified) is the most common large B-cell lymphoma, an additional 17 DLBCL subcategories are currently recognized. Morphologically and immunohistochemically DLBCL is characterized by large atypical CD3-negative and CD20-positive lymphocytes with a Ki-67 labeling index of greater than 80%. Within the WHO classification system DLBCL/high-grade B-cell lymphoma with *MYC* and *BCL2* rearrangements is recognized as a distinct entity and the double expressor phenotype can be verified by IHC [91]. EBV-positive DLBCL (EBV DLBCL) can be identified using EBV ISH [92, 93]. An immunohistochemically determined cell of origin (COO) can be determined using a panel of CD10, BCL-6, and MUM-1 antibodies and has been correlated with molecular gene signatures [94]. DLBCL in dogs is similarly morphologically and immunohistochemically diagnosed, with B-cell lineage determined most commonly using CD20 or CD79a antibodies. However, canine lymphomas are commonly diagnosed cytologically (+/− FC) and thus many canine patients do not have a WHO lymphoma type definitively determined. Using FC, the majority of large B-cell lymphomas are characterized by medium-sized CD21-positive cells with variable, but generally high, MHC class II expression. Cytologically, the cells can be variable in size with a large round nucleus, dispersed immature chromatin, often with multiple large round prominent nucleoli, and a small amount of deeply basophilic cytoplasm [65].

Molecular Characteristics

The molecular characteristics of DLBCL in people continue to be defined. Genomic approaches over the past 20 years have significantly increased our understanding of the molecular basis of DLBCL and have provided critical insight to understanding the heterogeneity of this disease and offers promise for developing more personalized and targeted therapies. Seminal in the advancement in our understanding of the molecular basis of lymphoma was the establishment of COO subclassification based on early transcriptional profiling studies that subclassified DLBCL based on gene signatures associated with a germinal center (GC) or activated B-cell (ABC) origin [95, 96]. COO subclassification was eventually incorporated into the WHO classification of DLBCL. Clinical translation of COO subclassification has proved challenging due to the technology required, thus surrogate IHC algorithms were developed as an alternative, but these do not replicate the classification as accurately as transcriptional methods [94, 97, 98]. There is tremendous genetic heterogeneity in DLBCL. In one study, whole-exome sequencing of 1001 DLBCL patients identified 150 genetic drivers with a mean number of 7.75 mutations per tumor [99]. More recently, multiple large studies have subclassified DLBCL based on the profile of mutations carried by individual tumors, with some groups associated with better or worse outcomes and other groups more variable in outcome [100–102]. Presumably, these genetically distinct groups explain some of the heterogeneity in response observed to different treatments. Notably, the current WHO classification recognizes the genetic subtype of DLBCL with *MYC* and *BCL6* rearrangements, as well as DLBCL/high-grade B-cell lymphoma (HBCL) with *MYC*, *BCL2*, and *BCL-6* rearrangements as a distinct entity referred to as double hit/triple hit high-grade B-cell lymphoma (DH/TH-HGBL). Thus, assessment of *MYC*, *BCL2*, and *BCL6* status is necessary to fully utilize the WHO classification. Typically, this is done using FISH on formalin-fixed paraffin-embedded sections [103].

The genomic characterization of canine DLBCL is more limited; however, several of the key molecular features of human DLBCL have been investigated in the dog. Canine DLBCL transcriptional profiles generally show the most similarity to the human ABC gene signature [104]. Most notably, within the ABC group both human and canine DLBCL are characterized by activation of the NFκB signaling pathway [104, 105]. As the ABC gene signature is associated with poorer outcomes in people, this appears to correlate with the poor long-term survival characteristic of canine DLBCL even when treated with relatively intensive multi-agent chemotherapy protocols. DNA sequencing and mutational analysis, although limited in extent, show some, but limited commonality in mutated genes shared between the two species [106]. Nonetheless, these mutations often result in perturbation of shared signaling pathways. This appears to be a common theme when comparing other human and canine cancers—similarities in dysregulation of signaling pathways, but differences in many of the most relevant mutations. In limited studies, the most common mutation in canine DLBCL is in *TRAF3*, whose inactivation results in activation of the NFκB pathway [106, 107]. Additional recurrently mutated genes reported to occur in >15% of tumors include *SETD2*, *POT1*, *TP53*, *MYC*, *FBXW7*, *DDX3X*, and *TBL1XR1*. In contrast, in humans, *MLL2*, *BCL2*, *MYD88*, *HIST1H1E*, *PIM1*, *CREBBP*, *CARD11*, and *SPEN* are the most commonly mutated genes in DLBCL [99]. Although there are differences in individual gene mutational frequency between the two species, there is overlap in which genes are mutated. In both species there is a high frequency of alterations in genes affecting NFκB signaling, chromatin regulation, and transcriptional regulation [106]. In humans, *MYC*, *BCL2*, and *BCL6* gene translocations contribute to lymphomagenesis, assignment of WHO classification, and have prognostic significance [108–110]. In dogs, *BCL6* is rarely expressed, consistent with a more common ABC-like phenotype [104, 111]. *BCL2* and *MYC* are both commonly expressed at high levels in canine DLBCL; however, expression is not predictive of outcome [112]. Further, there is an enrichment for genes in the MYC pathway in canine DLBCL and gain of part or all of chromosome 13, which carries *MYC*, and is the most common copy number variation (CNV) in canine B-cell lymphomas [113, 114]. Overall, the molecular evidence suggests that canine DLBCL is more similar to human ABC-DLBCL than GC-DLBCL.

1.4.2 Human and Canine Follicular and Marginal Zone Lymphoma

Follicular lymphoma (FL) and marginal zone lymphoma (MZL) are indolent mature B-cell malignancies. FL is the most common of the indolent lymphomas in people, representing about 12% of NHLs in the United States with an annual age-adjusted incidence of 3.5 per 100,000. The median age at diagnosis is 64 years and increases significantly with age [6]. In the United States, incidence rates are highest in non-Hispanic whites [115, 116]. MZL is the second most common B-cell indolent lymphoma, accounting for about 7% of all mature NHLs in the United States with an age-standardized incidence rate of 19.6 per 1,000,000 [117]. MZL is further divided into three subtypes based on anatomic origin: extranodal MZL (EMZL), splenic MZL (SMZL), and nodal MZL (NMZL) [1]. Collectively, the median age at diagnosis is 60 to 70 years and the incidence increases with age. There is no sex predisposition, except for some extranodal sites [118, 119]. EMZL is commonly referred to as MALT lymphoma as it resembles normal mucosa-associated lymphoid tissue (MALT) and is thought to arise from acquired mutations in response to various infectious, autoimmune, or other inflammatory stimuli [120]. The most common extranodal site for MZL is the stomach, followed by the adnexa of the eyes, lungs, skin, and salivary glands [118]. The etiology of EMZL is associated with chronic inflammation caused by infectious microorganisms, including *Helicobacter pylori*, *Chlamydia psittaci*, *Campylobacter jejuni*, *Borrelia burgdorferi*, and hepatitis C virus [21]. *H. pylori* infection in particular is closely associated with gastric EMZL [54, 121].

In contrast to humans, FL is a rare lymphoma type in dogs, where it comprises less than 1% of nodal lymphoma diagnoses [54, 122]. NMZL is the second most common nodal B-cell lymphoma in dogs, where it represents about 10% of diagnoses [54, 123, 124]. SMZL is a rare, poorly defined lymphoma in dogs that is described only in small case series [125–127]. Other histologic differential diagnoses for canine SMZL include mantle cell lymphoma (MCL)(an even rarer indolent lymphoma type in dogs), lymphoid nodular hyperplasia, and complex nodular hyperplasia [128, 129]. EMZL, or MALT, lymphomas are even more infrequently described, although EMZL of the uterus [130], third eyelid [131, 132], and urinary bladder [133] have been reported.

Pathology

FL is a B-cell malignancy originating from germinal center cells that morphologically appears as a mixture of cleaved centrocytes and noncleaved centroblasts. FL is a small B-cell lymphoma that expresses pan B-lymphocyte antigens (CD19, CD20, CD22, CD79a, PAX-5) and IgM with or without IgD and usually coexpresses CD10 and BCL2, with CD10 expression indicating germinal center origin, t(14;18) *BCL2* translocation causing aberrant expression of BCL2 and exhibits a follicular pattern of growth. Some higher-grade FLs may not express CD10 [134] and others lack the t(14;18) translocation [135], demonstrating molecular heterogeneity in this disease. Previously, FL was graded based on the number of centroblasts per high-power field; however, WHO-HAEM5 recognizes classic FL and follicular large B-cell lymphoma (FLBL). Additionally, FL with unusual diagnostic features and FL with predominantly diffuse growth pattern are recognized as distinct entities [1, 120]. Other differential diagnoses for small/low-grade B-cell lymphoma include chronic lymphocytic leukemia/small lymphocytic lymphoma (CLL/SLL), MCL, and MZL.

MZL originates in the follicular marginal zone. EMZL, SMZL, and NMZL share overlapping morphologic and phenotypic features; however, they differ in their clinical presentation, associated infectious microorganisms, and genetic features [120]. EMZL accounts for 70%, SMZL for 20%, and NMZL for 10% of MZL diagnoses [136]. In SMZL, small B cells surround and replace the normal white pulp nodules of the spleen, classically showing a biphasic appearance with central cores of small lymphocytes with mature chromatin and scant cytoplasm and a peripheral zone of cells with round to slightly irregular nuclei, slightly more open chromatin, and more abundant cytoplasm [120]. Patients present with splenomegaly, involvement of the bone marrow, and usually peripheral blood. Often diagnosis is made via bone marrow biopsy [137]. SMZL is a B-cell neoplasm lacking specific immunophenotypic markers. Neoplastic cells typically express CD19, CD20, CD22, CD79a, CD79b, FMC7, and IgM and lack expression of annexin A1, CD5, CD10, CD23, CD25, CD43, Cyclin D1, and LEF1. CD103 is usually negative [120, 138]. NMZL is a primary nodal B-cell lymphoma resembling SMZL and EMZL. In humans it is the least common form of

MZL. The morphologic appearance is quite heterogeneous. Neoplastic cells consist of small lymphocytes, monocytoid-appearing cells, and plasmacytoid cells in varying proportions. Like other MZLs, there is at least a partially nodular appearance, although some cases may be more diffuse. NMZL expresses pan B-cell antigens, and CD5 and CD10 are usually absent [120]. CD43 [139, 140], IRTA1, and MNDA are variably expressed [141]. The neoplastic cells of EMZL are small with mature chromatin, round to slightly irregular nuclear contours, and variable amounts of cytoplasm, although monocytoid features are typical at some anatomic locations. Tumor cells proliferate around the periphery of germinal centers, following a marginal distribution external to preserved mantle zones. Diffuse sheets of small neoplastic cells are typically present between germinal centers [120]. Immunophenotypically, EMZL neoplastic cells are positive for pan-B-cell antigens. They are generally negative for CD5, CD10, CD23, LEF1, Cyclin D1, and SOX11. Rarely, CD5- or CD10-positive cases have been described. CD43 is expressed in ~50% of cases [120].

Molecular Characteristics

Classic FL is characterized by *BCL2* rearrangements, most commonly t(14;18) (q32;q21); however, other variants including t(2;18) (p12;q21) and t(18;22)(q21;q11) occur, accounting for 85–90% of cases. Mutations in epigenetic regulators (e.g., *EZH2, ARID1A, MEF2B, KMT2C*) and chromatin remodeling genes (e.g., *KMT2D/MLL2, CREBBP, EP300*) are the most frequent in classic FL [142]. Genomic alterations in *TP53* or *CDKN2A* and *MYC* translocations are usually associated with high-grade features and/or risk of transformation [143]. *BCL2* rearrangement-negative FL represents 10–15% of FL cases and is heterogeneous both genetically and clinically [135]. In SMZL, the most common chromosomal abnormality is deletion of chromosome 7q found in approximately 30% of cases. In one study, two specific molecular subsets together accounted for 91% of SMZL tumors. The NNK subset was defined by mutations in NOTCH1, NFκB, and KLF2—pathways which regulate normal marginal zone development. The DMT subset was characterized by mutations in DNA damage repair (*TP53, ATM*) or the MAPK or TLR signaling pathways. The NNK subset was associated with poorer outcome. [144] Immunoglobulin heavy chain genes are clonally rearranged in EMZL. Within specific anatomic sites there is often biased usage of specific *IGH* variable gene families. Recurrent translocations have been identified and may be associated with specific anatomic sites [145, 146]. All lead to dysregulation of the NFκB signaling pathway. Recurrently mutated genes have been identified in EMZL and may vary across anatomic sites. As some of these translocations and mutations appear to be unique to EMZL, they can be useful in the differential diagnosis with other small B-cell diseases [147]. NMZL is comparatively rare, thus relatively little genetic data is available. The most highly recurrent mutation is in *KMT2D* at 20%. *TNFAIP3*, *CREBBP*, *FAS*, and *KLF2* mutations occur at frequencies of 12–14%, with other recurrent mutations being less frequent [147].

There is very little molecular data concerning canine FL and MZL. FL is rare and *BCL2* chromosomal translocations have not been found [148]. Integrated genomic analysis of 7 canine FL and 5 NMZL cases showed activation of BCR and TLR signaling pathways [123]. FL showed enrichment of E2F targets and MZL was characterized by MYC-driven transcriptional signals [123]. Importantly, no specific gene signatures differentiated canine NMZL and DLBCL [104, 123]. This finding is consistent with the typical biological behavior of MZL in dogs, where MZL more commonly has an aggressive clinical course in spite of being classified as an indolent lymphoma in people [124, 149].

1.4.3 Human and Canine Peripheral T-Cell Lymphoma

In humans, T-cell lymphomas comprise 10–15% of all NHL diagnoses, with peripheral T-cell lymphoma (PTCL) being the most common T-cell type accounting for 6% of cases [150] and the incidence of PTCL being 2.1 per 100,000 in the United States [151]. In contrast, PTCL represents 20–30% of NHL diagnoses in Asia, which is higher [152]. PTCL is a heterogeneous group of disease entities, currently grouped into nine mature T-cell and NK-cell types comprised of 34 defined entities [1]. PTCL-not otherwise specified (PTCL-NOS) is a T-cell lymphoma that does not meet any of the other specific subtype criteria and thus is a diagnosis of exclusion. PTCL-NOS is the most common subtype in Western countries and is the most common in dogs.

Pathology

PTCLs arise from post-thymic T lymphocytes. PTCL diagnosis is made from tumor biopsy with an IHC panel typically including T-cell markers (CD3, CD2, CD5, CD7, CD4, CD8), T-follicular helper subtype markers (CD10, BCL6, PD1/CD279, ICOS, CXCL13), CD30, ALK, CD56, TCRβ, TCRδ, Ki67, and EBV ISH [153], or incorporating corresponding FC panels where appropriate. Morphologically PTCL-NOS is characterized by paracortical infiltrates with effacement of the normal lymph node architecture. Immunophenotypically, PTCL-NOS is positive for CD3 and CD4 antigens and negative for CD7 and CD5. CD30 is variably expressed and EBV is present in about 30% of cases [154].

In dogs, beyond expression of the pan-leukocyte antigen CD45 and one or more pan-T-cell antigens (CD3 and/or CD5), further immunophenotypic characterization of canine PTCL has, to date, identified three flow cytometric subtypes, namely CD4+ disease, CD8+ disease, and CD4-/CD8- disease. Histologically, all three tumor types are characterized by an effacing population of intermediate to large cells demonstrating high nuclear pleomorphism and variable mitotic activity [72, 74, 155].

Molecular Characteristics

Transcriptional profiling of PTCL-NOS identifies two main groups. The first group, PTCL-TBX21 expresses T-box 21 (TBX21), a transcription factor which is associated with T_H1 and cytotoxic T-cell differentiation. This group is associated with NFκB and JAK/STAT pathway dysregulation. The second group, PTCL-GATA3, is characterized by overexpression of GATA3, a transcriptional regulator of T_H2 cell differentiation. This group is associated with PI3K/mTOR pathway enrichment, hyperactivated MYC, and genomic instability. [156, 157] Interestingly, the two groups were found to have different morphological features and can be further distinguished using a panel of four antibodies. TBX21 and CXCR3 (for PTCL-TBX21) and GATA3 and CCR4 (for PTCL-GATA3) can separate the molecularly defined groups in ~85% of cases [158]. The PTCL-GATA3 group has a poorer prognosis. Whole-exome and targeted capture mutation profiling have shown recurrent mutations in *RHOA*, *TP53*, *CDKN2A*, *PTEN*, *KMT2C*, *SETD1B*, *YTHDF2*, and *PDCD1* [159–161].

Canine T-cell lymphoma has not been well characterized molecularly. In one small study applying microarray-based transcriptional profiling to a heterogeneous sample set of 35 nodal lymphomas that included 13 T-cell lymphomas (PTCL = 3, lymphoblastic T-cell lymphoma (LBT) = 4, TZL = 6) the aggressive T-cell lymphomas (PTCL and LBT) segregated from TZL and B-cell lymphoma groups [162].

1.4.4 Human and Canine Cutaneous T-Cell Lymphoma

The majority of primary cutaneous lymphomas in humans are T cell in origin. Cutaneous T-cell lymphoma (CTCL) represents about 2–3% of all NHLs [163]. It constitutes a heterogeneous group of mature NHLs with mycosis fungoides (MF) being the most common, accounting for nearly 50% of CTCL diagnoses [163]. The median age at diagnosis is 55 to 60 years [164, 165]. Sézary syndrome (SS), a distinct clinical entity characterized by diffuse erythema and leukemic disease, is much rarer, accounting for less than 5% of primary CTCLs. MF has a higher incidence in the Black population where there is a female predominance, younger age of onset, and inferior outcomes [166, 167]. Patients with classic MF present with patches or plaques, which wax and wane and can be annular or arcuate, sharply demarcated, erythematous, and scaly. In advanced stages, tumors, erythroderma, and extracutaneous dissemination may occur.

Similarly, in dogs, most cutaneous lymphomas are T cell and most exhibit epitheliotropism, i.e., cutaneous epitheliotropic T-cell lymphoma (CETCL), and histopathologically resemble MF, pagetoid reticulosis, and SS in humans. The clinical presentation is highly variable and includes diffuse erythema, scaling, patches/plaques/nodules, focal hypopigmentation with mucocutaneous junctions or mucosa affected in ~50% of cases. Involvement of other organs can occur in later stages of the disease [168]. In general, the disease tends to be more aggressive and rapidly progressive in dogs.

Pathology

Primary cutaneous lymphomas are classified using the World Health Organization-European Organization for the Research and Treatment of Cancer (WHO-EORTC) consensus classification with recent updates from the WHO and International Consensus Classification [1, 61, 169]. Besides MF/SS the other CTCL disease entities are much less common; however, collectively they constitute about half of CTCLs [1, 61, 170, 171]. MF is an epitheliotropic, mature T-cell lymphoma composed of small- to medium-sized T cells with cerebriform nuclei. Histopathologically, lesions of MF vary from limited, epidermotropic, folliculotropic, and/or syringotropic lymphoid infiltrates in early disease, to dense, dermal to subcutaneous infiltrates without significant epidermotropism in advance disease [172]. IHC is important in the diagnosis of MF. In MF, the predominant cell population is typically CD3, CD4, and TCRBF1-positive with loss of one or more pan T-cell markers (CD2, CD5, CD7). Variant immunophenotypes may occur, including CD8-positive and/or λ/δTCRs, like dogs, and have a poorer prognosis [173, 174]. Demonstration of clonality by standard PCR or next generation sequencing can be helpful in diagnosis in selected cases but by itself is not diagnostic.

In canine CETCL neoplastic cells infiltrate the skin and mucosa. Different forms of this disease have been described as paralleling human MF, SS, and pagetoid reticulosis [175–179]. While the neoplastic cells in human MF are generally CD4-positive, in dogs CETCL cells are typically CD8-positive (80–90%) or CD4/CD8 negative [179, 180]. Although most human CTCL cases express the α/βTCR, canine CTCL cells express the λ/δTCR in greater than 60% of cases [180]. Neoplastic T cells demonstrate tropism for the epidermal or mucosal epithelium and adnexal structures. Neoplastic cells may be distributed throughout the epidermis or found as small discrete aggregates known as Pautrier's microabscesses. Neoplastic cells in patch and plaque lesions are often small-to-medium sized, whereas in the nodular/tumor stage they are usually intermediate to large.

Molecular Characteristics

MF/SS is characterized genomically by high rates of synonymous variants (SNVs) and CNVs. Pathway analysis indicates significant overlap between MF and SS in the pathways affected. Affected genes and pathways include: TCR signaling (*PLCG1*, *CARD11*, *CD28*, *RLTPR*), DNA damage response (*TP53*, *POT1*, *ATM*, *BRAC1*, *BRCA2*), chromatin modification (*ARID1A*, *TRRAO*, *DNMT3A*, *TET2*), JAK/STAT signaling (*STAT5B*, *JAK3*), and NKFκB signaling [181]. MF/SS exhibits a high mutational load and is linked to UV exposure. This high mutational load is unique among other types of T-cell lymphomas [181, 182].

Epitheliotropic lymphoma is the most common form of CTCL in dogs. Targeted transcriptomic analysis of six canine epitheliotropic lymphoma cases compared to healthy skin showed upregulation of genes involved in cytotoxic processes, including *GZMA*, *KLRB1*, *KLRD1*, *KLRK*1, *PRF1*, and *CPA3*, which is involved in proteolysis and degradation of endogenous proteins [183]. In another study, the transcriptomes of nine CETCL cases and 11 cases of immune-mediated dermatitis were compared. Among upregulated genes in CETCL, the top enriched pathways and gene ontology (GO) terms included genes related to ribosomes and protein translation (eIF2 signaling, ribosome, ribosomal subunits), and genes related to cell–matrix interactions (ILK signaling, integrin signaling, focal adhesion) and the interaction between cells and extracellular matrix (focal adhesion, ILK signaling and integrin signaling) [184]. It has been suggested, based on CD8 expression and expression of T_H1 type cytokines IL-12 and IFN-γ, that the canine form of CETCL may be more similar to human epidermotropic CD8+ T-cell lymphoma [174].

1.4.5 Other Lymphomas

Other lymphoma types recognized in dogs are either less clearly histologically defined and/or are infrequently diagnosed entities. Malignancies reported in both humans and canines are indicated in Table 1. T-zone lymphoma is a relatively common indolent lymphoma in dogs that does not have a clear human equivalent [5, 71]. Enteropathy-associated T-cell lymphoma (EATL)-like morphology has been described in dogs, but an association with celiac disease has not been documented [185]. In most cases the molecular similarity to humans, or lack thereof, of these less common lymphoma types and subtypes in the dog has not been defined.

1.5 Treatment and Prognosis

1.5.1 Treatment of Lymphoma in Humans

Treatment of lymphoma in humans is guided by consensus documents, the main ones being produced by the National Comprehensive Cancer Network (NCCN) [186, 187], the European Society for Medical Oncology (ESMO) [188], and the European Organization of Research and Treatment of Cancer (EORTC) [170] and are regularly updated. Treatment decisions generally follow these guidelines, especially for first-line treatment. Enrollment in clinical trials is often encouraged for diagnoses where generally effective first-line therapies do not exist and for relapsed/refractory patients. Treatment is very much driven by the specific lymphoma type, or subtype, diagnosis and then patient-specific criteria, including performance status. [189, 190] Treatment of lymphoma types of the most comparative interest are reviewed here.

Diffuse Large B-Cell Lymphoma

Multi-agent chemotherapy with CHOP became the standard of care for the treatment of aggressive lymphomas in the early 1990s [191] and remained the standard of care until the addition of CD20 antibody therapy, originally rituximab, and subsequently referred to as "R-CHOP" [192, 193]. R-CHOP immunochemotherapy remains a common primary first-line treatment for DLBCL. However, more recently, Pola-R-CHP (polatuzumab vedotin-piiq, rituximab, cyclophosphamide, doxorubicin, prednisone) was added as a first-line option for patients with an International Prognostic Index (IPI) of 2 or greater and has higher responses in non-GCB DLBCL [194]. Dose-adjusted EPOCH (etoposide, prednisone, vincristine, cyclophosphamide, doxorubicin) + rituximab is used for patients with double hit lymphoma or HIV associated lymphoma [195]. Polatuzumab vedotin-piiq is a CD79b antibody–drug conjugate with the cytotoxic agent being monomethyl auristatin E (MMAE), which disrupts microtubules [196–198] Other treatment regimens in which an anthracycline is replaced with an alternate agent, such as etoposide, are recommended for patients with poor left ventricular function [199]. For very frail patients and patients >80 years of age with comorbidities, reduced dosing of R-CHOP (R-miniCHOP) can be used [200]. Unlike dogs, in people DLBCL first-line treatment is used with the intent of cure. The 5-year survival rates range from 60% to 70% with first-line therapies; however, up to 50% of patients are refractory to therapy or eventually relapse. More than 50% of DLBCL are considered cured with R-CHOP [201].

Currently, recommendations for second-line therapy are based on the time interval from completion of chemotherapy and disease relapse. For patients relapsing greater than 1 year from chemotherapy, salvage therapy with a variety of combination chemotherapy regimens +/− rituximab followed by autologous stem cell transplant is a common approach [202]. For patients relapsing less than one year after completion of chemotherapy, CD19-directed CAR-T therapy is currently the standard of care based on the results of the ZUMA-5 trial showing the superiority of this approach [203]. In some circumstances, bridging therapy may be necessary until the CAR-T cell product is available, with better outcomes if the bridging therapy produces a deeper response [204]. Other therapy options for relapsed disease include polatuzumab vedotin-piiq+/-bendamustine +/-rituximab [205], tafasitamab-cxixl + lenalidomide [206], bispecific antibodies [207, 208], and loncastuximab tesirine [187, 209].

Marginal Zone Lymphoma

Treatment recommendations for MZL in humans differ depending on subtype, i.e., EMZL, NMZL, SMZL, or histologic transformation to DLBCL. NMZL is rare in humans and occurs most commonly as spread from extranodal sites. For localized disease, involved site radiation therapy (ISRT) is preferred. For advanced stage disease, either anti-CD20 monoclonal antibody as a monotherapy or in combination with chemotherapy are options depending on the overall burden of disease and patient performance status. First-line chemoimmunotherapy includes: bendamustine + rituximab, R-CHOP, and CVP (cyclophosphamide, vincristine, prednisone) + rituximab. Lenalidomide + rituximab is another chemotherapy-free option. For older or infirmed patients, rituximab monotherapy, chlorambucil + rituximab, and cyclophosphamide + rituximab can be considered. Second-line therapies include Bruton's tyrosine kinase (BTK) inhibitors, lenalidomide + rituximab, or chemoimmunotherapy with an alternate regimen. For third line and subsequent therapy, CD19-directed CAR-T cell therapy is now approved in this setting for patients who are candidates based on performance status and comorbidities.

EMZL is the most common MZL subtype in humans. Therapy differs somewhat for gastric, non-gastric, and cutaneous presentations [210]. For gastric EMZL patients that are *H. pylori* positive, initial treatment is antibiotic therapy for *H. pylori*. If *H. pylori* is negative, then ISRT is preferred. Alternatively, rituximab monotherapy is an option. Treatment response is monitored with endoscopy and second-line antibiotic treatment may be indicated [211]. For recurrent disease, observation or treatment may be indicated. If indicated, first- or second-line MZL treatment as described above are options [186]. For non-gastric EMZL, depending on clinical stage, ISRT (most often preferred), surgery (for certain sites), and rituximab or observation in selected cases are recommended. For systemic recurrence, if treatment is indicated, first- or second-line MZL treatment is indicated. For cutaneous EMZL patients with solitary/regional disease, local ISRT is generally preferred and can be curative. However, selected patients may be treated with surgical excision, skin-directed therapies, intralesional steroids, or observation. Patients with generalized skin disease or relapsed disease may be treated with rituximab and other systemic therapy. Patients with extracutaneous disease, or relapsed or progressive disease are managed as NMZL [186, 210].

SMZL patients are observed if they are asymptomatic. For patients with cytopenias or symptoms, the preferred treatment is rituximab monoclonal antibody therapy, as the alternative first-line option is splenectomy, which carries a greater future risk of increased susceptibility to infectious diseases. For recurrent disease, re-treatment with rituximab, rituximab + chemotherapy, or BTK inhibitors are all potential options given the duration of response to the initial rituximab monotherapy, burden of disease, and comorbidities.

Peripheral T-Cell Lymphoma Not Otherwise Specified

Treatment regimens, including CHOP, used for many aggressive B-cell lymphomas, are not as effective for T-cell lymphomas and approximately 70% of patients with PTCL develop relapsed or refractory disease after first-line therapy [212]. A large retrospective study of over 1000 patients with PTCL of different subtypes treated with CHOP-based induction chemotherapy had 2-year event-free survival and 3-year overall survival estimates of 46–52% and 58–61%, respectively [153]. Treatment is generally similar for different PTCL histologies using CHOP or CHOEP (cyclophosphamide, doxorubicin, vincristine, etoposide, prednisone). The exception is for anaplastic large cell lymphoma (ALCL) anaplastic lymphoma kinase (ALK)-positive tumors, for which the standard of care treatment is brentuximab vedotin + CHP which has demonstrated superior outcomes vs. CHOP therapy [213]. Enrollment in a clinical trial should always be considered, especially for patients with non-ALCL histologies. Often, these clinical trials incorporate novel agents to improve outcomes of first-line therapies. Unfortunately, most patients with PTCL will relapse after first-line therapy or will be refractory to treatment. The median time from end of treatment to relapse is 8–12 months [214, 215]. For relapsed/refractory patients there is no standard therapy. Patients are treated with a wide variety of single agents and combination regimens, either as the primary treatment, or with an intent to proceed to transplant, and it is recommended to consider a clinical trial when possible.

The potential benefit of allogeneic transplant was reported in large retrospective study where outcomes of 1942 patients with PTCL-NOS, AITL, and ALCL who underwent allogeneic transplant had 3-year PFS and OS of 48–52% and 60–64%, respectively [216]. Unfortunately, most patients with PTCL will die from lymphoma or treatment-related complications within a few years after diagnosis [217].

Cutaneous T-Cell lymphoma

Therapy for MF, the most common CTCL entity, is generally symptom-focused using a step-wise approach prioritizing quality of life [169]. Clinical stage I therapies include "watch and wait" and skin-directed therapies including topical corticosteroids [218], topical chlormethine [219, 220], and topical retinoids [221–223]. Ultraviolet (UV) phototherapy [224, 225], photodynamic therapy [226, 227], total skin electron beam therapy [169], and localized radiotherapy [169] are other therapies used for localized disease. Systemic therapies are recommended for early-stage disease refractory to skin directed therapy and for advanced stages of MF. Retinoids include all-trans retinoic acid, isotretinoin, etretinate, acitretin, and alitretinoin; however, bexarotene is the only one specifically developed and approved for CTCL [221]. Recombinant interferon-α (IFN-α), or pegylated IFN-α (peg-IFN-α) is used alone, or in combination therapy, with similar response rates of 50–66% [228–230]. Chemotherapy is generally used as single agent therapy with methotrexate, pegylated liposomal doxorubicin [231], gemcitabine [232], and chlorambucil [233] as potential options with activity. Targeted immunotherapy for MF includes mogamulizumab, a monoclonal antibody directed against C-C chemokine receptor 4 (CCR4), a chemokine involved in trafficking of lymphocytes to the skin [234] and brentuximab vedotin [235]. Allogeneic stem cell transplant may be considered for patients with advanced disease and poor prognosis [236, 237].

1.5.2 Treatment of Canine Lymphoma

Unlike treatment for lymphoma in people where NCCN and other consensus documents generally guide diagnosis, staging, and treatment, there are no widely accepted consensus documents guiding lymphoma treatment for veterinary patients. However, a general approach to lymphoma diagnosis, staging, and treatment in dogs is shared by most veterinary oncologists and is based on the published veterinary oncology literature and expert opinion. In practice, although an "ideal" diagnostic and staging approach and treatment is recommended by the veterinarian, something less than this is pursued frequently due to owner preference, often because of financial constraints.

Treatment of lymphoma in dogs is less nuanced than in people. This is in part because lymphoma WHO type often is not determined due to the widespread use of cytology for diagnosis. Further, clinical studies, both retrospective and prospective, often have not been restricted to a specific lymphoma type; therefore type-specific treatment response data is limited. Thus, treat-

Table 3 UW-Madison-19 canine CHOP protocol

Week 1	Vincristine (0.7/mg/m² IV)
	Prednisone (2 mg/m² PO, q24hr)
Week	Cyclophosphamide (250 mg/m² PO)
	Prednisone (1.5 mg/m² PO, q24hr)
Week 3:	Vincristine (0.7 mg/m² IV)
	Prednisone (1.0 mg/m² PO, q24hr)
Week 4	Doxorubicin (30 mg/m² IV)
	Prednisone (0.5 mg/m² PO, q24hr)
Week 6	Vincristine (0.7/mg/m² IV)
Week 7	Cyclophosphamide (250 mg/m² PO)
Week 8	Vincristine (0.7/mg/m² IV)
Week 9	Doxorubicin (30 mg/m² IV)
Week 11	Vincristine (0.7/mg/m² IV)
Week 12	Cyclophosphamide (250 mg/m² PO)
Week 13	Vincristine (0.7/mg/m² IV)
Week 14	Doxorubicin (30 mg/m² IV)
Week 16	Vincristine (0.7/mg/m² IV)
Week 17	Cyclophosphamide (250 mg/m² PO)
Week 18	Vincristine (0.7/mg/m² IV)
Week 19	Doxorubicin (30 mg/m² IV)

[a]All treatments are discontinued after week 19 if in complete remission.

[b]In dogs less than 15 kg in body weight, a dosage of 1 mg/kg doxorubicin is used.

[c]Alternatively, after week 9, all treatments may be given at every 2-week interval (UW-Madison-25).

ment of canine lymphoma is based primarily on whether the lymphoma diagnosis is determined to be aggressive or indolent and to some degree on the immunophenotype, i.e., whether B cell or T cell.

Aggressive Lymphoma

For first-line treatment of aggressive lymphomas in dogs there is general consensus that better response rates and remission durations are obtained with multi-agent chemotherapy protocols [238]. Although many different multi-agent chemotherapy protocols have been investigated, CHOP-based protocols, i.e., protocols incorporating the same drugs, cyclophosphamide, doxorubicin, vincristine, prednisone, as used in the human CHOP protocol, are the most widely used. Table 3 shows what is probably the most commonly used CHOP-based protocol to treat dogs with aggressive lymphomas. Note, that in this protocol the drugs are used sequentially. Unfortunately, there is no commercial anti-CD20, or other lymphoma-targeted therapeutic antibody, available currently for treating canine lymphoma, thus a dog equivalent of R-CHOP is not currently available for dogs. Several therapeutic antibodies for canine lymphoma have reached the market, but failed for different reasons, and others are currently being investigated. [239–246] CHOP-based chemotherapy is well-tolerated by most dogs with a response rate of 80–95% and an overall median survival time of 10–12 months; however, the response duration is generally significantly shorter for T-cell lymphomas [238].

CHOP chemotherapy is considered appropriate first-line therapy for dogs with aggres sive lymphoma regardless of immunophenotype; however, there are studies that suggest multi-agent chemotherapy protocols that incorporate more alkylating agents may have equivalent or superior outcomes for T-cell lymphomas [247–250]. Thus, for some veterinary oncologists, immunophenotype information dictates the choice of CHOP versus an alkylating agent intensive protocol, e.g., lomustine, vincristine, procarbazine, prednisone (LOPP), for initial treatment of aggressive T-cell lymphoma. Alternative to multi-agent chemotherapy for treatment of aggressive canine lymphoma is single-agent chemotherapy, or monotherapy. Monotherapy approaches are often chosen due to cost and convenience limitations. In general, the response rate and duration of response to monotherapy are inferior to combination chemotherapy for first-line treatment. The most commonly used single agents (often used with a corticosteroid) include doxorubicin, rabacfosadine, and lomustine [251–256]. Finally, for owners not interested in pursuing chemotherapy for their dog, prednisone alone is commonly prescribed. Most dogs will have an objective decrease in tumor size and improvement in clinical signs, if present. Nonetheless, responses are transient, with the median survival of dogs with lymphoma treated with prednisone alone being about 1–2 months [257].

Because canine lymphoma is usually incurable, i.e., dogs eventually die from their disease, treatment of relapsed/refractory (R/R) lymphoma is usually necessary to obtain maximum overall survival. In general, first-line treatment is given until completion of the induction protocol, provided an objective response is achieved. Ideally, at the completion of the protocol, the patient is restaged, although commonly complete restaging is not done, and the patient is re-evaluated for remission status (commonly lymph node palpation and caliper measurement alone if the dog had an initial multicentric presentation) on a regular basis until clinical progression is detected. Maintenance chemotherapy is thought to provide no additional benefit; however, no randomized prospective trials have been performed [258, 259]. There is no consensus regarding the choice of second-line and subsequent therapy, although in general, dogs that respond well to CHOP induction therapy often respond well, initially, to reintroduction of CHOP, or a modified CHOP protocol. After CHOP, the choice of "rescue" chemotherapy is dictated primarily by clinician preference, with any single-agent or multi-agent protocol that the dog has not previously received being considered. Single agents that are more commonly used after CHOP include rabacfosadine, lomustine, L-asparaginase, vinblastine, mitoxantrone, temozolomide, and others [260–264]. Combination rescue protocols include MOPP (mechlorethamine, vincristine, procarbazine, prednisone), DMAC (dexamethasone, melphalan, actinomycin D, cytosine arabinoside), and others [265] [266].

Indolent Lymphoma

Indolent lymphomas (NMZL, TZL, MCL) comprise only about 20% of canine lymphomas [4]. The most common indolent lymphoma in dogs is TZL. FL and small cell lymphoma are much more uncommon. Nodal MZL is problematic. As in humans, MZL it is considered an indolent lymphoma; however, in dogs MZL is commonly clinically aggressive [104, 124]. Treatment for indolent lymphomas is poorly defined. There are no prospective studies evaluating different treatment approaches for TZL or other indolent lymphomas. Retrospective analyses of canine indolent lymphomas suggest that many affected dogs do not die from their disease and outcomes are not improved with any particular treatment [127, 267–269]. However, the effect of treatment must be interpreted with caution due to the retrospective nature of these studies and the small number of dogs evaluated.

Because of the slower, less clinically aggressive course of disease for most cases of indolent lymphoma, a more conservative approach to treatment is recommended and is based primarily on the assessment of disease burden and rate of progression. For TZL, dogs with low numbers of circulating TZL cells and/or "mild" lymphadenopathy, generally confined to the mandibular lymph nodes, active monitoring/no treatment is often sufficient. For dogs with higher, or increasing, circulating TZL cell counts, or more extensive lymphadenopathy, treatment with an oral alkylating agent, most commonly chlorambucil, and corticosteroids may be indicated. Finally, for dogs with more extensive disease burden, especially if more rapidly progressing, or if systemic signs are present, treatment with more intensive chemotherapy, such as CHOP, is considered. Similarly, for dogs where MZL is clinically aggressive, treatment as for other aggressive lymphomas is indicated.

Cutaneous T-Cell Lymphoma

The most common first-line treatment for CTCL in dogs is lomustine, usually combined with prednisone. [270, 271] In one multi-institutional retrospective study of 46 dogs with treatment-naïve and previously treated cutaneous epitheliotropic lymphoma treated with lomustine +/− concurrent corticosteroids the ORR was 82.6% with an overall median duration of response of 94 days (range, 22–282) [270]. Another study had similar results, where a similar population of 36 dogs was enrolled. The ORR was 78% for a median duration of 106 days (95% CI, 75–182) [272]. Another common first-line therapy is rabacfosadine, based on a small study of 12 dogs with chemotherapy-naïve or relapsed

CTCL, where an ORR of 45% was observed with a PFS of 37.5 days [273]. Other therapies that have been reported include recombinant canine interferon-gamma (rCaIFN-λ) [274] and synthetic retinoids (isotretinoin, etretinate) [275, 276]. Additionally, total skin electron therapy has been explored [277].

2 Companion Animal Models and Comparative Oncology

Spontaneously occurring cancers in companion animals, especially dogs, have increasingly been used as a large animal model for drug and device development for human cancers. Advantages and characteristics of the companion animal spontaneous cancer model have been reviewed extensively, and include spontaneous occurrence of cancers in an immunocompetent host, tumor heterogeneity, shared tumor biology and genetics, an outbred animal population with a unique breed structure that facilitates genetic analyses, sharing of environmental exposures with humans, and similar physical size and physiology relative to humans [278–284]. Pet dogs with lymphoma have been used to investigate a wide variety of new anticancer therapies. Although canine trials potentially can inform all stages of the drug development process, the majority of studies are early-stage studies to establish drug dosage, toxicities, pharmacokinetics and pharmacokinetic/pharmacodynamic relationships, evaluate potential biomarkers, and evidence of potential efficacy. The incorporation of pet dog trials in the cancer drug development process has increased over the years and is now firmly established.

Compared to many other tumor types, lymphoma in dogs offers several additional advantages as a model. First, peripheral lymph nodes are readily accessible both for assessing response to treatment, often just requiring simple caliper measurements, and for sampling, either by tissue biopsy, or fine needle aspiration. Furthermore, because the tumor is so easily accessible, longitudinal sampling is relatively easy and straightforward. Thus, repeated sampling during the course of treatment is often much more practical than could be achieved in a human study, or in a rodent study where size restrictions may limit tumor and blood volumes that can be obtained. For any clinical trial patient accrual is an important consideration. Since lymphoma is one of the most common canine cancers, patient accrual is generally not a limitation.

Clinical trials reporting new anticancer therapies evaluated in dogs with lymphoma are summarized in Table 4 and discussed here. The safety of polyethylene glycol conjugated L-asparaginase was demonstrated in a double-blind randomized trial in dogs with lymphoma, representing one of the earliest comparative/translational canine cancer clinical trials [285]. In another early study, the safety of whole-body hyperthermia combined with doxorubicin chemotherapy was investigated [286]. The ability of concomitant pyridoxine to prevent palmar-plantar erythrodysesthesia (PPES) in patients treated with Doxil, a doxorubicin-containing pegylated liposome drug, was studied in a randomized, double-blind trial in 41 dogs with lymphoma. The relative risk was greater in the placebo group for developing severe PPES and for having to decrease or discontinue Doxil therapy [287]. Dolastatin-10, an inhibitor of tubulin polymerization, was evaluated in a dose escalation study of dogs with lymphoma and solid tumors. Neutropenia was dose limiting, and a complete response was achieved in one dog with relapsed high-grade lymphoma [288]. The toxicities, pharmacokinetics, tumor drug concentrations, pharmacodynamics, and activity of a class of peptide mimetics of thrombospondin-1 (ABT-510, ABT-526), alone or in combination with cytotoxic chemotherapy, were evaluated, documenting antitumor activity in several histologies, including lymphoma, and prolongation of lomustine median response duration when used in combination therapy [289, 290]. Tanovea® (VDC-1101, GS-9219, rabacfosadine), the first FDA-approved treatment for canine lymphoma, was first tested in dogs as part of the preclinical drug development for potential human use, with the initial clinical study demonstrating significant efficacy in five dogs with lymphoma [291]. A subsequent phase I/II clinical trial in 38 dogs

Table 4 Translational oncology clinical trials in dogs with lymphoma

Agent	Target/mechanism	Tumor histologies	Publication
Antibody 1E4-clgGB	Anti-canine CD20 antibody	DLBCL	McLinden, 2024
Antibody c4G12	Anti-PD-L1 antibody	Solid tumors, lymphoma	Maekawa, 2023 Igase, 2020
CB-5339	Valosin-containing protein (VCP)	Solid tumors, multiple myeloma, lymphoma	LeBlanc, 2022
EZN-3042	Anti-survivin locked nucleic acid oligo	Lymphoma	Thamm, 2020
F14512	Etoposide derivative topoisomerase II inhibitor targeting active polyamine transport	Lymphoma	Boye, 2020 Tierny, 2015
Antibody 10C6	Anti-canine CD22 antibody	DLBCL	Etienne, 2020
Verdinexor (KPT-335)	Nuclear export (SINE) inhibitor	Lymphoma, mast cell tumor, osteosarcoma	Sadowski, 2018 London, 2014
Indotecan (LMP400), indimitecan (LMP776), LMP744	Idenoisoquinoline topoisomerase I inhibitor	Lymphoma	Burton, 2018
RV1001	PI3Kδ inhibitor	Lymphoma	Gardner, 2018
VSV-IFNβ-NIS	Oncolytic virus	Solid tumors, lymphoma	Naik, 2018
PAC-1	Procaspase-3 activator	Osteosarcoma, lymphoma	Botham, 2016 Peterson, 2010
Acalabrutinib (ACP-196)	BTK inhibitor	B-cell lymphoma	Harrington, 2016
Canine CD20 CAR-T cells	CAR-T cell therapy	B-cell lymphoma DLBCL	Panjwani, 2016 Panjwani, 2020
HSPPCs-HA (heat shock protein-peptide complex hydroxyapatite)	Autologous vaccine	Indolent B-cell lymphoma DLBCL	Marconato, 2015 Marconato, 2014
Valspodar	ABCB1 inhibitor	Large B-cell lymphoma	Ito, 2017
Hydroxychloroquine	Autophagy inhibitor	Lymphoma	Barnard, 2014
NEMO-binding domain peptide	IKK inhibitor	DLBCL	Ndikuyeze, 2014 Gaurnier-Hausser, 2011
VDC-1101 (GS-9219)	Nuclear DNA polymerase α, δ, and ε inhibitor	Lymphoma	Vail, 2009 Reiser, 2008
dTERT vaccine (Ad6-dTERT$_{opt}$ and pV1J-dTERT.LTB$_{opt}$)	Telomerase reverse transcriptase adenovirus vaccine	B-cell lymphoma	Gavazza, 2013
^{111}In-DOTA-anti-*BCL2*-PNA-Tyr^{3}-octreotate	Radiolabeled peptide nucleic acid-peptide conjugate targeting BCL2 m RNA	B-cell lymphoma	Statham-Ringen, 2012
Autologous T-cells	T-cell therapy	B-cell lymphoma	O'Connor, 2012
Autologous RNA-loaded CD40-B vaccine	Cell-based CD40 cancer vaccination	Lymphoma	Sorenmo, 2011
Antigen-coated microbeads (large multivalent immunogen)	Autologous vaccine	B-cell lymphoma	Henson, 2010
Ibrutinib (PCI-32765)	BTK inhibitor	B-cell lymphoma	Honigberg, 2010

(continued)

Table 4 (continued)

Agent	Target/mechanism	Tumor histologies	Publication
pV1-dTERT.LTB$_{opt}$	Telomerase reverse transcriptase adenovirus vaccine	B-cell lymphoma	Peruzzi, 2010
ABT-526	Angiogenesis inhibitor	Lymphoma	Rusk, 2006
ABT-526, ABT-510	Angiogenesis inhibitor	Solid tumors, lymphoma	Rusk, 2006
Dolastatin-10	Tubulin polymerization inhibitor	Solid tumors, lymphoma	Thamm, 2002
Pyridoxine (vitamin B_6)	Unknown	Lymphoma	Vail, 1998
Whole-body hyperthermia + doxorubicin	Unknown	Lymphoma	Novotney, 1992
PEG-L-asparaginase	Asparagine depletion and inhibition of protein, RNA, DNA synthesis	Lymphoma	MacEwen, 1992

with lymphoma further assessed its pharmacokinetics, toxicities, and activity. Correlative studies demonstrated that the prodrug had a short plasma half-life but produced prolonged intracellular concentrations of the cytotoxic metabolite PMEG diphosphate in peripheral blood mononuclear cells. Objective responses were observed in 79% of dogs [292]. The differential efficacy, pharmacokinetics, pharmacodynamics, and toxicology of three novel topoisomerase I inhibitors (indenoisoquinolines) were evaluated in a phase I study enrolling 84 dogs with lymphoma in an NCI Comparative Oncology Trials Consortium (COTC) multi-institutional trial. Endpoints of the trial were achieved. Bone marrow toxicity was dose limiting. γH2AX induction was demonstrated in tumor samples and a decrease in TOP1 protein. Objective responses were seen with all indenoisoquinolines with efficacy (13/19 dogs) being the greatest for LMP744 [293]. F14512, a topoisomerase II inhibitor containing a spermine moiety that facilitates uptake by tumor cells, was investigated in phase I and randomized double-blind clinical trials in dogs with lymphoma. In the phase I trial, 23 dogs were enrolled. F14512 was well tolerated and demonstrated dose-dependent hematologic toxicity. A 91% (21/23) response rate was achieved with 10 complete responses (CRs) and 11 partial responses (PRs). Phosphorylation of histone H2AX was interrogated as a potential biomarker [294]. In the phase II trial, 42 dogs were enrolled and randomized to receive F14512 or single-agent etoposide. The ORR for the F14512-treated group was 76% (19/25, 12 CR, 7 PR). Dogs with p-glycoprotein overexpressing tumors had improved PFS compared to dogs treated with etoposide [295].

The feasibility and determination of dosing regimen for the procaspase-3 inhibitor, PAC-1, was evaluated in an initial study in six dogs with lymphoma. A feasible dosing regimen that achieved target steady-state plasma concentrations was determined and one dog had a partial response [296]. The synergistic activity of PAC-1 with doxorubicin was evaluated in ten dogs with metastatic osteosarcoma or lymphoma. Coadministration of PAC-1 did not appear to exacerbate doxorubicin-associated toxicity and all four lymphoma patients had partial, or complete responses [297]. The biological activity of the BTK inhibitors ibrutinib and acalabrutinib was demonstrated in canine B-cell lymphomas, and the utility of an affinity probe for BTK active site occupancy was validated [298, 299]. The toxicity and efficacy of the PI3Kδ inhibitor, RV1001, was evaluated in phase I and phase II clinical trials in dogs with treatment naïve and relapsed/refractory lymphoma. The primary toxicities observed were hepatobiliary and gastrointestinal, with hepatotoxicity being the primary dose-limiting toxicity. In the phase I study, the objective response rate was 62% (CR: 3/21, PR: 10/21), and in the phase II study, the objective response rate was 77% (CR: 1/35, PR: 26/35) [300]. A phase I study of the Selective Inhibitors of Nuclear Transport (SINE) compound, KPT-335 (verdinexor), was conducted in dogs with lymphoma, mast cell tumor, and osteosarcoma. Partial responses (*n* = 2/17) and stable disease (SD) (*n* = 7/17) were observed in the dogs with lymphoma. An expansion cohort of six dogs with lymphoma was evaluated. Two dogs had a PR, and four dogs had SD for greater than 28 days. Toxicities were primarily gastrointestinal and manageable with supportive care, dose modulation, and administration of low-dose prednisone [301]. In a subsequent phase II study, KPT-335 was evaluated in 58 dogs with treatment-naïve or relapsed/refractory lymphoma. Treatment as a single agent resulted in an objective response rate of 37% with the T-cell lymphoma dogs (*n* = 14) having an objective response rate of 71% [302]. CB-5083, a small molecule inhibitor of valosin-containing protein (VCP), which chaperones different proteins to the proteasome for degradation, was investigated in another COTC trial in dogs with a variety of solid tumors and lymphoma and enriched for multiple myeloma patients. The drug was well tolerated, and a PK/PD relationship was established between exposure and modulation of targets related to the unfolded protein response. Furthermore, clinical responses were seen in 33% (2/6) multiple myeloma patients [303]. In a phase I clinical trial of 18 dogs with peripheral nodal lymphoma, a novel anti-survivin locked nucleic acid antisense oligonucleotide, EZN-3042, was evaluated. No dose-limiting toxicities were observed, and a reduction in tumor-surviving mRNA and protein was observed [304].

The biological effects of the autophagy inhibitor hydroxychloroquine in combination with doxorubicin were evaluated in 30 dogs with lymphoma. Treatment was well tolerated. There was a 100-fold increase in hydroxychloroquine in tumors compared to plasma and a trend toward an increase in markers for autophagosomes after treatment. The overall response rate was greater than 93%, superior to historical single-agent doxorubicin [305]. Valspodar, a selective inhibitor of the ATP binding cassette B1 transporter (ABCB1), was evaluated in dogs with large B-cell lymphoma in the neoadjuvant setting followed by doxorubicin administration. Although well tolerated, there were no differences between groups in the progenitor cell population, event-free survival, or overall survival [306]. A novel radiolabeled peptide nucleic acid-peptide conjugate (RAPP) targeting B-cell leukemia-lymphoma 2 (BCL2) mRNA for scintigraphic detection of neoplastic B cell was conducted in eleven dogs with B-cell lymphoma. Increased uptake of the RaPP in mandibular and superficial cervical lymph nodes prior to the initiation of chemotherapy treatment was associated with increased risk of tumor progression [307].

A pilot trial of a NFκB Essential Modulator (NEMO) Binding Domain (NBD) peptide, a selective inhibitor of the IKK complex, enrolled six dogs with relapsed large B-cell lymphoma. Dogs were treated with intranodal injection of NBD into one lymph node and concurrent systemic chemotherapy. Four of the dogs had resulting decreased expression of NFκB target genes in the injected lymph node. [224] In a subsequent phase I study, NBD was administered intravenously to eleven dogs, where it was found to be safe and inhibited constitutive canonical NFκB activity in six of ten dogs. [225] Cancer vaccine strategies also have been evaluated using the canine lymphoma model. Telomerase reverse transcriptase (TERT) was evaluated as a target for immunotherapy using an adenovirus vector and DNA electroporation. dTERT-specific immune responses were induced, and survival times were increased when combined with chemotherapy compared to historical controls and in a randomized double-arm clinical trial. [308, 309] An autologous vaccination strategy showed presentation of autologous lymphoma cell membranes on cell-sized silica microbeads induced specific cell-mediated immunity in half of the dogs concurrently treated with induction chemotherapy [310]. A cell-based vaccination approach using autologous tumor RNA-loaded, CD40-activated B cells, acting as antigen-presenting cells, was evaluated in dogs with lymphoma where immunity was safely stimulated in dogs with lymphoma after remission was induced with chemotherapy [311]. Another vaccination approach evaluated using autologous tumor heat shock protein-peptide complex hydroxyapatite (HSPPC-HA). In a placebo-controlled double-blinded trial in dogs with DLBCL, evaluating

HSPPC-A + chemotherapy versus chemotherapy alone the vaccine was found to be safe and efficacious in prolonging time to progression and lymphoma-specific survival [312]. Using the same vaccination approach, HSPPC-HA vaccination was evaluated in non-randomized trial in dogs with indolent B-cell lymphomas. Dogs were treated with dose-intense chemotherapy or the same chemotherapy regimen and HSPPC-HA. The vaccinated group had significantly longer time to progression, although lymphoma-specific survival was not prolonged. Dogs that mounted a detectable immune response had significantly longer time to progression and lymphoma-specific survival than those without a detectable response [313]. Nine dogs with solid tumors and lymphomas were treated in a trial of an intravenous recombinant oncolytic vesicular stomatitis virus, VSV-IFNβ-NIS. Two dogs with high-grade PTCL had rapid, transient responses and transient hepatotoxicity (elevated transaminases). This study showed no shedding of infectious virus, elevated levels of VSV RNA in the blood of dogs having clinical responses, and that the virus was well-tolerated and safe [314].

A few cell therapies have been investigated in dogs with lymphoma. Autologous T cells from dogs with lymphoma expanded on artificial antigen-spresenting cells in the presence of human IL-2 and IL-21 were infused in dogs with lymphoma after CHOP chemotherapy. These cells persisted for 49 days, homed to the tumor, and significantly improved survival [315]. CAR-T approaches have been explored using CD20 CARs. In a first-in-canine study a first-generation canine CD20 CAR was expressed using mRNA electroporation in autologous expanded T cells and administered to a dog with relapsed B-cell lymphoma. Treatment was well tolerated in this single dog with modest, transient antitumor activity observed [316]. In a subsequent study, a second-generation CD20 CAR was expressed using a lentiviral vector and used to treat five dogs with DLBCL with CAR-T. CAR-T cells were well tolerated, detectable post-infusion, and appeared to exert selection pressure on CD20+ cells, followed by antigen escape and emergence of CD20- disease. From a translational model perspective, the model identified many of the key challenges in the development of effective CAR-T therapies, including poor expansion of the CAR-T-cell product, development of anti-CAR immunity, and antigen loss [317]. In both of these studies, canine anti-mouse antibodies (CAMA) were induced, suggesting the need for caninization of the scFV to prevent anti-CAR immunity.

Therapeutic antibodies have been investigated in dogs with lymphoma; both for translational and primary canine therapeutic purposes. Several of these efforts have focused on developing a canine equivalent of Rituximab, i.e., an anti-canine CD20 monoclonal antibody [242–244]; however, only one clinical trial using an anti-canine CD20 antibody has been published. In that trial, the canine chimeric anti-canine CD20 antibody (1E4-cIgGB) was given to dogs with DLBCL in combination with reduced dosage doxorubicin and one of three other immunomodulatory drugs. In this combination drug setting, the 1E4-cIgGB anti-CD20 monoclonal antibody appeared safe and depleted circulating B cells in dogs [246]. A murine monoclonal antibody targeting canine CD22 (10C6) and radiolabeled with indium-111 was successfully used for single-photon emission computed tomography (SPECT) imaging in three dogs with DLBCL where known and previously unknown disease was detected [318]. Antibodies for therapeutic immune checkpoint blockade in dogs have been developed [319–321], and some have been investigated in spontaneous canine tumors, including solid tumors and lymphoma. The safety and efficacy of a canine chimeric anti-PD-L1 antibody (c4G12) were evaluated in 12 dogs (11 solid tumors, 1 lymphoma) with an objective response rate of 25% and were found to be safe and tolerable [322]. A clinical study of chimeric (ch-4F12-E6) and caninized anti-canine PD-1 (ca-4F12-E6) monoclonal antibodies was conducted in 30 dogs with solid tumors [29] and lymphoma [1]. Treatment with the anti-PD-1 antibodies was relatively safe, and fewer adverse events were associated with the caninized antibody. Partial responses were observed in four cases of pulmonary metastatic oral melanoma [320].

3 Conclusions

Collectively, the lymphomas are relatively common cancers in both humans and dogs. They comprise a heterogeneous group of different disease entities characterized by unique histologies, molecular bases, and clinical behaviors, and many of these characteristics are shared between the two species, thus making spontaneous lymphoma in pet dogs a highly relevant and translationally useful preclinical large animal model for anticancer drug development.

References

1. Alaggio R, Amador C, Anagnostopoulos I, Attygalle AD, Araujo IBO, Berti E et al (2022) The 5th edition of the World Health Organization classification of haematolymphoid tumours: lymphoid neoplasms. Leukemia 36(7):1720–1748. https://doi.org/10.1038/s41375-022-01620-2. Epub 2022/06/23. PubMed PMID: 35732829; PubMed Central PMCID: PMCPMC9214472
2. Momotow J, Borchmann S, Eichenauer DA, Engert A, Sasse S (2021) Hodgkin lymphoma-review on pathogenesis, diagnosis, current and future treatment approaches for adult patients. J Clin Med 10(5). https://doi.org/10.3390/jcm10051125. Epub 2021/04/04. PubMed PMID: 33800409; PubMed Central PMCID: PMCPMC7962816
3. Kelly KM, Friedberg JW (2024) Classic hodgkin lymphoma in adolescents and young adults. J Clin Oncol 42(6):653–664. https://doi.org/10.1200/JCO.23.01799. Epub 2023/11/20. PubMed PMID: 37983570
4. Seelig DM, Avery AC, Ehrhart EJ, Linden MA (2016) The comparative diagnostic features of canine and human lymphoma. Vet Sci 3(2). https://doi.org/10.3390/vetsci3020011. Epub 2017/04/25. PubMed PMID: 28435836; PubMed Central PMCID: PMCPMC5397114
5. Hughes K, Conaway E, Blackwell E, Rout E, Yoshimoto J, Burnett R et al (2024) Canine T zone lymphoma is a tumor of mature, previously activated alphabeta T cells. Vet Immunol Immunopathol 269:110725. https://doi.org/10.1016/j.vetimm.2024.110725. Epub 2024/02/16. PubMed PMID: 38359755
6. National Cancer Institute Surveillance, Epidemiology, and End Results Program 2024 [cited 2024 June 9, 2024]. https://seer.cancer.gov/
7. Cronin KA, Scott S, Firth AU, Sung H, Henley SJ, Sherman RL et al (2022) Annual report to the nation on the status of cancer, part 1: national cancer statistics. Cancer 128(24):4251–4284. https://doi.org/10.1002/cncr.34479. Epub 2022/10/28. PubMed PMID: 36301149; PubMed Central PMCID: PMCPMC10092838
8. Wang SS (2023) Epidemiology and etiology of diffuse large B-cell lymphoma. Semin Hematol 60(5):255–266. https://doi.org/10.1053/j.seminhematol.2023.11.004. Epub 2024/01/20. PubMed PMID: 38242772; PubMed Central PMCID: PMCPMC10962251
9. Wolfe F, Michaud K (2004) Lymphoma in rheumatoid arthritis: the effect of methotrexate and anti-tumor necrosis factor therapy in 18,572 patients. Arthritis Rheum 50(6):1740–1751. https://doi.org/10.1002/art.20311. Epub 2004/06/10. PubMed PMID: 15188349
10. Cocco P, Vermeulen R, Flore V, Nonne T, Campagna M, Purdue M et al (2013) Occupational exposure to trichloroethylene and risk of non-Hodgkin lymphoma and its major subtypes: a pooled InterLymph [correction of IinterLlymph] analysis. Occup Environ Med 70(11):795–802. https://doi.org/10.1136/oemed-2013-101551. Epub 2013/07/25. PubMed PMID: 23881218
11. Mandel JH, Kelsh MA, Mink PJ, Alexander DD, Kalmes RM, Weingart M et al (2006) Occupational trichloroethylene exposure and non-Hodgkin's lymphoma: a meta-analysis and review. Occup Environ Med 63(9):597–607. https://doi.org/10.1136/oem.2005.022418. Epub 2006/04/29. PubMed PMID: 16644896; PubMed Central PMCID: PMCPMC2078160
12. Rana I, Dahlberg S, Steinmaus C, Zhang L (2021) Benzene exposure and non-Hodgkin lymphoma: a systematic review and meta-analysis of human studies. Lancet Planet Health 5(9):e633–ee43. https://doi.org/10.1016/S2542-5196(21)00149-2. Epub 2021/08/28. PubMed PMID: 34450064; PubMed Central PMCID: PMCPMC9109598
13. Yadlapati S, Efthimiou P (2016) Autoimmune/inflammatory arthritis associated lymphomas: who is at risk? Biomed Res Int 2016:8631061. https://doi.org/10.1155/2016/8631061. Epub 2016/07/20. PubMed PMID: 27429984; PubMed Central PMCID: PMCPMC4939344
14. Omar A, Marques N, Crawford N (2024) Cancer and HIV: the molecular mechanisms of the deadly duo. Cancers (Basel) 16(3). https://doi.org/10.3390/cancers16030546. Epub 2024/02/10. PubMed PMID: 38339297; PubMed Central PMCID: PMCPMC10854577
15. Huguet M, Navarro JT, Molto J, Ribera JM, Tapia G (2023) Diffuse large B-cell lymphoma in the HIV setting. Cancers (Basel) 15(12). https://doi.org/10.3390/cancers15123191. Epub 2023/06/28. PubMed PMID: 37370801; PubMed Central PMCID: PMCPMC10296551
16. Gibson TM, Engels EA, Clarke CA, Lynch CF, Weisenburger DD, Morton LM (2014) Risk of diffuse large B-cell lymphoma after solid organ transplantation in the United States. Am J

Hematol 89(7):714–720. https://doi.org/10.1002/ajh.23726. Epub 2014/04/23. PubMed PMID: 24753070; PubMed Central PMCID: PMCPMC4069221

17. Clarke CA, Morton LM, Lynch C, Pfeiffer RM, Hall EC, Gibson TM et al (2013) Risk of lymphoma subtypes after solid organ transplantation in the United States. Br J Cancer 109(1):280–288. https://doi.org/10.1038/bjc.2013.294. Epub 2013/06/13. PubMed PMID: 23756857; PubMed Central PMCID: PMCPMC3708563
18. Pradeep R, Shanmugam G, Rakshit S, Sarkar K (2024) Role of Wiskott Aldrich syndrome protein in haematological malignancies: genetics, molecular mechanisms and therapeutic strategies. Pathol Res Pract 253:155026. https://doi.org/10.1016/j.prp.2023.155026. Epub 2023/12/20. PubMed PMID: 38118219
19. Ekstrom Smedby K, Vajdic CM, Falster M, Engels EA, Martinez-Maza O, Turner J et al (2008) Autoimmune disorders and risk of non-Hodgkin lymphoma subtypes: a pooled analysis within the InterLymph Consortium. Blood 111(8):4029–4038. https://doi.org/10.1182/blood-2007-10-119974. Epub 2008/02/12. PubMed PMID: 18263783; PubMed Central PMCID: PMCPMC2288717
20. Anderson LA, Gadalla S, Morton LM, Landgren O, Pfeiffer R, Warren JL et al (2009) Population-based study of autoimmune conditions and the risk of specific lymphoid malignancies. Int J Cancer 125(2):398–405. https://doi.org/10.1002/ijc.24287. Epub 2009/04/15. PubMed PMID: 19365835; PubMed Central PMCID: PMCPMC2692814
21. Di Rocco A, Petrucci L, Assanto GM, Martelli M, Pulsoni A (2022) Extranodal marginal zone lymphoma: pathogenesis, diagnosis and treatment. Cancers (Basel) 14(7). https://doi.org/10.3390/cancers14071742. Epub 2022/04/13. PubMed PMID: 35406516; PubMed Central PMCID: PMCPMC8997163
22. Upadhyay R, Hammerich L, Peng P, Brown B, Merad M, Brody JD (2015) Lymphoma: immune evasion strategies. Cancers (Basel) 7(2):736–762. https://doi.org/10.3390/cancers7020736. Epub 2015/05/06. PubMed PMID: 25941795; PubMed Central PMCID: PMCPMC4491682
23. Gergely L, Udvardy M, Illes A (2024) The possible role of pathogens and chronic immune stimulation in the development of diffuse large B-cell lymphoma. Biomedicine 12(3). https://doi.org/10.3390/biomedicines12030648. Epub 2024/03/28. PubMed PMID: 38540261; PubMed Central PMCID: PMCPMC10967989
24. Engels EA (2007) Infectious agents as causes of non-Hodgkin lymphoma. Cancer Epidemiol Biomarkers Prev 16(3):401–404. https://doi.org/10.1158/1055-9965.EPI-06-1056. Epub 2007/03/06. PubMed PMID: 17337646
25. Boerkamp KM, Teske E, Boon LR, Grinwis GC, van den Bossche L, Rutteman GR (2014) Estimated incidence rate and distribution of tumours in 4,653 cases of archival submissions derived from the Dutch golden retriever population. BMC Vet Res 10:34. https://doi.org/10.1186/1746-6148-10-34. Epub 2014/02/04. PubMed PMID: 24484635; PubMed Central PMCID: PMCPMC3914708
26. Dorn CR, Taylor DO, Frye FL, Hibbard HH (1968) Survey of animal neoplasms in Alameda and Contra Costa Counties, California. I. Methodology and description of cases. J Natl Cancer Inst 40(2):295–305. Epub 1968/02/01. PubMed PMID: 5694271
27. Dorn CR, Taylor DO, Schneider R (1970) The epidemiology of canine leukemia and lymphoma. Bibl Haematol 1970(36):403–415. https://doi.org/10.1159/000391733. Epub 1970/01/01. PubMed PMID: 5538360
28. Merlo DF, Rossi L, Pellegrino C, Ceppi M, Cardellino U, Capurro C et al (2008) Cancer incidence in pet dogs: findings of the Animal Tumor Registry of Genoa, Italy. J Vet Intern Med 22(4):976–984. https://doi.org/10.1111/j.1939-1676.2008.0133.x. Epub 2008/06/20. PubMed PMID: 18564221
29. Rafalko JM, Kruglyak KM, McCleary-Wheeler AL, Goyal V, Phelps-Dunn A, Wong LK et al (2023) Age at cancer diagnosis by breed, weight, sex, and cancer type in a cohort of more than 3,000 dogs: Determining the optimal age to initiate cancer screening in canine patients. PLoS One 18(2):e0280795. https://doi.org/10.1371/journal.pone.0280795. Epub 2023/02/02. PubMed PMID: 36724177; PubMed Central PMCID: PMCPMC9891508 does not alter our adherence to PLOS ONE policies on sharing data and materials
30. Smith N, Luethcke KR, Craun K, Trepanier L (2022) Risk of bladder cancer and lymphoma in dogs is associated with pollution indices by county of residence. Vet Comp Oncol 20(1):246–255. https://doi.org/10.1111/vco.12771. Epub 2021/09/05. PubMed PMID: 34480391; PubMed Central PMCID: PMCPMC9969847
31. Gavazza A, Presciuttini S, Barale R, Lubas G, Gugliucci B (2001) Association between canine malignant lymphoma, living in industrial areas, and use of chemicals by dog owners. J Vet Intern Med 15(3):190–195. Epub 2001/05/31. PubMed PMID: 11380026
32. Schofield I, Stevens KB, Pittaway C, O'Neill DG, Fecht D, Dobson JM et al (2019) Geographic distribution and environmental risk factors of lymphoma in dogs under primary-care in the UK. J Small Anim Pract 60(12):746–754. https://doi.org/10.1111/jsap.13075. Epub 2019/11/12. PubMed PMID: 31709551
33. Takashima-Uebelhoer BB, Barber LG, Zagarins SE, Procter-Gray E, Gollenberg AL, Moore AS et al (2012) Household chemical exposures and the risk of canine malignant lymphoma, a model for human non-Hodgkin's lymphoma. Environ Res 112:171–176. https://doi.org/10.1016/j.envres.2011.12.003. Epub 2012/01/10. PubMed

PMID: 22222006; PubMed Central PMCID: PMCPMC3267855
34. Hayes HM, Tarone RE, Cantor KP (1995) On the association between canine malignant lymphoma and opportunity for exposure to 2,4-dichlorophenoxyacetic acid. Environ Res 70(2):119–125. https://doi.org/10.1006/enrs.1995.1056. Epub 1995/08/01. PubMed PMID: 8674480
35. Hayes HM, Tarone RE, Cantor KP, Jessen CR, McCurnin DM, Richardson RC (1991) Case-control study of canine malignant lymphoma: positive association with dog owner's use of 2,4-dichlorophenoxyacetic acid herbicides. J Natl Cancer Inst 83(17):1226–1231. https://doi.org/10.1093/jnci/83.17.1226. Epub 1991/09/04. PubMed PMID: 1870148
36. Pastor M, Chalvet-Monfray K, Marchal T, Keck G, Magnol JP, Fournel-Fleury C et al (2009) Genetic and environmental risk indicators in canine non-Hodgkin's lymphomas: breed associations and geographic distribution of 608 cases diagnosed throughout France over 1 year. J Vet Intern Med 23(2):301–310. https://doi.org/10.1111/j.1939--1676.2008.0255.x. Epub 2009/02/05. PubMed PMID: 19192140
37. Waugh EM, Gallagher A, McAulay KA, Henriques J, Alves M, Bell AJ et al (2015) Gammaherpesviruses and canine lymphoma: no evidence for direct involvement in commonly occurring lymphomas. J Gen Virol 96(Pt 7):1863–1872. https://doi.org/10.1099/vir.0.000106. Epub 2015/02/28. PubMed PMID: 25722346; PubMed Central PMCID: PMCPMC4635455
38. Jarosz AS, Pendleton AL, Lashbrook MJ, Cech E, Altieri M, Kunch A et al (2023) Expression and high levels of insertional polymorphism of an endogenous gammaretrovirus lineage in dogs. PLoS Genet 19(12):e1011083. https://doi.org/10.1371/journal.pgen.1011083. Epub 2023/12/06. PubMed PMID: 38055724; PubMed Central PMCID: PMCPMC10727363
39. Giannuzzi D, Aresu L (2020) A first NGS investigation suggests no association between viruses and canine cancers. Front Vet Sci 7:365. https://doi.org/10.3389/fvets.2020.00365. Epub 2020/08/09. PubMed PMID: 32766289; PubMed Central PMCID: PMCPMC7380080
40. Huang SH, Kozak PJ, Kim J, Habineza-Ndikuyeze G, Meade C, Gaurnier-Hausser A et al (2012) Evidence of an oncogenic gammaherpesvirus in domestic dogs. Virology 427(2):107–117. https://doi.org/10.1016/j.virol.2012.02.013. Epub 2012/03/13. PubMed PMID: 22405628; PubMed Central PMCID: PMCPMC4592777
41. Taillieu E, Chiers K, Amorim I, Gartner F, Maes D, Van Steenkiste C et al (2022) Gastric helicobacter species associated with dogs, cats and pigs: significance for public and animal health. Vet Res 53(1):42. https://doi.org/10.1186/s13567-022-01059-4. Epub 2022/06/13. PubMed PMID: 35692057; PubMed Central PMCID: PMCPMC9190127
42. Choi JK, Xiao W, Chen X, Loghavi S, Elenitoba-Johnson KS, Naresh KN et al (2024) 5(Th) edition of the World Health Organization classification of tumors of the hematopoietic and lymphoid tissues. Mod Pathol 2024:100466. https://doi.org/10.1016/j.modpat.2024.100466. Epub 2024/03/10. PubMed PMID: 38460674
43. Naresh KN, Medeiros LJ, Project WHOFEC (2023) Introduction to the fifth edition of the world health organization classification of tumors of hematopoietic and lymphoid tissues. Mod Pathol 36(12):100330. https://doi.org/10.1016/j.modpat.2023.100330. Epub 2023/09/17. PubMed PMID: 37716508
44. Cho J (2022) Basic immunohistochemistry for lymphoma diagnosis. Blood Res 57(S1):55–61. https://doi.org/10.5045/br.2022.2022037. Epub 2022/04/29. PubMed PMID: 35483927; PubMed Central PMCID: PMCPMC9057666
45. Rao IS (2010) Role of immunohistochemistry in lymphoma. Indian J Med Paediatr Oncol 31(4):145–147. https://doi.org/10.4103/0971-5851.76201. Epub 2011/05/18. PubMed PMID: 21584221; PubMed Central PMCID: PMCPMC3089924
46. Seegmiller AC, Hsi ED, Craig FE (2019) The current role of clinical flow cytometry in the evaluation of mature B-cell neoplasms. Cytometry B Clin Cytom 96(1):20–29. https://doi.org/10.1002/cyto.b.21756. Epub 2018/12/15. PubMed PMID: 30549186
47. Craig JW, Dorfman DM (2017) Flow cytometry of T cells and T-cell neoplasms. Clin Lab Med 37(4):725–751. https://doi.org/10.1016/j.cll.2017.07.002. Epub 2017/11/13. PubMed PMID: 29128066
48. Kroft SH, Harrington AM (2017) Flow cytometry of B-cell neoplasms. Clin Lab Med 37(4):697–723. https://doi.org/10.1016/j.cll.2017.07.001. Epub 2017/11/13. PubMed PMID: 29128065
49. van Dongen JJ, Lhermitte L, Bottcher S, Almeida J, van der Velden VH, Flores-Montero J et al (2012) EuroFlow antibody panels for standardized n-dimensional flow cytometric immunophenotyping of normal, reactive and malignant leukocytes. Leukemia 26(9):1908–1975. https://doi.org/10.1038/leu.2012.120. Epub 2012/05/04. PubMed PMID: 22552007; PubMed Central PMCID: PMCPMC3437410
50. Bottcher S, Engelmann R, Grigore G, Fernandez P, Caetano J, Flores-Montero J et al (2022) Expert-independent classification of mature B-cell neoplasms using standardized flow cytometry: a multicentric study. Blood Adv 6(3):976–992. https://doi.org/10.1182/bloodadvances.2021005725. Epub 2021/11/24. PubMed PMID: 34814179; PubMed Central PMCID: PMCPMC8945320
51. Comazzi S, Marconato L, Argyle DJ, Aresu L, Stirn M, Grant IA et al (2015) The European canine lymphoma network: a joining initiative to gener-

ate consensus guidelines for the diagnosis and therapy in canine lymphoma and research partnership. Vet Comp Oncol 13(4):494–497. https://doi.org/10.1111/vco.12128. Epub 2015/10/16. PubMed PMID: 26463403

52. Comazzi S, Guscetti F, Marconato L (2014) First meeting of the European canine lymphoma group. Workshop: state of the art and comparative aspects in canine lymphoma. CH-Lugano, 22 June 2013. Hematol Oncol 32(2):68–71. https://doi.org/10.1002/hon.2115. Epub 2013/11/07. PubMed PMID: 24193915
53. Vail DM, Michels GM, Khanna C, Selting KA, London CA (2010) Veterinary Cooperative Oncology G. Response evaluation criteria for peripheral nodal lymphoma in dogs (v1.0)–a Veterinary Cooperative Oncology Group (VCOG) consensus document. Vet Comp Oncol 8(1):28–37. https://doi.org/10.1111/j.1476-5829.2009.00200.x. Epub 2010/03/17. PubMed PMID: 20230579
54. Valli VE, San Myint M, Barthel A, Bienzle D, Caswell J, Colbatzky F et al (2011) Classification of canine malignant lymphomas according to the World Health Organization criteria. Vet Pathol 48(1):198–211. https://doi.org/10.1177/0300985810379428. Epub 2010/09/24. PubMed PMID: 20861499
55. Valli V, Jacobs RM, Parodi AL, Vernau W, Moore PF (2002) Classification of hematopoietic tumors of domestic animals. Washington DC, Armed Forces Institute of Pathology
56. Silva do Nascimento J, Maues T, da Silva Leite J, Reis Ferreira AM, Goncalves Ferreira ML (2021) Core-needle biopsy efficacy in histopathology diagnosis of canine multicentric lymphoma. Top Companion Anim Med 45:100561. https://doi.org/10.1016/j.tcam.2021.100561. Epub 2021/07/15. PubMed PMID: 34260990
57. Ku CK, Kass PH, Christopher MM (2017) Cytologic-histologic concordance in the diagnosis of neoplasia in canine and feline lymph nodes: a retrospective study of 367 cases. Vet Comp Oncol 15(4):1206–1217. https://doi.org/10.1111/vco.12256. Epub 2016/08/16. PubMed PMID: 27523399
58. Martini V, Marano G, Aresu L, Bonfanti U, Boracchi P, Caniatti M et al (2022) Performance of lymph node cytopathology in diagnosis and characterization of lymphoma in dogs. J Vet Intern Med 36(1):204–214. https://doi.org/10.1111/jvim.16326. Epub 2021/11/28. PubMed PMID: 34837263; PubMed Central PMCID: PMCPMC8783335
59. Teske E, Wisman P, Moore PF, van Heerde P (1994) Histologic classification and immunophenotyping of canine non-Hodgkin's lymphomas: unexpected high frequency of T cell lymphomas with B cell morphology. Exp Hematol 22(12):1179–1187. Epub 1994/11/01. PubMed PMID: 7925781
60. Comazzi S, Avery PR, Garden OA, Riondato F, Rutgen B, Vernau W et al (2017) European canine lymphoma network consensus recommendations for reporting flow cytometry in canine hematopoietic neoplasms. Cytometry B Clin Cytom 92(5):411–419. https://doi.org/10.1002/cyto.b.21382. Epub 2016/05/14. PubMed PMID: 27170500
61. Campo E, Jaffe ES, Cook JR, Quintanilla-Martinez L, Swerdlow SH, Anderson KC et al (2022) The international consensus classification of mature lymphoid neoplasms: a report from the Clinical Advisory Committee. Blood 140(11):1229–1253. https://doi.org/10.1182/blood.2022015851. Epub 2022/06/03. PubMed PMID: 35653592; PubMed Central PMCID: PMCPMC9479027
62. Evans SJM (2023) Flow cytometry in veterinary practice. Vet Clin North Am Small Anim Pract 53(1):89–100. https://doi.org/10.1016/j.cvsm.2022.07.008. Epub 2022/10/22. PubMed PMID: 36270838
63. Comazzi S, Riondato F (2021) Flow cytometry in the diagnosis of Canine T-cell lymphoma. Front Vet Sci 8:600963. https://doi.org/10.3389/fvets.2021.600963. Epub 2021/05/11. PubMed PMID: 33969027; PubMed Central PMCID: PMCPMC8096896
64. Riondato F, Comazzi S (2021) Flow cytometry in the diagnosis of Canine B-cell lymphoma. Front Vet Sci 8:600986. https://doi.org/10.3389/fvets.2021.600986. Epub 2021/04/20. PubMed PMID: 33869314; PubMed Central PMCID: PMCPMC8044988
65. Rout ED, Avery PR (2017) Lymphoid neoplasia: correlations between morphology and flow cytometry. Vet Clin North Am Small Anim Pract 47(1):53–70. https://doi.org/10.1016/j.cvsm.2016.07.004. Epub 2016/08/21. PubMed PMID: 27542692
66. Meichner K, Stokol T, Tarigo J, Avery A, Burkhard MJ, Comazzi S et al (2020) Multicenter flow cytometry proficiency testing of canine blood and lymph node samples. Vet Clin Pathol 49(2):249–257. https://doi.org/10.1111/vcp.12843. Epub 2020/04/05. PubMed PMID: 32246538
67. Wilkerson MJ, Dolce K, Koopman T, Shuman W, Chun R, Garrett L et al (2005) Lineage differentiation of canine lymphoma/leukemias and aberrant expression of CD molecules. Vet Immunol Immunopathol 106(3–4):179–196. https://doi.org/10.1016/j.vetimm.2005.02.020. Epub 2005/06/21. PubMed PMID: 15963817
68. Comazzi S, Gelain ME, Riondato F, Paltrinieri S (2006) Flow cytometric expression of common antigens CD18/CD45 in blood from dogs with lymphoid malignancies: a semi-quantitative study. Vet Immunol Immunopathol 112(3–4):243–252. https://doi.org/10.1016/j.vetimm.2006.03.004. Epub 2006/05/16. PubMed PMID: 16698089
69. Gelain ME, Mazzilli M, Riondato F, Marconato L, Comazzi S (2008) Aberrant phenotypes and

quantitative antigen expression in different subtypes of canine lymphoma by flow cytometry. Vet Immunol Immunopathol 121(3–4):179–188. https://doi.org/10.1016/j.vetimm.2007.09.018. Epub 2007/11/06. PubMed PMID: 17981339

70. Fogle JE, Tarigo JL, Thalheim L, Williams LE, English LB, Suter SE (2015) CD45+ and CD45- lymphocyte populations identified by flow cytometry from dogs with lymphoma exhibit similar morphology and the same clonal (B cell or T cell) lineage. Vet Immunol Immunopathol 168(3–4):242–248. https://doi.org/10.1016/j.vetimm.2015.10.004. Epub 2015/11/11. PubMed PMID: 26553299
71. Seelig DM, Avery P, Webb T, Yoshimoto J, Bromberek J, Ehrhart EJ et al (2014) Canine T-zone lymphoma: unique immunophenotypic features, outcome, and population characteristics. J Vet Intern Med 28(3):878–886. https://doi.org/10.1111/jvim.12343. Epub 2014/03/25. PubMed PMID: 24655022; PubMed Central PMCID: PMCPMC4895451
72. Harris LJ, Hughes KL, Ehrhart EJ, Labadie JD, Yoshimoto J, Avery AC (2019) Canine CD4+ T-cell lymphoma identified by flow cytometry exhibits a consistent histomorphology and gene expression profile. Vet Comp Oncol 17(3):253–264. https://doi.org/10.1111/vco.12460. Epub 2019/01/27. PubMed PMID: 30684308
73. Deravi N, Berke O, Woods JP, Bienzle D (2017) Specific immunotypes of canine T cell lymphoma are associated with different outcomes. Vet Immunol Immunopathol 191:5–13. https://doi.org/10.1016/j.vetimm.2017.07.008. Epub 2017/09/13. PubMed PMID: 28895866
74. Harris LJ, Rout ED, Labadie JD, Avery PR, Fernandez M, Yoshimoto J et al (2020) Clinical features of canine nodal T-cell lymphomas classified as CD8+ or CD4-CD8- by flow cytometry. Vet Comp Oncol 18(3):416–427. https://doi.org/10.1111/vco.12568. Epub 2020/01/18. PubMed PMID: 31951040
75. Keller SM, Vernau W, Moore PF (2016) Clonality testing in veterinary medicine: a review with diagnostic guidelines. Vet Pathol 53(4):711–725. https://doi.org/10.1177/0300985815626576. Epub 2016/03/05. PubMed PMID: 26933096
76. Aresu L, Arico A, Ferraresso S, Martini V, Comazzi S, Riondato F et al (2014) Minimal residual disease detection by flow cytometry and PARR in lymph node, peripheral blood and bone marrow, following treatment of dogs with diffuse large B-cell lymphoma. Vet J 200(2):318–324. https://doi.org/10.1016/j.tvjl.2014.03.006. Epub 2014/04/05. PubMed PMID: 24698669
77. Yamazaki J, Baba K, Goto-Koshino Y, Setoguchi-Mukai A, Fujino Y, Ohno K et al (2008) Quantitative assessment of minimal residual disease (MRD) in canine lymphoma by using real-time polymerase chain reaction. Vet Immunol Immunopathol 126(3–4):321–331. https://doi.org/10.1016/j.vetimm.2008.09.004. Epub 2008/11/04. PubMed PMID: 18977540
78. Yamazaki J, Takahashi M, Setoguchi A, Fujino Y, Ohno K, Tsujimoto H (2010) Monitoring of minimal residual disease (MRD) after multidrug chemotherapy and its correlation to outcome in dogs with lymphoma: a proof-of-concept pilot study. J Vet Intern Med 24(4):897–903. https://doi.org/10.1111/j.1939--1676.2010.0536.x. Epub 2010/05/25. PubMed PMID: 20492493
79. Sato M, Yamzaki J, Goto-Koshino Y, Takahashi M, Fujino Y, Ohno K et al (2013) The prognostic significance of minimal residual disease in the early phases of chemotherapy in dogs with high-grade B-cell lymphoma. Vet J 195(3):319–324. https://doi.org/10.1016/j.tvjl.2012.07.013. Epub 2012/08/23. PubMed PMID: 22909955
80. Owen LN (1980) TNM classification of tumours in domestic animals, Veterinary Public Health Unit & WHO Collaborating Center for Comparative Oncology. World Health Organization, Geneva
81. Watton TC, Purzycka K, Fitzgerald E (2021) Computed tomographic findings and clinical features in dogs with canine cutaneous lymphoma: 10 cases (2007-2018). J Am Vet Med Assoc 259(12):1433–1440. https://doi.org/10.2460/javma.20.11.0635. Epub 2021/11/11. PubMed PMID: 34757940
82. Tanaka T, Yamazaki H, Ashida K, Iimori Y, Mie K, Nishida H et al (2021) Computed tomography may detect liver infiltration of canine diffuse hepatic lymphoma. Vet Med Sci 7(6):2172–2177. https://doi.org/10.1002/vms3.598. Epub 2021/08/15. PubMed PMID: 34390546; PubMed Central PMCID: PMCPMC8604121
83. Mesquita L, Finotello R, Ferreira A, Maddox T (2022) Comparison between computed tomographic and ultrasonographic findings of the liver and spleen in dogs with confirmed hepatic or splenic lymphoma involvement. Vet Rec 190(2):e780. https://doi.org/10.1002/vetr.780. Epub 2021/08/06. PubMed PMID: 34352128
84. Jones ID, Daniels AD, Lara-Garcia A, Peters LM, Mantis P (2017) Computed tomographic findings in 12 cases of canine multi-centric lymphoma with splenic and hepatic involvement. J Small Anim Pract 58(11):622–628. https://doi.org/10.1111/jsap.12714. Epub 2017/08/02. PubMed PMID: 28762504
85. Seiler SM, Baumgartner C, Hirschberger J, Beer AJ, Bruhschwein A, Kreutzmann N et al (2015) Comparative oncology: evaluation of 2-Deoxy-2-[18F]fluoro-D-glucose (FDG) positron emission tomography/computed tomography (PET/CT) for the staging of dogs with malignant tumors. PLoS One 10(6):e0127800. https://doi.org/10.1371/

journal.pone.0127800. Epub 2015/06/13. PubMed PMID: 26068641; PubMed Central PMCID: PMCPMC4466332

86. Lawrence J, Vanderhoek M, Barbee D, Jeraj R, Tumas DB, Vail DM (2009) Use of 3′-deoxy-3′-[18F] fluorothymidine PET/CT for evaluating response to cytotoxic chemotherapy in dogs with non-Hodgkin's lymphoma. Vet Radiol Ultrasound 50(6):660–668. https://doi.org/10.1111/j.1740-8261.2009.01612.x. Epub 2009/12/17. PubMed PMID: 19999354
87. Flory AB, Rassnick KM, Stokol T, Scrivani PV, Erb HN (2007) Stage migration in dogs with lymphoma. J Vet Intern Med 21(5):1041–1047. https://doi.org/10.1892/0891-6640(2007)21[1041:smidwl]2.0.co;2. Epub 2007/10/18. PubMed PMID: 17939562
88. Barber LG, Weishaar KM (2016) Criteria for designation of clinical substage in canine lymphoma: a survey of veterinary oncologists. Vet Comp Oncol 14(Suppl 1):32–39. https://doi.org/10.1111/vco.12086. Epub 2016/08/11. PubMed PMID: 27508350
89. Valli VE (2007) Veterinary comparative hematopathology, 1st edn. Blackwell, Ames
90. Campo E, Harris NL, Jaffe ES, Pileri SA, Stein H, Thiele J, Vardiman JW (2008) WHO classification of tumours of haematopoietic and lymphoid tissues. France International Agency for Research on Cancer, Lyon
91. Riedell PA, Smith SM (2018) Double hit and double expressors in lymphoma: definition and treatment. Cancer 124(24):4622–4632. https://doi.org/10.1002/cncr.31646. Epub 2018/09/27. PubMed PMID: 30252929
92. AbuSalah MAH, Gan SH, Al-Hatamleh MAI, Irekeola AA, Shueb RH, Yean C (2020) Recent advances in diagnostic approaches for Epstein-Barr virus. Pathogens 9(3). https://doi.org/10.3390/pathogens9030226. Epub 2020/03/22. PubMed PMID: 32197545; PubMed Central PMCID: PMCPMC7157745
93. Hwang J, Suh CH, Won Kim K, Kim HS, Armand P, Huang RY et al (2021) The incidence of Epstein-Barr Virus-positive diffuse large B-cell lymphoma: a systematic review and meta-analysis. Cancers (Basel) 13(8). https://doi.org/10.3390/cancers13081785. Epub 2021/05/01. PubMed PMID: 33917961; PubMed Central PMCID: PMCPMC8068359
94. Hans CP, Weisenburger DD, Greiner TC, Gascoyne RD, Delabie J, Ott G et al (2004) Confirmation of the molecular classification of diffuse large B-cell lymphoma by immunohistochemistry using a tissue microarray. Blood 103(1):275–282. https://doi.org/10.1182/blood-2003-05-1545. Epub 2003/09/25. PubMed PMID: 14504078
95. Alizadeh AA, Eisen MB, Davis RE, Ma C, Lossos IS, Rosenwald A et al (2000) Distinct types of diffuse large B-cell lymphoma identified by gene expression profiling. Nature 403(6769):503–511. https://doi.org/10.1038/35000501. Epub 2000/02/17. PubMed PMID: 10676951
96. Shipp MA, Ross KN, Tamayo P, Weng AP, Kutok JL, Aguiar RC et al (2002) Diffuse large B-cell lymphoma outcome prediction by gene-expression profiling and supervised machine learning. Nat Med 8(1):68–74. https://doi.org/10.1038/nm0102-68. Epub 2002/01/12. PubMed PMID: 11786909
97. Meyer PN, Fu K, Greiner TC, Smith LM, Delabie J, Gascoyne RD et al (2011) Immunohistochemical methods for predicting cell of origin and survival in patients with diffuse large B-cell lymphoma treated with rituximab. J Clin Oncol 29(2):200–207. https://doi.org/10.1200/JCO.2010.30.0368. Epub 2010/12/08. PubMed PMID: 21135273; PubMed Central PMCID: PMCPMC3058275 are found at the end of this article
98. Swerdlow SH, Campo E, Pileri SA, Harris NL, Stein H, Siebert R et al (2016) The 2016 revision of the World Health Organization classification of lymphoid neoplasms. Blood 127(20):2375–2390. https://doi.org/10.1182/blood-2016-01-643569. Epub 2016/03/17. PubMed PMID: 26980727; PubMed Central PMCID: PMCPMC4874220
99. Reddy A, Zhang J, Davis NS, Moffitt AB, Love CL, Waldrop A et al (2017) Genetic and functional drivers of diffuse large B cell lymphoma. Cell 171(2):481–94 e15. https://doi.org/10.1016/j.cell.2017.09.027. Epub 2017/10/07. PubMed PMID: 28985567; PubMed Central PMCID: PMCPMC5659841
100. Chapuy B, Stewart C, Dunford AJ, Kim J, Kamburov A, Redd RA et al (2018) Molecular subtypes of diffuse large B cell lymphoma are associated with distinct pathogenic mechanisms and outcomes. Nat Med 24(5):679–690. https://doi.org/10.1038/s41591-018-0016-8. Epub 2018/05/02. PubMed PMID: 29713087; PubMed Central PMCID: PMCPMC6613387
101. Schmitz R, Wright GW, Huang DW, Johnson CA, Phelan JD, Wang JQ et al (2018) Genetics and pathogenesis of diffuse large B-cell lymphoma. N Engl J Med 378(15):1396–1407. https://doi.org/10.1056/NEJMoa1801445. Epub 2018/04/12. PubMed PMID: 29641966; PubMed Central PMCID: PMCPMC6010183
102. Lacy SE, Barrans SL, Beer PA, Painter D, Smith AG, Roman E et al (2020) Targeted sequencing in DLBCL, molecular subtypes, and outcomes: a Haematological Malignancy Research Network report. Blood 135(20):1759–1771. https://doi.org/10.1182/blood.2019003535. Epub 2020/03/19. PubMed PMID: 32187361; PubMed Central PMCID: PMCPMC7259825 Therapeutics, OncoDNA, and Everything Genetic. D.J.H. received research funding from Gilead International; and reports consultancy for Karus. The remaining authors declare no competing financial interests
103. Larson DP, Peterson JF, Nowakowski GS, McPhail ED (2020) A practical approach to FISH test-

ing for MYC rearrangements and brief review of MYC in aggressive B-cell lymphomas. J Hematop 13(3):127–135. https://doi.org/10.1007/s12308-020-00404-w
104. Richards KL, Motsinger-Reif AA, Chen HW, Fedoriw Y, Fan C, Nielsen DM et al (2013) Gene profiling of canine B-cell lymphoma reveals germinal center and postgerminal center subtypes with different survival times, modeling human DLBCL. Cancer Res 73(16):5029–5039. https://doi.org/10.1158/0008-5472.CAN-12-3546. Epub 2013/06/21.PubMed PMID: 23783577; PubMed Central PMCID: PMCPMC3755352
105. Seelig DM, Ito D, Forster CL, Yoon UA, Breen M, Burns LJ et al (2017) Constitutive activation of alternative nuclear factor kappa B pathway in canine diffuse large B-cell lymphoma contributes to tumor cell survival and is a target of new adjuvant therapies. Leuk Lymphoma 58(7):1702–1710. https://doi.org/10.1080/10428194.2016.1260122. Epub 2016/12/10. PubMed PMID: 27931134; PubMed Central PMCID: PMCPMC6198319
106. Giannuzzi D, Marconato L, Fanelli A, Licenziato L, De Maria R, Rinaldi A et al (2022) The genomic landscape of canine diffuse large B-cell lymphoma identifies distinct subtypes with clinical and therapeutic implications. Lab Anim (NY) 51(7):191–202. https://doi.org/10.1038/s41684-022-00998-x. Epub 2022/06/22. PubMed PMID: 35726023
107. Bushell KR, Kim Y, Chan FC, Ben-Neriah S, Jenks A, Alcaide M et al (2015) Genetic inactivation of TRAF3 in canine and human B-cell lymphoma. Blood 125(6):999–1005. https://doi.org/10.1182/blood-2014-10-602714. Epub 2014/12/04. PubMed PMID: 25468570
108. Salam D, Thit EE, Teoh SH, Tan SY, Peh SC, Cheah SC (2020) C-MYC, BCL2 and BCL6 translocation in B-cell non-hodgkin lymphoma cases. J Cancer 11(1):190–198. https://doi.org/10.7150/jca.36954. Epub 2020/01/02. PubMed PMID: 31892985; PubMed Central PMCID: PMCPMC6930405
109. Horn H, Ziepert M, Becher C, Barth TF, Bernd HW, Feller AC et al (2013) MYC status in concert with BCL2 and BCL6 expression predicts outcome in diffuse large B-cell lymphoma. Blood 121(12):2253–2263. https://doi.org/10.1182/blood-2012-06-435842. Epub 2013/01/22. PubMed PMID: 23335369
110. Kurz KS, Ott M, Kalmbach S, Steinlein S, Kalla C, Horn H et al (2023) Large B-cell lymphomas in the 5th edition of the WHO-classification of haematolymphoid neoplasms-updated classification and new concepts. Cancers (Basel) 15(8). https://doi.org/10.3390/cancers15082285. Epub 2023/05/16. PubMed PMID: 37190213; PubMed Central PMCID: PMCPMC10137297
111. Sato M, Kanemoto H, Kagawa Y, Kobayashi T, Goto-Koshino Y, Mochizuki H et al (2012) Evaluation of the prognostic significance of BCL6 gene expression in canine high-grade B-cell lymphoma. Vet J 191(1):108–114. https://doi.org/10.1016/j.tvjl.2010.12.006. Epub 2011/02/01. PubMed PMID: 21277811
112. Curran KM, Schaffer PA, Frank CB, Lana SE, Hamil LE, Burton JH et al (2017) BCL2 and MYC are expressed at high levels in canine diffuse large B-cell lymphoma but are not predictive for outcome in dogs treated with CHOP chemotherapy. Vet Comp Oncol 15(4):1269–1279. https://doi.org/10.1111/vco.12263. Epub 2016/08/16. PubMed PMID: 27514648
113. Thomas R, Smith KC, Ostrander EA, Galibert F, Breen M (2003) Chromosome aberrations in canine multicentric lymphomas detected with comparative genomic hybridisation and a panel of single locus probes. Br J Cancer 89(8):1530–1537. https://doi.org/10.1038/sj.bjc.6601275. Epub 2003/10/17. PubMed PMID: 14562028; PubMed Central PMCID: PMCPMC2394339
114. Thomas R, Seiser EL, Motsinger-Reif A, Borst L, Valli VE, Kelley K et al (2011) Refining tumor-associated aneuploidy through 'genomic recoding' of recurrent DNA copy number aberrations in 150 canine non-Hodgkin lymphomas. Leuk Lymphoma 52(7):1321–1335. https://doi.org/10.3109/10428194.2011.559802. Epub 2011/03/08. PubMed PMID: 21375435; PubMed Central PMCID: PMCPMC4304668
115. Cerhan JR (2020) Epidemiology of follicular lymphoma. Hematol Oncol Clin North Am 34(4):631–646. https://doi.org/10.1016/j.hoc.2020.02.001. Epub 2020/06/27. PubMed PMID: 32586570; PubMed Central PMCID: PMCPMC7323888
116. Teras LR, DeSantis CE, Cerhan JR, Morton LM, Jemal A, Flowers CR (2016) 2016 US lymphoid malignancy statistics by World Health Organization subtypes. CA Cancer J Clin 66(6):443–459. https://doi.org/10.3322/caac.21357. Epub 2016/09/13. PubMed PMID: 27618563
117. Cerhan JR, Habermann TM (2021) Epidemiology of marginal zone lymphoma. Ann Lymphoma 5. https://doi.org/10.21037/aol-20-28. Epub 2021/04/09. PubMed PMID: 33829216; PubMed Central PMCID: PMCPMC8020862
118. Khalil MO, Morton LM, Devesa SS, Check DP, Curtis RE, Weisenburger DD et al (2014) Incidence of marginal zone lymphoma in the United States, 2001-2009 with a focus on primary anatomic site. Br J Haematol 165(1):67–77. https://doi.org/10.1111/bjh.12730. Epub 2014/01/15. PubMed PMID: 24417667; PubMed Central PMCID: PMCPMC3967856
119. Nakamura S, Ponzoni M (2020) Marginal zone B-cell lymphoma: lessons from Western and Eastern diagnostic approaches. Pathology 52(1):15–29. https://doi.org/10.1016/j.pathol.2019.08.012. Epub 2019/11/24. PubMed PMID: 31757436

120. Laurent C, Cook JR, Yoshino T, Quintanilla-Martinez L, Jaffe ES (2023) Follicular lymphoma and marginal zone lymphoma: how many diseases? Virchows Arch 482(1):149–162. https://doi.org/10.1007/s00428-022-03432-2. Epub 2022/11/18. PubMed PMID: 36394631; PubMed Central PMCID: PMCPMC9852150
121. Ishikawa E, Nakamura M, Satou A, Shimada K, Nakamura S (2022) Mucosa-Associated Lymphoid Tissue (MALT) lymphoma in the gastrointestinal tract in the modern era. Cancers (Basel) 14(2). https://doi.org/10.3390/cancers14020446. Epub 2022/01/22. PubMed PMID: 35053607; PubMed Central PMCID: PMCPMC8773811
122. Ponce F, Marchal T, Magnol JP, Turinelli V, Ledieu D, Bonnefont C et al (2010) A morphological study of 608 cases of canine malignant lymphoma in France with a focus on comparative similarities between canine and human lymphoma morphology. Vet Pathol 47(3):414–433. Epub 2010/05/18. PubMed PMID: 20472804. https://doi.org/10.1177/0300985810363902
123. Giannuzzi D, Giudice L, Marconato L, Ferraresso S, Giugno R, Bertoni F et al (2020) Integrated analysis of transcriptome, methylome and copy number aberrations data of marginal zone lymphoma and follicular lymphoma in dog. Vet Comp Oncol 18(4):645–655. Epub 2020/03/11. PubMed PMID: 32154977. https://doi.org/10.1111/vco.12588
124. Cozzi M, Marconato L, Martini V, Aresu L, Riondato F, Rossi F et al (2018) Canine nodal marginal zone lymphoma: descriptive insight into the biological behaviour. Vet Comp Oncol 16(2):246–252. Epub 2017/12/06. PubMed PMID: 29205839. https://doi.org/10.1111/vco.12374
125. O'Brien D, Moore PF, Vernau W, Peauroi JR, Rebhun RB, Rodriguez CO Jr et al (2013) Clinical characteristics and outcome in dogs with splenic marginal zone lymphoma. J Vet Intern Med 27(4):949–954. https://doi.org/10.1111/jvim.12116. Epub 2013/06/06. PubMed PMID: 23734665; PubMed Central PMCID: PMCPMC5012422
126. Stefanello D, Valenti P, Zini E, Comazzi S, Gelain ME, Roccabianca P et al (2011) Splenic marginal zone lymphoma in 5 dogs (2001-2008). J Vet Intern Med 25(1):90–93. https://doi.org/10.1111/j.1939--1676.2010.0639.x. Epub 2010/11/26. PubMed PMID: 21092007
127. Valli VE, Vernau W, de Lorimier LP, Graham PS, Moore PF (2006) Canine indolent nodular lymphoma. Vet Pathol 43(3):241–256. https://doi.org/10.1354/vp.43-3-241. Epub 2006/05/05. PubMed PMID: 16672571
128. Sabattini S, Lopparelli RM, Rigillo A, Giantin M, Renzi A, Matteo C et al (2018) Canine splenic nodular lymphoid lesions: immunophenotyping, proliferative activity, and clonality assessment. Vet Pathol 55(5):645–653. https://doi.org/10.1177/0300985818777035. Epub 2018/05/29. PubMed PMID: 29807508
129. Stein L, Bacmeister C, Ylaya K, Fetsch P, Wang Z, Hewitt SM et al (2019) Immunophenotypic characterization of canine splenic follicular-derived B-cell lymphoma. Vet Pathol 56(3):350–357. https://doi.org/10.1177/0300985818823668. Epub 2019/01/15. PubMed PMID: 30636524; PubMed Central PMCID: PMCPMC8191390
130. Ko JS, Kim HJ, Han S, Do SH (2013) Primary lymphoma of the uterine horn in a Lhasa Apso dog. Ir Vet J 66(1):24. https://doi.org/10.1186/2046-0481-66-24. Epub 2013/12/12. PubMed PMID: 24325894; PubMed Central PMCID: PMCPMC4028852
131. Hong IH, Bae SH, Lee SG, Park JK, Ji AR, Ki MR et al (2011) Mucosa-associated lymphoid tissue lymphoma of the third eyelid conjunctiva in a dog. Vet Ophthalmol 14(1):61–65. https://doi.org/10.1111/j.1463-5224.2010.00843.x. Epub 2011/01/05. PubMed PMID: 21199281
132. Pereira VC, Henker LC, Menegatt JCO, Vielmo A, Bertolini M, Legramanti WM et al (2024) Primary third eyelid lymphoma with aggressive local behavior in a dog. Top Companion Anim Med 100864. https://doi.org/10.1016/j.tcam.2024.100864. Epub 2024/03/22. PubMed PMID: 38513794
133. Kessler M, Kandel-Tschiederer B, Pfleghaar S, Tassani-Prell M (2008) Primary malignant lymphoma of the urinary bladder in a dog: longterm remission following treatment with radiation and chemotherapy. Schweiz Arch Tierheilkd 150(11):565–569. https://doi.org/10.1024/0036-7281.150.11.565. Epub 2008/11/04. PubMed PMID: 18979422
134. Randall C, Fedoriw Y (2020) Pathology and diagnosis of follicular lymphoma and related entities. Pathology 52(1):30–39. https://doi.org/10.1016/j.pathol.2019.09.010. Epub 2019/12/04. PubMed PMID: 31791624
135. Nann D, Ramis-Zaldivar JE, Muller I, Gonzalez-Farre B, Schmidt J, Egan C et al (2020) Follicular lymphoma t(14;18)-negative is genetically a heterogeneous disease. Blood Adv 4(22):5652–5665. https://doi.org/10.1182/bloodadvances.2020002944. Epub 2020/11/20. PubMed PMID: 33211828; PubMed Central PMCID: PMCPMC7686888 interests
136. Zucca E, Arcaini L, Buske C, Johnson PW, Ponzoni M, Raderer M et al (2020) Marginal zone lymphomas: ESMO Clinical Practice Guidelines for diagnosis, treatment and follow-up. Ann Oncol 31(1):17–29. https://doi.org/10.1016/j.annonc.2019.10.010. Epub 2020/01/09. PubMed PMID: 31912792
137. Cook JR (2010) Splenic B-cell lymphomas/leukemias. Surg Pathol Clin 3(4):933–954. https://doi.org/10.1016/j.path.2010.09.004. Epub 2010/12/01. PubMed PMID: 26839295
138. Santos TSD, Tavares RS, Farias DLC (2017) Splenic marginal zone lymphoma: a literature review of diagnostic and therapeutic challenges. Rev Bras

Hematol Hemoter 39(2):146–154. https://doi.org/10.1016/j.bjhh.2016.09.014. Epub 2017/06/05. PubMed PMID: 28577652; PubMed Central PMCID: PMCPMC5457460
139. Salama ME, Lossos IS, Warnke RA, Natkunam Y (2009) Immunoarchitectural patterns in nodal marginal zone B-cell lymphoma: a study of 51 cases. Am J Clin Pathol 132(1):39–49. https://doi.org/10.1309/AJCPZQ1GXBBNG8OG. Epub 2009/10/30. PubMed PMID: 19864232; PubMed Central PMCID: PMCPMC2894708
140. Lai R, Weiss LM, Chang KL, Arber DA (1999) Frequency of CD43 expression in non-Hodgkin lymphoma. A survey of 742 cases and further characterization of rare CD43+ follicular lymphomas. Am J Clin Pathol 111(4):488–494. https://doi.org/10.1093/ajcp/111.4.488. Epub 1999/04/07. PubMed PMID: 10191768
141. Wang Z, Cook JR (2019) IRTA1 and MNDA expression in marginal zone lymphoma: utility in differential diagnosis and implications for classification. Am J Clin Pathol 151(3):337–343. https://doi.org/10.1093/ajcp/aqy144. Epub 2018/10/23. PubMed PMID: 30346478
142. Pastore A, Jurinovic V, Kridel R, Hoster E, Staiger AM, Szczepanowski M et al (2015) Integration of gene mutations in risk prognostication for patients receiving first-line immunochemotherapy for follicular lymphoma: a retrospective analysis of a prospective clinical trial and validation in a population-based registry. Lancet Oncol 16(9):1111–1122. https://doi.org/10.1016/S1470-2045(15)00169-2. Epub 2015/08/11. PubMed PMID: 26256760
143. Pasqualucci L, Khiabanian H, Fangazio M, Vasishtha M, Messina M, Holmes AB et al (2014) Genetics of follicular lymphoma transformation. Cell Rep 6(1):130–140. https://doi.org/10.1016/j.celrep.2013.12.027. Epub 2014/01/07. PubMed PMID: 24388756; PubMed Central PMCID: PMCPMC4100800
144. Bonfiglio F, Bruscaggin A, Guidetti F, Terzi di Bergamo L, Faderl M, Spina V et al (2022) Genetic and phenotypic attributes of splenic marginal zone lymphoma. Blood 139(5):732–747. https://doi.org/10.1182/blood.2021012386. Epub 2021/10/16. PubMed PMID: 34653238
145. Remstein ED, Dogan A, Einerson RR, Paternoster SF, Fink SR, Law M et al (2006) The incidence and anatomic site specificity of chromosomal translocations in primary extranodal marginal zone B-cell lymphoma of mucosa-associated lymphoid tissue (MALT lymphoma) in North America. Am J Surg Pathol 30(12):1546–1553. https://doi.org/10.1097/01.pas.0000213275.60962.2a. Epub 2006/11/24. PubMed PMID: 17122510
146. Streubel B, Simonitsch-Klupp I, Mullauer L, Lamprecht A, Huber D, Siebert R et al (2004) Variable frequencies of MALT lymphoma-associated genetic aberrations in MALT lymphomas of different sites. Leukemia 18(10):1722–1726. https://doi.org/10.1038/sj.leu.2403501. Epub 2004/09/10. PubMed PMID: 15356642
147. Vela V, Juskevicius D, Dirnhofer S, Menter T, Tzankov A (2022) Mutational landscape of marginal zone B-cell lymphomas of various origin: organotypic alterations and diagnostic potential for assignment of organ origin. Virchows Arch 480(2):403–413. https://doi.org/10.1007/s00428-021-03186-3. Epub 2021/09/09. PubMed PMID: 34494161; PubMed Central PMCID: PMCPMC8986713
148. Thomas R, Demeter Z, Kennedy KA, Borst L, Singh K, Valli VE et al (2017) Integrated immunohistochemical and DNA copy number profiling analysis provides insight into the molecular pathogenesis of canine follicular lymphoma. Vet Comp Oncol 15(3):852–867. https://doi.org/10.1111/vco.12227. Epub 2016/05/03. PubMed PMID: 27135201
149. Aresu L, Martini V, Rossi F, Vignoli M, Sampaolo M, Arico A et al (2015) Canine indolent and aggressive lymphoma: clinical spectrum with histologic correlation. Vet Comp Oncol 13(4):348–362. https://doi.org/10.1111/vco.12048. Epub 2013/06/21. PubMed PMID: 23782432
150. Thandra KC, Barsouk A, Saginala K, Padala SA, Barsouk A, Rawla P (2021) Epidemiology of non-Hodgkin's lymphoma. Med Sci (Basel) 9(1). https://doi.org/10.3390/medsci9010005. Epub 2021/02/13. PubMed PMID: 33573146; PubMed Central PMCID: PMCPMC7930980
151. Zain JM, Hanona P (2021) Aggressive T-cell lymphomas: 2021 Updates on diagnosis, risk stratification and management. Am J Hematol 96(8):1027–1046. https://doi.org/10.1002/ajh.26270. Epub 2021/06/11. PubMed PMID: 34111312
152. Wudhikarn K, Bennani NN (2021) How to sequence therapies in peripheral T cell lymphoma. Curr Treat Options in Oncol 22(9):74. https://doi.org/10.1007/s11864-021-00873-w. Epub 2021/07/03. PubMed PMID: 34213653
153. Ong SY, Zain JM (2024) Aggressive T-cell lymphomas: 2024: Updates on diagnosis, risk stratification, and management. Am J Hematol 99(3):439–456. https://doi.org/10.1002/ajh.27165. Epub 2024/02/02. PubMed PMID: 38304959
154. Broccoli A, Zinzani PL (2017) Peripheral T-cell lymphoma, not otherwise specified. Blood 129(9):1103–1112. https://doi.org/10.1182/blood-2016-08-692566. Epub 2017/01/25. PubMed PMID: 28115372
155. Avery PR, Burton J, Bromberek JL, Seelig DM, Elmslie R, Correa S et al (2014) Flow cytometric characterization and clinical outcome of CD4+ T-cell lymphoma in dogs: 67 cases. J Vet Intern Med 28(2):538–546. https://doi.org/10.1111/jvim.12304. Epub 2014/02/06. PubMed PMID: 24495161; PubMed Central PMCID: PMCPMC4857986
156. Iqbal J, Wright G, Wang C, Rosenwald A, Gascoyne RD, Weisenburger DD et al (2014) Gene expression signatures delineate biological and prognostic

subgroups in peripheral T-cell lymphoma. Blood 123(19):2915–2923. https://doi.org/10.1182/blood-2013-11-536359. Epub 2014/03/19. PubMed PMID: 24632715; PubMed Central PMCID: PMCPMC4014836

157. Heavican TB, Bouska A, Yu J, Lone W, Amador C, Gong Q et al (2019) Genetic drivers of oncogenic pathways in molecular subgroups of peripheral T-cell lymphoma. Blood 133(15):1664–1676. https://doi.org/10.1182/blood-2018-09-872549. Epub 2019/02/21. PubMed PMID: 30782609; PubMed Central PMCID: PMCPMC6460420 interests

158. Amador C, Greiner TC, Heavican TB, Smith LM, Galvis KT, Lone W et al (2019) Reproducing the molecular subclassification of peripheral T-cell lymphoma-NOS by immunohistochemistry. Blood 134(24):2159–2170. https://doi.org/10.1182/blood.2019000779. Epub 2019/09/29. PubMed PMID: 31562134; PubMed Central PMCID: PMCPMC6908831 interests

159. Watatani Y, Sato Y, Miyoshi H, Sakamoto K, Nishida K, Gion Y et al (2019) Molecular heterogeneity in peripheral T-cell lymphoma, not otherwise specified revealed by comprehensive genetic profiling. Leukemia 33(12):2867–2883. https://doi.org/10.1038/s41375-019-0473-1. Epub 2019/05/17. PubMed PMID: 31092896

160. Maura F, Agnelli L, Leongamornlert D, Bolli N, Chan WC, Dodero A et al (2019) Integration of transcriptional and mutational data simplifies the stratification of peripheral T-cell lymphoma. Am J Hematol 94(6):628–634. https://doi.org/10.1002/ajh.25450. Epub 2019/03/05.PubMed PMID: 30829413; PubMed Central PMCID: PMCPMC6684242

161. Huang Y-H, Qiu Y-R, Zhang Q-L, Cai M-C, Yu H, Zhang J-M et al (2024) Genomic and transcriptomic profiling of peripheral T cell lymphoma reveals distinct molecular and microenvironment subtypes. Cell Rep Med 5(2). https://doi.org/10.1016/j.xcrm.2024.101416

162. Frantz AM, Sarver AL, Ito D, Phang TL, Karimpour-Fard A, Scott MC et al (2013) Molecular profiling reveals prognostically significant subtypes of canine lymphoma. Vet Pathol 50(4):693–703. https://doi.org/10.1177/0300985812465325. Epub 2012/11/06. PubMed PMID: 23125145; PubMed Central PMCID: PMCPMC4683027

163. Bradford PT, Devesa SS, Anderson WF, Toro JR (2009) Cutaneous lymphoma incidence patterns in the United States: a population-based study of 3884 cases. Blood 113(21):5064–5073. https://doi.org/10.1182/blood-2008-10-184168. Epub 2009/03/13. PubMed PMID: 19279331; PubMed Central PMCID: PMCPMC2686177

164. Cai ZR, Chen ML, Weinstock MA, Kim YH, Novoa RA, Linos E (2022) Incidence trends of primary cutaneous T-Cell lymphoma in the US From 2000 to 2018: A SEER population data analysis. JAMA Oncol 8(11):1690–1692. https://doi.org/10.1001/jamaoncol.2022.3236. Epub 2022/09/02. PubMed PMID: 36048455; PubMed Central PMCID: PMCPMC9437821

165. Criscione VD, Weinstock MA (2007) Incidence of cutaneous T-cell lymphoma in the United States, 1973-2002. Arch Dermatol 143(7):854–859. https://doi.org/10.1001/archderm.143.7.854. Epub 2007/07/20. PubMed PMID: 17638728

166. Huang AH, Kwatra SG, Khanna R, Semenov YR, Okoye GA, Sweren RJ (2019) Racial disparities in the clinical presentation and prognosis of patients with mycosis fungoides. J Natl Med Assoc 111(6):633–639. https://doi.org/10.1016/j.jnma.2019.08.006. Epub 2019/10/19. PubMed PMID: 31623818

167. Johnson WT, Kartan S, Sokol K, Nikbakht N, Porcu P (2021) Clinical characteristics and outcomes of black patients with mycosis fungoides and Sezary syndrome: a subgroup analysis of the phase III MAVORIC trial. Leuk Lymphoma 62(8):1877–1883. https://doi.org/10.1080/10428194.2021.1888376. Epub 2021/02/24. PubMed PMID: 33618592; PubMed Central PMCID: PMCPMC9931803

168. Fontaine J, Heimann M, Day MJ (2010) Canine cutaneous epitheliotropic T-cell lymphoma: a review of 30 cases. Vet Dermatol 21(3):267–275. https://doi.org/10.1111/j.1365-3164.2009.00793.x. Epub 2010/02/10. PubMed PMID: 20141606

169. Latzka J, Assaf C, Bagot M, Cozzio A, Dummer R, Guenova E et al (2023) EORTC consensus recommendations for the treatment of mycosis fungoides/Sezary syndrome – update 2023. Eur J Cancer 195:113343. https://doi.org/10.1016/j.ejca.2023.113343. Epub 2023/10/28. PubMed PMID: 37890355

170. Willemze R, Jaffe ES, Burg G, Cerroni L, Berti E, Swerdlow SH et al (2005) WHO-EORTC classification for cutaneous lymphomas. Blood 105(10):3768–3785. https://doi.org/10.1182/blood-2004-09-3502. Epub 2005/02/05. PubMed PMID: 15692063

171. Willemze R, Cerroni L, Kempf W, Berti E, Facchetti F, Swerdlow SH et al (2019) The 2018 update of the WHO-EORTC classification for primary cutaneous lymphomas. Blood 133(16):1703–1714. https://doi.org/10.1182/blood-2018-11-881268. Epub 2019/01/13. PubMed PMID: 30635287; PubMed Central PMCID: PMCPMC6473500 Board of Takeda. The remaining authors declare no competing financial interests

172. Saleh JS, Subtil A, Hristov AC (2023) Primary cutaneous T-cell lymphoma: a review of the most common entities with focus on recent updates. Hum Pathol 140:75–100. https://doi.org/10.1016/j.humpath.2023.09.009. Epub 2023/10/07. PubMed PMID: 37802757

173. Diwan H, Ivan D (2009) CD8-positive mycosis fungoides and primary cutaneous aggressive epidermotropic CD8-positive cytotoxic T-cell lym-

phoma. J Cutan Pathol 36(3):390–392. https://doi.org/10.1111/j.1600-0560.2008.01259.x. Epub 2009/02/18. PubMed PMID: 19220641

174. Berti E, Tomasini D, Vermeer MH, Meijer CJ, Alessi E, Willemze R (1999) Primary cutaneous CD8-positive epidermotropic cytotoxic T cell lymphomas. A distinct clinicopathological entity with an aggressive clinical behavior. Am J Pathol 155(2):483–492. https://doi.org/10.1016/S0002-9440(10)65144-9. Epub 1999/08/06. PubMed PMID: 10433941; PubMed Central PMCID: PMCPMC1866866
175. Thrall MA, Macy DW, Snyder SP, Hall RL (1984) Cutaneous lymphosarcoma and leukemia in a dog resembling Sezary syndrome in man. Vet Pathol 21(2):182–186. https://doi.org/10.1177/030098588402100209. Epub 1984/03/01. PubMed PMID: 6610244
176. Ghernati I, Auger C, Chabanne L, Corbin A, Bonnefont C, Magnol JP et al (1999) Characterization of a canine long-term T cell line (DLC 01) established from a dog with Sezary syndrome and producing retroviral particles. Leukemia 13(8):1281–1290. https://doi.org/10.1038/sj.leu.2401480. Epub 1999/08/18. PubMed PMID: 10450758
177. Rutgen BC, Flickinger I, Wolfesberger B, Litschauer B, Fuchs-Baumgartinger A, Hammer SE et al (2016) Cutaneous T-cell lymphoma – sezary syndrome in a boxer. Vet Clin Pathol 45(1):172–178. https://doi.org/10.1111/vcp.12311. Epub 2015/12/29. PubMed PMID: 26709607
178. Johnson JA, Patterson JM (1981) Canine epidermotropic lymphoproliferative disease resembling pagetoid reticulosis in man. Vet Pathol 18(4):487–493. https://doi.org/10.1177/030098588101800407. Epub 1981/07/01. PubMed PMID: 7257090
179. Moore PF, Affolter VK, Graham PS, Hirt B (2009) Canine epitheliotropic cutaneous T-cell lymphoma: an investigation of T-cell receptor immunophenotype, lesion topography and molecular clonality. Vet Dermatol 20(5–6):569–576. https://doi.org/10.1111/j.1365-3164.2009.00814.x. Epub 2010/02/25. PubMed PMID: 20178496
180. Moore PF, Olivry T, Naydan D (1994) Canine cutaneous epitheliotropic lymphoma (mycosis fungoides) is a proliferative disorder of CD8+ T cells. Am J Pathol 144(2):421–429. Epub 1994/02/01. PubMed PMID: 7906096; PubMed Central PMCID: PMCPMC1887150
181. Bakr FS, Whittaker SJ (2022) Advances in the understanding and treatment of Cutaneous T-cell lymphoma. Front Oncol 12:1043254. https://doi.org/10.3389/fonc.2022.1043254. Epub 2022/12/13. PubMed PMID: 36505788; PubMed Central PMCID: PMCPMC9729763
182. Jones CL, Degasperi A, Grandi V, Amarante TD, Genomics England Research C, Mitchell TJ et al (2021) Spectrum of mutational signatures in T-cell lymphoma reveals a key role for UV radiation in cutaneous T-cell lymphoma. Sci Rep 11(1):3962. https://doi.org/10.1038/s41598-021-83352-4. Epub 2021/02/19. PubMed PMID: 33597573; PubMed Central PMCID: PMCPMC7889847 conceptualization, design, data collection, analysis, decision to publish, or preparation of the manuscript
183. Olayinka JT, Nagarkar A, Ma DJ, Wong NB, Romasco A, Piedra-Mora C et al (2023) Cathepsin W, T-cell receptor-associated transmembrane adapter 1, lymphotactin and killer cell lectin like receptor K1 are sensitive and specific RNA biomarkers of canine epitheliotropic lymphoma. Front Vet Sci 10:1225764. https://doi.org/10.3389/fvets.2023.1225764. Epub 2023/11/29. PubMed PMID: 38026637; PubMed Central PMCID: PMCPMC10654980
184. Gerber N, Brunner MAT, Jagannathan V, Leeb T, Gerhards NM, Welle MM et al (2021) Transcriptional differences between canine cutaneous epitheliotropic lymphoma and immune-mediated dermatoses. Genes (Basel) 12(2). https://doi.org/10.3390/genes12020160. Epub 2021/01/29. PubMed PMID: 33504055; PubMed Central PMCID: PMCPMC7912288
185. Kojima K, Chambers JK, Nakashima K, Goto-Koshino Y, Uchida K (2022) Immunophenotyping of intraepithelial lymphocytes in canine chronic enteropathy and intestinal T-cell lymphoma using endoscopic samples. Vet Pathol 59(2):227–235. https://doi.org/10.1177/03009858211057220. Epub 2021/11/20. PubMed PMID: 34794367
186. B-Cell Lymphomas, Version 1.2024-January 18, 2024, NCCN clinical practice guidelines in oncology (NCCN Guidelines): National Comprehensive Cancer Network; [updated January 18, 2024; cited 2024 April, 2024]. Available from: https://www.nccn.org/professionals/physician_gls/pdf/b-cell.pdf
187. T-Cell Lymphomas, Version 4.2024-May 28, 2024, NCCN clinical practice guidelines in oncology (NCCN Guidelines) [cited 2024 June 2024]. Available from: https://www.nccn.org/professionals/physician_gls/pdf/t-cell.pdf
188. ESMO Clinical Practice Guidelines: Haematological Malignancies [November 5, 2024]. Available from: https://www.esmo.org/guidelines/guidelines-by-topic/esmo-clinical-practice-guidelines-haematological-malignancies
189. Ziepert M, Hasenclever D, Kuhnt E, Glass B, Schmitz N, Pfreundschuh M et al (2010) Standard International prognostic index remains a valid predictor of outcome for patients with aggressive CD20+ B-cell lymphoma in the rituximab era. J Clin Oncol 28(14):2373–2380. https://doi.org/10.1200/JCO.2009.26.2493. Epub 2010/04/14. PubMed PMID: 20385988
190. Oken MM, Creech RH, Tormey DC, Horton J, Davis TE, McFadden ET et al (1982) Toxicity and response criteria of the Eastern Cooperative Oncology Group. Am J Clin Oncol 5(6):649–655. Epub 1982/12/01. PubMed PMID: 7165009

191. Fisher RI, Gaynor ER, Dahlberg S, Oken MM, Grogan TM, Mize EM et al (1993) Comparison of a standard regimen (CHOP) with three intensive chemotherapy regimens for advanced non-Hodgkin's lymphoma. N Engl J Med 328(14):1002–1006. https://doi.org/10.1056/NEJM199304083281404. Epub 1993/04/08. PubMed PMID: 7680764
192. Ngo L, Hee SW, Lim LC, Tao M, Quek R, Yap SP et al (2008) Prognostic factors in patients with diffuse large B cell lymphoma: Before and after the introduction of rituximab. Leuk Lymphoma 49(3):462–469. https://doi.org/10.1080/10428190701809156. Epub 2008/02/26. PubMed PMID: 18297522
193. Pfreundschuh M, Trumper L, Osterborg A, Pettengell R, Trneny M, Imrie K et al (2006) CHOP-like chemotherapy plus rituximab versus CHOP-like chemotherapy alone in young patients with good-prognosis diffuse large-B-cell lymphoma: a randomised controlled trial by the MabThera International Trial (MInT) Group. Lancet Oncol 7(5):379–391. https://doi.org/10.1016/S1470-2045(06)70664-7. Epub 2006/05/02. PubMed PMID: 16648042
194. Tilly H, Morschhauser F, Sehn LH, Friedberg JW, Trneny M, Sharman JP et al (2022) Polatuzumab vedotin in previously untreated diffuse large B-cell lymphoma. N Engl J Med 386(4):351–363. https://doi.org/10.1056/NEJMoa2115304. Epub 2021/12/15. PubMed PMID: 34904799
195. Major A, Smith SM (2021) DA-R-EPOCH vs R-CHOP in DLBCL: how do we choose? Clin Adv Hematol Oncol 19(11):698–709. Epub 2021/11/23. PubMed PMID: 34807015; PubMed Central PMCID: PMCPMC9036549
196. Doronina SO, Toki BE, Torgov MY, Mendelsohn BA, Cerveny CG, Chace DF et al (2003) Development of potent monoclonal antibody auristatin conjugates for cancer therapy. Nat Biotechnol 21(7):778–784. https://doi.org/10.1038/nbt832. Epub 2003/06/05. PubMed PMID: 12778055
197. Francisco JA, Cerveny CG, Meyer DL, Mixan BJ, Klussman K, Chace DF et al (2003) cAC10-vcMMAE, an anti-CD30-monomethyl auristatin E conjugate with potent and selective antitumor activity. Blood 102(4):1458–1465. https://doi.org/10.1182/blood-2003-01-0039. Epub 2003/04/26. PubMed PMID: 12714494
198. Abdur Raqib M, Haseeb A, Shafique MA, Fadlalla Ahmed TK, Mustafa MS (2023) Advances in polatuzumab vedotin-PIIQ therapy: a review of treatment efficacy in diffuse large B cell lymphoma and high-grade B cell lymphoma. Pediatric Health Med Ther 14:323–331. https://doi.org/10.2147/PHMT.S429252. Epub 2023/10/23. PubMed PMID: 37867604; PubMed Central PMCID: PMCPMC10589404
199. Al-Sarayfi D, Meeuwes FO, Durmaz M, Issa DE, Brouwer RE, Beeker A et al (2022) R-CEOP as first-line treatment for anthracycline-ineligible patients with diffuse large B-cell lymphoma. Blood Cancer J 12(9):125. https://doi.org/10.1038/s41408-022-00723-4
200. Peyrade F, Jardin F, Thieblemont C, Thyss A, Emile JF, Castaigne S et al (2011) Attenuated immunochemotherapy regimen (R-miniCHOP) in elderly patients older than 80 years with diffuse large B-cell lymphoma: a multicentre, single-arm, phase 2 trial. Lancet Oncol 12(5):460–468. https://doi.org/10.1016/S1470-2045(11)70069-9. Epub 2011/04/13. PubMed PMID: 21482186
201. Crump M, Neelapu SS, Farooq U, Van Den Neste E, Kuruvilla J, Westin J et al (2017) Outcomes in refractory diffuse large B-cell lymphoma: results from the international SCHOLAR-1 study. Blood 130(16):1800–1808. https://doi.org/10.1182/blood-2017-03-769620. Epub 2017/08/05. PubMed PMID: 28774879; PubMed Central PMCID: PMCPMC5649550 as a consultant and an advisory board member for Kite Pharma. U.F. received research funding from Kite Pharma. J.K. received research funding from Celgene, Roche, and Karyopharm; served as a consultant for Bristol-Myers Squibb, Gilead, Janssen, Hoffman LaRoche, and Seattle Genetics; and received honoraria from Amgen, Bristol-Myers Squibb, Celgene, Gilead, Roche, Janssen, Lundbeck, Merck, and Seattle Genetics. J.W. served on advisory boards for ProNAi Therapeutics, Celgene, and Genentech and received research funding from Janssen, Celgene, Genentech, Kite, and Novartis. B.K.L., J.R.C., and M.J.M. received research funding from Kite Pharma. L.N., J.W., and W.Y.G. are employed by and have equity ownership in Kite Pharma. The remaining authors declare no competing financial interests
202. Chen H, Zhao J, Zhao D, Wang W, Wei C, Wang Z et al (2024) Lymphoma relapse 1 year or later after immunochemotherapy in DLBCL patients: clinical features and outcome. Clin Exp Med 24(1):48. https://doi.org/10.1007/s10238-024-01306-2. Epub 2024/03/01. PubMed PMID: 38427082; PubMed Central PMCID: PMCPMC10907456
203. Jacobson CA, Chavez JC, Sehgal AR, William BM, Munoz J, Salles G et al (2022) Axicabtagene ciloleucel in relapsed or refractory indolent non-Hodgkin lymphoma (ZUMA-5): a single-arm, multicentre, phase 2 trial. Lancet Oncol 23(1):91–103. Epub 2021/12/14. PubMed PMID: 34895487. https://doi.org/10.1016/S1470-2045(21)00591-X
204. Roddie C, Neill L, Osborne W, Iyengar S, Tholouli E, Irvine D et al (2023) Effective bridging therapy can improve CD19 CAR-T outcomes while maintaining safety in patients with large B-cell lymphoma. Blood Adv 7(12):2872–2883. https://doi.org/10.1182/bloodadvances.2022009019. Epub 2023/02/02. PubMed PMID: 36724512; PubMed Central PMCID: PMCPMC10300297 advisory boards and received honoraria from Kite/Gilead, Novartis, and Bristol Myers Squibb. A.A.K. received honoraria from Kite/Gilead. R.S., D.I., B.U., E.T., C.J., and M.O. have

served on advisory boards and received honoraria from Kite/Gilead and Novartis. W.O. has served on advisory boards and received honoraria from Kite/Gilead, Novartis, Bristol Myers Squibb, Janssen, Roche, Servier, and Pfizer. W.T. has received honoraria and consultancy fees from Kite, Bristol Myers Squibb, and Roche. The remaining authors declare no competing financial interests

205. Sehn LH, Hertzberg M, Opat S, Herrera AF, Assouline S, Flowers CR et al (2022) Polatuzumab vedotin plus bendamustine and rituximab in relapsed/refractory diffuse large B-cell lymphoma (R/R DLBCL): final results of a phase Ib/II randomized study and single-arm extension (Ext) study. Blood 140:9464–9467. https://doi.org/10.1182/blood-2022-157679

206. Salles G, Duell J, Gonzalez Barca E, Tournilhac O, Jurczak W, Liberati AM et al (2020) Tafasitamab plus lenalidomide in relapsed or refractory diffuse large B-cell lymphoma (L-MIND): a multicentre, prospective, single-arm, phase 2 study. Lancet Oncol 21(7):978–988. https://doi.org/10.1016/S1470-2045(20)30225-4. Epub 2020/06/09. PubMed PMID: 32511983

207. Dickinson MJ, Carlo-Stella C, Morschhauser F, Bachy E, Corradini P, Iacoboni G et al (2022) Glofitamab for relapsed or refractory diffuse large B-cell lymphoma. N Engl J Med 387(24):2220–2231. https://doi.org/10.1056/NEJMoa2206913. Epub 2022/12/13. PubMed PMID: 36507690

208. Thieblemont C, Phillips T, Ghesquieres H, Cheah CY, Clausen MR, Cunningham D et al (2023) Epcoritamab, a novel, subcutaneous CD3xCD20 bispecific T-cell-engaging antibody, in relapsed or refractory large B-Cell lymphoma: dose expansion in a phase I/II trial. J Clin Oncol 41(12):2238–2247. https://doi.org/10.1200/JCO.22.01725. Epub 2022/12/23. PubMed PMID: 36548927; PubMed Central PMCID: PMCPMC10115554 IN RELAPSED OR REFRACTORY LARGE B-CELL LYMPHOMA: DOSE EXPANSION IN A PHASE I/II TRIAL: The following represents disclosure information provided by authors of this manuscript. All relationships are considered compensated unless otherwise noted. Relationships are self-held unless noted. I = Immediate Family Member, Inst = My Institution. Relationships may not relate to the subject matter of this manuscript. For more information about ASCO's conflict of interest policy, please refer to www.asco.org/rwc or ascopubs.org/jco/authors/author-center. Open Payments is a public database containing information reported by companies about payments made to US-licensed physicians (Open Payments). CATHERINE THIEBLEMONT: Honoraria: Celgene, AbbVie, Bayer, Janssen, Roche, Incyte, Novartis, Gilead Sciences Research Funding: Roche Travel, Accommodations, Expenses: Roche, Janssen-Cilag, Kite/Gilead, Novartis, AbbVie TYCEL PHILLIPS: Honoraria: Seattle Genetics, Lymphoma & Myeloma Connect Consulting or Advisory Role: Seattle Genetics, Pharmacyclics, Incyte, Genentech, Bayer, Gilead Sciences, Curis, Kite/Gilead, Celgene, Genmab, TG Therapeutics, ADC Therapeutics, Lilly Research Funding: AbbVie, Pharmacyclics/Janssen, Bayer, Genentech HERVE GHESQUIERES: Honoraria: Gilead Sciences, Roche, Takeda Consulting or Advisory Role: Gilead Sciences, Roche Travel, Accommodations, Expenses: AbbVie CHAN Y. CHEAH: Honoraria: Roche/Genentech, Janssen-Cilag, TG Therapeutics, Loxo/Lilly, AstraZeneca, Bristol Myers Squibb, Gilead Sciences, BeiGene, Novartis Consulting or Advisory Role: Janssen-Cilag, Roche/Genentech (Inst), TG Therapeutics, Loxo/Lilly, Gilead Sciences, AstraZeneca, Bristol Myers Squibb, Ascentage Pharma, Merck Research Funding: Roche/Genentech (Inst), Bristol Myers Squibb (Inst), AbbVie (Inst), Merck (Inst) Travel, Accommodations, Expenses: Roche MICHAEL ROOST CLAUSEN: Consulting or Advisory Role: AbbVie, Janssen, Kite, a Gilead company, Genmab Speakers' Bureau: AbbVie, Janssen Travel, Accommodations, Expenses: AstraZeneca/Merck, Janssen, Genmab, AbbVie DAVID CUNNINGHAM: Stock and Other Ownership Interests: OVIBIO Consulting or Advisory Role: OVIBIO Research Funding: Celgene (Inst), MedImmune (Inst), Bayer (Inst), 4SC (Inst), Clovis Oncology (Inst), Lilly (Inst), Roche (Inst), Leap Oncology (Inst) TATYANA FELDMAN: Honoraria: Seattle Genetics, Pharmacyclics/Janssen, AbbVie, Bristol Myers Squibb, Kite, a Gilead company, Bayer, Takeda Consulting or Advisory Role: Seattle Genetics, Bristol Myers Squibb, Genmab, ADC Therapeutics, AstraZeneca Speakers' Bureau: Seattle Genetics, Kite, a Gilead company Research Funding: Bristol Myers Squibb (Inst), Seattle Genetics (Inst), Portola Pharmaceuticals (Inst), Eisai (Inst), Kyowa Hakko Kirin (Inst), Amgen (Inst), Viracta Therapeutics (Inst), Cell Medica (Inst), Roche (Inst), Trillium Therapeutics (Inst), Pfizer (Inst) Travel, Accommodations, Expenses: Seattle Genetics, Takeda ROBIN GASIOROWSKI: Honoraria: MSD, AbbVie, Astellas Pharma, Janssen, Novartis, Otsuka WOJCIECH JURCZAK: Consulting or Advisory Role: Roche, AstraZeneca, BeiGene Research Funding: Acerta Pharma, TG Therapeutics, Sandoz-Novartis, Roche, Takeda, Epizyme, Janssen-Cilag, BeiGene, MorphoSys, MEI Pharma TAE MIN KIM: Consulting or Advisory Role: Hanmi, AstraZeneca/MedImmune, Janssen Oncology, Novartis, Takeda, Yuhan Speakers' Bureau: Takeda, Roche/Genentech Research Funding: AstraZeneca Uncompensated Relationships: AstraZeneca/MedImmune, Novartis, Bayer, Sanofi, Boryung, Roche/Genentech DAVID JOHN LEWIS: Consulting or Advisory Role: Janssen Oncology, Kite/Gilead, BeiGene Travel, Accommodations, Expenses: Kite, a Gilead company MARJOLEIN VAN DER POEL: Consulting or Advisory Role: Takeda Travel, Accommodations,

Expenses: Jazz Pharmaceuticals, Daiichi Sankyo, AbbVie MARIANA COTA STIRNER: Employment: AbbVie Stock and Other Ownership Interests: AbbVie Travel, Accommodations, Expenses: AbbVie NURGUL KILAVUZ: Employment: ADC Therapeutics, Genmab Stock and Other Ownership Interests: Bristol Myers Squibb/Celgene, Genmab, ADC Therapeutics CHRISTOPHER CHIU: Employment: Janssen Research & Development, Genmab Stock and Other Ownership Interests: Genmab Patents, Royalties, Other Intellectual Property: Related to Daratumumab with Janssen, Related to Epcoritamab with Genmab MENGHUI CHEN: Employment: Genmab, Janssen Stock and Other Ownership Interests: Genmab, Merck/Schering Plough MARIANA SACCHI: Employment: Genmab Leadership: Genmab Stock and Other Ownership Interests: Genmab BRIAN ELLIOTT: Employment: Genmab, Novartis Stock and Other Ownership Interests: Novartis, Genmab Patents, Royalties, Other Intellectual Property: Patents pending related to Genmab development of epcoritamab Travel, Accommodations, Expenses: Genmab, Novartis TAHAMTAN AHMADI: Employment: Genmab Leadership: Genmab Stock and Other Ownership Interests: Genmab MARTIN HUTCHINGS: Consulting or Advisory Role: Takeda, Roche, Genmab, Janssen, AbbVie Research Funding: Celgene (Inst), Genmab (Inst), Roche (Inst), Takeda (Inst), Novartis (Inst), Janssen (Inst), Merck (Inst), AbbVie (Inst), AstraZeneca (Inst) PIETERNELLA J. LUGTENBURG: Consulting or Advisory Role: Takeda, Roche/Genentech, Genmab, Celgene, Regeneron, Incyte, AbbVie, Y-mAbs Therapeutics Research Funding: Takeda (Inst), Servier (Inst) Travel, Accommodations, Expenses: Celgene No other potential conflicts of interest were reported

209. Caimi PF, Ai W, Alderuccio JP, Ardeshna KM, Hamadani M, Hess B et al (2021) Loncastuximab tesirine in relapsed or refractory diffuse large B-cell lymphoma (LOTIS-2): a multicentre, open-label, single-arm, phase 2 trial. Lancet Oncol 22(6):790–800. https://doi.org/10.1016/S1470-2045(21)00139-X
210. Peters A, Keating MM, Nikonova A, Doucette S, Prica A (2023) Management of marginal zone lymphoma: a Canadian perspective. Curr Oncol 30(2):1745–1759. https://doi.org/10.3390/curroncol30020135. Epub 2023/02/25. PubMed PMID: 36826096; PubMed Central PMCID: PMCPMC9955247
211. Kaddu-Mulindwa D, Thurner L, Christofyllakis K, Bewarder M, Kos IA (2022) Management of extranodal marginal zone lymphoma: present and upcoming perspectives. Cancers (Basel) 14(12). https://doi.org/10.3390/cancers14123019. Epub 2022/06/25. PubMed PMID: 35740684; PubMed Central PMCID: PMCPMC9220961
212. Armitage JO, Vose JM, Weisenburger DD (2004) Towards understanding the peripheral T-cell lymphomas. Ann Oncol 15(10):1447–1449. https://doi.org/10.1093/annonc/mdh409. Epub 2004/09/16. PubMed PMID: 15367401
213. Horwitz S, O'Connor OA, Pro B, Illidge T, Fanale M, Advani R et al (2019) Brentuximab vedotin with chemotherapy for CD30-positive peripheral T-cell lymphoma (ECHELON-2): a global, double-blind, randomised, phase 3 trial. Lancet 393(10168):229–240. https://doi.org/10.1016/S0140-6736(18)32984-2
214. Bellei M, Foss FM, Shustov AR, Horwitz SM, Marcheselli L, Kim WS et al (2018) The outcome of peripheral T-cell lymphoma patients failing first-line therapy: a report from the prospective, International T-Cell Project. Haematologica 103(7):1191–1197. https://doi.org/10.3324/haematol.2017.186577. Epub 2018/03/31. PubMed PMID: 29599200; PubMed Central PMCID: PMCPMC6029527
215. Lansigan F, Horwitz SM, Pinter-Brown LC, Rosen ST, Pro B, Hsi ED et al (2020) Outcomes for relapsed and refractory peripheral T-cell lymphoma patients after front-line therapy from the COMPLETE registry. Acta Haematol 143(1):40–50. https://doi.org/10.1159/000500666. Epub 2019/07/18. PubMed PMID: 31315113
216. Foley NC, Mehta-Shah N (2022) Management of peripheral T-cell lymphomas and the role of transplant. Curr Oncol Rep 24(11):1489–1499. https://doi.org/10.1007/s11912-022-01310-3. Epub 2022/08/11. PubMed PMID: 35947286; PubMed Central PMCID: PMCPMC9901943
217. Bachow SH, O'Connor OA (2015) Emerging therapies in relapsed and refractory peripheral T-cell lymphoma. Clin Adv Hematol Oncol 13(12):837–846. Epub 2016/04/09. PubMed PMID: 27058850
218. Zackheim HS, Kashani-Sabet M, Amin S (1998) Topical corticosteroids for mycosis fungoides. Experience in 79 patients. Arch Dermatol 134(8):949–954. https://doi.org/10.1001/archderm.134.8.949. Epub 1998/09/02. PubMed PMID: 9722724
219. Querfeld C, Scarisbrick JJ, Assaf C, Guenova E, Bagot M, Ortiz-Romero PL et al (2022) Post hoc analysis of a randomized, controlled, phase 2 study to assess response rates with chlormethine/mechlorethamine gel in patients with stage IA-IIA mycosis fungoides. Dermatology 238(2):347–357. https://doi.org/10.1159/000516138. Epub 2021/06/07. PubMed PMID: 34091453; PubMed Central PMCID: PMCPMC8985008
220. Geskin LJ, Kim EJ, Angello JT, Kim YH (2021) Evaluating the treatment patterns of chlormethine/mechlorethamine gel in patients with stage I-IIA mycosis fungoides: by-time reanalysis of a randomized controlled phase 2 study. Clin Lymphoma Myeloma Leuk 21(2):119–124. e4. Epub

2020/12/29. PubMed PMID: 33358692. https://doi.org/10.1016/j.clml.2020.11.022

221. Hamada T, Morita A, Suga H, Boki H, Fujimura T, Hirai Y et al (2022) Safety and efficacy of bexarotene for Japanese patients with cutaneous T-cell lymphoma: real-world experience from post-marketing surveillance. J Dermatol 49(2):253–262. https://doi.org/10.1111/1346-8138.16201. Epub 2021/10/19. PubMed PMID: 34658060
222. Besner Morin C, Roberge D, Turchin I, Petrogiannis-Haliotis T, Popradi G, Pehr K (2016) Tazarotene 0.1% cream as monotherapy for early-stage cutaneous T-cell lymphoma. J Cutan Med Surg 20(3):244–248. https://doi.org/10.1177/1203475415626686. Epub 2016/01/09. PubMed PMID: 26742957
223. Apisarnthanarax N, Talpur R, Ward S, Ni X, Kim HW, Duvic M (2004) Tazarotene 0.1% gel for refractory mycosis fungoides lesions: an open-label pilot study. J Am Acad Dermatol 50(4):600–607. https://doi.org/10.1016/j.jaad.2003.09.005. Epub 2004/03/23. PubMed PMID: 15034511
224. Olsen EA, Hodak E, Anderson T, Carter JB, Henderson M, Cooper K et al (2016) Guidelines for phototherapy of mycosis fungoides and Sezary syndrome: a consensus statement of the United States Cutaneous Lymphoma Consortium. J Am Acad Dermatol 74(1):27–58. https://doi.org/10.1016/j.jaad.2015.09.033. Epub 2015/11/09. PubMed PMID: 26547257
225. Phan K, Ramachandran V, Fassihi H, Sebaratnam DF (2019) Comparison of narrowband UV-B with psoralen-UV-A phototherapy for patients with early-stage mycosis fungoides: a systematic review and meta-analysis. JAMA Dermatol 155(3):335–341. https://doi.org/10.1001/jamadermatol.2018.5204. Epub 2019/01/31. PubMed PMID: 30698622; PubMed Central PMCID: PMCPMC6439931
226. Hooper M, Hatch L, Seminario-Vidal L (2021) Photodynamic therapy of mycosis fungoides: a systematic review of case studies. Photodermatol Photoimmunol Photomed 37(6):549–552. https://doi.org/10.1111/phpp.12698. Epub 2021/05/21. PubMed PMID: 34013563
227. Liu WT, Wang HT, Yeh YH, Wong TW (2023) An update on recent advances of photodynamic therapy for primary cutaneous lymphomas. Pharmaceutics 15(5). https://doi.org/10.3390/pharmaceutics15051328. Epub 2023/05/27. PubMed PMID: 37242570; PubMed Central PMCID: PMCPMC10223676
228. Olsen EA (2003) Interferon in the treatment of cutaneous T-cell lymphoma. Dermatol Ther 16(4):311–321. https://doi.org/10.1111/j.1396--0296.2003.01643.x. Epub 2003/12/23. PubMed PMID: 14686974
229. Patsatsi A, Papadavid E, Kyriakou A, Georgiou E, Koletsa T, Avgeros C et al (2022) The use of pegylated interferon a-2a in a cohort of Greek patients with mycosis fungoides. J Eur Acad Dermatol Venereol 36(4):e291–e2e3. https://doi.org/10.1111/jdv.17795. Epub 2021/11/10. PubMed PMID: 34753217
230. Schiller M, Tsianakas A, Sterry W, Dummer R, Hinke A, Nashan D et al (2017) Dose-escalation study evaluating pegylated interferon alpha-2a in patients with cutaneous T-cell lymphoma. J Eur Acad Dermatol Venereol 31(11):1841–1847. https://doi.org/10.1111/jdv.14366. Epub 2017/05/31. PubMed PMID: 28557110
231. Falkenhain-Lopez D, Fulgencio-Barbarin J, Puerta-Pena M, Montero-Menarguez J, Sanchez-Velazquez A, Ortiz-Romero PL (2022) Single-centre experience of using pegylated liposomal doxorubicin as maintenance treatment in mycosis fungoides. Br J Dermatol 186(2):363–365. https://doi.org/10.1111/bjd.20757. Epub 2021/09/17. PubMed PMID: 34528240
232. Blazejak C, Stranzenbach R, Gosman J, Gambichler T, Wehkamp U, Stendel S et al (2022) Clinical outcomes of advanced-stage cutaneous lymphoma under low-dose gemcitabine treatment: real-life data from the german cutaneous lymphoma network. Dermatology 238(3):498–506. https://doi.org/10.1159/000517830. Epub 2021/09/03. PubMed PMID: 34474414
233. Trautinger F, Eder J, Assaf C, Bagot M, Cozzio A, Dummer R et al (2017) European Organisation for research and treatment of cancer consensus recommendations for the treatment of mycosis fungoides/Sezary syndrome – update 2017. Eur J Cancer 77:57–74. https://doi.org/10.1016/j.ejca.2017.02.027. Epub 2017/04/04. PubMed PMID: 28365528
234. Kim YH, Bagot M, Pinter-Brown L, Rook AH, Porcu P, Horwitz SM et al (2018) Mogamulizumab versus vorinostat in previously treated cutaneous T-cell lymphoma (MAVORIC): an international, open-label, randomised, controlled phase 3 trial. Lancet Oncol 19(9):1192–1204. https://doi.org/10.1016/S1470-2045(18)30379-6. Epub 2018/08/14. PubMed PMID: 30100375
235. Prince HM, Kim YH, Horwitz SM, Dummer R, Scarisbrick J, Quaglino P et al (2017) Brentuximab vedotin or physician's choice in CD30-positive cutaneous T-cell lymphoma (ALCANZA): an international, open-label, randomised, phase 3, multicentre trial. Lancet 390(10094):555–566. https://doi.org/10.1016/S0140-6736(17)31266-7. Epub 2017/06/11. PubMed PMID: 28600132
236. Iqbal M, Reljic T, Ayala E, Sher T, Murthy H, Roy V et al (2020) Efficacy of allogeneic hematopoietic cell transplantation in cutaneous T cell lymphoma: results of a systematic review and meta-analysis. Biol Blood Marrow Transplant 26(1):76–82. https://doi.org/10.1016/j.bbmt.2019.08.019. Epub 2019/09/09. PubMed PMID: 31494227
237. de Masson A, Beylot-Barry M, Ram-Wolff C, Mear JB, Dalle S, d'Incan M et al (2023) Allogeneic transplantation in advanced cutaneous T-cell lymphomas (CUTALLO): a propensity score matched controlled

prospective study. Lancet 401(10392):1941–1950. https://doi.org/10.1016/S0140-6736(23)00329-X. Epub 2023/04/28. PubMed PMID: 37105210
238. Vail DM, Pinkerton ME, Young KM (2020) Canine lymphoma and lymphocytic leukemias. In: Vail DM, Thamm DH, Liptak JM (eds) Withrow & MacEwen's small animal clinical oncology. Elsevier, St. Louis, pp 688–715
239. Weiskopf K, Anderson KL, Ito D, Schnorr PJ, Tomiyasu H, Ring AM et al (2016) Eradication of canine diffuse large B-cell lymphoma in a murine xenograft model with CD47 blockade and anti-CD20. Cancer Immunol Res 4(12):1072–1087. https://doi.org/10.1158/2326-6066.CIR-16-0105. Epub 2016/11/20. PubMed PMID: 27856424; PubMed Central PMCID: PMCPMC5454476
240. Rosales C, Jeglum KA, Obrocka M, Steplewski Z (1988) Cytolytic activity of murine anti-dog lymphoma monoclonal antibodies with canine effector cells and complement. Cell Immunol 115(2):420–428. https://doi.org/10.1016/0008-8749(88)90194-3. Epub 1988/09/01. PubMed PMID: 3409330
241. Jeglum KA (1996) Chemoimmunotherapy of canine lymphoma with adjuvant canine monoclonal antibody 231. Vet Clin North Am Small Anim Pract 26(1):73–85. https://doi.org/10.1016/s0195-5616(96)50007-0. Epub 1996/01/01. PubMed PMID: 8825567
242. Ito D, Brewer S, Modiano JF, Beall MJ (2015) Development of a novel anti-canine CD20 monoclonal antibody with diagnostic and therapeutic potential. Leuk Lymphoma 56(1):219–225. https://doi.org/10.3109/10428194.2014.914193. Epub 2014/04/15. PubMed PMID: 24724777; PubMed Central PMCID: PMCPMC5002357
243. Rue SM, Eckelman BP, Efe JA, Bloink K, Deveraux QL, Lowery D et al (2015) Identification of a candidate therapeutic antibody for treatment of canine B-cell lymphoma. Vet Immunol Immunopathol 164(3–4):148–159. https://doi.org/10.1016/j.vetimm.2015.02.004. Epub 2015/03/15. PubMed PMID: 25764941
244. Jain S, Aresu L, Comazzi S, Shi J, Worrall E, Clayton J et al (2016) The development of a recombinant scFv monoclonal antibody targeting canine CD20 for use in comparative medicine. PLoS One 11(2):e0148366. https://doi.org/10.1371/journal.pone.0148366. Epub 2016/02/20. PubMed PMID: 26894679; PubMed Central PMCID: PMCPMC4760772 Mologic. Mologic have not funded the project nor are they currently working on or have they worked on the CD20 project. There are no patents or products in development with this project with Mologic. Mologic scientists are co-authors as they have performed the Kd determination of the antibody (according to the methods sections using Octet Red). In addition, Mologic advised the Edinburgh authors on how to clone and use non-commercially sensitive CPG2 vectors for production of chimeric antibodies. Mologic as co-authors do not alter the authors' adherence to all PLOS ONE policies on sharing data and materials
245. Mizuno T, Kato Y, Kaneko MK, Sakai Y, Shiga T, Kato M et al (2020) Generation of a canine anti-canine CD20 antibody for canine lymphoma treatment. Sci Rep 10(1):11476. https://doi.org/10.1038/s41598-020-68470-9. Epub 2020/07/12. PubMed PMID: 32651429; PubMed Central PMCID: PMCPMC7351721 The rest of authors declare no other potential conflicts of interest
246. McLinden GP, Avery AC, Gardner HL, Hughes K, Rodday AM, Liang K et al (2024) Safety and biologic activity of a canine anti-CD20 monoclonal antibody in dogs with diffuse large B-cell lymphoma. J Vet Intern Med. https://doi.org/10.1111/jvim.17080. Epub 2024/04/25. PubMed PMID: 38662527
247. Moore AS (2016) Treatment of T cell lymphoma in dogs. Vet Rec 179(11):277. https://doi.org/10.1136/vr.103456. Epub 2016/09/17. PubMed PMID: 27634860
248. Brown PM, Tzannes S, Nguyen S, White J, Langova V (2018) LOPP chemotherapy as a first-line treatment for dogs with T-cell lymphoma. Vet Comp Oncol 16(1):108–113. https://doi.org/10.1111/vco.12318. Epub 2017/05/17. PubMed PMID: 28508557
249. Goodman IH, Moore AS, Frimberger AE (2016) Treatment of canine non-indolent T cell lymphoma using the VELCAP-TSC protocol: A retrospective evaluation of 70 dogs (2003-2013). Vet J 211:39–44. https://doi.org/10.1016/j.tvjl.2016.03.003. Epub 2016/03/28. PubMed PMID: 27017053
250. Brodsky EM, Maudlin GN, Lachowicz JL, Post GS (2009) Asparaginase and MOPP treatment of dogs with lymphoma. J Vet Intern Med 23(3):578–584. https://doi.org/10.1111/j.1939-1676.2009.0289.x. Epub 2009/08/04. PubMed PMID: 19645842
251. Mutsaers AJ, Glickman NW, DeNicola DB, Widmer WR, Bonney PL, Hahn KA et al (2002) Evaluation of treatment with doxorubicin and piroxicam or doxorubicin alone for multicentric lymphoma in dogs. J Am Vet Med Assoc 220(12):1813–1817. https://doi.org/10.2460/javma.2002.220.1813. Epub 2002/07/03. PubMed PMID: 12092954
252. Valerius KD, Ogilvie GK, Mallinckrodt CH, Getzy DM (1997) Doxorubicin alone or in combination with asparaginase, followed by cyclophosphamide, vincristine, and prednisone for treatment of multicentric lymphoma in dogs: 121 cases (1987-1995). J Am Vet Med Assoc 210(4):512–516. Epub 1997/02/15. PubMed PMID: 9040837
253. Al-Nadaf S, Rebhun RB, Curran KM, Venable RO, Skorupski KA, Willcox JL et al (2018) Retrospective analysis of doxorubicin and prednisone as first-line therapy for canine B-cell lymphoma. BMC Vet Res 14(1):356. https://doi.org/10.1186/

s12917-018-1688-5. Epub 2018/11/22. PubMed PMID: 30458771; PubMed Central PMCID: PMCPMC6245930
254. Weishaar KM, Wright ZM, Rosenberg MP, Post GS, McDaniel JA, Clifford CA et al (2022) Multicenter, randomized, double-blinded, placebo-controlled study of rabacfosadine in dogs with lymphoma. J Vet Intern Med 36(1):215–226. https://doi.org/10.1111/jvim.16341. Epub 2021/12/26. PubMed PMID: 34952995; PubMed Central PMCID: PMCPMC8783351
255. Saba CF, Clifford C, Burgess K, Phillips B, Vail D, Wright Z et al (2020) Rabacfosadine for naive canine intermediate to large cell lymphoma: efficacy and adverse event profile across three prospective clinical trials. Vet Comp Oncol 18(4):763–769. https://doi.org/10.1111/vco.12605. Epub 2020/04/30. PubMed PMID: 32346934; PubMed Central PMCID: PMCPMC7754483
256. Sauerbrey ML, Mullins MN, Bannink EO, Van Dorp TE, Kaneene JB, Obradovich JE (2007) Lomustine and prednisone as a first-line treatment for dogs with multicentric lymphoma: 17 cases (2004-2005). J Am Vet Med Assoc 230(12):1866–1869. https://doi.org/10.2460/javma.230.12.1866. Epub 2007/06/19. PubMed PMID: 17571992
257. Rassnick KM, Bailey DB, Kamstock DA, LeBlanc CJ, Berger EP, Flory AB et al (2021) Survival time for dogs with previously untreated, peripheral nodal, intermediate- or large-cell lymphoma treated with prednisone alone: the Canine Lymphoma Steroid Only trial. J Am Vet Med Assoc 259(1):62–71. https://doi.org/10.2460/javma.259.1.62. Epub 2021/06/15. PubMed PMID: 34125606
258. Garrett LD, Thamm DH, Chun R, Dudley R, Vail DM (2002) Evaluation of a 6-month chemotherapy protocol with no maintenance therapy for dogs with lymphoma. J Vet Intern Med 16(6):704–709. https://doi.org/10.1892/0891-6640(2002)016<0704:eoacpw>2.3.co;2. Epub 2002/12/06. PubMed PMID: 12465768
259. Lautscham EM, Kessler M, Ernst T, Willimzig L, Neiger R (2017) Comparison of a CHOP-LAsp-based protocol with and without maintenance for canine multicentric lymphoma. Vet Rec 180(12):303. https://doi.org/10.1136/vr.104077. Epub 2017/01/20. PubMed PMID: 28100766
260. Saba CF, Vickery KR, Clifford CA, Burgess KE, Phillips B, Vail DM et al (2018) Rabacfosadine for relapsed canine B-cell lymphoma: efficacy and adverse event profiles of 2 different doses. Vet Comp Oncol 16(1):E76–E82. https://doi.org/10.1111/vco.12337. Epub 2017/09/12. PubMed PMID: 28891260
261. Moore AS, London CA, Wood CA, Williams LE, Cotter SM, L'Heureux DA et al (1999) Lomustine (CCNU) for the treatment of resistant lymphoma in dogs. J Vet Intern Med 13(5):395–398. https://doi.org/10.1892/0891-6640(1999)013<0395:lfttor>2.3.co;2. Epub 1999/09/28. PubMed PMID: 10499719
262. Lenz JA, Robat CS, Stein TJ (2016) Vinblastine as a second rescue for the treatment of canine multicentric lymphoma in 39 cases (2005 to 2014). J Small Anim Pract 57(8):429–434. https://doi.org/10.1111/jsap.12500. Epub 2016/06/03. PubMed PMID: 27251593
263. Moore AS, Ogilvie GK, Ruslander D, Rand WS, Cotter SM, Getzy DM et al (1994) Evaluation of mitoxantrone for the treatment of lymphoma in dogs. J Am Vet Med Assoc 204(12):1903–1905. Epub 1994/06/15. PubMed PMID: 8077132
264. Treggiari E, Elliott JW, Baines SJ, Blackwood L (2018) Temozolomide alone or in combination with doxorubicin as a rescue agent in 37 cases of canine multicentric lymphoma. Vet Comp Oncol 16(2):194–201. https://doi.org/10.1111/vco.12335. Epub 2017/08/03. PubMed PMID: 28766920
265. Rassnick KM, Mauldin GE, Al-Sarraf R, Mauldin GN, Moore AS, Mooney SC (2002) MOPP chemotherapy for treatment of resistant lymphoma in dogs: a retrospective study of 117 cases (1989-2000). J Vet Intern Med 16(5):576–580. https://doi.org/10.1892/0891-6640(2002)016<0576:mcftor>2.3.co;2. Epub 2002/09/27. PubMed PMID: 12322709
266. Alvarez FJ, Kisseberth WC, Gallant SL, Couto CG (2006) Dexamethasone, melphalan, actinomycin D, cytosine arabinoside (DMAC) protocol for dogs with relapsed lymphoma. J Vet Intern Med 20(5):1178–1183. https://doi.org/10.1892/0891-6640(2006)20[1178:dmadca]2.0.co;2. Epub 2006/10/27. PubMed PMID: 17063713
267. Flood-Knapik KE, Durham AC, Gregor TP, Sanchez MD, Durney ME, Sorenmo KU (2013) Clinical, histopathological and immunohistochemical characterization of canine indolent lymphoma. Vet Comp Oncol 11(4):272–286. https://doi.org/10.1111/j.1476-5829.2011.00317.x. Epub 2012/02/03. PubMed PMID: 22296667
268. Martini V, Marconato L, Poggi A, Riondato F, Aresu L, Cozzi M et al (2016) Canine small clear cell/T--zone lymphoma: clinical presentation and outcome in a retrospective case series. Vet Comp Oncol 14(Suppl 1):117–126. https://doi.org/10.1111/vco.12155. Epub 2015/06/05. PubMed PMID: 26040658
269. Mizutani N, Goto-Koshino Y, Takahashi M, Uchida K, Tsujimoto H (2016) Clinical and histopathological evaluation of 16 dogs with T-zone lymphoma. J Vet Med Sci 78(8):1237–1244. https://doi.org/10.1292/jvms.15-0688. Epub 2016/04/22. PubMed PMID: 27098109; PubMed Central PMCID: PMCPMC5053923
270. Risbon RE, de Lorimier LP, Skorupski K, Burgess KE, Bergman PJ, Carreras J et al (2006) Response of canine cutaneous epitheliotropic lymphoma to lomustine (CCNU): a retrospective

study of 46 cases (1999-2004). J Vet Intern Med 20(6):1389–1397. https://doi.org/10.1892/0891-6640(2006)20[1389:roccel]2.0.co;2. Epub 2006/12/26. PubMed PMID: 17186855

271. Laprais A, Olivry T (2017) Is CCNU (lomustine) valuable for treatment of cutaneous epitheliotropic lymphoma in dogs? A critically appraised topic. BMC Vet Res 13(1):61. https://doi.org/10.1186/s12917-017-0978-7. Epub 2017/02/23. PubMed PMID: 28222789; PubMed Central PMCID: PMCPMC5320629
272. Williams LE, Rassnick KM, Power HT, Lana SE, Morrison-Collister KE, Hansen K et al (2006) CCNU in the treatment of canine epitheliotropic lymphoma. J Vet Intern Med 20(1):136–143. https://doi.org/10.1892/0891-6640(2006)20[136:cittoc]2.0.co;2. Epub 2006/02/25. PubMed PMID: 16496933
273. Morges MA, Burton JH, Saba CF, Vail DM, Burgess KE, Thamm DH (2014) Phase II evaluation of VDC-1101 in canine cutaneous T-cell lymphoma. J Vet Intern Med 28(5):1569–1574. https://doi.org/10.1111/jvim.12429. Epub 2014/10/03. PubMed PMID: 25274443; PubMed Central PMCID: PMCPMC4895598
274. Hoshino T, Murayama N, Yamagishi K, Okado Y, Iwai H, Shirai K et al (2023) Clinical efficacy of recombinant canine interferon-gamma therapy in dogs with cutaneous epitheliotropic T-cell lymphoma. Vet Dermatol 34(5):460–467. https://doi.org/10.1111/vde.13161. Epub 2023/04/04. PubMed PMID: 37006127.
275. Ramos SC, Macfarlane MJ, Polton G (2022) Isotretinoin treatment of 12 dogs with epitheliotropic lymphoma. Vet Dermatol 33(4):345–e80. https://doi.org/10.1111/vde.13079. Epub 2022/06/01. PubMed PMID: 35637167
276. White SD, Rosychuk RA, Scott KV, Trettien AL, Jonas L, Denerolle P (1993) Use of isotretinoin and etretinate for the treatment of benign cutaneous neoplasia and cutaneous lymphoma in dogs. J Am Vet Med Assoc 202(3):387–391. Epub 1993/02/01. PubMed PMID: 8440627
277. Rechner KN, Weeks KJ, Pruitt AF (2011) Total skin electron therapy technique for the canine patient. Vet Radiol Ultrasound 52(3):345–352. https://doi.org/10.1111/j.1740-8261.2011.01799.x. Epub 2011/02/24. PubMed PMID: 21342305
278. Ramos-Cardona XE, Luo W, Mohammed SI (2022) Advances and challenges of CAR T therapy and suitability of animal models (review). Mol Clin Oncol 17(3):134. https://doi.org/10.3892/mco.2022.2567. Epub 2022/08/12.PubMed PMID: 35949897; PubMed Central PMCID: PMCPMC9353808
279. Dias JNR, Andre AS, Aguiar SI, Gil S, Tavares L, Aires-da-Silva F (2021) Immunotherapeutic strategies for canine lymphoma: changing the odds against non-Hodgkin lymphoma. Front Vet Sci 8:621758. https://doi.org/10.3389/fvets.2021.621758. Epub 2021/09/14. PubMed PMID: 34513964; PubMed Central PMCID: PMCPMC8427286
280. Villarnovo D, McCleary-Wheeler AL, Richards KL (2017) Barking up the right tree: advancing our understanding and treatment of lymphoma with a spontaneous canine model. Curr Opin Hematol 24(4):359–366. https://doi.org/10.1097/MOH.0000000000000357. Epub 2017/04/21. PubMed PMID: 28426554; PubMed Central PMCID: PMCPMC5553274
281. Schiffman JD, Breen M (2015) Comparative oncology: what dogs and other species can teach us about humans with cancer. Philos Trans R Soc Lond Ser B Biol Sci 370(1673). https://doi.org/10.1098/rstb.2014.0231. Epub 2015/06/10. PubMed PMID: 26056372; PubMed Central PMCID: PMCPMC4581033
282. Richards KL, Suter SE (2015) Man's best friend: what can pet dogs teach us about non-Hodgkin's lymphoma? Immunol Rev 263(1):173–191. https://doi.org/10.1111/imr.12238. Epub 2014/12/17. PubMed PMID: 25510277; PubMed Central PMCID: PMCPMC4269254
283. Ito D, Frantz AM, Modiano JF (2014) Canine lymphoma as a comparative model for human non-Hodgkin lymphoma: recent progress and applications. Vet Immunol Immunopathol 159(3–4):192–201. https://doi.org/10.1016/j.vetimm.2014.02.016. Epub 2014/03/20. PubMed PMID: 24642290; PubMed Central PMCID: PMCPMC4994713
284. Marconato L, Gelain ME, Comazzi S (2013) The dog as a possible animal model for human non-Hodgkin lymphoma: a review. Hematol Oncol 31(1):1–9. https://doi.org/10.1002/hon.2017. Epub 2012/06/08. PubMed PMID: 22674797
285. MacEwen EG, Rosenthal RC, Fox LE, Loar AS, Kurzman ID (1992) Evaluation of L-asparaginase: polyethylene glycol conjugate versus native L-asparaginase combined with chemotherapy. A randomized double-blind study in canine lymphoma. J Vet Intern Med 6(4):230–234. https://doi.org/10.1111/j.1939-1676.1992.tb00344.x. Epub 1992/07/01. PubMed PMID: 1522554
286. Novotney CA, Page RL, Macy DW, Dewhirst MW, Ogilvie GK, Withrow SJ et al (1992) Phase I evaluation of doxorubicin and whole-body hyperthermia in dogs with lymphoma. J Vet Intern Med 6(4):245–249. https://doi.org/10.1111/j.1939-1676.1992.tb00346.x. Epub 1992/07/01. PubMed PMID: 1522556
287. Vail DM, Chun R, Thamm DH, Garrett LD, Cooley AJ, Obradovich JE (1998) Efficacy of pyridoxine to ameliorate the cutaneous toxicity associated with doxorubicin containing pegylated (Stealth) liposomes: a randomized, double-blind clini-

cal trial using a canine model. Clin Cancer Res 4(6):1567–1571. Epub 1998/06/17. PubMed PMID: 9626479

288. Thamm DH, MacEwen EG, Phillips BS, Hershey AE, Burgess KM, Pettit GR et al (2002) Preclinical study of dolastatin-10 in dogs with spontaneous neoplasia. Cancer Chemother Pharmacol 49(3):251–255. https://doi.org/10.1007/s00280-001-0402-6. Epub 2002/04/06. PubMed PMID: 11935218
289. Rusk A, Cozzi E, Stebbins M, Vail D, Graham J, Valli V et al (2006) Cooperative activity of cytotoxic chemotherapy with antiangiogenic thrombospondin-I peptides, ABT-526 in pet dogs with relapsed lymphoma. Clin Cancer Res 12(24):7456–7464. https://doi.org/10.1158/1078-0432.CCR-06-0110. Epub 2006/12/26. PubMed PMID: 17189419
290. Rusk A, McKeegan E, Haviv F, Majest S, Henkin J, Khanna C (2006) Preclinical evaluation of antiangiogenic thrombospondin-1 peptide mimetics, ABT-526 and ABT-510, in companion dogs with naturally occurring cancers. Clin Cancer Res 12(24):7444–7455. https://doi.org/10.1158/1078-0432.CCR-06-0109. Epub 2006/12/26. PubMed PMID: 17189418
291. Reiser H, Wang J, Chong L, Watkins WJ, Ray AS, Shibata R et al (2008) GS-9219–a novel acyclic nucleotide analogue with potent antineoplastic activity in dogs with spontaneous non-Hodgkin's lymphoma. Clin Cancer Res 14(9):2824–2832. https://doi.org/10.1158/1078-0432.CCR-07-2061. Epub 2008/05/03. PubMed PMID: 18451250
292. Vail DM, Thamm DH, Reiser H, Ray AS, Wolfgang GH, Watkins WJ et al (2009) Assessment of GS-9219 in a pet dog model of non-Hodgkin's lymphoma. Clin Cancer Res 15(10):3503–3510. https://doi.org/10.1158/1078-0432.CCR-08-3113. Epub 2009/05/07. PubMed PMID: 19417014
293. Burton JH, Mazcko C, LeBlanc A, Covey JM, Ji J, Kinders RJ et al (2018) NCI comparative oncology program testing of non-camptothecin indenoisoquinoline topoisomerase I inhibitors in naturally occurring canine lymphoma. Clin Cancer Res 24(23):5830–5840. https://doi.org/10.1158/1078-0432.CCR-18-1498. Epub 2018/08/01. PubMed PMID: 30061364; PubMed Central PMCID: PMCPMC6312717
294. Tierny D, Serres F, Segaoula Z, Bemelmans I, Bouchaert E, Petain A et al (2015) Phase I clinical pharmacology study of F14512, a new polyamine-vectorized anticancer drug, in naturally occurring canine lymphoma. Clin Cancer Res 21(23):5314–5323. https://doi.org/10.1158/1078-0432.CCR-14-3174. Epub 2015/07/15. PubMed PMID: 26169968
295. Boye P, Floch F, Serres F, Segaoula Z, Hordeaux J, Pascal Q et al (2020) Randomized, double-blind trial of F14512, a polyamine-vectorized anticancer drug, compared with etoposide phosphate, in dogs with naturally occurring lymphoma. Oncotarget 11(7):671–686. https://doi.org/10.18632/oncotarget.27461. Epub 2020/03/07. PubMed PMID: 32133044; PubMed Central PMCID: PMCPMC7041934
296. Peterson QP, Hsu DC, Novotny CJ, West DC, Kim D, Schmit JM et al (2010) Discovery and canine preclinical assessment of a nontoxic procaspase-3-activating compound. Cancer Res 70(18):7232–7241. https://doi.org/10.1158/0008-5472.CAN-10-0766. Epub 2010/09/09. PubMed PMID: 20823163; PubMed Central PMCID: PMCPMC3113694
297. Botham RC, Roth HS, Book AP, Roady PJ, Fan TM, Hergenrother PJ (2016) Small-molecule procaspase-3 activation sensitizes cancer to treatment with diverse chemotherapeutics. ACS Cent Sci 2(8):545–559. https://doi.org/10.1021/acscentsci.6b00165. Epub 2016/09/10. PubMed PMID: 27610416; PubMed Central PMCID: PMCPMC4999974 of Illinois has filed patents on compounds in this manuscript
298. Honigberg LA, Smith AM, Sirisawad M, Verner E, Loury D, Chang B et al (2010) The Bruton tyrosine kinase inhibitor PCI-32765 blocks B-cell activation and is efficacious in models of autoimmune disease and B-cell malignancy. Proc Natl Acad Sci USA 107(29):13075–13080. https://doi.org/10.1073/pnas.1004594107. Epub 2010/07/10. PubMed PMID: 20615965; PubMed Central PMCID: PMCPMC2919935
299. Harrington BK, Gardner HL, Izumi R, Hamdy A, Rothbaum W, Coombes KR et al (2016) Preclinical evaluation of the novel BTK inhibitor acalabrutinib in canine models of B-cell non-Hodgkin lymphoma. PLoS One 11(7):e0159607. https://doi.org/10.1371/journal.pone.0159607. Epub 2016/07/21. PubMed PMID: 27434128; PubMed Central PMCID: PMCPMC4951150 Hamdy, Allard Kaptein, Michael Gulrajani, Bart Van Lith, Todd Covey, Wayne Rothbaum, and Cecile Krejsa are employed by Acerta Pharma. This does not alter the authors' adherence to PLOS ONE policies on sharing data and materials. The remaining authors have no conflicts of interest to disclose
300. Gardner HL, Rippy SB, Bear MD, Cronin KL, Heeb H, Burr H et al (2018) Phase I/II evaluation of RV1001, a novel PI3Kdelta inhibitor, in spontaneous canine lymphoma. PLoS One 13(4):e0195357. https://doi.org/10.1371/journal.pone.0195357. Epub 2018/04/25. PubMed PMID: 29689086; PubMed Central PMCID: PMCPMC5915681 of this manuscript have the following competing interests: Kumar Penmetsa, Srikant Viswanadha, and Swaroop Vakkalanka are employees of Rhizen Pharmaceuticals SA/Incozen Therapeutics Pvt. Ltd., which provided financial support for the study. Kim Cronin is employed by New England Oncology Group, Heather Heeb is employed by Blue Pearl Kansas City, and Holly Burr is employed by Las Vegas Veterinary Specialists. Cheryl London is also

a consultant for Rhizen Pharmaceuticals. This does not alter the authors' adherence to PLOS ONE policies on sharing data and materials

301. London CA, Bernabe LF, Barnard S, Kisseberth WC, Borgatti A, Henson M et al (2014) Preclinical evaluation of the novel, orally bioavailable Selective Inhibitor of Nuclear Export (SINE) KPT-335 in spontaneous canine cancer: results of a phase I study. PLoS One 9(2):e87585. https://doi.org/10.1371/journal.pone.0087585. Epub 2014/02/08. PubMed PMID: 24503695; PubMed Central PMCID: PMCPMC3913620 conflicts. J S-M, DM, MK, and SS are all employees of Karyopharm Therapeutics. The clinical trial work was funded by Karyopharm therapeutics. CAL has received honoraria from Karyopharm Therapeutics. This does not alter our adherence to all the PLOS ONE policies on sharing data and materials
302. Sadowski AR, Gardner HL, Borgatti A, Wilson H, Vail DM, Lachowicz J et al (2018) Phase II study of the oral selective inhibitor of nuclear export (SINE) KPT-335 (verdinexor) in dogs with lymphoma. BMC Vet Res 14(1):250. https://doi.org/10.1186/s12917-018-1587-9. Epub 2018/08/26. PubMed PMID: 30143046; PubMed Central PMCID: PMCPMC6109271
303. LeBlanc AK, Mazcko CN, Fan TM, Vail DM, Flesner BK, Bryan JN et al (2022) Comparative oncology assessment of a novel inhibitor of valosin-containing protein in tumor-bearing dogs. Mol Cancer Ther 21(10):1510–1523. https://doi.org/10.1158/1535-7163.MCT-22-0167. Epub 2022/07/26. PubMed PMID: 35876604; PubMed Central PMCID: PMCPMC9538592
304. Thamm DH, Joseph JK, Rose BJ, Meuten TK, Weishaar KM (2020) Phase-I trial of survivin inhibition with EZN-3042 in dogs with spontaneous lymphoma. BMC Vet Res 16(1):97. https://doi.org/10.1186/s12917-020-02317-3. Epub 2020/03/27. PubMed PMID: 32209084; PubMed Central PMCID: PMCPMC7092583
305. Barnard RA, Wittenburg LA, Amaravadi RK, Gustafson DL, Thorburn A, Thamm DH (2014) Phase I clinical trial and pharmacodynamic evaluation of combination hydroxychloroquine and doxorubicin treatment in pet dogs treated for spontaneously occurring lymphoma. Autophagy 10(8):1415–1425. https://doi.org/10.4161/auto.29165. Epub 2014/07/06. PubMed PMID: 24991836; PubMed Central PMCID: PMCPMC4203518
306. Ito D, Childress M, Mason N, Winter A, O'Brien T, Henson M et al (2015) A double blinded, placebo-controlled pilot study to examine reduction of CD34 (+)/CD117 (+)/CD133 (+) lymphoma progenitor cells and duration of remission induced by neoadjuvant valspodar in dogs with large B-cell lymphoma. F1000Res 4:42. https://doi.org/10.12688/f1000research.6055.3. Epub 2015/02/11. PubMed PMID: 28357033; PubMed Central PMCID: PMCPMC5357040
307. Statham-Ringen KA, Selting KA, Lattimer JC, Henry CJ, Green JA, Bryan JN et al (2012) Evaluation of a B-cell leukemia-lymphoma 2-specific radiolabeled peptide nucleic acid-peptide conjugate for scintigraphic detection of neoplastic lymphocytes in dogs with B-cell lymphoma. Am J Vet Res 73(5):681–688. https://doi.org/10.2460/ajvr.73.5.681. Epub 2012/04/27. PubMed PMID: 22533400.
308. Peruzzi D, Gavazza A, Mesiti G, Lubas G, Scarselli E, Conforti A et al (2010) A vaccine targeting telomerase enhances survival of dogs affected by B-cell lymphoma. Mol Ther 18(8):1559–1567. https://doi.org/10.1038/mt.2010.104. Epub 2010/06/10. PubMed PMID: 20531395; PubMed Central PMCID: PMCPMC2927056
309. Gavazza A, Lubas G, Fridman A, Peruzzi D, Impellizeri JA, Luberto L et al (2013) Safety and efficacy of a genetic vaccine targeting telomerase plus chemotherapy for the therapy of canine B-cell lymphoma. Hum Gene Ther 24(8):728–738. https://doi.org/10.1089/hum.2013.112. Epub 2013/08/02. PubMed PMID: 23902422; PubMed Central PMCID: PMCPMC3746211
310. Henson MS, Curtsinger JM, Larson VS, Klausner JS, Modiano JF, Mescher MF et al (2011) Immunotherapy with autologous tumour antigen-coated microbeads (large multivalent immunogen), IL-2 and GM-CSF in dogs with spontaneous B-cell lymphoma. Vet Comp Oncol 9(2):95–105. https://doi.org/10.1111/j.1476-5829.2010.00234.x. Epub 2011/05/17. PubMed PMID: 21569195
311. Sorenmo KU, Krick E, Coughlin CM, Overley B, Gregor TP, Vonderheide RH et al (2011) CD40-activated B cell cancer vaccine improves second clinical remission and survival in privately owned dogs with non-Hodgkin's lymphoma. PLoS One 6(8):e24167. https://doi.org/10.1371/journal.pone.0024167. Epub 2011/09/10. PubMed PMID: 21904611; PubMed Central PMCID: PMCPMC3164165
312. Marconato L, Frayssinet P, Rouquet N, Comazzi S, Leone VF, Laganga P et al (2014) Randomized, placebo-controlled, double-blinded chemoimmunotherapy clinical trial in a pet dog model of diffuse large B-cell lymphoma. Clin Cancer Res 20(3):668–677. https://doi.org/10.1158/1078-0432.CCR-13-2283. Epub 2013/12/05. PubMed PMID: 24300788
313. Marconato L, Stefanello D, Sabattini S, Comazzi S, Riondato F, Laganga P et al (2015) Enhanced therapeutic effect of APAVAC immunotherapy in combination with dose-intense chemotherapy in dogs with advanced indolent B-cell lymphoma. Vaccine 33(39):5080–5086. https://doi.org/10.1016/j.vaccine.2015.08.017. Epub 2015/08/25. PubMed PMID: 26296495

314. Naik S, Galyon GD, Jenks NJ, Steele MB, Miller AC, Allstadt SD et al (2018) Comparative oncology evaluation of intravenous recombinant oncolytic vesicular stomatitis virus therapy in spontaneous canine cancer. Mol Cancer Ther 17(1):316–326. https://doi.org/10.1158/1535-7163.MCT-17-0432. Epub 2017/11/22. PubMed PMID: 29158470; PubMed Central PMCID: PMCPMC5752571
315. O'Connor CM, Sheppard S, Hartline CA, Huls H, Johnson M, Palla SL et al (2012) Adoptive T-cell therapy improves treatment of canine non-Hodgkin lymphoma post chemotherapy. Sci Rep 2:249. https://doi.org/10.1038/srep00249. Epub 2012/02/23. PubMed PMID: 22355761; PubMed Central PMCID: PMCPMC3278154
316. Panjwani MK, Smith JB, Schutsky K, Gnanandarajah J, O'Connor CM, Powell DJ Jr et al (2016) Feasibility and safety of RNA-transfected CD20-specific chimeric antigen receptor T cells in dogs with spontaneous B cell lymphoma. Mol Ther 24(9):1602–1614. https://doi.org/10.1038/mt.2016.146. Epub 2016/07/13. PubMed PMID: 27401141; PubMed Central PMCID: PMCPMC5113111
317. Panjwani MK, Atherton MJ, MaloneyHuss MA, Haran KP, Xiong A, Gupta M et al (2020) Establishing a model system for evaluating CAR T cell therapy using dogs with spontaneous diffuse large B cell lymphoma. Onco Targets Ther 9(1):1676615. https://doi.org/10.1080/2162402X.2019.1676615. Epub 2020/02/01. PubMed PMID: 32002286; PubMed Central PMCID: PMCPMC6959441
318. Etienne F, Berthaud M, Nguyen F, Bernardeau K, Maurel C, Bodet-Milin C et al (2020) SPECT-CT imaging of dog spontaneous diffuse large B-cell lymphoma targeting CD22 for the implementation of a relevant preclinical model for human. Front Oncol 10:20. https://doi.org/10.3389/fonc.2020.00020. Epub 2020/03/03. PubMed PMID: 32117707; PubMed Central PMCID: PMCPMC7018706
319. Maekawa N, Konnai S, Takagi S, Kagawa Y, Okagawa T, Nishimori A et al (2017) A canine chimeric monoclonal antibody targeting PD-L1 and its clinical efficacy in canine oral malignant melanoma or undifferentiated sarcoma. Sci Rep 7(1):8951. https://doi.org/10.1038/s41598-017-09444-2. Epub 2017/08/23. PubMed PMID: 28827658; PubMed Central PMCID: PMCPMC5567082 covering materials and techniques described in this paper (Japanese patent, application number 2016-159088)
320. Igase M, Nemoto Y, Itamoto K, Tani K, Nakaichi M, Sakurai M et al (2020) A pilot clinical study of the therapeutic antibody against canine PD-1 for advanced spontaneous cancers in dogs. Sci Rep 10(1):18311. https://doi.org/10.1038/s41598-020-75533-4. Epub 2020/10/29. PubMed PMID: 33110170; PubMed Central PMCID: PMCPMC7591904 authors declare no other potential conflicts of interest
321. Yoshimoto S, Chester N, Xiong A, Radaelli E, Wang H, Brillantes M et al (2023) Development and pharmacokinetic assessment of a fully canine anti-PD-1 monoclonal antibody for comparative translational research in dogs with spontaneous tumors. MAbs 15(1):2287250. https://doi.org/10.1080/19420862.2023.2287250. Epub 2023/12/04. PubMed PMID: 38047502; PubMed Central PMCID: PMCPMC10793675
322. Maekawa N, Konnai S, Hosoya K, Kim S, Kinoshita R, Deguchi T et al (2023) Safety and clinical efficacy of an anti-PD-L1 antibody (c4G12) in dogs with advanced malignant tumours. PLoS One 18(10):e0291727. https://doi.org/10.1371/journal.pone.0291727. Epub 2023/10/04. PubMed PMID: 37792729; PubMed Central PMCID: PMCPMC10550157 Kagawa, ST, YS, TO, SM, and KO are the authors of patent applications covering materials and techniques described in this paper (PCT/JP2017/029055, PCT/JP2018/011895). All other authors declare no competing interests. This does not alter our adherence to PLOS ONE policies on sharing data and materials

Invasive Urinary Bladder Cancer

Deborah W. Knapp, Noah M. Hahn,
Christopher M. Fulkerson, and Deepika Dhawan

1 Overview of Human and Canine Urinary Bladder Cancer

1.1 Introduction

Urinary bladder cancer is a major human health concern worldwide, with more than 600,000 new cases and 200,000 deaths per year [327]. In the United States alone, bladder cancer represents the sixth most common cancer diagnosis annually, with 82,290 new cases and 16,710 deaths projected in 2023 [284]. Bladder cancer comprises 1.5–2% of all naturally occurring cancers in dogs, a rate similar to that in humans [151, 284]. An estimated 20,000 to 40,000 dogs will develop bladder cancer in the United States each year [289]. It is acknowledged that many of these canine cases currently go undiagnosed and untreated.

More than 90% of bladder neoplasia in humans and companion dogs consists of urothelial carcinoma (UC), also referred to as transitional cell carcinoma (TCC) [63, 151]. UC can arise from the urothelium throughout the urinary tract including the bladder, renal pelvises, ureters, and urethra. Clinical problems that can be associated with UC include hematuria and dysuria, urinary tract obstruction, and regional and distant metastasis. In humans, UC of the bladder represents the second most common class of genitourinary cancers, only being surpassed by prostatic adenocarcinoma in men [268]. Other cancers that can affect the bladder include squamous cell carcinoma, adenocarcinoma, small-cell carcinoma, carcinosarcoma, undifferentiated carcinoma, rhabdomyosarcoma, lymphoma, hemangiosarcoma, fibroma, and other mesenchymal tumors [8, 15, 63, 97, 127, 140, 151, 163, 168, 204, 207, 240, 269, 283, 324].

Approximately two-thirds of humans with UC present with noninvasive tumors, with low-grade tumors being the most common [217]. Low-grade tumors can be managed initially by resection alone. If low-grade tumors recur, then intravesical therapy with chemotherapy or Bacillus Calmette-Guérin (BCG) is usually recommended [110]. High-grade superficial UC, e.g., carcinoma in situ, is typically treated with resection and BCG [110]. Recurrence of superficial tumors, however,

D. W. Knapp (✉) · C. M. Fulkerson
Department of Veterinary Clinical Sciences, College of Veterinary Medicine, Purdue University, West Lafayette, IN, USA

Purdue University Institute for Cancer Research, West Lafayette, IN, USA
e-mail: knappd@purdue.edu

N. M. Hahn
Department of Oncology and Urology, Johns Hopkins University School of Medicine, and Sidney Kimmel Comprehensive Cancer Center, Baltimore, MD, USA

D. Dhawan
Department of Veterinary Clinical Sciences, College of Veterinary Medicine, Purdue University, West Lafayette, IN, USA

M. W. Nolan et al. (eds.), *Comparative Oncology*, https://doi.org/10.1007/978-3-032-04454-9_11

is frequent, with progression to invasive cancer being a persistent risk, thus necessitating lifelong monitoring [217]. Interestingly, when a patient with low-grade superficial UC "progresses" to high-grade UC, it can occur through the development of new primary tumors which are high-grade, or through the transformation of the low-grade lesion to high-grade cancer resulting from the acquisition of additional molecular variants [26, 145]. Muscle-invasive bladder cancer in humans is less common at initial presentation and is uniformly high-grade. It is a much more aggressive cancer with a guarded prognosis [63, 170]. Muscle-invasive UC (InvUC) metastasizes to distant sites in approximately 50% of patients, and metastatic disease is almost uniformly lethal over time [63, 165]. Interestingly, the vast majority of UC that occurs in companion dogs is the high-grade invasive form of the cancer [107, 151, 289]. In a series of 226 canine UCs, >95% were intermediate to high-grade [154 . Low-grade superficial tumors are uncommon in dogs [67, 153]. It is recognized that in humans, low-grade superficial noninvasive UCs are largely driven by Ras-MAPK (mitogen-activated protein kinase) signaling with activating *FGFR3* mutations or gene fusions present in 60–80% of patients [63, 95, 208, 209]. InvUC is typically driven by deleterious mutations in *TP53* and *RB1*, alterations in *CDH1* (E-cadherin), and increased expression of *VEGFR2* [63, 95, 208, 209]. It is likely that the activation pathways leading to low-grade tumors in humans are not usually active in dogs.

The need for better therapies for UC in humans, especially for InvUC, is unquestioned. It is encouraging that substantial progress has been made in the last few years in the development of new targeted therapies and immunotherapies [99, 142, 202, 265]. In addition to new drugs, there is evidence for differential treatment responses based on molecular subtypes of InvUC, i.e., luminal, basal, and other molecular targets [136, 260]. Exploiting these findings along with combinations of new drugs could lead to substantial improvement in patient outcomes in the future [48, 63, 136, 196]. Bench-to-bedside research is essential to capitalize on these discoveries and advance UC management.

In research in UC and other types of human cancer, the flow of information to develop better therapies has traditionally started with discoveries in basic science, followed by safety studies in animals, and studies of anticancer activity in experimental animal models of cancer [295]. Following these steps, a limited number of drugs are selected for human clinical trials [295]. Substantial improvements have been made at each step of this bench-to-bedside research approach [336]. Yet, even with improvements in the "drug development pipeline," and with unprecedented advances in drug development and technologies, nine out of ten human clinical trials of new cancer therapies fail [188, 295]. A major reason for the high failure rate in human trials is that the currently available experimental models do not accurately predict treatment outcomes in humans [155, 188]. Although in vitro systems, carcinogen-induced models, engraftment, and genetically-engineered mouse models are essential in bladder cancer research, they do not possess important collective features such as cancer heterogeneity, molecular complexity, invasion, metastasis, and immune cell responses that are essential to predicting the success or failure of emerging therapies in humans [55, 117, 133, 155, 234, 338]. With the surge in interest in developing new immunotherapies and the recognition that the immune system plays a critical role in the outcomes of multiple types of therapies [65, 94, 196, 244, 246, 262, 291], it is especially important that animal models have a similar level of immunocompetence to humans. Thus, while experimental models remain essential in cancer research, complementary animal models that more accurately recapitulate human cancer are crucially needed. There is compelling evidence that dogs with naturally occurring InvUC can provide such a model for muscle-invasive bladder cancer in humans [93, 153, 289]. Canine and human InvUC are very similar in cellular and molecular features, molecular subtypes, tumor heterogeneity, immune cell responses, aggressive local cancer behavior, sites and frequency of distant metastases, and response to therapy [153]. It is important to note that the naturally occurring canine model of InvUC is meant to complement, not replace, experimental model systems in which more controlled experiments are possible.

Studies of dogs with naturally occurring cancer are especially important in bladder cancer because the number of human patients available for trials of new drugs and combinations of drugs is limited. There are especially limitations in the number of patients with metastases who would still be eligible for trials after failing multiple standard therapies. This increases the importance of pre-clinical animal studies to identify the most promising therapies to move forward to human clinical trials.

This chapter will focus on InvUC as this is the form of bladder cancer where there is the greatest need for better therapies and management in humans, and this is the form of bladder cancer where dogs can offer a highly relevant naturally occurring animal model for translational research. The chapter will provide an overview of canine and human InvUC, summarize the similarities and differences between the species, and offer examples of areas in which the canine model could be most useful in translational research.

1.2 Clinical Epidemiology and Risk Factors for Bladder Cancer

1.2.1 Human Bladder Cancer

Bladder cancer typically occurs in older patients with a median age at diagnosis of 73 years. Men are four times more likely to develop bladder cancer than women, and white people are affected more than Asian people [63, 134]. Women typically have more advanced bladder cancer at diagnosis [160]. Several factors and mechanisms have been proposed to account for the sex differences in bladder cancer development and progression. Over the last several decades, men have been more likely to smoke and have had occupational exposures that increase bladder cancer risk [160]. Differences in the timing and level of health care between men and women could also have a role [303]. Several biological mechanisms for the sex differences have also been proposed including (1) the protective effects of estrogens and the cancer-promoting effects of androgens through enhanced cell signaling and dampened immune response, (2) sex-biasing factors related to the makeup of the X and Y chromosomes, (3) sex-specific differences in post-translational modification and chromatin organization, (4) sex-related effects on the metabolic reprogramming of cancer cells, and (5) sex differences in carcinogen metabolism [160, 303].

Related to other risk, patients with Cowden disease driven by *PTEN* mutations, or retinoblastoma driven by *RB1* mutations, have a higher risk for UC of the bladder [88, 227]. Other inheritable germline genetic risk factors have been identified in more than 10% of patients with InvUC. Germline variants which were classified as pathogenic or likely pathogenic (P/LP) were identified in 80 (14%) of 586 individuals with UC in one study [37]. In high- or moderate-penetrance genes, the most common variants were in *BRCA2* (n = 9; 1.5%), *MSH2* (n = 8; 1.4%), *BRCA1* (n = 8; 1.4%), *CHEK2* (n = 6; 1.0%), *ERCC3* (n = 4; 0.7%), and *NBN* and *RAD50* (n = 3; 0.5% each). Sixty-six patients (83%) had germline P/LP variants in DNA-damage repair (DDR) genes, and 28 patients (42%) had biallelic inactivation [37]. In studies to date, there is not a sole germline genetic alteration that explains the risk across the majority of patients, and there is much research still to be done. The impact of germline genetic alterations on family members of patients with InvUC is also not yet well defined.

The most important known risk factor for InvUC in humans is exposure to tobacco products (cigarettes, cigars, pipes, etc.), accounting for >50% of cases over the last several decades [63, 134, 157]. This is not surprising as there are an estimated 70 or more carcinogenic substances in tobacco smoke [39]. Carcinogens in tobacco smoke include 4-(methylnitrosamino)-1-(3-pyridyl)-1-butanone (NNK), beta-naphthylamine, and polycyclic aromatic hydrocarbons [22, 268]. These are filtered through the kidneys and bathe the urothelium, leading to inflammation, DNA-adduct formation, and acquired genetic variants that drive cancer development [22, 268]. Second-hand smoke exposure has also been reported as a risk factor for human InvUC, although results vary across studies [22, 61, 268, 308]. Inherited genetic variants related to detoxification enzymes have been reported to increase the risk of the cancer with smoke exposure in humans [61].

Other risk factors for InvUC include occupational exposure to carcinogens, such as aromatic amines, polycyclic aromatic hydrocarbons, and chlorinated hydrocarbons that are used in the production of paint, dyes, rubber, and petroleum products [35, 63, 134, 268, 337]. Firefighters have also been found to be at higher risk for InvUC as they can be exposed to compounds in smoke including acetaldehyde, formaldehyde, sulfur dioxide, benzene, toluene, and ethylbenzene [132, 134]. Exposure to herbicides, agricultural chemicals, and hair style products has also been implicated in some, although not all, studies (Babić et al. 2022; [178, 268]). Exposure to arsenic is also a strong risk factor for InvUC in humans [134]. Additional risk factors include exposure to opium through smoking or ingestion, and exposure to radiation such as through the treatment of gynecologic cancers [134, 279, 319]. Additional concern has been raised for a potentially higher risk for bladder cancer in patients taking pioglitazone, a drug used in the treatment of diabetes, although extensive reviews and meta analyses have yielded inconsistent results [134]. There is sufficient evidence, however, for a small risk with long-term pioglitazone use, and bladder cancer is currently listed as a risk in the pioglitazone prescribing information. An association between chronic inflammatory states and the development of squamous bladder cancer clearly exists. One example of this is inflammation caused by Schistosomiasis, which is a major risk for squamous cell carcinoma of the bladder in Africa [268]. Bladder cancer risk is also higher in patients with paraplegia and long-term indwelling catheters [134].

With the growing knowledge of risk factors, it is estimated that at least one-third of bladder cancer cases in humans could be prevented, such as through smoking cessation and avoiding environmental causes. It is also noted that many human InvUC patients have no known risk factors, highlighting the need to identify additional risks, especially modifiable ones.

1.2.2 Canine Bladder Cancer

As in humans, canine InvUC is typically a disease of older dogs, with median age at diagnosis ranging from 9 to 11 years across studies [107, 153, 289]. An intriguing finding in canine InvUC is the very strong breed-associated risk including a 21-fold higher risk in Scottish Terriers compared to dogs in other breeds (Table 1) [151]. Unlike the situation in humans, female dogs are more likely to develop InvUC than male dogs. The female:male ratio of dogs with InvUC has been reported to range from 1.71:1 to 1.95:1, although the sex predilection is less pronounced in dogs in high-risk breeds [151]. Many dogs in these studies, however, had been neutered, and the effects of this on the sex predisposition for InvUC and mechanisms involved are not yet known. Furthermore, there is an approximately two fold higher risk for InvUC in neutered dogs than intact dogs of both sexes, as is the case with some other canine cancers, although the reasons for this are not yet known [31, 151, 159, 304, 311].

The etiology of InvUC in dogs is thought to be multifactorial. Known risk factors include female sex; history of ovariohysterectomy or orchiectomy; obesity; exposure to older types of flea dips and sprays, lawn herbicides and pesticides, tap water contaminants, airborne environmental pollutants, and cigarette smoke; living within a mile of a marsh or wetland; and possibly exposure to cyclophosphamide [102, 103, 107, 153, 154, 223, 287]. In a case-control study including dogs of many breeds, dogs in the highest risk group (overweight female dogs) were 28 times more likely to develop InvUC when exposed to the old-generation flea dips, shampoos, or sprays than normal-weight male dogs not exposed to the insecticides [102].

In a case-control study in 166 Scottish Terriers, the risk of InvUC was significantly higher in the dogs that had been exposed to lawn herbicides and insecticides (OR, 7.19; 95% CI 2.15–24.07; $P < 0.001$) compared to the dogs that had not been exposed [103]. In a follow-up study, at least one of

Table 1 Breed and risk of invasive urothelial carcinoma (InvUC) in pet dogs [151]

Breed	Number of dogs in that breed in the data base	InvUC cases in that breed in the data base	OR compared to mixed breed	95% confidence intervals
Mixed-breed dog (reference category)	42,777	269	1.0	NA
Scottish Terrier	670	79	21.12	16.23–27.49
Eskimo Dog	225	9	6.58	3.34–12.96
Shetland Sheepdog	2521	93	6.05	4.76–7.69
West Highland White Terrier	1234	44	5.84	4.23–8.08
Keeshond	381	10	4.26	2.25–8.07
Samoyed	471	10	3.43	1.81–6.49
Beagle	3236	62	3.09	2.34–4.08
Dalmatian	1253	19	2.43	1.52–3.89

The odds ratios (ORs) of InvU risk compared with the risk in mixed-breed dogs are included for breeds with an OR $\geq$ 2.0 and at least nine cases of InvUC in the breed

three commonly used chemicals in lawn treatments [2,4-dichlorophenoxyacetic acid, 2,4-D; 4-chloro-2methylphenoxypropionic acid, MCPP; dimethyl 2-(difluoromethyl)-4-(2-methylpropyl)-6-(trifluoromethyl) pyridine-3,5-dicarbothioate, dithiopyr)] was detected in the urine of dogs in 19 of 25 households that used lawn chemicals [150]. Of greater concern, chemicals were also detected in the urine of dogs in 14 of 25 households before the lawn was treated, and in dogs in 4 of 8 control households that did not apply lawn chemicals [150]. The detection of lawn chemicals in grass residues from treated and untreated lawns and in the urine of the dogs confirms the potential widespread exposure of the dogs to these chemicals.

Interestingly, in a case-control study in Scottish Terriers, the risk for InvUC was significantly lower in dogs that consumed vegetables at least three times per week in addition to their dog food (OR, 0.30; 95% CI 0.01–0.97; $P < 0.001$) [251]. The specific type of vegetable offering the most benefit could not be determined, but carrots were the most frequently fed vegetable. In contrast to the risk of exposure to older types of flea dips, in the more recent case-control study, the exposure to spot-on products containing fipronil was not associated with InvUC risk [250].

A recent cohort study in Scottish Terriers provides additional insight into the risk factors for InvUC in dogs [78]. In this early detection–early intervention study, 32 of 120 dogs developed biopsy-confirmed UC which was detected through screening in the absence of clinical signs. The cancer consisted of: InvUC ($n = 29$, three starting as dysplasia), grade 1 noninvasive cancer ($n = 2$), and carcinoma in situ ($n = 1$). In this study, the factors significantly associated with the development of UC in the final multivariable model included: living in households with cigarette smokers (OR 6.34, 95% CI 1.16–34.69, $P = 0.033$), living within a mile of a marsh or wetland (OR 21.23, 95% CI 3.64–123.69, $P = 0.001$), living away from a crop farm (OR for living near the crop farm 0.09, 95% CI 0.02–0.38, $P = 0.001$), history of prior urinary tract infection (UTI) (OR 3.87, 95% CI 1.0–14.98, $P = 0.050$), and older age at enrollment (OR 1.38, 95% CI 1.05–1.82, $P = 0.024$) [78, 154]. Although the number of dogs living with cigarette smokers was small ($n = 15$), the association between cigarette smoke exposure and UC risk was further supported by the analysis of the nicotine metabolite, cotinine, in the urine of the dogs [141, 154, 292]. Cotinine was present in the urine of dogs that were not reported to live with cigarette smokers, indicating other sources of smoke exposure. UC developed in 18 of 51 dogs (35.3%) with quantifiable cotinine concentrations in their urine, and in 6 of 40 dogs (15.0%) without quantifiable cotinine concentrations in their urine ($P = 0.0165$) [154]. There was also a trend for an association between the pack-years smoked by the dog owners and UC development in the dogs that lived with cigarette smokers ($P = 0.052$).

The higher risk for InvUC in dogs living near a wetland or marsh noted in the cohort study has been reported in earlier studies, and could be potentially related to exposure to insecticide spraying or trapped pollutants in the marsh [102, 109]. The higher risk of living away from a crop farm has also been previously reported and has been postulated to represent a surrogate for living closer to an urban environment and pollutants there [287]. The association between previous UTIs and the development of UC observed in the dogs in the Scottish Terrier cohort study has also been reported in humans, although with mixed results across studies [19].

In another study by Smith et al., the home addresses of dogs with InvUC (n = 66) and dogs without InvUC (n = 70) were compiled along with known levels of air and water pollutants in the counties where the dogs lived [287]. The water disinfection by-products, trihalomethanes, in the tap water were more than three times higher in the counties where dogs with InvUC resided compared to counties where the control dogs resided ($P < 0.0001$) [287]. Additionally, a higher proportion of dogs with InvUC (41.8%) lived in counties where the ozone limits exceeded EPA ozone limits compared to the control dogs in which 13.6% of the dogs lived in counties with the higher ozone ($P = 0.0008$) [287]. These findings support the investigators' hypothesis that tap water contaminants and airborne environmental pollutants contribute to the risk of InvUC in dogs.

Multiple studies have been conducted to measure chemical exposures shared between dogs and humans. In a study by Craun et al. [58] the concentrations of acrolein (assessed as its metabolite 3-HPMA), arsenic species, 4-aminobiphenyl, and 4-chlorophenol (a metabolite of the phenoxy-herbicide 2,4-D) were measured in the urine of pet dogs and their owners. Arsenic, 3-HPMA, and 4-chlorophenol were found in the urine of the dogs and their owners, and the concentrations were three to six fold higher in the dogs than in the humans [58]. In a study using silicone passive samplers in the form of wristbands for people and silicone tags for dogs, significant correlations were noted between measures of chemicals on the dog tags and the wristbands (rs = 0.38–0.90; $P < 0.05$) [322]. A correlation between chemicals measured with the silicone dog tags and the same chemicals in the urine was noted, especially for exposure to organophosphate esters in the dogs [322]. In another study using silicone detectors, multiple pesticides were detected in >70% of silicone samplers in dogs and humans, including permethrin, N,N-diethyl-meta-toluamide (DEET), chlorpyrifos, and fipronil [323]. Significant and positive correlations were observed between silicone sampler levels of permethrin and DEET with their corresponding urinary metabolites (rs = 0.50–0.96, $P < 0.05$) in both species [323]. These studies confirm that people and their dogs have similar chemical exposures, and mutagenic chemicals are shared between the species.

1.3 Clinical Presentation and Diagnostic Workup

1.3.1 Human Bladder Cancer

In the majority of patients, gross or microscopic hematuria, in the absence of pain, represents the initial indication of an underlying urinary tract cancer [110]. Occasionally, patients present with flank pain associated with hydronephrosis due to renal pelvic or ureteral obstruction. It is rare for patients to present with cachexia and widespread metastatic disease. The initial clinical evaluation in men and women includes urine cytology and examination of the bladder by cystoscopy [110]. The detection of small tumors, particularly flat noninvasive tumors of the bladder, can be facilitated with the use of blue light cystoscopy or narrowband imaging cystoscopy. It is important to note, however, that cytology is successful in identifying cancer in only 50% of patients with high-grade bladder cancers. Evaluation of the urinary tract with computed tomography or magnetic resonance imaging is also indicated, as well as imaging to detect metastases in patients found to have InvUC [110].

Additional urine tests to assess cancer-associated chromosomal changes by fluorescent in situ hybridization, increased levels of nuclear mitotic proteins, increased bladder tumor-associated antigens, or higher levels of staining in immunocytochemistry of cells shed in the urine can assist in the detection of some cancers that are not picked up by traditional tests, but these additional tests can also have false-positive results [110]. Currently, these adjunct molecular tests are mainly used to detect cancer recurrence in patients that already have a diagnosis of urinary tract cancer and who are undergoing or have completed therapy [110]. When abnormalities are found in the bladder or upper tract (renal pelvis, ureter), endoscopic resection for histologic diagnosis and for cancer staging is performed by transurethral resection of bladder tumor (TURBT) or endoscopic resection of upper tract tumors [110].

1.3.2 Canine Bladder Cancer

In dogs with InvUC, the clinical signs commonly noted by dog owners include hematuria, dysuria, and pollakiuria [92, 107]. Nonpainful hematuria often goes unnoticed by dog owners, with the exception of gross hematuria observed when the dog urinates on snow on the ground, rather than when the dog urinates on the grass. Less commonly, lameness due to bone metastasis or hypertrophic osteopathy is part of the presenting complaint [92]. The combination of hematuria and stranguria mimics those of dogs with cystoliths or UTIs, and may resolve temporarily with antibiotic therapy if a concurrent UTI is present. Suspicion for InvUC increases in older dogs, especially those in breeds with high risk for the cancer. A rectal exam may reveal a thickened urethra, firm mass in the trigone region of the bladder, enlargement of lymph nodes, or prostatomegaly in male dogs. However, a normal physical examination does not rule out InvUC.

In dogs with confirmed or suspected InvUC, the evaluation typically includes an assessment of overall health (complete blood count, serum biochemistry profile, urinalysis, ± urine culture) and cancer staging with ultrasonography and radiography, or with computed tomography [92, 125, 182, 258]. It is also important to image the urinary tract using a consistent imaging protocol to monitor the subsequent response to therapy [125, 164, 258]. Clinical signs are not an accurate indicator of change in tumor size, and detailed imaging is important. A definitive diagnosis of InvUC is made through histopathologic examination of tumor tissues [30, 92, 151]. Immunohistochemistry for uroplakin III (UPK3) and potentially GATA-3 can be used to help detect the urothelial origin of the cancer in cases with unclear histology [151]. Methods for obtaining tissue for histopathologic diagnosis include cystotomy, cystoscopy, and catheter biopsy [47, 153]. Percutaneous biopsy methods can lead to tumor seeding and are therefore best avoided. Commercially-available molecularly-based urine tests for bladder cancer detection include tests to detect a proprietary bladder tumor antigen, and to detect the presence of the $BRAF^{V595E}$ mutation in urine sediment, but both of these approaches are associated with false-negative and false-positive results [70, 78, 120, 210].

1.4 Histopathology and Cancer Staging

1.4.1 Human Bladder Cancer

The staging of bladder cancer is defined by the depth of invasion within the bladder wall, involvement of lymph nodes, and spread to surrounding and distant organs. The different stages of UC in humans are summarized in Fig. 1 with this chapter focused on InvUC. In humans, InvUC is more often referred to as "muscle-invasive bladder cancer" and is defined as UC that has invaded into the muscularis propria (T2), through the muscularis propria to involve the surrounding serosa (T3), or into immediately adjacent pelvic organs such as the rectum, prostate, vagina, or cervix (T4) (Table 2) [110].

Interestingly, within parts of InvUC masses in the bladder, variations in histology can be found. These "variant histologies" include squamous, glandular, micropapillary, plasmacytoid, sarcomatoid, and other variant features [91, 110, 215, 216]. It is rare, however, for these variant features to make up the entire mass. The presence of some areas of variant histologies within the mass, such as micropapillary and plasmacytoid variants, has been associated with worse outcomes following surgery compared to the more typical UC [110].

UCs can be found in any part of the bladder without one site being overrepresented across patients [63]. In patients with InvUC of the bladder, prostate involvement has been reported in cystoprostatectomy sections in 15–48% of cases across multiple studies [13]. Not surprisingly, higher rates of prostatic involvement have been reported in studies with more detailed pathologic examination of the tissues. Primary urothelial carcinoma of the prostatic urethra and ducts, in the absence of bladder disease, is rare in humans [340]. Prostatic adenocarcinoma arising from glandular tissue is much more common. Upper tract, e.g., renal pelvic, urothelial carcinoma is reported to occur in 5–10% of humans with InvUC [90].

Tumor staging is very important in selecting therapy and assessing the prognosis in human InvUC. The primary cause of death from InvUC in humans is metastasis [110]. The 5-year survival rate is 70% for patients with InvUC confined to the bladder, but decreases to 34% for patients with cancer that has spread locally beyond the bladder. The 5-year survival rate for patients with distant metastasis is only 5%. In an autopsy study involving 367 patients with InvUC, metastases were identified in 251 of 367 patients (68%), with the most common sites including regional lymph nodes (90%), liver (47%), lung (45%), bone (32%), peritoneum (19%), pleura (16%), kidney (14%), adrenal gland (14%), and the intestine (13%) [315].

1.4.2 Canine Bladder Cancer

As mentioned above, the vast majority of UC in dogs consists of high-grade invasive cancer [151]. Canine InvUC progresses through multiple genetic and pathologic changes including

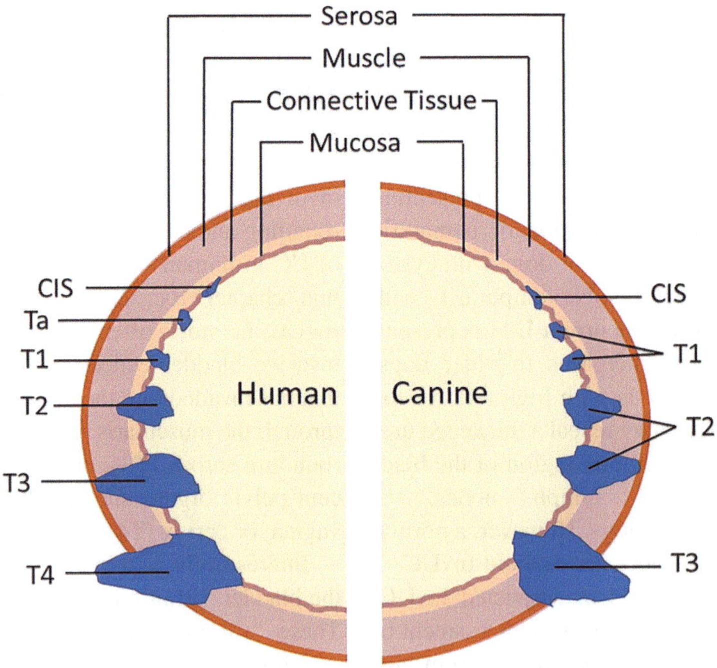

Fig. 1 Diagram of the cross section through the urinary bladder wall. Note the layers of the bladder wall and the assigned T stages for human (left) and canine (right) urothelial carcinoma. Carcinoma in situ (CIS) is a high-grade flat lesion that has not yet invaded the lamina propria (connective tissue below the mucosa). Ta tumors are noninvasive papillary tumors. T1 tumors invade the lamina propria. Note that the definition of T2, T3, and T4 tumors differ between dogs and humans. While T2 tumors invade the muscle layer in both species, in dogs, tumors that penetrate the deep muscle layers are also classified as T2, whereas in human bladder cancer, these are classified as T3. Tumors that have spread through the serosa and invade perivesical tissues or organs are classified as T4 tumors in humans, whereas in dogs these are classified as T3 tumors

Table 2 TNM staging system for human bladder cancer [46]

T—Primary tumor	
TX	Primary tumor cannot be assessed
T0	No evidence of primary tumor
Ta	Noninvasive papillary carcinoma
Tis	Carcinoma in situ
T1	Tumor invades subepithelial connective tissue (lamina propria)
T2	Tumor invades musclularis propria bladder wall
T2a	Tumor invades superficial muscle (inner half)
T2b	Tumor invades deep muscle (outer half)
T3	Tumor invades perivesical tissue
T3a	Microscopically
T3b	Macroscopically (extravesical mass)
T4	Tumor invades any of the following: prostate, uterus, vagina, pelvic wall, and abdominal wall
T4a	Tumor invades prostate, uterus, or vagina
T4b	Tumor invades pelvic or abdominal wall
N—Regional lymph nodes	
NX	Regional lymph nodes cannot be assessed
N0	No regional lymph node metastasis
N1	Metastases in a single lymph node, 2 cm or less in greatest dimension
N2	Metastases in a single lymph node, more than 2 cm but not more than 5 cm in greatest dimension, or multiple lymph nodes, none more than 5 cm in greatest dimension
N3	Metastasis in a lymph node more than 5 cm in greatest dimension
M—Distant metastasis	
MX	Distant metastasis cannot be assessed
M0	No distant metastasis
M1	Distant metastasis

dysplasia, carcinoma in situ (CIS), local invasion, regional spread, and distant metastasis [151]. Common histologic features of canine InvUC include lack of normal urothelial cell maturation, polygonal to columnar epithelial cells, marked nuclear atypia with vesicular chromatin and central nucleoli, and mitotic figures with some being bizarre (Fig. 2). Cytoplasmic vacuoles within the neoplastic cells are common, although these vary from case to case and are not unique to InvUC [151]. Marked desmoplastic reaction to invasion in the primary and metastatic lesions is also commonly observed, especially in surgical biopsies. Infiltrates of leukocytes are also observed in the tumors, although the immune infiltration varies considerably from dog to dog.

Several classification and grading schemes for canine InvUC have been published [84, 220, 243, 307], and these have been summarized in prior reviews [30, 151]. When considering growth patterns, UCs are divided into papillary (50%) or nonpapillary (50%) tumors, and infiltrating (≥90%) or noninfiltrating (<10%) tumors [151]. Distant metastases are more common in anaplastic tumors, followed by nonpapillary and infiltrating variants. When tumor specimens from surgery are examined, there is typically ample tissue to assess growth pattern, depth of invasion, vascular invasion, and desmoplastic reaction. In contrast to surgical biopsies, biopsies obtained by cystoscopy in dogs are often small. A nuclear grading scheme has been established as one of the few constant features that can be evaluated even in small tissue samples [151]. In a retrospective study in which nuclear grade was applied to assign tumor grade, of 226 canine InvUC specimens collected by biopsy or during a necropsy, two tumors were grade I; 67 were grade II; and 163 were grade III [151]. Although this earlier work utilized a three-tier grading system, a four-tier grading system is currently in use in dogs, reflecting that used in humans [46].

Some of the urothelial carcinoma histologic variants that have been reported in humans have also been reported in dogs including plasmacytoid and rhabdoid types [167]. Although the study of such variants in relation to clinical outcomes has been limited, canine InvUC with fibromyxoid stroma has been associated with invasion of the muscle layer, suggesting a more aggressive behavior in one study [68].

The TNM staging system used in canine bladder cancer is summarized in Fig. 1. It is important to note that the TNM staging system for canine bladder cancer differs somewhat from that used in humans [236]. There are three designated T stages for the canine tumors and four T stages defined in human tumors (Fig. 1, Table 3).

The metastatic behavior of InvUC has been investigated in multiple studies including a necropsy study of 137 dogs with InvUC [151]. In this study, 67% of the dogs had metastases in at least one site. Nodal metastases alone (in the absence of distant metastases) were detected in

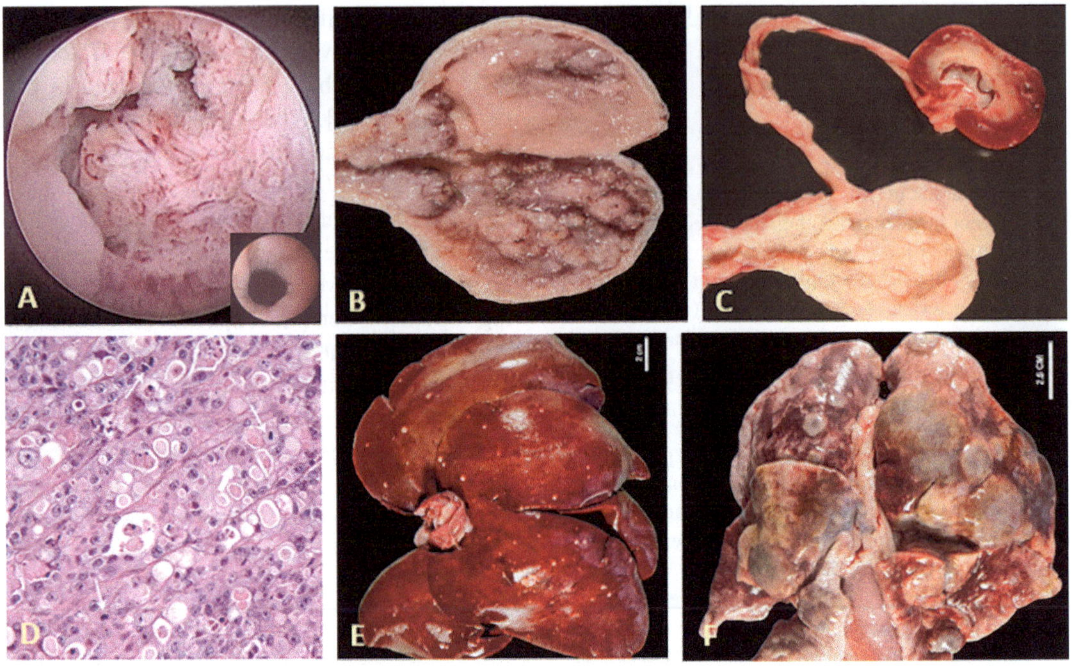

Fig. 2 Canine invasive urothelial carcinoma (InvUC). Canine InvUC often produces papillary lesions extending into the lumen of the urethra (as seen in the cystoscopic image in **a**) and bladder (as seen on post mortem specimen in **b**, and **c**), along with deep invasion into the bladder wall. For comparison, in **a**, the inset demonstrates the normal appearance of the urethra in the absence of cancer. In **c**, note the infiltration of the cancer into the ureter and hydronephrosis of the right kidney resulting from ureteral obstruction. Hydronephrosis was also present in the left kidney (not shown). The photomicrograph in **d** (H&E 40X) is typical of high-grade InvUC. There is lack of normal cell maturation and marked nuclear atypia with some binucleated and multinucleated cells, and mitotic figures. Note the presence of cytoplasmic vacuoles within neoplastic cells, a common but not unique finding to InvUC. Canine InvUC is locally aggressive and metastasizes to distant sites in more than 50% of cases. Note metastases to the liver (**e**) and lung (**f**). The gross appearance of metastases varies from single to multiple nodules that can become confluent as observed in the lung (**f**). (Photos courtesy of J. Ramos-Vara, Purdue University)

9% of dogs, distant metastases alone were identified in 25% of dogs, and a combination of nodal and distant metastases was found in 33% of the dogs. The frequency of metastasis and the sites involved were similar between dogs and humans (Table 4) with lung and liver being common sites of distant metastasis in both species [151, 315]. In a series of 12 dogs with cutaneous InvUC metastases, gross lesions consisted of plaques, papules, and nodules [255]. Bone metastases represent another important metastatic site in dogs and humans [42, 200, 333]. To assess the frequency of bone metastases in dogs, 188 dogs with InvUC undergoing necropsy were retrospectively studied [42], and 17 dogs (9%) had histologically confirmed skeletal metastasis, mainly to the vertebrae. This was followed by a prospective study of 21 dogs with InvUC that underwent total body CT at the time of euthanasia, followed by a standardized pathologic examination [42]. In four dogs, skeletal lesions suspicious for bone metastases were detected on CT, and were confirmed to be InvUC metastases histologically in three (14%) dogs. Interestingly, in another report of 65 dogs with InvUC that had whole body computed tomography (CT) performed at diagnosis, iliosacral lymphadenomegaly, sternal lymphadenomegaly, bone metastasis, and lung metastasis were suspected in 48%, 18%, 25%, and 35% of the dogs, respectively [130]. These rates of metastases at diagnosis appear higher than those reported in other studies [153]. In addition to visceral and nodal metastasis, InvUC also spreads to the abdominal wall through spread on instru-

Table 3 TNM staging system for canine bladder cancer [236]

T—primary tumor	
T_{is} (CIS)	Carcinoma in situ
T_0	No evidence of a primary tumor
T_1	Superficial papillary tumor
T_2	Tumor invading the bladder wall, with induration
T_3	Tumor invading neighboring organs (prostate, uterus, vagina, and pelvic canal)
N—Regional lymph node (internal and external iliac lymph node)	
N_0	No regional lymph node involvement
N_1	Regional lymph node involved
N_2	Regional lymph node and juxtaregional lymph node involved
M—Distant metastases	
M_0	No evidence of metastasis
M_1	Distant metastasis present

Table 4 Sites of metastases identified in 137 dogs with invasive urothelial carcinoma undergoing necropsy at Purdue University between 2005 and 2013 with comparison to published autopsy findings from humans [151, 315]

Location of metastases	Number of dogs with metastases in that location (% of 137 dogs undergoing necropsy)	Number of humans with metastases in that location (% of 308 humans undergoing autopsy)
Any metastases	92 (67%)	214 (69%)
Any nodal metastases	57 (42%)	180 (58%)
Regional nodes (abdominal, pelvic inguinal nodes)[a]	40 (29%)	158 (51%)
Thoracic nodes[b]	17 (12%)	80 (26%)
Other nodes	1 (1%)	8 (3%)
Any distant metastases	80 (58%)	147 (48%)
Lung	69 (50%)	96 (31%)
Bone	15 (11%)	71 (23%)
Liver	10 (7%)	103 (33%)
Kidney[c]	10 (7%)	30 (10%)
Adrenal gland	8 (6%)	28 (10%)
Skin	8 (6%)	4 (1.5%)
Spleen	6 (4%)	11 (3.6%)
Gastrointestinal[d]	3 (2%)	45 (15%)
Heart	5 (4%)	13 (4%)
Brain	2 (1.5%)	8 (2.5%)

[a]Nodes included 32 iliac, sacral, and other "sub lumbar," 3 inguinal, 2 mesenteric, 2 pancreatic, and 1 hypogastric node in dogs

[b]Nodes included 9 tracheobronchial, 4 sternal, 3 mediastinal, and 1 hilar node in dogs

[c]It was not always possible to determine if the InvUC represented a second primary site in the kidney or a metastatic lesion

[d]Tumor location included stomach in 1 dog, jejunum in 1 dog, and pancreas in 1 dog

ments and needles used in surgical and nonsurgical procedures, and through natural spread along ligaments that support the bladder [122, 126, 201, 310]. Once detected in the abdominal wall, the cancer typically grows aggressively and responds poorly to medical therapy [122, 201].

An additional interesting finding from the necropsy study in 137 dogs with InvUC was the presence of a second primary tumor in 18 dogs (13%). The second primary tumors included hemangiosarcoma (3), marginal zone lymphoma (3), hepatocholangiocarcinoma (2), follicular thyroid carcinoma (2), B-cell lymphoma (2), and 1 each of the following: adrenal adenocarcinoma, meningioma, nasal adenocarcinoma, cutaneous squamous cell carcinoma, oral melanoma, pancreatic adenocarcinoma, undifferentiated neuroendocrine tumor, histiocytic sarcoma, and splenic sarcoma [151]. In an autopsy study of 376 humans with InvUC, second primary tumors were found in 20% of the patients with most being carcinomas arising from other primary sites [315].

The majority of InvUCs in dogs are found in the trigone region of the bladder, and extension into the urethra occurs in >50% of cases [151]. The trigonal location in dogs is in contrast to human InvUC in which the cancer is located fairly evenly over different parts of the bladder. In male dogs, 29% of InvUC cases have been reported to have prostatic involvement based on evidence from imaging studies or pathology [151]. Primary urothelial carcinoma of the prostatic urethra and ducts, in the absence of bladder disease, is not uncommon in dogs. The possible effects of the common practice of neutering male pet dogs, especially when <6 months of age, on the development of UC of the prostatic ducts versus adenocarcinoma in the glandular tissue require further study. Renal pelvic urothelial carcinoma has been observed in dogs undergoing necropsy, but the frequency at which this occurs is unknown.

As in humans, tumor staging is very important in guiding therapy and assessing prognosis [92, 151]. Survival has been strongly associated with the TNM stage at the time of diagnosis. Factors associated with a more advanced TNM stage at diagnosis include younger age (increased risk of nodal metastasis), prostate involvement (increased risk of distant metastasis), and higher T stage (increased risk of nodal and distant metastasis) [151].

The cause of death often differs between dogs and humans with InvUC. In humans, local tumor control is accomplished through cystectomy or bladder-sparing protocols, and metastases are the usual cause of death. In dogs, cystectomy is rarely performed, and other local therapies are usually not curative. Therefore, the typical cause of death in the majority of dogs is growth of the primary tumor resulting in urinary obstruction or other issues in renal and urinary function. Regional and distant metastases do occur, however, in more than half of cases, and these can contribute to morbidity and mortality.

1.5 Molecular Features

1.5.1 Human Bladder Cancer

1.5.1.1 Chromosomes, Genes, and Pathways

In InvUC, as well as in superficial UC in humans, the loss of portions of chromosomes 9q and 9p by loss of heterozygosity is an early molecular event, although the precise mechanisms and effects of this are not well defined. Potential candidate regulatory genes in these genomic regions include *CDNK2A*, a cyclin-dependent kinase inhibitor, and *TSC1*, a gene encoding hamartin mutated in tuberous sclerosis [110]. In 2017, the analyses of the bladder cancer data in The Cancer Genome Atlas (TCGA) at that time were published [260]. This provided a comprehensive analysis of gene mutations, fusions, expression, copy number variations, methylation, and microRNA across the genome of patients with InvUC treated with surgery. Some of the main findings included (1) alterations in druggable target genes in more than 70% of the patients including *FGFR3*, *EGFR*, *ERBB2*, *ERBB3*, *PIK3CA/AKT/mTOR*, *TSC1*, and others; (2) alterations in chromatin-modifying genes such as *KMT2D*, *KDM6A*, *KMT2C*, *EP300*, and *CREBBP*, in the majority of patients; (3) hypermethylation and epigenetic silencing of gene expression in ~25% of the patients; and (4) the identification of five distinct intrinsic molecular subtypes (luminal papillary, luminal infiltrated, luminal, basal squamous, and neuronal) through RNA-sequence analyses that closely resemble luminal and basal subtypes in human breast cancers [260]. Consistent with earlier studies, the p53 cell cycle pathway was inactivated in 89% of tumors, and *TP53* mutations were identified in 48% of cases [260]. Other findings included upregulation of the CDKN2A/CDK4/CCND1 and RTK/RAS pathways. These TCGA findings have led to clinical trial designs aimed at enriching enrollment for patients with specific gene mutation profiles and further study of biomarkers related to the intrinsic molecular subtypes.

As in other cancers, mutation signatures have also been detected in InvUC. Using apolipoprotein B mRNA-editing enzyme, catalytic polypeptide (APOBEC)-mediated mutagenesis was identified as the principal mutation signature in InvUC [4, 169, 219, 260]. The activity of the APOBEC family enzymes leads to DNA editing caused by the deamination of cytidines (C) to uridines (U), which are repaired to guanines (G) or thymidines (T) [199, 219, 231, 260]. There is strong evidence for the role of *APOBEC* mutations in UC especially during the evolution from early stage to InvUC and in further tumor progression [36, 260]. In the TCGA analysis, *APOBEC3A* and *APOBEC3B* signatures were present in 67% of single-nucleotide variations (SNVs) among patients with InvUC [199, 260]. Recent work has specifically implicated *APOBEC3G* for a role in the mutagenesis and clonal evolution in bladder cancer [169].

Another feature of importance in cancer, including InvUC, is the tumor mutation burden (TMB). The TMB is quantified as the number of coding somatic mutations per megabase (MB) of DNA [332]. A higher number of mutations increases the chances of generating tumor neoantigens, which can be recognized by the host immune system as new immunogenic proteins [259, 288, 332]. In tumors with high TMB, the microenvironment is often rich in immune cells and associated cytokines [81]. It is important to note that UC is one of the cancer types with the highest mutation burden, and the TMB has been linked to positive responses with immunotherapies in InvUC [5, 21, 271].

1.5.1.2 Molecular Subtypes

Another advancement in the understanding of bladder cancer over the last several years has been the identification of tumor RNA expression patterns that segregate InvUC into molecular subtypes including basal, luminal, and others initially described in human breast cancer [48, 49, 63, 65, 89, 136, 197, 260]. Interestingly, the gene expression patterns for the basal and luminal subtypes are already present early in the cancer development process [26]. Basal tumors are enriched for STAT3, TP63, KRT5/6A, CD44, NFkB, c-Myc, and HIF signaling [48, 63, 65, 197, 260]. Luminal tumors are enriched for ER, TRIM24, FOXA1, GATA3, PPARG, and activating FGFR3 mutations (with good response to FGFR inhibitors) [48, 65, 254, 298]. Importantly, the cancer behavior and treatment responses differ between subtypes, and this information could help develop better predictors of patient outcomes and optimize the selection of the therapy for individual patients in the future [63, 136, 196]. The molecular subtypes of InvUC are defined at the highest level as luminal and basal, also referred to as "nonluminal" tumors [196, 260, 285]. When grouping InvUC at the highest level of luminal or basal, women with InvUC have a higher prevalence of basal subtype cancer, and basal tumors are inherently more aggressive. Basal InvUC is often associated with more advanced cancer within the bladder and metastases at presentation, and shorter overall survival [197, 285]. There is evidence that patients with basal tumors receive more clinical benefit from platinum-based neoadjuvant chemotherapy when compared to patients with luminal tumors [196, 275, 285]. Basal InvUC also has higher levels of immune infiltration [124, 196, 256, 275, 285], and is typically more responsive to immunotherapies than luminal tumors [197, 225]. Luminal InvUC is inherently less aggressive, and is enriched with *FGFR3* mutations that can be targeted for therapy [23, 197, 285].

Going beyond the two major subtypes, different groups have published schemes including up to six subtypes and seven tumor clusters in InvUC, with variation in the classification schemes between research groups [136]. In an attempt to reach an international consensus on the molecular subtypes in InvUC, 1750 InvUC transcriptomic profiles from 16 published datasets and two additional cohorts were examined using a network-based analysis and multivariable Cox models to examine relationships between subtypes and clinical outcomes [136]. In this consensus, six molecular classes were identified: luminal papillary (24%), luminal nonspecified (8%), luminal unstable (15%), stroma-rich (15%), basal/squamous (35%), and neuroendocrine-like (3%) [136]. These consensus classes differed in underlying oncogenic mechanisms, infiltration by stromal and immune cells, histological and clinical characteristics, and patient outcomes [136]. In this six-class consensus scheme, basal/squamous tumors were overrepresented in women ($P < 0.001$) and were associated with higher clinical stages ($P < 0.001$), similar to earlier reports [65, 136, 254, 260, 285]. Basal/squamous tumors were also associated with a poor prognosis (HRBaSq/LumP = 1.83, IC = [1.30, 2.58], $P < 0.001$), consistent with previous studies. Neuroendocrine tumors, however, were associated with the worst prognosis (HRNE-like/LumP = 2.34, IC = [1.09, 5.05], $P < 0.03$).

There is interest in exploiting information about the molecular subtypes to develop strategies to select therapies and assign prognoses in a more personalized manner, and to better understand UC development and progression.

1.5.2 Canine Bladder Cancer

1.5.2.1 Chromosomes, Genes, and Pathways

In canine InvUC, gain of dog chromosome (CFA) 13 and 36 and loss of CFA 19 are commonly found [277]. Although there is not yet a TCGA for canine bladder tumors, multiple publications have addressed the alterations in genes and pathways, and the presence of molecular subtypes in canine InvUC [60, 70, 76, 153, 161, 183, 210, 237, 276, 280, 290, 305, 312, 326]. The data from some of these studies have been deposited in the National Cancer Institute's Integrated Canine Data Commons (NCI, ICDC). The ICDC was launched in 2020 to advance research on human cancers by facilitating comparative analyses with canine cancer, including bladder cancer [225]. The ICDC contains data related to genomics, pathology, imaging, clinical features, treatment, and case outcomes for naturally occurring canine cancers, and can be mined to address new hypotheses [172]. The ICDC is well integrated with the Cancer Research Data Commons (CRDC) which contains human cancer data. This facilitates the analysis and comparison of canine and human cancer patient data within cloud-based resources.

Several reports have focused on one to a few genes of interest in canine InvUC. Some of the early work included studies of cyclooxygenese-2 (COX-2) which is overexpressed in both canine and human InvUC [38, 211, 281, 314], the apoptosis-inhibiting protein survivin which is also expressed in canine and human InvUC and has been negatively associated with prognosis [253, 278], and telomerase which has also been detected in dogs and humans with InvUC [195, 235, 320]. Other findings related to fatty acid metabolism include the expression of lipoxygenase-5 detected by immunohistochemistry and the detection of the prostaglandin EP4 receptor by RNA in situ hybridization [87, 222]. An interesting scenario in which activation of the RAF/MEK/ERK pathway drives an increase in the expression of COX-2 has also been described [334], as well as an association between the presence of the $BRAF^{V595E}$ mutation and COX-2 expression [106]. Other reports describe the expression of other genes in canine InvUC including PDGFR-β, VEGFR2, Caveolin-1, and GATA-3 [105, 276, 316].

One of the molecular features that has attracted attention because of its potential for therapeutic targeting is the epidermal growth factor receptor (EGFR, also called ERBB1 or HER-1) [44, 51, 75, 113, 131]. EGFR is overexpressed in more than 70% of canine InvUC, which is a rate comparable to that reported in humans [44, 51, 75, 113, 131]. Inhibitors of EGFR family proteins have been evaluated in multiple human bladder cancer trials with varying success [218, 245, 249, 329]. In humans, EGFR inhibitors have had the best activity in patients who have not yet received chemotherapy, and in tumors that overexpress EGFR or ERBB2 [218]. Multiple approaches to target EGFR are under investigation including EGFR targeting of a photoimmunotherapy conjugate (Can225-IR700 conjugate), an approach with promising results in canine InvUC cell lines in vitro and in rodent models [224]. In another approach, EGF conjugated to anthrax toxin promoted its own cellular uptake and induced apoptosis in low nanomolar concentrations in vitro and had good antitumor activity in mice and dogs with InvUC [131]. Near-infrared imaging of canine and human InvUC cells expressing EGFR has also been described [1].

EGFR2 (also called ERBB2 or HER-2/NEU) is also significantly overexpressed in canine InvUC samples when compared to nonneoplastic urothelium, as is the case in human InvUC [53, 59, 85, 183, 205, 270, 306]. In multiple studies, HER-2 was overexpressed in 35–60% of canine InvUC [205, 270, 306]. The drug lapatinib, which inhibits EGFR and HER2 and blocks the MAPK/ERK and the PI3K/AKT pathways, has been evaluated in dogs. Following studies of dosing, safety, and pharmacokinetics in lab dogs, pet dogs with InvUC were treated with lapatinib plus the COX inhibitor piroxicam or with piroxicam alone [184]. The dogs treated with the two drugs together were more likely to have remission and to have longer progression-free survival and overall survival than dogs treated with piroxicam alone [184].

Another gene of interest in InvUC is the *p53* tumor suppressor gene, a gene with an important role in the differentiation of the urothelium [318]. Loss of p53 expression has been associated with lymph node metastasis, advanced TNM stage, and shorter survival times in human InvUC [43, 318]. Similar to the studies in humans, the expression of p63, a homolog of p53, as well as the p63 isoform ΔNp63 has been reported to be significantly lower in InvUC in dogs when compared to polypoid cystitis and to normal urothelium [114, 229]. Expression of p53, the *p53* inducible gene 14-3-3σ protein, and vimentin has been documented in canine InvUC in vitro and in vivo [72, 294]. In human InvUC, vimentin expression has been associated with epithelial-mesenchymal transition, cancer progression, and metastasis, and in dogs a higher vimentin score was associated with shorter survival [17, 280]. Recently, a vaccination approach against extracellular vimentin in dogs with InvUC has been reported [83]. The 14-3-3σ protein, which is expressed in human and canine bladder cancer, has also been linked to tumorigenesis [158, 203].

Mutations in several other genes that have been implicated in the development and progression of InvUC and other cancers in humans have also been identified in canine InvUC, especially in next-generation sequencing studies [75, 252]. Examples include *CDKN2B*, *PIK3CA*, *BRCA2*, *NFkB*, *ARHGEF4*, *XPA*, *NCOA4*, *MDC1*, *UBR5*, *RB1CC1*, *RPS6*, *CIITA*, *MITF*, and *WT1* [24, 75, 82, 162, 196, 252, 263,317, 339]. In a study that included tumor samples from 87 dogs with InvUC, amplification and deletion of genes involved in the regulation of the cell cycle, chromatin remodeling, and mismatch repair were identified in the tumors along with driver genes such as *ARID1A*, *KDM6A*, *TP53*, *FAT1*, and *NRAS* [326]. In this study, the analyses were performed to identify differences between tumor tissues and "normal" tissues from the bladder or other organs from the same dog. With the knowledge that the mucosal field effect can lead to altered gene expression throughout the urothelium [26], it would be interesting to consider additional analyses of the data from this study with comparison to normal bladder mucosa from nontumor-bearing dogs. Interestingly, across studies, while MAPK activation is more common in canine InvUC than in human InvUC, the cancer in the two species converges into the same two major intrinsic molecular subtypes, i.e., luminal and basal [63, 70, 76, 153, 173, 210, 290].

In addition to bulk RNA-sequencing studies, the microRNAs involved in bladder cancer have also been reported [139, 309]. Kent reported significant differences in miR-103b and miR-16 in the urine between dogs with InvUC and dogs with other lower urinary tract diseases [139]. In a study by Varvil, the miRNAs that were differentially expressed between canine InvUC and normal bladder tissues were ones often associated with gene silencing by miRNA, with other miRNAs in cancer, and miRNAs involved in DNA damage responses [309]. The proteins involved included HRAS, KRAS, ARAF, RAF1, MAPK1, MAP2K1, MAPK3, FGFR3, EGFR, HBEGF, RASSF1, E2F2, E2F3, ERBB2, SRC, MMP1, and UPK3A [309].

There is an intriguing difference between canine and human InvUC. The majority (67–85%) of canine InvUCs harbor a $BRAF^{V595E}$ mutation, which is the dog homolog of the $BRAF^{V600E}$ mutation in humans [70, 96, 98, 106, 210]. A variety of methods have been reported to detect the mutation including traditional tumor sequencing, PCR-RFLP (PCR-Restriction Fragment Length Polymorphism) detection, immunohistochemistry and cytochemistry, droplet digital PCR on tumor or urine sediment, and analysis of circulating cell-free tumor DNA (cfDNA) [12, 70, 144, 210, 300, 301, 331]. Recently, an artificial intelligence approach to predict the presence of the $BRAF^{V595E}$ mutation in histologic sections was described [156]. This mutation leads to constitutive activation of the MAPK pathway and is considered a driver mutation in 8% of all human cancer across cancer types [70, 210]. While *BRAF* mutations are common in certain forms of human cancer, such as metastatic melanoma, these mutations are very uncommon in human InvUC and are largely limited to the most aggressive InvUC cases [173]. Other mutations within the MAPK pathway, however, occur in approximately 30% of human InvUC cases [260]. It is again noted that although *BRAF* mutations are common in canine InvUC and that different molecular drivers are responsible for most human InvUC, the cancer in dogs and humans still converges into the same two major intrinsic molecular subtypes [153].

Additional reports have started to address the drivers of InvUC in dogs that do not have the $BRAF^{V595E}$ mutation. In one study, RNA-sequencing analyses were performed on 15 InvUC samples, four with wild-type *BRAF* and 11 with $BRAF^{V595E}$, and five adjoining histologically normal bladder tissue samples [241]. Two expression clusters were defined by the presence or absence of the $BRAF^{V595E}$ mutation with 398 genes differentiating the two clusters. The genomic site with the highest number of dysregulated genes overall corresponded to the human chromosome 8q24, a region frequently amplified in human UC [241]. In another study of the urine sediment from 28 dogs with wild-type *BRAF*, 13 dogs (46%) had short in-frame deletions in other parts of the *BRAF* gene or mutations in *MAP2K1* exons 2 and 3, suggesting alternative MAPK-pathway-activating events [301]. In a different study, the presence of phospho Erk1/2, indicating MAPK-pathway activation, was noted in dogs in which $BRAF^{V595E}$ was not detected in the tumors [331].

1.5.2.2 Molecular Subtypes

As in human InvUC, canine InvUC can also be segregated into two major intrinsic molecular subtypes based on RNA expression patterns. The presence of luminal and basal subtypes was described in an initial group of 29 dogs [75], followed by a report of a larger group of dogs ($n = 56$) along with the clinical and pathological features associated with the subtypes [76]. Briefly, RNA-seq analyses were performed using Strand NGS, and pairwise comparisons were made between normal and InvUC samples [176, 261]. In addition to unsupervised analyses, the differentially expressed genes in the RNA-seq data were also specifically interrogated for genes used to assign canine InvUC into molecular subtypes, e.g., luminal and basal using a previously reported 60-gene prediction panel [76]. The data were also interrogated for genes used to characterize the tumor immune status [296], and other gene panels of importance in human UC [76, 137, 241, 256, 296] using the canine orthologs. The results of the study are summarized in the heatmap in Fig. 3. In this study, 29 tumors were classified as luminal and 27 tumors as basal subtype. In RNA-seq analyses, basal tumors were strongly associated with immune infiltration (OR 52.22, 95% CI 4.68–582.38, $P = 0.001$), cancer progression signatures, more advanced clinical stage, and earlier onset of distant metastases in exploratory analyses, consistent with findings in human basal InvUC. Luminal tumors were strongly associated with breeds at high risk for InvUC (OR 0.06, 95% CI 0.01–0.37, $P = 0.002$), nonimmune infiltrative signatures, and less advanced clinical stage. There was an association between the $BRAF^{V595E}$ mutation and the luminal subtype, and between wild-type *BRAF* and the basal subtype (OR 0.27 for basal tumors having $BRAF^{V595E}$, 95% CI 0.07–1.01, $P = 0.0424$).

1.5.2.3 Other Cross-Species Comparisons

Other methods have been used to compare the cellular and molecular features of canine and human InvUC. One example of this is the application of imaging mass spectrometry methods that combine chemical information collected for multiple analytes using mass spectrometry with spatial information in the analysis of histological tissue sections including InvUC. In initial work, desorption electrospray ionization (DESI) and microprobe imaging procedures were applied to tissue sections while recording mass spectra under ambient conditions [79]. Differences in lipid patterns involving glycerophospholipids, free fatty acids, and other lipid species were found between canine InvUC and normal bladder sections. After the successful proof of concept work in canine InvUC, similar methods were applied to human InvUC sections with similarities in the spectra noted between dogs and humans [80]. In follow-up studies, a newer ambient ionization MS approach, touch spray MS (TS-MS), was applied in canine tissues, and this technique rapidly identified lipid patterns that

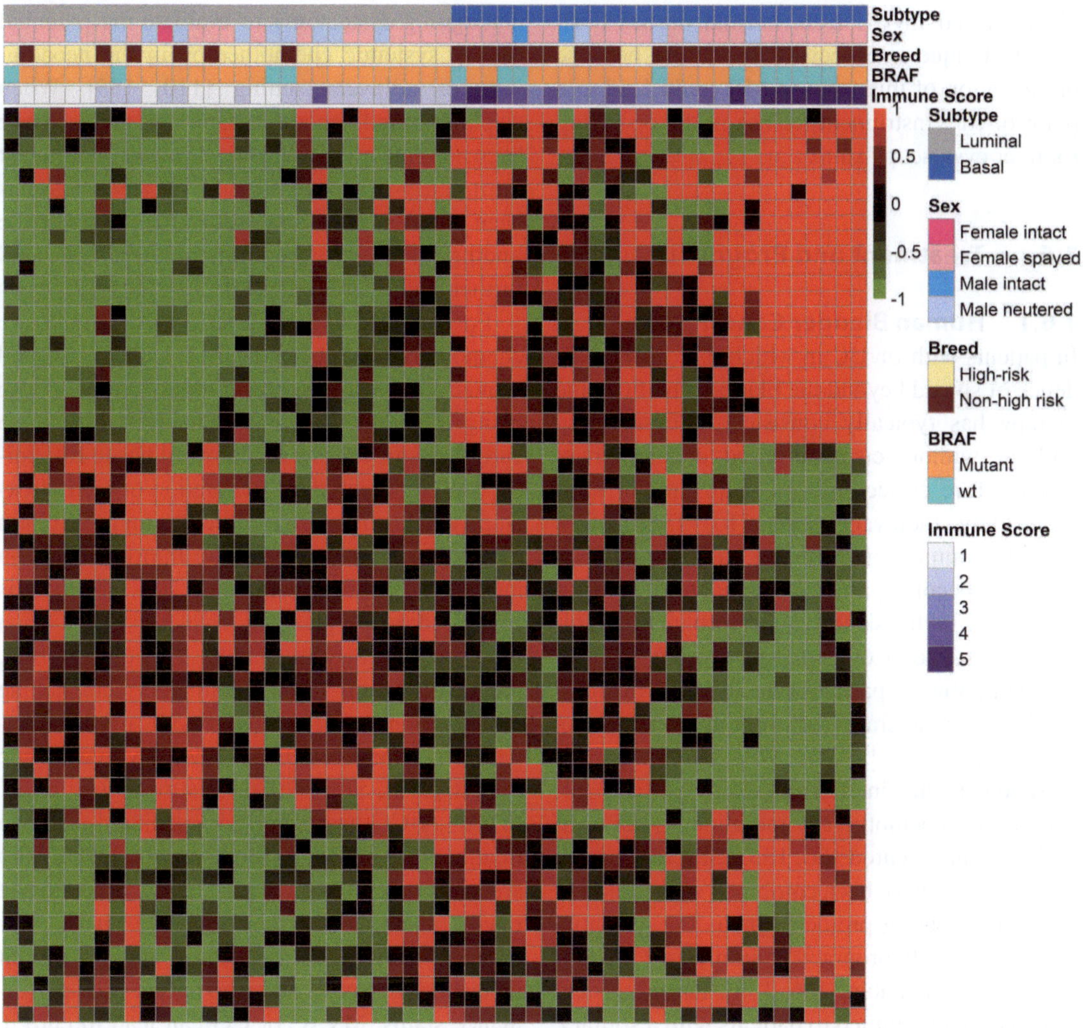

Fig. 3 Heatmap generated from canine InvUC RNA-seq analyses demonstrating the presence of luminal (n = 29 cases) and basal (n = 27 cases) subtypes. A published 60-gene class prediction model was used for subtype assignment [76]. Canine InvUC samples (n = 56) were compared to canine normal bladder mucosa samples from dogs with no evidence of bladder disease (n = 4). In the heatmap, each column represents data from one sample, and each row represents data for a specific gene. Information related to the subtype, sex, breed, *BRAF* status (mutated or not), and immune score is provided in the color bars above the heatmap. Note the segregation of tumor samples into two main groups identified as luminal and basal subtype, with multiple subgroups within each subtype. Dogs in breeds with high inherited risk for InvUC were more likely to have luminal tumors, and dogs in other breeds were more likely to have basal tumors (OR 0.06 for basal tumors in high-risk breeds, 95% CI 0.01–0.37, $P = 0.002$). Basal tumors were strongly associated with immune infiltration (OR 52.22, 95% CI 4.68–582.38, $P = 0.001$) as indicated by purple bars, with darker shades indicating higher T-cell infiltration. There was an association between the *BRAF*^{V595E} mutation and the luminal subtype, and between wild-type *BRAF* and the basal subtype (OR 0.27 for basal tumors having *BRAF*^{V595E}, 95% CI 0.07–1.01, P = 0.0424) [290]. Reprinted from Sommer BC et al. Basal and luminal molecular subtypes in naturally-occurring canine urothelial carcinoma are associated with tumor immune signatures and dog breed. Bladder Cancer 2021; 7:317–33 with permission from IOS Press. (The publication is available at IOS Press through https://doi.org/10.3233/BLC-201523)

distinguished InvUC from normal tissues [64]. This technique is especially intriguing because optimization of this form of MS could lead to a point-of-care instrument for use in the operating room or cystoscopy suite.

1.6 Treatment and Prognosis

1.6.1 Human Bladder Cancer

In patients with InvUC in which there is no evidence of spread beyond the bladder, the first-line therapy has typically consisted of cystectomy with or without cisplatin-based chemotherapy given before cystectomy (neoadjuvant) or after cystectomy (adjuvant) [99, 110, 135]. More recently, immune checkpoint inhibitors (ICIs) have also become part of the standard of care for patients at high risk for cancer progression following cystectomy or nephroureterotomy [16]. In selected patients, partial cystectomy or bladder-sparing chemotherapy-radiation approaches can also be considered [135]. With careful patient selection and maximal debulking by TURBT followed by chemotherapy-radiation, ~65% of patients can be cured [66, 135]. Several chemotherapy drugs have been combined with radiation in bladder-sparing protocols including cisplatin, carboplatin, 5-fluorouracil, mitomycin C, paclitaxel, and gemcitabine [66, 135]. Partial cystectomy is usually limited to patients with a solitary, clinical T2 tumor in the dome of the bladder.

In the majority of patients with organ-confined disease, resection of the entire bladder is pursued [99, 110]. In men, cystoprostatectomy with removal of the bladder, prostate, and pelvic lymph nodes is performed. In women, the bladder and pelvic lymph nodes are removed. Removal of the uterus, ovaries, and cervix has also been performed with cystectomy in women, although the value of this is being re-evaluated. Various urinary diversion surgical techniques are then employed. Despite this aggressive surgery, only half of the patients are cured by surgery alone [110]. In half of the patients, distant metastases emerge over a year or two following cystectomy, and sometimes later [170, 202]. Several clinical trials have been performed in patients undergoing cystectomy to evaluate the potential role of systemic chemotherapy in the neoadjuvant or adjuvant setting [110, 135]. When cisplatin-based chemotherapy protocols have been administered in the neoadjuvant or adjuvant setting, a 5–10% overall survival advantage has been noted in meta analyses [110]. Some of the findings, however, are from older reports, and further studies are indicated.

For patients with metastatic InvUC, systemic chemotherapy has been the most well-established standard of care, with immunotherapies also being included in recent years [99, 110]. One early key study was a randomized phase III clinical trial, in which the combination of methotrexate, vinblastine, doxorubicin, and cisplatin (MVAC) demonstrated an improvement in median overall survival from 8.2 to 12.5 months compared to singleagent cisplatin [171]. In a head-to-head randomized phase III clinical trial, the combination of cisplatin and gemcitabine (CG) demonstrated similar overall survival compared to MVAC with considerably fewer side effects [313]. Since 2000, treatment with either MVAC or CG has remained a standard frontline treatment for patients with metastatic InvUC who are candidates for cisplatin, based on adequate renal function and performance status. For patients with nodal metastases and no distant metastases detected, and who have a good performance status, MVAC or CG can lead to cure in 15–20% of these cases [110, 135]. Unfortunately, only ~5% of patients with metastases, however, have the cancer limited to the nodes and also have good functional status. Furthermore, approximately half of patients with InvUC have impaired renal function, significant comorbidities, or poor functional status, and are therefore not candidates for cisplatin treatment. In patients who are not eligible for cisplatin, carboplatin-based chemotherapy regimens have typically been used, but these regimens are not as effective [110].

One of the most promising advances in the treatment of metastatic InvUC is the development of ICIs, especially those that block programmed cell death protein 1 (PD-1) or programmed death ligand 1 (PD-L1) [110, 135, 272]. The ICIs have become additional standard options for patients with metastatic InvUC including frontline therapy in patients who have not yet received chemotherapy (atezolizumab, pembrolizumab), frontline maintenance therapy (avelumab), and secondline therapy in patients who have failed platinum-based chemotherapy protocols (pembrolizumab, nivolumab, and avelumab) [272]. Although these agents only result in remission (complete or partial) in 10–30% of patients, they are attractive because of better safety profiles compared to traditional chemotherapy and the prolonged length of remission in some patients. ICIs were developed to allow the reactivation of the patient's own immune system to recognize and eliminate their cancer. ICIs have unique side effects related to the release of the immune response and autoimmune consequences [272]. Serious adverse events are rare, but when they occur, they can include colitis, pneumonitis, hepatitis, nephritis, myocarditis, GuillainBarré syndrome, and idiopathic thrombocytopenic purpura. Other adverse events can include rash, hypothyroidism, and adrenal insufficiency.

Targeted agents are also showing promise in patients with InvUC. Activating mutations or fusions in tumor fibroblast growth factor 2 or 3 (FGFR2/3) are important emerging targets in InvUC therapy (reviewed in [11]). In patients that have failed platinum-based therapies, for example, the oral FGFR tyrosine kinase inhibitor erdafitinib is another option that has been associated with remission in 32% of patients with a median duration of response of 5.4 months [11]. Another targeted drug, the nectin4-targeting antibodydrug conjugate enfortumab vedotin, provides an additional option for patients with progression after both platinum-based therapy and PD-1/PD-L1 immune checkpoint therapy independent of tumor mutation status [248]. Good tumor responses have been observed in 44% of patients, including patients with liver metastases, with a median response duration of 7.6 months.

1.6.2 Canine Bladder Cancer

As in humans, the treatment of InvUC in dogs can include surgery, radiation therapy, chemotherapy and other drugs, or combinations of these, although surgery and radiation therapy are used less often than drug therapy in dogs [93, 107, 151, 289]. Partial and complete cystectomy has been described in dogs [27, 29, 69, 71, 194, 206, 257, 267, 286, 293], although in contrast to the management of human InvUC, cystectomy, especially complete cystectomy, is rarely performed in dogs. There are multiple reasons for this. Canine InvUC frequently arises in the trigone region of the bladder and extends down the urethra, and in this setting, cystectomy is unlikely to be curative. Recurrence of the primary tumor is common even following complete cystectomy [27, 257, 267, 286]. The development of distant metastases is also a lifelong risk. The morbidity and complications of the procedure are a concern for most pet owners and veterinarians, and the expense of cystectomy exceeds what most pet owners can afford [93, 151, 206, 267, 286, 289]. The fact that cystectomy is not typically performed is a plus and a minus. Leaving the primary tumor intact will lead to the continued emergence of cells with metastatic potential. In addition, because the primary InvUC mass is left in place in dogs, the placement of ureteral or urethral stents or other procedures to restore patency of the urinary tract can become necessary if urinary obstruction occurs [143, 180, 192, 274]. From a comparative oncology research perspective, however, dogs can be used to study new therapies for organ-confined disease, metastases, or both. It is also possible to obtain samples of the tumor tissue multiple times via cystoscopy over the course of therapy for parallel mechanistic studies in canine clinical trials.

Radiation therapy is also used in dogs with InvUC, although the optimal regimens and level of benefit have not yet been defined. Early attempts to treat InvUC with radiation therapy in dogs were fraught with unacceptable side effects [9], although newer radiation therapy approaches are better tolerated, allowing further study [52, 54, 189, 230].

Currently, drugs are the mainstay for the treatment of InvUC in dogs [93]. It should be noted that pet owners insist that the drug protocols be well tolerated, and anything beyond mild side effects is not considered acceptable. This means that dogs are less often treated with multi-drug or higher-dose protocols compared to people. Although InvUC is not usually curable in dogs with current therapies, the cancer can be controlled in 80% or more of dogs, and the dogs can enjoy many months to beyond a year with good quality of life [93]. Exceptional responders can live for 3 years or more.

The responses to chemotherapy for InvUC are similar between dogs and humans. Cisplatin is considered to be the most active agent in dogs, as well as in humans [99, 151]. The remission rate with single-agent cisplatin has been reported to be 12–20% in dogs and 17–34% in humans [110, 151], although the remission rate increases to 50–70% when cisplatin is combined with a COX inhibitor in dogs [148]. Cisplatin, however, is not often used in dogs because of side effects considered unacceptable to the pet owner or attending veterinarian [121, 149]. Carboplatin has activity in canine InvUC, although as is the case in humans, carboplatin appears less active than cisplatin [99, 151]. In one study, carboplatin combined with piroxicam induced partial remission in 38% of dogs. The MVAC protocol that is used in humans is not used in dogs due to unacceptable toxicities. One of the drugs, however, in this protocol, vinblastine, has emerged as the preferred chemotherapy agent in dogs with InvUC due to very good antitumor activity and a favorable safety profile [93]. As is the case with platinum therapy in dogs with InvUC, the antitumor activity of vinblastine is enhanced when it is combined with a COX inhibitor [152]. Following promising results in a single-arm vinblastine trial in dogs with advanced resistant InvUC, a follow-up trial was performed in which dogs were randomly assigned to receive vinblastine combined with the COX inhibitor piroxicam or vinblastine alone [152]. Remission (partial) occurred in 58% of dogs receiving vinblastine plus piroxicam ($n = 24$) and in 22% of dogs treated with vinblastine alone ($n = 27$) ($P < 0.02$). When cancer progression occurred in dogs receiving vinblastine alone, the pet owners were given the option to pursue treatment for their dog with piroxicam alone or other therapy off study. Interestingly, the median survival time was significantly longer ($P < 0.03$) in dogs receiving vinblastine alone followed by piroxicam alone ($n = 20$, 531 days) than in dogs treated with the two drugs given concurrently ($n = 24$, 299 days) [152]. Another chemotherapy commonly used in dogs with InvUC is mitoxantrone, although this drug is not typically used in humans with InvUC. Mitoxantrone combined with piroxicam has resulted in remission (most partial) in 35% of dogs with InvUC with a median survival time of 291 days ($n = 55$) [93, 119]. Building on these studies, the dogs with the longest survival are usually those that receive more than one treatment protocol, sequentially, over the course of their disease. Gemcitabine also has antitumor activity in dogs and in humans [99, 190, 191]. In dogs treated with gemcitabine, remission was reported in 8 of 16 and 10 of 38 dogs, respectively, in two studies [100, 190]. Although intravenous paclitaxel is not given to dogs due to severe hypersensitivity reactions to the cremophor carrier, an oral formulation of paclitaxel has been evaluated in a pilot study in dogs [40]. Other oral drugs that have been evaluated in dogs with InvUC include the targeted drugs toceranib [108, 258] and lapatinib [184], and metronomic chemotherapy [92, 273]. The activity of toceranib has been modest in studies to date with 7% of dogs having remission in one study [108], and failure to enhance the activity of vinblastine in another study [258]. Lapatinib may have more promise. In a study including 44 dogs with InvUC treated with lapatinib and piroxicam, remission was reported in 54% of the dogs [184]. Localized therapies have also been investigated including intravesical mitomycin C and photodynamic therapy (PDT), although both have been limited by toxicities [2, 179]. Of note, systemic absorption of mitomycin from the bladder occurred in two dogs in one study [2] resulting in serious bone marrow suppression and gastrointestinal toxicity.

Drugs in another class that are often administered to dogs with InvUC are the COX inhibitors, including the nonselective COX inhibitor, piroxicam, and more COX-2 selective inhibitors such as deracoxib and firocoxib [93, 151]. In 76 dogs treated with piroxicam, the tumor responses included 3% complete remission, 18% partial remission, 59% stable disease, and 20% progressive disease. The median progression-free interval was 120 days (range 17–1256 days), and the median survival time was 244 days (range 6–1256 days) [151]. This median survival time compared favorably to that of 55 dogs in the Purdue Comparative Oncology Program Tumor Registry that were treated with cytoreductive surgery alone (median survival 109 days) prior to studies to determine which drugs had activity [151]. Antitumor activity has also been observed in dogs treated with firocoxib or deracoxib, although further study is needed to determine if nonselective COX inhibitors or COX-2 inhibitors possibly have more activity than the other drugs [149, 198]. The benefit of giving COX inhibitors following partial cystectomy has also been reported [151, 194].

2 Unique Opportunities in Canine Studies

There are several areas in InvUC research in which dog studies are expected to ultimately lead to advances that can improve the outlook for human patients with InvUC. A few examples are provided here.

2.1 Cancer Prevention Research

2.1.1 Primary Cancer Prevention

Cancer prevention can be implemented at multiple levels. Primary cancer prevention refers to the prevention of even the earliest stages of cancer. Secondary cancer prevention refers to early cancer detection and early intervention, typically accomplished through screening when cancer is more responsive to intervention [78, 174]. Both primary and secondary prevention research in InvUC can be facilitated by the very high breed-associated risk for InvUC in dogs. Some of the prominent breeds include Scottish Terriers which have over a 20-fold higher risk, and West Highland White Terriers, Shetland sheepdogs, and Beagles which have a three to six fold higher risk for InvUC than dogs in other breeds [151]. As discussed in further detail below, a bladder cancer screening study in a cohort of Scottish Terriers confirmed the benefit of secondary prevention, with early detection and intervention improving the dogs' outcomes [78].

To develop primary prevention strategies, it is essential to understand the risk factors for InvUC, especially modifiable risks. While exposure to tobacco and carcinogens in the workplace has been well documented as risks for InvUC in humans, approximately half of patients with InvUC have no known risk factors, and thus, it is important to continue to determine other factors involved. In work related to environmental risk factors, it is expected that dog studies can reveal previously unknown environmental risks that could contribute to InvUC development in humans, and to do so in a timely manner. The latency period between chemical exposure and InvUC development can be as short as a year in dogs (range 1–10 years) [233], whereas latency periods in humans can extend to several decades [28, 268]. It is expected that dogs could have a role as sentinels for environmental exposures in humans that could lead to higher InvUC risk if not addressed soon enough. Dogs have already been identified as sentinels for the risk of other cancers. One of the best examples is mesothelioma caused by exposure to asbestos [101, 138]. In another example, higher genotoxic changes (micronuclei in cultured peripheral blood lymphocytes) were identified in dogs living near toxic Superfund sites than in dogs living in other areas [14]. Examples of risk factors already identified in dogs with InvUC that warrant further study in humans include exposure to marshes, wetlands, and air and water pollutants.

2.1.2 Secondary Cancer Prevention

Secondary cancer prevention in the form of early detection and early intervention is expected to save countless numbers of lives. One of the best examples of this in humans is the implementation of colonoscopy for the detection of colonic polyps and adenomas before these could progress to cancer, and to detect early cancer before it has spread. Detection allows early surgery to remove the lesions before they can progress and spread. Colorectal cancer screening has been reported to reduce the overall incidence of the cancer by 69% and mortality from the cancer by 68% [321]. Early detection and early intervention research in human bladder cancer, however, has been held back because groups of people with known high risk for the cancer are limited, with the exception being current and former smokers and potentially those with a family risk. Early detection and early prevention research in dogs, however, is quite feasible because of the very high breed-associated risk for InvUC. The expectation is that valuable information can be learned from the dogs that can be applied in humans as high-risk cohorts in humans are defined. It is also important to note that with the compressed life span in dogs compared to humans, a physiological period of 15–20 years in humans could be studied in 2–3 years in dogs [151]. As this field develops, timely dog studies could be conducted to select the most promising strategies to carry forward into the much more lengthy and costly human trials.

The strongest evidence for the value of early detection and early intervention for InvUC in dogs comes from a recent cohort study in Scottish Terriers [78]. Briefly, 120 Scottish Terriers that were at least 6 years old and that had no outward evidence of urinary disease were enrolled. The dogs were screened for bladder cancer at 6-month intervals for 3 years by physical exam with digital rectal exam, urinary tract ultrasonography, and urinalysis with sediment exam. When positive screening tests occurred, cystoscopy with biopsy was performed to make a definitive diagnosis. The pathological, clinical, and molecular characteristics of the "early" cancer detected through screening were assessed. The transcriptomic signatures were compared between the "early" cancer and published findings in human InvUC and to more advanced "later" cancer from Scottish Terriers who had the typical clinical presentation of hematuria and urinary dysfunction. For dogs with early cancer, the dog owners were offered the option for the dogs to participate in the early intervention trial of an oral COX inhibitor, deracoxib, or to receive other therapy off study.

Biopsy-confirmed UC in the absence of clinical signs was detected in 32 (27%) of the 120 Scottish Terriers including InvUC ($n = 29$, with three that started as dysplasia), grade 1 noninvasive cancer ($n = 2$), and carcinoma in situ ($n = 1$) [78]. Another feature discovered in the study was a nonprogressive nodule in the bladder apex in seven dogs that appears to represent an anatomic variant in the breed [118]. The transcriptomic analyses in the early tumors included the finding of several pathways of importance in human bladder cancer. These included MAPK, Notch, PI3K-AKT-mTOR, EGF / EGFR, TP53, MYC, and E2F targets; G2M checkpoint; apoptosis pathways; DNA repair including Base Excision Repair; and Kinetochore Metaphase Signaling [78]. Of note, druggable targets were found including EGFR and the PI3K-AKT-mTOR pathway, that were very similar between canine and human InvUC, especially within the context of molecular subtypes.

As anticipated, there were marked transcriptomic differences between the early and later canine tumors, especially within luminal subtype tumors [78]. The basal subtype tumors had numerous gene and pathway aberrations even from the early stages of detection, while the luminal tumors were much less advanced at the molecular level when detected early. This would indicate that luminal tumors detected early should be especially more sensitive to therapy. This was in line with the results of the intervention part of the study. The remission rate with deracoxib (42% CR + PR) compared very favorably to that with single-agent COX inhibitor use in more advanced canine InvUC (17–25%). The median progression-free interval (304 days) and overall survival (615 days) when the InvUC was found by screening also compared favorably to those in dogs that presented later with the more advanced tumors (101–133 days and 146–323 days, respectively) across multiple studies, but these were considered secondary endpoints as they could be affected by lead-time bias [57].

In humans, there are a variety of molecular tests performed on urine that have been investigated for a role in detection and disease monitoring. These include cancer-associated chromosomal changes assessed by fluorescent in situ hybridization, changes in the levels of nuclear mitotic proteins, the presence of bladder tumor-associated antigens, and higher levels of various immunocytochemical markers on cells shed into the urine [110]. Because these tests can all lead to false-negative and false-positive results, the potential role of these tests in humans is thought to be limited to the detection of cancer recurrence in patients that have been rendered free of cancer such as by cystectomy. Findings consistent with this were observed in the Scottish Terriers in the early detection–early intervention study in which two molecular-based urine tests were evaluated. The first test was a commercial Veterinary Bladder Tumor Antigen test (V-BTA, PolyMedco Inc. Seattle, Washington) [120] which was performed on 434 urine samples from 118 dogs. As is the case with more advanced InvUC, false positives were common, limiting the utility of the test [78]. The second test focused on the detection of the $BRAF^{V595E}$ mutation in the urine by droplet digital PCR, and this test was run on 383 urine sediment samples from 117 dogs. The $BRAF^{V595E}$ mutation was found in the majority of dogs with high-grade cancer, in 4 of 5 dogs with lower grade cancer, in 2 of 3 dogs with dysplasia, and in 3 dogs that later developed InvUC [78]. Unexpectedly, the mutation was also detected in the urine of dogs that did not have cancer and that did not develop detectable cancer over a median follow-up period of 18 months [78]. This finding is in line with molecular tests in human bladder cancer [110]. While these findings place limitations on the value of applying these tests in InvUC detection in dogs, the findings open up important avenues to understanding key aspects of cancer biology such as why the *BRAF* mutation, which is a somatic mutation, occurs, and what other factors determine if individuals with the mutation will develop cancer or not. This could have important implications for humans with *BRAF*-driven cancer across cancer types.

2.2 Understanding Cancer Biology in InvUC

Dogs offer many opportunities to study the biology of InvUC. With the primary tumor intact, cystoscopy and cancer biopsy can be performed multiple times in the cancer development process and over the course of treatment. As an example, in a clinical trial of the *BRAF* inhibitor vemurafenib, tumor samples were collected prior to treatment, 1 month into treatment, and at the time of cancer progression [264]. As expected, the upregulation of genes in the classical and alternative MAPK-related pathways in the cancer was noted in subsets of dogs at the time of cancer progression. A more interesting finding was that the most consistent transcriptomic changes observed were an increase in patterns of T lymphocyte infiltration during the first month of vemurafenib and patterns of immune failure at the time of cancer progression, suggesting the immunologic effects of the drug are crucial in positive and negative tumor responses [264]. In addition to collecting biopsies during cystoscopy, the majority of pet owners, when requested, will permit a necropsy of their dog when the dog dies, and this allows the collection of tissue samples from multiple parts of the primary tumor and multiple sites of metastases for mechanism studies [151].

Another area of increasing awareness and research in the biology of bladder cancer is the effects of the commensal urinary microbiome on InvUC development and response to therapy, especially related to therapies that work at least in part through immunomodulatory effects [10]. The microbiome is defined as the collection of microbes, their products, and their surrounding environment. There is convincing evidence that has discredited the long-held view that the urine and bladder are sterile in healthy individuals [10, 33, 34, 56, 62, 166, 325]. Better culture techniques, 16S ribosomal RNA (rRNA) sequencing studies, and whole-genome shotgun sequencing analyses have demonstrated the presence of a commensal urinary microbiome with bacteria that are not routinely cultivated by clinical microbiology laboratories [3, 10, 123, 335]. It is clear that there is a microbiome in the bladder wall and in the urine, and that these differ between normal people and patients with InvUC. Studies have revealed an increased abundance of Acinetobacter, Anaerococcus, Fusobacterium, Campylobacter, and others in the urine of bladder cancer patients [32–34, 134, 328]. Sex-related differences in the microbiome between men and women with bladder cancer have also been reported [25]. Details related to how the microbiome affects InvUC development are not yet defined, but one possibility is how certain organisms affect the metabolism of carcinogens like polycyclic aromatic hydrocarbons (PAHs). Microbes that degrade PAHs, such as Acinetobacter, Micrococcus, and Pseudomonas, could be linked to bladder cancer development through potent PAH intermediates formed by the bacteria [33, 34, 134]. The presence of Lactobacillus has been linked to reduced risk for bladder cancer, although differences in in vitro versus in vivo studies exist [193]. In addition to the urinary microbiome, the gut microbiome may also have a role in InvUC development, but research in this area related to bladder cancer is in the beginning stages [134]. In other cancers, there is concern that the gut microbiome can have a substantial effect on the efficacy of immunotherapies, including those targeting PD-1 [10].

There is also interest in the study of the microbiome in canine InvUC. In a pilot study, the urine and fecal microbiota of dogs with UC were compared to that of matched healthy controls [221]. Dogs with InvUC had a significant reduction in microbial diversity ($P = 0.048$) and altered microbial composition (PERMANOVA: Unweighted UniFrac, $P = 0.011$) in urine, but not in fecal samples. The relative abundance of Fusobacterium was increased, although not significantly, in urine and fecal samples of dogs with InvUC [221]. The canine and human urine microbiota were compared, and additional similarities between the species were noted in the dominant microbial taxa [221].

2.3 Therapy Trials

An initial point to make related to therapy trials is that clinical trials in dogs are feasible, and they are considered to be a "win–win–win" scenario [151, 161]. The expectation is that each individual dog will potentially benefit from a new treatment made available to them in the trial, and that the findings from the study will help other dogs and will ultimately be of benefit to humans with InvUC. Clinical trials are also typically subsidized, making them a source of "hope" for pet owners who are financially limited and cannot afford other therapies. In addition to clinical endpoints, parallel studies of drug mechanisms and cancer biology are feasible in dogs. Some of the key areas for scientific rigor in trials of dogs with InvUC include an accurate diagnosis, i.e., histopathology; complete tumor staging; a well-defined treatment protocol; and careful monitoring of tumor response with a standardized imaging protocol at set intervals [93]. The investigator designing trials should give careful consideration to whether to allow COX inhibitors or not in a trial, and to be consistent across cases throughout the trial as COX inhibitors will enhance the antitumor activity of other therapies [153].

It is encouraging that there are multiple studies reported in the literature of drugs tested in dogs in which the findings have implications for human InvUC, and a few examples are summarized here.

2.3.1 Demethylating Agents

The role of epigenetic events in cancer development and progression has become widely recognized including aberrant methylation in the promoter region of tumor suppressor genes, resulting in silencing of the genes [18, 302]. A key enzyme in DNA methylation (DNMT1) is overexpressed in human and canine InvUC [74], and this has been associated with more aggressive cancer in humans. Canine studies were undertaken to help determine the level of effectiveness, safety, and treatment schedule of a demethylating agent prior to human trials. Briefly, the demethylating agent, 5-azacitidine (5-AzaC) in dogs with InvUC was evaluated in which doses were escalated in two different dose schedules (daily treatment for 5 days once per month, or daily treatment for 5 days twice per month) [111]. The safety, pharmacokinetics, antitumor activity, and effects on epigenetic targets were assessed [111]. Of 18 dogs evaluable for tumor response, partial remission, stable disease, and progressive disease were observed in 4 (22.2%), 9 (50.0%), and 4 (22.2%) dogs, respectively, and consistent 5-AzaC concentrations (205–857 ng/mL) were detected in urine [111]. This study demonstrated promising activity of a demethylating agent in dogs with InvUC, justifying the continued study of this treatment approach to apply in human InvUC.

2.3.2 Cyclooxygenase (COX) Inhibitors

An example of an older class of drugs being repurposed in the cancer field is the COX inhibitors. An early unexpected discovery was made in dogs with other cancers and then in dogs with InvUC [146, 151]. Briefly, dramatic remission was documented of a poorly differentiated sarcoma of the thoracic wall in a dog receiving the nonselective COX inhibitor, piroxicam, alone and no other drugs [151]. Complete remission confirmed at necropsy also occurred in a dog with advanced metastatic carcinoma of unknown primary when the dog was receiving piroxicam alone [151]. These initial observations led to phase I, II, and III clinical trials of COX inhibitors in dogs which confirmed the antitumor effects and defined a safe dose range of the drug [146–148]. In 76 dogs with InvUC treated with single-agent piroxicam, tumor responses included two (3%) complete remission, 14 (18%) partial remission, 45 (59%) stable disease, and 15 (20%) progressive disease [151]. With the results of these trials and others [6, 54, 149, 152, 198], COX inhibitors are part of the standard of care for InvUC in dogs.

Antitumor effects of COX inhibitors have also been observed in experimentally induced bladder tumors in rodents [177, 214, 228, 330]. It would be expected that COX inhibitors would also have beneficial effects in human InvUC, and there is support for this in the limited studies to date. In a neoadjuvant trial of celecoxib in patients with InvUC, the biological effects associated with COX inhibitor-induced remission in dogs (e.g., induction of apoptosis) were found to occur to the same degree in humans with InvUC receiving celecoxib which was prescribed between initial diagnosis and cystectomy [73, 212, 213]. No residual invasive cancer was identified in 3 of 13 patients at the time of cystectomy (post celecoxib). Of the remaining ten patients, seven had induction of apoptosis in the tumor, demonstrating a similar biological effect to that observed in dogs with InvUC. Reduction in VEGF was also significantly more frequent in patients receiving celecoxib (four of nine patients) than in untreated patients (0 of 11) ($P < 0.027$). In further analyses of the tumor samples from this trial, the number of tumor-infiltrating lymphocytes (TILs) increased multifold in 73% of patients receiving celecoxib, compared to 38% of control cases. COX inhibitors have also reduced the recurrence of superficial bladder tumors in humans in some, but not all studies [242, 266]. In another study, aspirin use at least three times per week was associated with increased survival among human bladder cancer patients [175], and aspirin use was associated with lower cancer-specific mortality specifically in patients that had undergone radical cystectomy [181]. Further studies of the effects of COX inhibitors in InvUC treatment are indicated.

2.3.3 Targeted Therapies

There are examples of targeted therapies that have been tested in dogs with InvUC with the goal to not only help dogs, but to generate new information that could be incorporated into new therapy strategies for humans with InvUC. One type of targeted therapy that has been tested in dogs with InvUC is folate-targeted therapy, or more specifically drug-folate conjugates that are taken up by the high-affinity folate receptor alpha [297, 77]. Briefly, folate receptor alpha expression has been identified in 78% of canine InvUC tissues as well as in a subset of human InvUC. Folate uptake in the tumors has been confirmed in vivo by scintigraphy studies in dogs. Two folate-targeted drugs were tested in dogs with InvUC including folate-vinblastine (EC0905) and folate-tubulysin (EC0531) [297, 77]. While both had good activity, folate-tubulysin has the advantage of not being a substrate for the P-glycoprotein drug efflux pump. These studies suggest a potential role of folate-targeted therapy in human InvUC.

In another targeted therapy approach, EGF was conjugated to anthrax toxin (EGF-toxin). This unique agent was developed to overcome some of the limitations of other EGF-based technologies and other toxin derivatives [131]. One advantage was the EGF-toxin conjugate promoted its own uptake via receptor microclustering, and this occurred even in the presence of HER2 expression. In vitro, the EGF-toxin induced cell death with a $LC_{50} < 1$ nM in a short time frame, taking ~3 minutes to commit human, mouse, and canine bladder cancer cells to undergo apoptosis [131]. The EGF-toxin was administered intravesically to dogs with InvUC that expressed EGFR with the treatment given daily for up to five days (1 hour dwell time). The EGF-toxin was well tolerated, and up to 30% regression in the tumor masses was observed [131]. EGFR-targeted therapies in the form of small-molecule inhibitors, monoclonal antibodies, and drug conjugates continue to be of strong interest in human InvUC [45].

2.3.4 Immunotherapy

Immunotherapy has been labeled the "fourth pillar of cancer therapy" after surgery, radiation therapy, and chemotherapy [128]. The medical oncology community has witnessed impressive remissions in patients with advanced chemotherapy-refractory cancer, especially in studies of immune checkpoint blockade, i.e., ICIs [20, 21, 112, 142, 239]. Immune checkpoints such as PD-L1, PD-1, CTLA-4, and B7x are regulatory components of the immune system. These are essential for maintaining self-tolerance and dampening the physiological immune responses in peripheral tissues at the appropriate time to minimize collateral tissue damage from the immune attack on microbes and other targets [239]. Cancer, however, exploits these immune checkpoints to evade immune attack [239]. In patients with InvUC, PD-1/PD-L1 blockade therapy has induced complete and durable remissions, but unfortunately, this only occurs in 10–30% of patients. Thus, while there is clear promise for ICIs, research to improve the success rate of these agents is crucial.

With their shared cancer features and their level of immunocompetence mirroring that of human cancer patients, dogs with naturally occurring cancer are an attractive animal model for research to improve immunotherapies in humans. There are multiple reports of the expression of immune checkpoints in InvUC and other cancers in dogs [7, 41, 86, 115, 116, 185, 186, 226, 247, 282, 299], and the scientific community is eagerly waiting to test ICIs in cancer-bearing dogs pending further access to these drugs. Because human ICIs are monoclonal antibodies developed specifically for people, they are not suitable for dogs. Although the availability of ICIs for dogs is limited as of the writing of this chapter, there are emerging drugs in this class that are expected to impact immunotherapy research in dogs. There are reports of canine PD-L1 (cPD-L1) antibodies developed by academic laboratories [129, 185–187, 226, 232]. In one report, a canine chimeric PD-L1 antibody was developed which had excellent activity in binding and blocking PD-L1 and enhancing cytotoxic T cell killing of tumor cell targets in vitro, and strong antitumor activity in a syngeneic mouse bladder tumor system [232]. This antibody was also found to have a good safety profile in laboratory dogs, and clinical trials in pet dogs are ongoing [232]. Another chimera antibody to canine PD-L1 has been developed and tested in pet dogs with naturally occurring oral melanoma and soft tissue sarcomas, and tumor regression was reported in two dogs [186]. In other work, anti-canine PD-1 and PD-L1 antibodies were developed for diagnostic applications, although the therapeutic use of these has not been reported [50].

Another form of immunotherapy gaining attention consists of chimeric antigen receptor T cells (CAR T cells) in which T lymphocytes are engineered to express a specific chimeric antigen receptor [104, 238]. CAR T cell therapy has been successfully developed and administered to dogs with naturally occurring lymphoma [238].

3 Conclusions

In conclusion, there is strong evidence that dogs with naturally occurring InvUC can provide a highly relevant animal model to complement experimental models of InvUC in humans. Dogs can fill a unique niche in research in the cancer biology of InvUC, early detection and early intervention strategies, therapies including repurposed drugs and new drugs, and opportunities to individualize and personalize the management of the cancer.

References

1. Aayush A, Darji S, Dhawan D, Enstrom A, Broman MM, Idrees MT et al (2022) Targeted elastin-like polypeptide fusion protein for near-infrared imaging of human and canine urothelial carcinoma. Oncotarget 13:1004–1016
2. Abbo AH, Jones DR, Masters AR, Stewart JC, Fourez L, Knapp DW (2010) Phase I clinical trial and pharmacokinetics of intravesical mitomycin C in dogs with localized transitional cell carcinoma of the urinary bladder. J Vet Intern Med 24(5):1124–1130
3. Akram A, Maley M, Gosbell I, Nguyen T, Chavada R (2017) Utility of 16S rRNA PCR performed on clinical specimens in patient management. Int J Infect Dis 57:144–149
4. Al-Ahmadie H, Iyer G (2018) Updates on the genetics and molecular subtypes of urothelial carcinoma and select variants. Surg Pathol Clin 11(4):713–723
5. Alexandrov LB, Nik-Zainal S, Wedge DC, Aparicio SAJR, Behjati S, Biankin AV et al (2013) Signatures of mutational processes in human cancer. Nature 500(7463):415–421
6. Allstadt SD, Rodriguez CO, Boostrom B, Rebhun RB, Skorupski KA (2015) Randomized phase III trial of piroxicam in combination with mitoxantrone or carboplatin for first-line treatment of urogenital tract transitional cell carcinoma in dogs. J Vet Intern Med 29(1):261–267
7. Ambrosius LA, Dhawan D, Ramos-Vara JA, Ruple A, Knapp DW, Childress MO (2018) Quantification and prognostic value of programmed cell death ligand-1 expression in dogs with diffuse large B-cell lymphoma. Am J Vet Res 79(6):643–649
8. Amores-Fuster I, Elliott JW, Freeman AI, Blackwood L (2011) Histiocytic sarcoma of the urinary bladder in a dog. J Small Anim Pract 52(12):665
9. Anderson CR, McNiel EA, Gillette EL, Powers BE, LaRue SM (2002) Late complications of pelvic irradiation in 16 dogs. Vet Radiol Ultrasound 43(2):187–192
10. Andolfi C, Bloodworth JC, Papachristos A, Sweis RF (2020) The urinary microbiome and bladder cancer: susceptibility and immune responsiveness. Bladder Cancer 6(3):225–235
11. Ascione CM, Napolitano F, Esposito D, Servetto A, Belli S, Santaniello A et al (2023) Role of FGFR3 in bladder cancer: Treatment landscape and future challenges. Cancer Treat Rev 115:102530
12. Aupperle-Lellbach H, Grassinger J, Hohloch C, Kehl A, Pantke P (2018) Diagnostic value of the BRAF variant V595E in urine samples, smears and biopsies from canine transitional cell carcinoma. Tierarztl Prax Ausg K Kleintiere Heimtiere 46(5):289–295
13. Autorino R, Di Lorenzo G, Damiano R, Giannarini G, De Sio M, Cheng L et al (2009) Pathology of the prostate in radical cystectomy specimens: a critical review. Surg Oncol 18(1):73–84
14. Backer LC, Grindem CB, Corbett WT, Cullins L, Hunter JL (2001) Pet dogs as sentinels for environmental contamination. Sci Total Environ 274(1–3):161–169
15. Bae IH, Kim Y, Pakhrin B, You MH, Hwang CY, Kim JH et al (2007) Genitourinary rhabdomyosarcoma with systemic metastasis in a young dog. Vet Pathol 44(4):518–520
16. Bajorin DF, Witjes JA, Gschwend JE, Schenker M, Valderrama BP, Tomita Y et al (2021) Adjuvant nivolumab versus placebo in muscle-invasive urothelial carcinoma. N Engl J Med 384(22):2102–2114
17. Baumgart E, Cohen MS, Silva Neto B, Jacobs MA, Wotkowicz C, Rieger-Christ KM et al (2007) Identification and prognostic significance of an epithelial-mesenchymal transition expression profile in human bladder tumors. Clin Cancer Res 13(6):1685–1694
18. Baylin SB, Jones PA (2011) A decade of exploring the cancer epigenome – biological and translational implications. Nat Rev Cancer 11(10):726–734
19. Bayne CE, Farah D, Herbst KW, Hsieh MH (2018) Role of urinary tract infection in bladder cancer: a systematic review and meta-analysis. World J Urol 36(8):1181–1190
20. Bellmunt J, Powles T, Vogelzang NJ (2017) A review on the evolution of PD-1/PD-L1 immunotherapy for bladder cancer: The future is now. Cancer Treat Rev 54:58–67
21. Bellmunt J, de Wit R, Fradet Y, Climent M, Petrylak D, Lee J-L, Fong L, Necchi A, Sternberg C, Grivas P et al (2020) 747P Association of TMB with efficacy of pembrolizumab (pembro) in patients (pts) with advanced urothelial cancer (UC): Results from KEYNOTE-045 and KEYNOTE-052. Ann Oncol 31:S580–S581. https://doi.org/10.1016/j.annonc.2020.08.819
22. Benowitz N, Goniewicz ML, Eisner MD, Lazcano-Ponce E, Zielinska-Danch W, Koszowski B et al (2010) Urine cotinine underestimates exposure to the tobacco-derived lung carcinogen 4-(methylnitrosamino)-1-(3-pyridyl)-1-butanone in passive compared with active smokers. Cancer Epidemiol Biomarkers Prev 19(11):2795–2800
23. Bernardo C, Eriksson P, Marzouka NAD, Liedberg F, Sjödahl G, Höglund M (2019) Molecular pathol-

ogy of the luminal class of urothelial tumors. J Pathol 249(3):308–318
24. Bilgrami SM, Qureshi SA, Pervez S, Abbas F (2014) Promoter hypermethylation of tumor suppressor genes correlates with tumor grade and invasiveness in patients with urothelial bladder cancer. Springerplus 3:178
25. Bilski K, Dobruch J, Kozikowski M, Skrzypczyk MA, Oszczudłowski M, Ostrowski J (2020) Urobiome in gender-related diversities of bladder cancer. Int J Mol Sci 21(12):4488
26. Bondaruk J, Jaksik R, Wang Z, Cogdell D, Lee S, Chen Y et al (2022) The origin of bladder cancer from mucosal field effects. iScience 25(7):104551
27. Boston S, Singh A (2014) Total cystectomy for treatment of transitional cell carcinoma of the urethra and bladder trigone in a dog. Vet Surg 43(3):294–300
28. Böthig R, Kowald B, Fiebag K, Balzer O, Tiburtius C, Thietje R et al (2021) Bladder management, severity of injury and period of latency: a descriptive study on 135 patients with spinal cord injury and bladder cancer. Spinal Cord 59(9):971–977
29. Bradbury ML, Mullin CM, Gillian SD, Weisse C, Bergman PJ, Morges MA et al (2021) Clinical outcomes of dogs with transitional cell carcinoma receiving medical therapy, with and without partial cystectomy. Can Vet J 62(2):133–140
30. Brambilla E, Govoni VM, Cavalca AMB, Laufer-Amorim R, Fonseca-Alves CE, Grieco V (2022) Grading systems for canine urothelial carcinoma of the bladder: a comparative overview. Animals (Basel) 12(11):1455
31. Bryan JN, Keeler MR, Henry CJ, Bryan ME, Hahn AW, Caldwell CW (2007) A population study of neutering status as a risk factor for canine prostate cancer. Prostate 67(11):1174–1181
32. Bučević Popović V, Šitum M, Chow CET, Chan LS, Roje B, Terzić J (2018) The urinary microbiome associated with bladder cancer. Sci Rep 8(1):12157
33. Bukavina L, Ginwala R, Sindhani M, Prunty M, Geynisman D, Pooja G et al (2023a) Role of gut microbiome in neoadjuvant chemotherapy response in urothelial carcinoma: a multi-institutional prospective cohort evaluation. bioRxiv. 2023.01.21.525021
34. Bukavina L, Isali I, Ginwala R, Sindhani M, Calaway A, Magee D et al (2023b) Global meta-analysis of urine microbiome: colonization of polycyclic aromatic hydrocarbon-degrading bacteria among bladder cancer patients. Eur Urol Oncol 6(2):190–203
35. Burger M, Catto JWF, Dalbagni G, Grossman HB, Herr H, Karakiewicz P et al (2013) Epidemiology and risk factors of urothelial bladder cancer. Eur Urol 63(2):234–241
36. Burns MB, Temiz NA, Harris RS (2013) Evidence for APOBEC3B mutagenesis in multiple human cancers. Nat Genet 45(9):977–983
37. Carlo MI, Ravichandran V, Srinavasan P, Bandlamudi C, Kemel Y, Ceyhan-Birsoy O et al (2020) Cancer susceptibility mutations in patients with urothelial malignancies. J Clin Oncol 38(5):406–414
38. Cekanova M, Uddin MJ, Bartges JW, Callens A, Legendre AM, Rathore K, Wright L, Carter A, Marnett LJ (2013) Molecular imaging of cyclooxygenase-2 in canine transitional cell carcinomas in vitro and in vivo. Cancer Prev Res (Phila) 6:466–476
39. Centers for Disease Control and Prevention, Tobacco and Cancer (2023). https://www.cdc.gov/cancer/tobacco/index.htm#:~:text=Smoke%20from%20cigarettes%2C%20cigars%2C%20and,all%20parts%20of%20your%20body. Accessed 07/30/23
40. Chae HK, Yang JI, An JH, Lee IH, Son MH, Song WJ et al (2020) Use of oral paclitaxel for the treatment of bladder tumors in dogs. J Vet Med Sci 82(5):527–530
41. Chand D, Dhawan D, Sankin A, Ren X, Lin J, Schoenberg M et al (2019) Immune checkpoint B7x (B7-H4/B7S1/VTCN1) is over expressed in spontaneous canine bladder cancer: the first report and its implications in a preclinical model. Bladder Cancer 5(1):63–71
42. Charney VA, Miller MA, Heng HG, Weng HY, Knapp DW (2017) Skeletal metastasis of canine urothelial carcinoma: pathologic and computed tomographic features. Vet Pathol 54(3):380–386
43. Chatterjee SJ, Datar R, Youssefzadeh D, George B, Goebell PJ, Stein JP et al (2004) Combined effects of p53, p21, and pRb expression in the progression of bladder transitional cell carcinoma. J Clin Oncol 22(6):1007–1013
44. Chaux A, Cohen JS, Schultz L, Albadine R, Jadallah S, Murphy KM et al (2012) High epidermal growth factor receptor immunohistochemical expression in urothelial carcinoma of the bladder is not associated with EGFR mutations in exons 19 and 21: a study using formalin-fixed, paraffin-embedded archival tissues. Hum Pathol 43(10):1590–1595
45. Chen D, Ye Y, Guo S, Yao K (2021) Progress in the research and targeted therapy of ErbB/HER receptors in urothelial bladder cancer. Front Mol Biosci 8:800945
46. Cheng L, MacLennan GT, Lopez-Beltran A (2012) Histologic grading of urothelial carcinoma: a reappraisal. Hum Pathol 43(12):2097–2108
47. Childress MO, Adams LG, Ramos-Vara JA, Freeman LJ, He S, Constable PD et al (2011) Results of biopsy via transurethral cystoscopy and cystotomy for diagnosis of transitional cell carcinoma of the urinary bladder and urethra in dogs: 92 cases (2003-2008). J Am Vet Med Assoc 239(3):350–356
48. Choi W, Porten S, Kim S, Willis D, Plimack ER, Hoffman-Censits J et al (2014) Identification of distinct basal and luminal subtypes of muscle-invasive bladder cancer with different sensitivities to frontline chemotherapy. Cancer Cell 25(2):152–165
49. Choi W, Ochoa A, McConkey DJ, Aine M, Höglund M, Kim WY et al (2017) Genetic alterations in the molecular subtypes of bladder cancer: illustration in The Cancer Genome Atlas Dataset. Eur Urol 72(3):354–365

50. Choi JW, Withers SS, Chang H, Spanier JA, De La Trinidad VL, Panesar H, et al (2020) Development of canine PD-1/PD-L1 specific monoclonal antibodies and amplification of canine T cell function. PLoS One 15(7):e0235518
51. Chow NH, Chan SH, Tzai TS, Ho CL, Liu HS (2001) Expression profiles of ErbB family receptors and prognosis in primary transitional cell carcinoma of the urinary bladder. Clin Cancer Res 7(7):1957–1962
52. Choy K, Fidel J (2016) Tolerability and tumor response of a novel low-dose palliative radiation therapy protocol in dogs with transitional cell carcinoma of the bladder and urethra. Vet Radiol Ultrasound 57(3):341–351
53. Cimpean AM, Tarlui V, Cumpănaş AA, Bolintineanu S, Cumpănaş A, Raica M (2017) Critical overview of HER2 assessement in bladder cancer: what is missing for a better therapeutic approach? Anticancer Res 37(9):4935–4942
54. Clerc-Renaud B, Gieger TL, LaRue SM, Nolan MW (2021) Treatment of genitourinary carcinoma in dogs using nonsteroidal anti-inflammatory drugs, mitoxantrone, and radiation therapy: A retrospective study. J Vet Intern Med 35(2):1052–1061
55. Constantin T, Păvălean M, Bucur Ştefana, Constantin MM, Nicolescu AC, Pacu I, et al. Animal models in bladder cancer. Biomedicines 2021;9(12):1762
56. Cosma CL, Sherman DR, Ramakrishnan L (2003) The secret lives of the pathogenic mycobacteria. Ann Rev Microbiol 57:641–676
57. Cox B, Sneyd MJ (2013) Bias in breast cancer research in the screening era. Breast 22(6):1041–1045
58. Craun K, Luethcke KR, Shafer M, Stanton N, Zhang C, Schauer J et al (2020) Environmental chemical exposures in the urine of dogs and people sharing the same households. J Clin Transl Sci 5(1):e54
59. Cronise KE, Hernandez BG, Gustafson DL, Duval DL (2019) Identifying the ErbB/MAPK signaling cascade as a therapeutic target in canine bladder cancer. Mol Pharmacol 96(1):36–46
60. Cronise KE, Das S, Hernandez BG, Regan DP, Dailey DD, McGeachan RI et al (2022) Characterizing the molecular and immune landscape of canine bladder cancer. Vet Comp Oncol 20(1):69–81
61. Cumberbatch MGK, Noon AP (2019) Epidemiology, aetiology and screening of bladder cancer. Transl Androl Urol 8(1):5–11
62. Curtiss N, Balachandran A, Krska L, Peppiatt-Wildman C, Wildman S, Duckett J (2018) Age, menopausal status and the bladder microbiome. Eur J Obstet Gynecol Reprod Biol 228:126–129
63. Czerniak B, Dinney C, McConkey D (2016) Origins of bladder cancer. Annu Rev Pathol 11:149–174
64. D'Hue CA, Dhawan D, Peat T, Ramos-Vara J, Jarmusch A, Knapp DW et al (2018) Fatty acid patterns detected by ambient ionization mass spectrometry in canine invasive urothelial carcinoma from dogs of different breeds. Bladder Cancer 4(3):283–291
65. Damrauer JS, Hoadley KA, Chism DD, Fan C, Tiganelli CJ, Wobker SE et al (2014) Intrinsic subtypes of high-grade bladder cancer reflect the hallmarks of breast cancer biology. Proc Natl Acad Sci USA 111(8):3110–3115
66. de Angelis M, Basile G, Scornajenghi CM, Asero V, Del Giudice F, Moschini M (2023) Bladder-sparing strategies in patients with clinically localized muscle-invasive bladder cancer. Curr Opin Urol 33(5):354–359
67. de Brot S, Robinson BD, Scase T, Grau-Roma L, Wilkinson E, Boorjian SA et al (2018) The dog as an animal model for bladder and urethral urothelial carcinoma: comparative epidemiology and histology. Oncol Lett 16(2):1641–1649
68. de Brot S, Grau-Roma L, Stirling-Stainsby C, Dettwiler M, Guscetti F, Meier D et al (2019) A Fibromyxoid Stromal response is associated with muscle invasion in canine urothelial carcinoma. J Comp Pathol 169:35–46
69. de Vlaming A, Mathews KG, Hash JA, Keenihan EK, Sommer S, Borst L et al (2022) Creation of a continent urinary bladder reservoir vascularized by omentum as a possible surgical option for canine trigonal/urethral urothelial carcinoma. J Investig Surg 35(3):481–495
70. Decker B, Parker HG, Dhawan D, Kwon EM, Karlins E, Davis BW et al (2015) Homologous mutation to human BRAF V600E is common in naturally occurring canine bladder cancer–evidence for a relevant model system and urine-based diagnostic test. Mol Cancer Res 13(6):993–1002
71. Delaune T, Bernard F, Matres-Lorenzo L, Bernardé A (2018) Radical cystectomy and subsequent uretero-hysterostomy in a bitch. Vet Surg 47(8):1106–1111
72. Dhawan D, Ramos-Vara JA, Stewart JC, Zheng R, Knapp DW (2009) Canine invasive transitional cell carcinoma cell lines: in vitro tools to complement a relevant animal model of invasive urinary bladder cancer. Urol Oncol 27(3):284–292
73. Dhawan D, Craig BA, Cheng L, Snyder PW, Mohammed SI, Stewart JC et al (2010) Effects of short-term celecoxib treatment in patients with invasive transitional cell carcinoma of the urinary bladder. Mol Cancer Ther 9(5):1371–1377
74. Dhawan D, Ramos-Vara JA, Hahn NM, Waddell J, Olbricht GR, Zheng R et al (2013) DNMT1: an emerging target in the treatment of invasive urinary bladder cancer. Urol Oncol 31(8):1761–1769
75. Dhawan D, Paoloni M, Shukradas S, Choudhury DR, Craig BA, Ramos-Vara JA et al (2015) Comparative gene expression analyses identify luminal and basal subtypes of canine invasive urothelial carcinoma that mimic patterns in human invasive bladder cancer. PLoS One 10(9):e0136688
76. Dhawan D, Hahn NM, Ramos-Vara JA, Knapp DW (2018) Naturally-occurring canine invasive urothelial carcinoma harbors luminal and basal transcriptional subtypes found in human muscle invasive bladder cancer. PLoS Genet 14(8):e1007571

77. Dhawan D, Ramos-Vara JA, Naughton JF, Cheng L, Low PS, Rothenbuhler R et al (2013) Targeting folate receptors to treat invasive urinary bladder cancer. Cancer Res 73(2):875–884
78. Dhawan D, Ramos-Vara JA, Utturkar SM, Ruple A, Tersey SA, Nelson JB et al (2022) Identification of a naturally-occurring canine model for early detection and intervention research in high grade urothelial carcinoma. Front Oncol 12:1011969
79. Dill AL, Ifa DR, Manicke NE, Costa AB, Ramos-Vara JA, Knapp DW et al (2009) Lipid profiles of canine invasive transitional cell carcinoma of the urinary bladder and adjacent normal tissue by desorption electrospray ionization imaging mass spectrometry. Anal Chem 81(21):8758–8764
80. Dill AL, Eberlin LS, Costa AB, Zheng C, Ifa DR, Cheng L et al (2011) Multivariate statistical identification of human bladder carcinomas using ambient ionization imaging mass spectrometry. Chemistry 17(10):2897–2902
81. Dolcetti R, Viel A, Doglioni C, Russo A, Guidoboni M, Capozzi E et al (1999) High prevalence of activated intraepithelial cytotoxic T lymphocytes and increased neoplastic cell apoptosis in colorectal carcinomas with microsatellite instability. Am J Pathol 154(6):1805–1813
82. Eissa S, Matboli M, Awad N, Kotb Y (2017) Identification and validation of a novel autophagy gene expression signature for human bladder cancer patients. Tumour Biol 39(4):1010428317698360
83. Engbersen DJM, van Beijnum JR, Roos A, van Beelen M, de Haan JD, Grinwis GCM et al (2023) Vaccination against extracellular vimentin for treatment of urothelial cancer of the bladder in client-owned dogs. Cancers (Basel) 15(15):3958
84. Epstein JI (2010) Diagnosis and classification of flat, papillary, and invasive urothelial carcinoma: the WHO/ISUP consensus. Int J Surg Pathol 18(3 Suppl):106S–111S
85. Eriksson P, Sjödahl G, Chebil G, Liedberg F, Höglund M (2017) HER2 and EGFR amplification and expression in urothelial carcinoma occurs in distinct biological and molecular contexts. Oncotarget 8(30):48905–48914
86. Filley A, Henriquez M, Bhowmik T, Tewari BN, Rao X, Wan J et al (2018) Immunologic and gene expression profiles of spontaneous canine oligodendrogliomas. J Neuro-Oncol 137(3):469–479
87. Finotello R, Schiavo L, Ressel L, Frohmader A, Silvestrini P, Verin R (2019) Lipoxygenase-5 expression in canine urinary bladder: normal urothelium, cystitis and transitional cell carcinoma. J Comp Pathol 170:1–9
88. Fletcher O, Easton D, Anderson K, Gilham C, Jay M, Peto J (2004) Lifetime risks of common cancers among retinoblastoma survivors. J Natl Cancer Inst 96(5):357–363
89. Fong MHY, Feng M, McConkey DJ, Choi W (2020) Update on bladder cancer molecular subtypes. Transl Androl Urol 9(6):2881–2889
90. Froemming A, Potretzke T, Takahashi N, Kim B (2018) Upper tract urothelial cancer. Eur J Radiol 98:50–60
91. Fu M, Klose C, Sparks A, Whalen M (2022) Impact of variant histology on occult nodal metastasis after neoadjuvant chemotherapy for muscle-invasive bladder cancer: a review of the national cancer database. Clin Genitourin Cancer 20(2):e135–e139
92. Fulkerson CM, Knapp DW (2015) Management of transitional cell carcinoma of the urinary bladder in dogs: a review. Vet J 205(2):217–225
93. Fulkerson CM, Dhawan D, Ratliff TL, Hahn NM, Knapp DW (2017) Naturally occurring canine invasive urinary bladder cancer: a complementary animal model to improve the success rate in human clinical trials of new cancer drugs. Int J Genomics 2017:6589529
94. Galluzzi L, Zitvogel L, Kroemer G (2016) Immunological Mechanisms underneath the efficacy of cancer therapy. Cancer Immunol Res 4(11):895–902
95. Gamblin RM, Sagartz JE, Couto CG (1997) Overexpression of p53 tumor suppressor protein in spontaneously arising neoplasms of dogs. Am J Vet Res 58(8):857–863
96. Gedon J, Kehl A, Aupperle-Lellbach H, von Bomhard W, Schmidt JM (2022) BRAF mutation status and its prognostic significance in 79 canine urothelial carcinomas: A retrospective study (2006-2019). Vet Comp Oncol 20(2):449–457
97. Gelberg HB (2010) Urinary bladder mass in a dog. Vet Pathol 47(1):181–184
98. Gentilini F, Palgrave CJ, Neta M, Tornago R, Furlanello T, McKay JS et al (2022) Validation of a liquid biopsy protocol for canine BRAFV595E variant detection in dog urine and its evaluation as a diagnostic test complementary to cytology. Front Vet Sci 9:909934
99. Ghatalia P, Kaur J, Sonpavde G (2023) Muscle invasive bladder cancer: where is the field headed? Expert Opin Biol Ther 1–15
100. Ghisoni G, Foglia A, Sabattini S, Agnoli C, Dondi F, Perfetti S et al (2023) A retrospective clinicopathologic study of 35 dogs with urethral transitional cell carcinoma undergoing treatment. Animals (Basel) 13(14):2395
101. Glickman LT, Domanski LM, Maguire TG, Dubielzig RR, Churg A (1983) Mesothelioma in pet dogs associated with exposure of their owners to asbestos. Environ Res 32(2):305–313
102. Glickman LT, Schofer FS, McKee LJ, Reif JS, Goldschmidt MH (1989) Epidemiologic study of insecticide exposures, obesity, and risk of bladder cancer in household dogs. J Toxicol Environ Health 28(4):407–414
103. Glickman LT, Raghavan M, Knapp DW, Bonney PL, Dawson MH (2004) Herbicide exposure and the risk of transitional cell carcinoma of the urinary bladder in Scottish Terriers. J Am Vet Med Assoc 224(8):1290–1297

104. Gomes-Silva D, Ramos CA (2018) Cancer immunotherapy using car-t cells: from the research bench to the assembly line. Biotechnol J 13(2)
105. Govoni VM, Pigoli C, Brambilla E, Ruiz Sueiro FA, Torres Neto R, Laufer-Amorim R et al (2022) Caveolin-1, GATA-3, and Ki67 expressions and their correlation with pathological findings in canine bladder urothelial carcinoma. Front Vet Sci 9:986269
106. Grassinger JM, Merz S, Aupperle-Lellbach H, Erhard H, Klopfleisch R (2019) Correlation of BRAF variant V595E, breed, histological grade and cyclooxygenase-2 expression in canine transitional cell carcinomas. Vet Sci 6(1):31
107. Griffin MA, Culp WTN, Rebhun RB (2018) Lower urinary tract neoplasia. Vet Sci 5(4):96
108. Gustafson TL, Biller B (2019) Use of toceranib phosphate in the treatment of canine bladder tumors: 37 Cases. J Am Anim Hosp Assoc 55(5):243–248
109. Haarstad K, Bavor HJ, Mæhlum T (2012) Organic and metallic pollutants in water treatment and natural wetlands: a review. Water Sci Technol 65(1):76–99
110. Hahn NM (2022) Cancer of the bladder and urinary tract. In: Loscalzo J, Fauci A, Kasper D, Hauser S, Longo D, Jameson J (eds) Harrison's principles of internal medicine, 21th edn. McGraw Hill. Accessed 30 Jul 2023. https://accessmedicine.mhmedical.com/content.aspx?bookid=3095&sectionid=263362878
111. Hahn NM, Bonney PL, Dhawan D, Jones DR, Balch C, Guo Z et al (2012) Subcutaneous 5-azacitidine treatment of naturally occurring canine urothelial carcinoma: a novel epigenetic approach to human urothelial carcinoma drug development. J Urol 187(1):302–309
112. Hahn AW, Gill DM, Agarwal N, Maughan BL (2017) PD-1 checkpoint inhibition: Toxicities and management. Urol Oncol 35(12):701–707
113. Hanazono K, Fukumoto S, Kawamura Y, Endo Y, Kadosawa T, Iwano H et al (2015) Epidermal growth factor receptor expression in canine transitional cell carcinoma. J Vet Med Sci 77(1):1–6
114. Hanazono K, Nishimori T, Fukumoto S, Kawamura Y, Endo Y, Kadosawa T et al (2016) Immunohistochemical expression of p63, Ki67 and β-catenin in canine transitional cell carcinoma and polypoid cystitis of the urinary bladder. Vet Comp Oncol 14(3):263–269
115. Hartley G, Faulhaber E, Caldwell A, Coy J, Kurihara J, Guth A et al (2017) Immune regulation of canine tumour and macrophage PD-L1 expression. Vet Comp Oncol 15(2):534–549
116. Hartley G, Elmslie R, Dow S, Guth A (2018) Checkpoint molecule expression by B and T cell lymphomas in dogs. Vet Comp Oncol 16(3):352–360
117. He Z, Kosinska W, Zhao ZL, Wu XR, Guttenplan JB (2012) Tissue-specific mutagenesis by N-butyl-N-(4-hydroxybutyl)nitrosamine as the basis for urothelial carcinogenesis. Mutat Res 742(1–2):92–95
118. Heng HG, Ramos-Vara JA, Fulkerson CM, Fourez LM, Knapp DW (2022) Ultrasonographic detection of apex nodules in the urinary bladder of Scottish Terriers. Vet Radiol Ultrasound 63(2):234–239
119. Henry CJ, McCaw DL, Turnquist SE, Tyler JW, Bravo L, Sheafor S et al (2003a) Clinical evaluation of mitoxantrone and piroxicam in a canine model of human invasive urinary bladder carcinoma. Clin Cancer Res 9(2):906–911
120. Henry CJ, Tyler JW, McEntee MC, Stokol T, Rogers KS, Chun R et al (2003b) Evaluation of a bladder tumor antigen test as a screening test for transitional cell carcinoma of the lower urinary tract in dogs. Am J Vet Res 64(8):1017–1020
121. Henry CJ, Flesner BK, Bechtel SA, Bryan JN, Tate DJ, Selting KA et al (2018) Clinical evaluation of tavocept to decrease diuresis time and volume in dogs with bladder cancer receiving cisplatin. J Vet Intern Med 32(1):370–376
122. Higuchi T, Burcham GN, Childress MO, Rohleder JJ, Bonney PL, Ramos-Vara JA et al (2013) Characterization and treatment of transitional cell carcinoma of the abdominal wall in dogs: 24 cases (1985-2010). J Am Vet Med Assoc 242(4):499–506
123. Hilt EE, McKinley K, Pearce MM, Rosenfeld AB, Zilliox MJ, Mueller ER et al (2014) Urine is not sterile: use of enhanced urine culture techniques to detect resident bacterial flora in the adult female bladder. J Clin Microbiol 52(3):871–876
124. Hodgson A, Liu SK, Vesprini D, Xu B, Downes MR (2018) Basal-subtype bladder tumours show a "hot" immunophenotype. Histopathology 73(5):748–757
125. Honkisz SI, Naughton JF, Weng HY, Fourez LM, Knapp DW (2018) Evaluation of two-dimensional ultrasonography and computed tomography in the mapping and measuring of canine urinary bladder tumors. Vet J 232:23–26
126. Hosoya K, Takagi S, Okumura M (2013) Iatrogenic tumor seeding after ureteral stenting in a dog with urothelial carcinoma. J Am Anim Hosp Assoc 49(4):262–266
127. Hu SP, Zhang Z, Xiao F, Huang JN, Jiang Y, Mao DS et al (2022) Paraganglioma of the urinary bladder in a dog. J Comp Pathol 195:1–6
128. Hunter P (2017) The fourth pillar: Despite some setbacks in the clinic, immunotherapy has made notable progress toward becoming an additional therapeutic option against cancer. EMBO Rep 18(11):1889–1892
129. Igase M, Nemoto Y, Itamoto K, Tani K, Nakaichi M, Sakurai M et al (2020) A pilot clinical study of the therapeutic antibody against canine PD-1 for advanced spontaneous cancers in dogs. Sci Rep 10(1):18311
130. Iwasaki R, Shimosato Y, Yoshikawa R, Goto S, Yoshida K, Murakami M et al (2019) Survival analysis in dogs with urinary transitional cell carcinoma that underwent whole-body computed tomography at diagnosis. Vet Comp Oncol 17(3):385–393
131. Jack S, Madhivanan K, Ramadesikan S, Subramanian S, Edwards DF, Elzey BD et al (2020) A novel, safe, fast and efficient treatment for Her2-positive and

negative bladder cancer utilizing an EGF-anthrax toxin chimera. Int J Cancer 146(2):449–460
132. Jalilian H, Ziaei M, Weiderpass E, Rueegg CS, Khosravi Y, Kjaerheim K (2019) Cancer incidence and mortality among firefighters. Int J Cancer 145(10):2639–2646
133. John BA, Said N (2017) Insights from animal models of bladder cancer: recent advances, challenges, and opportunities. Oncotarget 8(34):57766–57781
134. Jubber I, Ong S, Bukavina L, Black PC, Compérat E, Kamat AM et al (2023) Epidemiology of bladder cancer in 2023: a systematic review of risk factors. Eur Urol 84(2):176–190
135. Kamat AM, Hahn NM, Efstathiou JA, Lerner SP, Malmström PU, Choi W et al (2016) Bladder cancer. Lancet 388(10061):2796–2810
136. Kamoun A, de Reyniès A, Allory Y, Sjödahl G, Robertson AG, Seiler R et al (2020) A Consensus molecular classification of muscle-invasive bladder cancer. Eur Urol 77(4):420–433
137. Kanehisa M, Goto S (2000) KEGG: kyoto encyclopedia of genes and genomes. Nucleic Acids Res 28(1):27–30
138. Kelsey JL, Moore AS, Glickman LT (1998) Epidemiologic studies of risk factors for cancer in pet dogs. Epidemiol Rev 20(2):204–217
139. Kent MS, Zwingenberger A, Westropp JL, Barrett LE, Durbin-Johnson BP, Ghosh P et al (2017) MicroRNA profiling of dogs with transitional cell carcinoma of the bladder using blood and urine samples. BMC Vet Res 13(1):339
140. Kessler M, Kandel-Tschiederer B, Pfleghaar S, Tassani-Prell M (2008) Primary malignant lymphoma of the urinary bladder in a dog: longterm remission following treatment with radiation and chemotherapy. Schweiz Arch Tierheilkd 150(11):565–569
141. Kim S (2016) Overview of cotinine cutoff values for smoking status classification. Int J Environ Res Public Health 13(12):1236
142. Kim HS, Seo HK (2018) Immune checkpoint inhibitors for urothelial carcinoma. Investig Clin Urol 59(5):285–296
143. Kim S, Hosoya K, Takagi S, Okumura M (2019) Outcomes following balloon dilation for management of urethral obstruction secondary to urothelial carcinoma in dogs: 12 cases (2010-2015). J Am Vet Med Assoc 255(3):330–335
144. Kim JH, Ahn DH, Moon JS, Han HJ, Bae K, Yoon KA (2021) Longitudinal assessment of B-RAF V595E levels in the peripheral cell-free tumor DNA of a 10-year-old spayed female Korean Jindo dog with unresectable metastatic urethral transitional cell carcinoma for monitoring the treatment response to a RAF inhibitor (sorafenib). Vet Q 41(1):153–162
145. Kittler R, Shiang C, Hutchinson R, Kollipara RK, Kapur P, Franto F et al (2018) Grade progression in urothelial carcinoma can occur with high or low mutational homology: a first-step toward tumor-specific care in initial low-grade bladder cancer. Oncotarget 9(10):9415–9424
146. Knapp DW, Richardson RC, Bottoms GD, Teclaw R, Chan TC (1992) Phase I trial of piroxicam in 62 dogs bearing naturally occurring tumors. Cancer Chemother Pharmacol 29(3):214–218
147. Knapp DW, Richardson RC, Chan TC, Bottoms GD, Widmer WR, DeNicola DB et al (1994) Piroxicam therapy in 34 dogs with transitional cell carcinoma of the urinary bladder. J Vet Intern Med 8(4):273–278
148. Knapp DW, Glickman NW, Widmer WR, DeNicola DB, Adams LG, Kuczek T et al (2000) Cisplatin versus cisplatin combined with piroxicam in a canine model of human invasive urinary bladder cancer. Cancer Chemother Pharmacol 46(3):221–226
149. Knapp DW, Henry CJ, Widmer WR, Tan KM, Moore GE, Ramos-Vara JA et al (2013a) Randomized trial of cisplatin versus firocoxib versus cisplatin/firocoxib in dogs with transitional cell carcinoma of the urinary bladder. J Vet Intern Med 27(1):126–133
150. Knapp DW, Peer WA, Conteh A, Diggs AR, Cooper BR, Glickman NW et al (2013b) Detection of herbicides in the urine of pet dogs following home lawn chemical application. Sci Total Environ 456–457:34–41
151. Knapp DW, Ramos-Vara JA, Moore GE, Dhawan D, Bonney PL, Young KE (2014) Urinary bladder cancer in dogs, a naturally occurring model for cancer biology and drug development. ILAR J 55(1):100–118
152. Knapp DW, Ruple-Czerniak A, Ramos-Vara JA, Naughton JF, Fulkerson CM, Honkisz SI (2016) A nonselective cyclooxygenase inhibitor enhances the activity of vinblastine in a naturally-occurring canine model of invasive urothelial carcinoma. Bladder Cancer 2(2):241–250
153. Knapp DW, Dhawan D, Ramos-Vara JA, Ratliff TL, Cresswell GM, Utturkar S et al (2019) Naturally-occurring invasive urothelial carcinoma in dogs, a unique model to drive advances in managing muscle invasive bladder cancer in humans. Front Oncol 9:1493
154. Knapp DW, Dhawan D, Ruple A, Cooper BR, Zhang M, Liu D, Ramos-Vara JA, Bonney PL, Fourez LM, Enstrom AW, Lahrman SA, Tullius JA (2024) Association between cigarette smoke exposure and urinary bladder cancer in Scottish terriers in a cohort study. Vet J 303:106044
155. Kobayashi T, Owczarek TB, McKiernan JM, Abate-Shen C (2015) Modelling bladder cancer in mice: opportunities and challenges. Nat Rev Cancer 15(1):42–54
156. Küchler L, Posthaus C, Jäger K, Guscetti F, van der Weyden L, von Bomhard W et al (2023) Artificial intelligence to predict the BRAF V595E mutation in canine urinary bladder urothelial carcinomas. Animals (Basel) 13(15):2404
157. Kumar R, Matulewicz R, Mari A, Moschini M, Ghodoussipour S, Pradere B et al (2023) Impact of

smoking on urologic cancers: a snapshot of current evidence. World J Urol 41(6):1473–1479
158. Kunze E, Wendt M, Schlott T (2006) Promoter hypermethylation of the 14-3-3 sigma, SYK and CAGE-1 genes is related to the various phenotypes of urinary bladder carcinomas and associated with progression of transitional cell carcinomas. Int J Mol Med 18(4):547–557
159. Kutzler MA (2020) Possible relationship between long-term adverse health effects of gonad-removing surgical sterilization and luteinizing hormone in dogs. Animals (Basel) 10(4):599
160. Lam CM, Li Z, Theodorescu D, Li X (2022) Mechanism of sex differences in bladder cancer: evident and elusive sex-biasing factors. Bladder Cancer 8(3):241–254
161. LeBlanc AK, Mazcko CN (2020) Improving human cancer therapy through the evaluation of pet dogs. Nat Rev Cancer 20(12):727–742
162. Lee JH, Park SJ, Kim SW, Hariharasudhan G, Jung SM, Jun S et al (2017) c-Fos-dependent miR-22 targets MDC1 and regulates DNA repair in terminally differentiated cells. Oncotarget 8(29):48204–48221
163. Lee SW, Baek SM, Lee AR, Kim TU, Kim D, Kwon YS et al (2020) Malignant peripheral nerve sheath tumour in the urinary bladder of a dog. J Comp Pathol 175:64–68
164. Leffler AJ, Hostnik ET, Warry EE, Habing GG, Auld DM, Green EM et al (2018) Canine urinary bladder transitional cell carcinoma tumor volume is dependent on imaging modality and measurement technique. Vet Radiol Ultrasound 59(6):767–776
165. Lenis AT, Lec PM, Chamie K, Mshs MD (2020) Bladder cancer: a review. JAMA 324(19):1980–1991
166. Lewis DA, Brown R, Williams J, White P, Jacobson SK, Marchesi JR et al (2013) The human urinary microbiome; bacterial DNA in voided urine of asymptomatic adults. Front Cell Infect Microbiol 3:41
167. Lin SJH, Kao CF, Wang FI, Jeng CR, Lee JJ, Wang LY et al (2018) Urothelial carcinomas of the urinary bladder with plasmacytoid or rhabdoid features and tendency of epithelial-mesenchymal transition in 3 dogs. Vet Pathol 55(5):673–677
168. Liptak JM, Dernell WS, Withrow SJ (2004) Haemangiosarcoma of the urinary bladder in a dog. Aust Vet J 82(4):215–217
169. Liu W, Newhall KP, Khani F, Barlow L, Nguyen D, Gu L et al (2023) The cytidine deaminase APOBEC3G contributes to cancer mutagenesis and clonal evolution in bladder cancer. Cancer Res 83(4):506–520
170. Lobo N, Mount C, Omar K, Nair R, Thurairaja R, Khan MS (2017) Landmarks in the treatment of muscle-invasive bladder cancer. Nat Rev Urol 14(9):565–574
171. Loehrer PJ, Einhorn LH, Elson PJ, Crawford ED, Kuebler P, Tannock I et al (1992) A randomized comparison of cisplatin alone or in combination with methotrexate, vinblastine, and doxorubicin in patients with metastatic urothelial carcinoma: a cooperative group study. J Clin Oncol 10(7):1066–1073
172. Long J, Ganakammal SR, Jones SE, Kothandaraman H, Dhawan D, Ogas J et al (2023) cTULIP: application of a human-based RNA-seq primary tumor classification tool for cross-species primary tumor classification in canine. Front Oncol 13:1216892
173. Longo T, McGinley KF, Freedman JA, Etienne W, Wu Y, Sibley A et al (2016) Targeted exome sequencing of the cancer genome in patients with very high-risk bladder cancer. Eur Urol 70(5):714–717
174. Loomans-Kropp HA, Umar A (2019) Cancer prevention and screening: the next step in the era of precision medicine. NPJ Precis Oncol 3:3
175. Loomans-Kropp HA, Pinsky P, Umar A (2021) Evaluation of aspirin use with cancer incidence and survival among older adults in the prostate, lung, colorectal, and ovarian cancer screening trial. JAMA Netw Open 4(1):e2032072
176. Love MI, Huber W, Anders S (2014) Moderated estimation of fold change and dispersion for RNA-seq data with DESeq2. Genome Biol 15(12):550
177. Lubet RA, Scheiman JM, Bode A, White J, Minasian L, Juliana MM et al (2015) Prevention of chemically induced urinary bladder cancers by naproxen: protocols to reduce gastric toxicity in humans do not alter preventive efficacy. Cancer Prev Res (Phila) 8(4):296–302
178. Lucchesi CA, Vasilatis DM, Mantrala S, Chandrasekar T, Mudryj M, Ghosh PM (2023) Pesticides and bladder cancer: mechanisms leading to anti-cancer drug chemoresistance and new chemosensitization strategies. Int J Mol Sci 24(14):11395
179. Lucroy MD, Ridgway TD, Peavy GM, Krasieva TB, Higbee RG, Campbell GA et al (2003) Preclinical evaluation of 5-aminolevulinic acid-based photodynamic therapy for canine transitional cell carcinoma. Vet Comp Oncol 1(2):76–85
180. Lulich JP (2022) Evaluation of temporary urethral stents in the management of malignant and nonmalignant urethral diseases in dogs. Vet Sci 9(2):63
181. Lyon TD, Frank I, Shah PH, Tarrell R, Cheville JC, Karnes RJ et al (2018) The association of aspirin use with survival following radical cystectomy. J Urol 200(5):1014–1021
182. Macrì F, Di Pietro S, Mangano C, Pugliese M, Mazzullo G, Iannelli NM et al (2018) Quantitative evaluation of canine urinary bladder transitional cell carcinoma using contrast-enhanced ultrasonography. BMC Vet Res 14(1):84
183. Maeda S, Tomiyasu H, Tsuboi M, Inoue A, Ishihara G, Uchikai T et al (2018) Comprehensive gene expression analysis of canine invasive urothelial bladder carcinoma by RNA-Seq. BMC Cancer 18:472
184. Maeda S, Sakai K, Kaji K, Iio A, Nakazawa M, Motegi T et al (2022) Lapatinib as first-line treatment for muscle-invasive urothelial carcinoma in dogs. Sci Rep 12(1):4

185. Maekawa N, Konnai S, Okagawa T, Nishimori A, Ikebuchi R, Izumi Y et al (2016) Immunohistochemical analysis of PD-L1 expression in canine malignant cancers and PD-1 expression on lymphocytes in canine oral melanoma. PLoS One 11(6):e0157176
186. Maekawa N, Konnai S, Takagi S, Kagawa Y, Okagawa T, Nishimori A et al (2017) A canine chimeric monoclonal antibody targeting PD-L1 and its clinical efficacy in canine oral malignant melanoma or undifferentiated sarcoma. Sci Rep 7(1):8951
187. Maekawa N, Konnai S, Nishimura M, Kagawa Y, Takagi S, Hosoya K et al (2021) PD-L1 immunohistochemistry for canine cancers and clinical benefit of anti-PD-L1 antibody in dogs with pulmonary metastatic oral malignant melanoma. NPJ Precis Oncol 5(1):10
188. Mak IW, Evaniew N, Ghert M (2014) Lost in translation: animal models and clinical trials in cancer treatment. Am J Transl Res 6(2):114–118
189. Malfassi L, Fidanzio F, Sala M, Marcarini S, Mazza G, Carrara N et al (2021) A combined protocol with piroxicam, chemotherapy, and whole pelvic irradiation with simultaneous boost volumetric modulated arc radiotherapy for muscle-invasive canine urinary transitional cell carcinoma: First clinical experience. J Vet Med Sci 83(4):695–704
190. Marconato L, Zini E, Lindner D, Suslak-Brown L, Nelson V, Jeglum AK (2011) Toxic effects and antitumor response of gemcitabine in combination with piroxicam treatment in dogs with transitional cell carcinoma of the urinary bladder. J Am Vet Med Assoc 238(8):1004–1010
191. Marconato L, Finotello R, Bonfanti U, Dacasto M, Beatrice L, Pizzoni S et al (2015) An open-label phase 1 dose-escalation clinical trial of a single intravenous administration of gemcitabine in dogs with advanced solid tumors. J Vet Intern Med 29(2):620–625
192. Marie Butty E, Forsyth B, Labato MA (2022) Irreversible electroporation balloon therapy for palliative treatment of obstructive urethral transitional cell carcinoma in dogs. J Am Anim Hosp Assoc 58(5):231–239
193. Martin A, Woolbright BL, Umar S, Ingersoll MA, Taylor JA (2022) Bladder cancer, inflammageing and microbiomes. Nat Rev Urol 19(8):495–509
194. Marvel SJ, Séguin B, Dailey DD, Thamm DH (2017) Clinical outcome of partial cystectomy for transitional cell carcinoma of the canine bladder. Vet Comp Oncol 15(4):1417–1427
195. McCleary-Wheeler AL, Williams LE, Hess PR, Suter SE (2010) Evaluation of an in vitro telomeric repeat amplification protocol assay to detect telomerase activity in canine urine. Am J Vet Res 71(12):1468–1474
196. McConkey DJ, Choi W (2018) Molecular Subtypes of Bladder Cancer. Curr Oncol Rep 20(10):77
197. McConkey DJ, Choi W, Shen Y, Lee IL, Porten S, Matin SF et al (2016) A Prognostic gene expression signature in the molecular classification of chemotherapy-naïve urothelial cancer is predictive of clinical outcomes from neoadjuvant chemotherapy: a phase 2 trial of dose-dense methotrexate, vinblastine, doxorubicin, and cisplatin with bevacizumab in urothelial cancer. Eur Urol 69(5):855–862
198. McMillan SK, Boria P, Moore GE, Widmer WR, Bonney PL, Knapp DW (2011) Antitumor effects of deracoxib treatment in 26 dogs with transitional cell carcinoma of the urinary bladder. J Am Vet Med Assoc 239(8):1084–1089
199. Meeks JJ, Al-Ahmadie H, Faltas BM, Taylor JA, Flaig TW, DeGraff DJ et al (2020) Genomic heterogeneity in bladder cancer: challenges and possible solutions to improve outcomes. Nat Rev Urol 17(5):259–270
200. Melilli A (2020) Uncommon skeletal metastasis secondary to transitional cell carcinoma. Open Vet J 9(4):313–316
201. Merickel JL, Lawrence J, Young SJ, Thomson CB (2021) Cutaneous seeding of transitional cell carcinoma of the urinary bladder after placement of a subcutaneous ureteral bypass device in a dog with bilateral ureteral obstruction. J Am Vet Med Assoc 258(8):877–882
202. Merseburger AS, Apolo AB, Chowdhury S, Hahn NM, Galsky MD, Milowsky MI et al (2019) SIU-ICUD recommendations on bladder cancer: systemic therapy for metastatic bladder cancer. World J Urol 37(1):95–105
203. Mhawech P, Benz A, Cerato C, Greloz V, Assaly M, Desmond JC et al (2005) Downregulation of 14-3-3sigma in ovary, prostate and endometrial carcinomas is associated with CpG island methylation. Mod Pathol 18(3):340–348
204. Michishita M, Ishizaki Y, Konnai M, Machida Y, Nakahira R, Hatakeyama H et al (2020) Primary lymphangiosarcoma of the urinary bladder in a dog. J Comp Pathol 179:31–35
205. Millanta F, Impellizeri J, McSherry L, Rocchigiani G, Aurisicchio L, Lubas G (2018) Overexpression of HER-2 via immunohistochemistry in canine urinary bladder transitional cell carcinoma – a marker of malignancy and possible therapeutic target. Vet Comp Oncol 16(2):297–300
206. Milovancev M, Scharf VF, Townsend KL, Singh A, Tremolada G, Worley D et al (2020) Partial cystectomy with a bipolar sealing device in seven dogs with naturally occurring bladder tumors. Vet Surg 49(4):794–799
207. Mineshige T, Kawarai S, Yauchi T, Segawa K, Neo S, Sugahara G et al (2016) Cutaneous epitheliotropic T-cell lymphoma with systemic dissemination in a dog. J Vet Diagn Invest 28(3):327–331
208. Mitra AP, Datar RH, Cote RJ (2006) Molecular pathways in invasive bladder cancer: new insights into mechanisms, progression, and target identification. J Clin Oncol 24(35):5552–5564
209. Mitra AP, Hansel DE, Cote RJ (2012) Prognostic value of cell-cycle regulation biomarkers in bladder cancer. Semin Oncol 39(5):524–533

210. Mochizuki H, Shapiro SG, Breen M (2015) Detection of BRAF mutation in urine dna as a molecular diagnostic for canine urothelial and prostatic carcinoma. PLoS One 10(12):e0144170
211. Mohammed SI, Knapp DW, Bostwick DG, Foster RS, Khan KN, Masferrer JL et al (1999) Expression of cyclooxygenase-2 (COX-2) in human invasive transitional cell carcinoma (TCC) of the urinary bladder. Cancer Res 59(22):5647–5650
212. Mohammed SI, Bennett PF, Craig BA, Glickman NW, Mutsaers AJ, Snyder PW et al (2002) Effects of the cyclooxygenase inhibitor, piroxicam, on tumor response, apoptosis, and angiogenesis in a canine model of human invasive urinary bladder cancer. Cancer Res 62(2):356–358
213. Mohammed SI, Dhawan D, Abraham S, Snyder PW, Waters DJ, Craig BA et al (2006) Cyclooxygenase inhibitors in urinary bladder cancer: in vitro and in vivo effects. Mol Cancer Ther 5(2):329–336
214. Mohammed A, Miller MS, Lubet RA, Suen CS, Sei S, Shoemaker RH et al (2020) Combination of erlotinib and naproxen employing pulsatile or intermittent dosing profoundly inhibits urinary bladder cancers. Cancer Prev Res (Phila) 13(3):273–282
215. Mohanty SK, Lobo A, Cheng L (2023a) The 2022 revision of the World Health Organization classification of tumors of the urinary system and male genital organs: advances and challenges. Hum Pathol 136:123–143
216. Mohanty SK, Lobo A, Mishra SK, Cheng L (2023b) Precision medicine in bladder cancer: present challenges and future directions. J Pers Med 13(5):756
217. Monteiro LL, Witjes JA, Agarwal PK, Anderson CB, Bivalacqua TJ, Bochner BH et al (2019) ICUD-SIU International Consultation on Bladder Cancer 2017: management of non-muscle invasive bladder cancer. World J Urol 37(1):51–60
218. Mooso BA, Vinall RL, Mudryj M, Yap SA, deVere White RW, Ghosh PM (2015) The role of EGFR family inhibitors in muscle invasive bladder cancer: a review of clinical data and molecular evidence. J Urol 193(1):19–29
219. Moris A, Murray S, Cardinaud S (2014) AID and APOBECs span the gap between innate and adaptive immunity. Front Microbiol 5:534
220. Mostofi K, Ito N, Weinstein R, Denis L (1986) Pathology: the need for standardization of pathological examination and reporting, developments in bladder cancer. Alan R. Liss, New York, pp 67–83
221. Mrofchak R, Madden C, Evans MV, Kisseberth WC, Dhawan D, Knapp DW, Hale VL (2022) Urine and fecal microbiota in a canine model of bladder cancer and comparison of canine and human urine microbiota. All. Life 15:1245–1263
222. Musser ML, Viall AK, Phillips RL, Hostetter JM, Johannes CM (2020) Gene expression of prostaglandin EP4 receptor in three canine carcinomas. BMC Vet Res 16(1):213
223. Mutsaers AJ, Widmer WR, Knapp DW (2003) Canine transitional cell carcinoma. J Vet Intern Med 17(2):136–144
224. Nagaya T, Okuyama S, Ogata F, Maruoka Y, Knapp DW, Karagiannis SN et al (2018) Near infrared photoimmunotherapy targeting bladder cancer with a canine anti-epidermal growth factor receptor (EGFR) antibody. Oncotarget 9(27):19026–19038
225. London CA, Gardner H, Zhao S, Knapp DW, Utturkar SM, Duval DL, Chambers MR, Ostrander E, Trent JM, Kuffel G (2023) Leading the pack: best practices in comparative canine cancer genomics to inform human oncology. Vet Comp Oncol 21(4):565–577. https://doi.org/10.1111/vco.12935. Epub 2023 Oct 1. PMID: 37778398; PMCID: PMC12065084
226. Necchi A, Raggi D, Gallina A, Ross JS, Farè E, Giannatempo P et al (2020) Impact of molecular subtyping and immune infiltration on pathological response and outcome following neoadjuvant pembrolizumab in muscle-invasive bladder cancer. Eur Urol 77(6):701–710
227. Nemoto Y, Shosu K, Okuda M, Noguchi S, Mizuno T (2018) Development and characterization of monoclonal antibodies against canine PD-1 and PD-L1. Vet Immunol Immunopathol 198:19–25
228. Ngeow J, Stanuch K, Mester JL, Barnholtz-Sloan JS, Eng C (2014) Second malignant neoplasms in patients with Cowden syndrome with underlying germline PTEN mutations. J Clin Oncol 32(17):1818–1824
229. Nicastro HL, Grubbs CJ, Margaret Juliana M, Bode AM, Kim MS, Lu Y et al (2014) Preventive effects of NSAIDs, NO-NSAIDs, and NSAIDs plus difluoromethylornithine in a chemically induced urinary bladder cancer model. Cancer Prev Res (Phila) 7(2):246–254
230. Nishimori T, Hanazono K, Matsuda K, Kawamura Y, Kadosawa T, Endo Y et al (2021) Prognostic role of ΔNp63 expression in canine transitional cell carcinoma of the urinary bladder. Open Vet J 11(4):700–706
231. Nolan MW, Kogan L, Griffin LR, Custis JT, Harmon JF, Biller BJ et al (2012) Intensity-modulated and image-guided radiation therapy for treatment of genitourinary carcinomas in dogs. J Vet Intern Med 26(4):987–995
232. Nordentoft I, Lamy P, Birkenkamp-Demtröder K, Shumansky K, Vang S, Hornshøj H et al (2014) Mutational context and diverse clonal development in early and late bladder cancer. Cell Rep 7(5):1649–1663
233. Oh W, Kim AMJ, Dhawan D, Kirkham PM, Ostafe R, Franco J et al (2023) Development of an anti-canine PD-L1 antibody and caninized PD-L1 mouse model as translational research tools for the study of immunotherapy in humans. Cancer Res Commun 3(5):860–873
234. Okajima E, Hiramatsu T, Hirao K, Ijuin M, Hirao Y, Babaya K et al (1981) Urinary bladder tumors induced by N-butyl-N-(4-hydroxybutyl)nitrosamine in dogs. Cancer Res 41(5):1958–1966
235. Oliveira PA, Gil da Costa RM, Vasconcelos-Nóbrega C, Arantes-Rodrigues R, Pinto-Leite R (2016)

Challenges with in vitro and in vivo experimental models of urinary bladder cancer for novel drug discovery. Expert Opin Drug Discov 11(6):599–607
236. Orlando C, Gelmini S, Selli C, Pazzagli M (2001) Telomerase in urological malignancy. J Urol 166(2):666–673
237. Owen LN (1980) TNM classification of tumours in domestic animals. World Health Organization, Geneva
238. Packeiser EM, Taher L, Kong W, Ernst M, Beck J, Hewicker-Trautwein M et al (2022) RNA-seq of nine canine prostate cancer cell lines reveals diverse therapeutic target signatures. Cancer Cell Int 22(1):54
239. Panjwani MK, Smith JB, Schutsky K, Gnanandarajah J, O'Connor CM, Powell DJ et al (2016) Feasibility and safety of RNA-transfected CD20-specific chimeric antigen receptor t cells in dogs with spontaneous B cell lymphoma. Mol Ther 24(9):1602–1614
240. Pardoll DM (2012) The blockade of immune checkpoints in cancer immunotherapy. Nat Rev Cancer 12(4):252–264
241. Park S, Reuter VE, Hansel DE (2019) Non-urothelial carcinomas of the bladder. Histopathology 74(1):97–111
242. Parker HG, Dhawan D, Harris AC, Ramos-Vara JA, Davis BW, Knapp DW et al (2020) RNAseq expression patterns of canine invasive urothelial carcinoma reveal two distinct tumor clusters and shared regions of dysregulation with human bladder tumors. BMC Cancer 20(1):251
243. Pastore A, Palleschi G, Fuschi A, Silvestri L, Al Salhi Y, Costantini E et al (2015) Can daily intake of aspirin and/or statins influence the behavior of non-muscle invasive bladder cancer? A retrospective study on a cohort of patients undergoing transurethral bladder resection. BMC Cancer 15:120
244. Patrick DJ, Fitzgerald SD, Sesterhenn IA, Davis CJ, Kiupel M (2006) Classification of canine urinary bladder urothelial tumours based on the World Health Organization/International Society of Urological Pathology consensus classification. J Comp Pathol 135(4):190–199
245. Peng J, Hamanishi J, Matsumura N, Abiko K, Murat K, Baba T et al (2015) Chemotherapy induces programmed cell death-ligand 1 overexpression via the nuclear factor-κB to foster an immunosuppressive tumor microenvironment in ovarian cancer. Cancer Res 75(23):5034–5045
246. Petrylak DP, Tangen CM, Van Veldhuizen PJ, Goodwin JW, Twardowski PW, Atkins JN et al (2010) Results of the Southwest Oncology Group phase II evaluation (study S0031) of ZD1839 for advanced transitional cell carcinoma of the urothelium. BJU Int 105(3):317–321
247. Pfirschke C, Engblom C, Rickelt S, Cortez-Retamozo V, Garris C, Pucci F et al (2016) Immunogenic chemotherapy sensitizes tumors to checkpoint blockade therapy. Immunity 44(2):343–354
248. Pinard CJ, Stegelmeier AA, Bridle BW, Mutsaers AJ, Wood RD, Wood GA et al (2022) Evaluation of lymphocyte-specific programmed cell death protein 1 receptor expression and cytokines in blood and urine in canine urothelial carcinoma patients. Vet Comp Oncol 20(2):427–436
249. Powles T, Rosenberg JE, Sonpavde GP, Loriot Y, Durán I, Lee JL et al (2021) Enfortumab vedotin in previously treated advanced urothelial carcinoma. N Engl J Med 384(12):1125–1135
250. Pruthi RS, Nielsen M, Heathcote S, Wallen EM, Rathmell WK, Godley P et al (2010) A phase II trial of neoadjuvant erlotinib in patients with muscle-invasive bladder cancer undergoing radical cystectomy: clinical and pathological results. BJU Int 106(3):349–354
251. Raghavan M, Knapp DW, Dawson MH, Bonney PL, Glickman LT (2004) Topical flea and tick pesticides and the risk of transitional cell carcinoma of the urinary bladder in Scottish Terriers. J Am Vet Med Assoc 225(3):389–394
252. Raghavan M, Knapp DW, Bonney PL, Dawson MH, Glickman LT (2005) Evaluation of the effect of dietary vegetable consumption on reducing risk of transitional cell carcinoma of the urinary bladder in Scottish Terriers. J Am Vet Med Assoc 227(1):94–100
253. Ramsey SA, Xu T, Goodall C, Rhodes AC, Kashyap A, He J et al (2017) Cross-species analysis of the canine and human bladder cancer transcriptome and exome. Genes Chromosomes Cancer 56(4):328–343
254. Rankin WV, Henry CJ, Turnquist SE, Turk JR, Beissenherz ME, Tyler JW et al (2008) Identification of survivin, an inhibitor of apoptosis, in canine urinary bladder transitional cell carcinoma. Vet Comp Oncol 6(3):141–150
255. Rebouissou S, Bernard-Pierrot I, de Reyniès A, Lepage ML, Krucker C, Chapeaublanc E et al (2014) EGFR as a potential therapeutic target for a subset of muscle-invasive bladder cancers presenting a basal-like phenotype. Sci Transl Med 6(244):244ra91
256. Reed LT, Knapp DW, Miller MA (2013) Cutaneous metastasis of transitional cell carcinoma in 12 dogs. Vet Pathol 50(4):676–681
257. Ren R, Tyryshkin K, Graham CH, Koti M, Siemens DR (2017) Comprehensive immune transcriptomic analysis in bladder cancer reveals subtype specific immune gene expression patterns of prognostic relevance. Oncotarget 8(41):70982–71001
258. Ricardo Huppes R, Crivellenti LZ, Barboza De Nardi A, Roque Lima B, Alves Cintra C, Luiz Costa Castro J et al (2017) Radical cystectomy and cutaneous ureterostomy in 4 dogs with trigonal transitional cell carcinoma: description of technique and case series. Vet Surg 46(1):111–119
259. Rippy SB, Gardner HL, Nguyen SM, Warry EE, Portela RA, Drost WT et al (2016) A pilot study of toceranib/vinblastine therapy for canine transitional cell carcinoma. BMC Vet Res 12(1):257
260. Rizvi NA, Hellmann MD, Snyder A, Kvistborg P, Makarov V, Havel JJ et al (2015) Cancer immunology. Mutational landscape determines sensitivity

to PD-1 blockade in non-small cell lung cancer. Science 348(6230):124–128
261. Robertson AG, Kim J, Al-Ahmadie H, Bellmunt J, Guo G, Cherniack AD et al (2017) Comprehensive molecular characterization of muscle-invasive bladder cancer. Cell 171(3):540–556.e25
262. Robinson MD, Oshlack A (2010) A scaling normalization method for differential expression analysis of RNA-seq data. Genome Biol 11(3):R25
263. Rosenberg JE, Hoffman-Censits J, Powles T, van der Heijden MS, Balar AV, Necchi A et al (2016) Atezolizumab in patients with locally advanced and metastatic urothelial carcinoma who have progressed following treatment with platinum-based chemotherapy: a single-arm, multicentre, phase 2 trial. Lancet 387(10031):1909–1920
264. Ross JS, Wang K, Al-Rohil RN, Nazeer T, Sheehan CE, Otto GA et al (2014) Advanced urothelial carcinoma: next-generation sequencing reveals diverse genomic alterations and targets of therapy. Mod Pathol 27(2):271–280
265. Rossman P, Zabka TS, Ruple A, Tuerck D, Ramos-Vara JA, Liu L et al (2021) Phase I/II Trial of vemurafenib in dogs with naturally occurring, BRAF-mutated urothelial carcinoma. Mol Cancer Ther 20(11):2177–2188
266. Rouanne M, Loriot Y, Lebret T, Soria JC (2016) Novel therapeutic targets in advanced urothelial carcinoma. Crit Rev Oncol Hematol 98:106–115
267. Sabichi AL, Lee JJ, Grossman HB, Liu S, Richmond E, Czerniak BA et al (2011) A randomized controlled trial of celecoxib to prevent recurrence of nonmuscle-invasive bladder cancer. Cancer Prev Res (Phila) 4(10):1580–1589
268. Saeki K, Fujita A, Fujita N, Nakagawa T, Nishimura R (2015) Total cystectomy and subsequent urinary diversion to the prepuce or vagina in dogs with transitional cell carcinoma of the trigone area: a report of 10 cases (2005-2011). Can Vet J 56(1):73–80
269. Saginala K, Barsouk A, Aluru JS, Rawla P, Padala SA, Barsouk A (2020) Epidemiology of bladder cancer. Med Sci (Basel) 8(1):15
270. Sakai H, Yonemaru K, Takeda M, Niimi K, Murakami M, Hirata A et al (2011) Ganglioneuroma in the urinary bladder of a dog. J Vet Med Sci 73(6):801–803
271. Sakai K, Maeda S, Saeki K, Yoshitake R, Goto-Koshino Y, Nakagawa T et al (2020) ErbB2 copy number aberration in canine urothelial carcinoma detected by a digital polymerase chain reaction assay. Vet Pathol 57(1):56–65
272. Samstein RM, Lee CH, Shoushtari AN, Hellmann MD, Shen R, Janjigian YY et al (2019) Tumor mutational load predicts survival after immunotherapy across multiple cancer types. Nat Genet 51(2):202–206
273. Santopietro AL, Einstein D, Bellmunt J (2021) Advances in the management of urothelial carcinoma: is immunotherapy the answer? Expert Opin Pharmacother 22(13):1743–1759
274. Schrempp DR, Childress MO, Stewart JC, Leach TN, Tan KM, Abbo AH et al (2013) Metronomic administration of chlorambucil for treatment of dogs with urinary bladder transitional cell carcinoma. J Am Vet Med Assoc 242(11):1534–1538
275. Schwartz P (2022) Current concepts in urinary surgery. Vet Clin North Am Small Anim Pract 52(2):387–417
276. Seiler R, Ashab HAD, Erho N, van Rhijn BWG, Winters B, Douglas J et al (2017) Impact of molecular subtypes in muscle-invasive bladder cancer on predicting response and survival after neoadjuvant chemotherapy. Eur Urol 72(4):544–554
277. Setyo LC, Donahoe SL, Shearer PL, Wang P, Krockenberger MB (2023) Immunohistochemical analysis of expression of VEGFR2, KIT, PDGFR-β, and CDK4 in canine urothelial carcinoma. J Vet Diagn Invest 35(2):109–115
278. Shapiro SG, Raghunath S, Williams C, Motsinger-Reif AA, Cullen JM, Liu T et al (2015) Canine urothelial carcinoma: genomically aberrant and comparatively relevant. Chromosom Res 23(2):311–331
279. Shariat SF, Karakiewicz PI, Godoy G, Karam JA, Ashfaq R, Fradet Y et al (2009) Survivin as a prognostic marker for urothelial carcinoma of the bladder: a multicenter external validation study. Clin Cancer Res 15(22):7012–7019
280. Sheikh M, Shakeri R, Poustchi H et al (2020) Opium use and subsequent incidence of cancer: results from the Golestan Cohort Study. Lancet Glob Health 8:e649–e660
281. Shinada M, Saeki K, Yoshitake R, Eto S, Tsuboi M, Chambers JK et al (2020) Evaluation of epithelial and mesenchymal cell markers in canine urinary bladder transitional cell carcinoma. Vet J 266:105571
282. Shirahama T (2000) Cyclooxygenase-2 expression is up-regulated in transitional cell carcinoma and its preneoplastic lesions in the human urinary bladder. Clin Cancer Res 6(6):2424–2430
283. Shosu K, Sakurai M, Inoue K, Nakagawa T, Sakai H, Morimoto M et al (2016) Programmed cell death ligand 1 expression in canine cancer. In Vivo 30(3):195–204
284. Shrader S, Lauridson J, King Z, Loch J (2016) Urachal adenocarcinoma in a dog. J Comp Pathol 154(4):304–308
285. Siegel RL, Miller KD, Wagle NS, Jemal A (2023) Cancer statistics, 2023. CA Cancer J Clin 73(1):17–48
286. Sjödahl G, Jackson CL, Bartlett JM, Siemens DR, Berman DM (2019) Molecular profiling in muscle-invasive bladder cancer: more than the sum of its parts. J Pathol 247(5):563–573
287. Skinner OT, Boston SE, Maxwell PL (2020) Interventions and experience after complicated total cystectomy in a dog with transitional cell carcinoma. Vet Surg 49(4):811–817
288. Smith N, Luethcke KR, Craun K, Trepanier L (2022) Risk of bladder cancer and lymphoma in dogs is associated with pollution indices by county of residence. Vet Comp Oncol 20(1):246–255
289. Snyder A, Makarov V, Merghoub T, Yuan J, Zaretsky JM, Desrichard A et al (2014) Genetic basis for clini-

cal response to CTLA-4 blockade in melanoma. N Engl J Med 371(23):2189–2199
290. Sommer BC, Dhawan D, Ratliff TL, Knapp DW (2018) Naturally-occurring canine invasive urothelial carcinoma: a model for emerging therapies. Bladder Cancer 4(2):149–159
291. Sommer BC, Dhawan D, Ruple A, Ramos-Vara JA, Hahn NM, Utturkar SM et al (2021) Basal and luminal molecular subtypes in naturally-occurring canine urothelial carcinoma are associated with tumor immune signatures and dog breed. Bladder Cancer 7:317–333
292. Soria F, Krabbe LM, Todenhöfer T, Dobruch J, Mitra AP, Inman BA et al (2019) Molecular markers in bladder cancer. World J Urol 37(1):31–40
293. Stolker ALAM, Niesing W, Hogendoorn EA, Bisoen Rambali A, Vleeming W (2003) Determination of nicotine and cotinine in rat plasma by liquid chromatography-tandem mass spectrometry. J Chromatogr A 1020(1):35–43
294. Stone EA, George TF, Gilson SD, Page RL (1996) Partial cystectomy for urinary bladder neoplasia: surgical technique and outcome in 11 dogs. J Small Anim Pract 37(10):480–485
295. Suárez-Bonnet A, Herráez P, Aguirre M, Suárez-Bonnet E, Andrada M, Rodríguez F et al (2015) Expression of cell cycle regulators, 14-3-3σ and p53 proteins, and vimentin in canine transitional cell carcinoma of the urinary bladder. Urol Oncol 33(7):332.e1–332.e7
296. Sun D, Gao W, Hu H, Zhou S (2022) Why 90% of clinical drug development fails and how to improve it? Acta Pharm Sin B 12(7):3049–3062
297. Sweis RF, Spranger S, Bao R, Paner GP, Stadler WM, Steinberg G et al (2016) Molecular drivers of the non-T-cell-Inflamed tumor microenvironment in urothelial bladder cancer. Cancer Immunol Res 4(7):563–568
298. Szigetvari NM, Dhawan D, Ramos-Vara JA, Leamon CP, Klein PJ, Ruple AA et al (2018) Phase I/II clinical trial of the targeted chemotherapeutic drug, folate-tubulysin, in dogs with naurally-occurring invasive urothelial carcinoma. Oncotarget 9(97):37042–37053
299. Tabernero J, Bahleda R, Dienstmann R, Infante JR, Mita A, Italiano A et al (2015) Phase I dose-escalation study of JNJ-42756493, an oral pan-fibroblast growth factor receptor inhibitor, in patients with advanced solid tumors. J Clin Oncol 33(30):3401–3408
300. Tagawa M, Kurashima C, Takagi S, Maekawa N, Konnai S, Shimbo G et al (2018) Evaluation of costimulatory molecules in dogs with B cell high grade lymphoma. PLoS One 13(7):e0201222
301. Tagawa M, Tambo N, Maezawa M, Tomihari M, Watanabe KI, Inokuma H et al (2020) Quantitative analysis of the BRAF V595E mutation in plasma cell-free DNA from dogs with urothelial carcinoma. PLoS One 15(4):e0232365
302. Thomas R, Wiley CA, Droste EL, Robertson J, Inman BA, Breen M (2023) Whole exome sequencing analysis of canine urothelial carcinomas without BRAF V595E mutation: Short in-frame deletions in BRAF and MAP2K1 suggest alternative mechanisms for MAPK pathway disruption. PLoS Genet 19(4):e1010575
303. Thompson D, Lawrentschuk N, Bolton D (2023) New approaches to targeting epigenetic regulation in bladder cancer. Cancers (Basel) 15(6):1856
304. Toren P, Wilkins A, Patel K, Burley A, Gris T, Kockelbergh R et al (2023) The sex gap in bladder cancer survival – a missing link in bladder cancer care? Nat Rev Urol. https://doi.org/10.1038/s41585--023-00806-2. Epub ahead of print
305. Torres de la Riva G, Hart BL, Farver TB, Oberbauer AM, Messam LLM, Willits N et al (2013) Neutering dogs: effects on joint disorders and cancers in golden retrievers. PLoS One 8(2):e55937
306. Tsamouri MM, Steele TM, Mudryj M, Kent MS, Ghosh PM (2021) Comparative cancer cell signaling in muscle-invasive urothelial carcinoma of the bladder in dogs and humans. Biomedicine 9(10):1472
307. Tsuboi M, Sakai K, Maeda S, Chambers JK, Yonezawa T, Matsuki N et al (2019) Assessment of HER2 expression in canine urothelial carcinoma of the urinary bladder. Vet Pathol 56(3):369–376
308. Valli VE, Norris A, Jacobs RM, Laing E, Withrow S, Macy D et al (1995) Pathology of canine bladder and urethral cancer and correlation with tumour progression and survival. J Comp Pathol 113(2):113–130
309. van Osch FHM, Jochems SHJ, Wesselius A, van Schooten FJ, Bryan RT, Zeegers MP (2018) A stratified meta-analysis of the association between exposure to environmental tobacco smoke during childhood and adulthood and urothelial bladder cancer risk. Int J Environ Res Public Health 15(4):569
310. Varvil MS, Bailey T, Dhawan D, Knapp DW, Ramos-Vara JA, Dos Santos AP (2022) The miRNome of canine invasive urothelial carcinoma. Front Vet Sci 9:945638
311. Vignoli M, Rossi F, Chierici C, Terragni R, De Lorenzi D, Stanga M et al (2007) Needle tract implantation after fine needle aspiration biopsy (FNAB) of transitional cell carcinoma of the urinary bladder and adenocarcinoma of the lung. Schweiz Arch Tierheilkd 149(7):314–318
312. Villamil JA, Henry CJ, Hahn AW, Bryan JN, Tyler JW, Caldwell CW (2009) Hormonal and sex impact on the epidemiology of canine lymphoma. J Cancer Epidemiol 2009:591753
313. Vitti Gambim V, Laufer-Amorim R, Fonseca Alves RH, Grieco V, Fonseca-Alves CE (2020) A comparative Meta-analysis and in silico analysis of differentially expressed genes and proteins in canine and human bladder cancer. Front Vet Sci 7:558978
314. von der Maase H, Hansen SW, Roberts JT, Dogliotti L, Oliver T, Moore MJ et al (2000) Gemcitabine and cisplatin versus methotrexate, vinblastine, doxo-

rubicin, and cisplatin in advanced or metastatic bladder cancer: results of a large, randomized, multinational, multicenter, phase III study. J Clin Oncol 18(17):3068–3077
315. Wadhwa P, Goswami AK, Joshi K, Sharma SK (2005) Cyclooxygenase-2 expression increases with the stage and grade in transitional cell carcinoma of the urinary bladder. Int Urol Nephrol 37(1):47–53
316. Wallmeroth A, Wagner U, Moch H, Gasser TC, Sauter G, Mihatsch MJ (1999) Patterns of metastasis in muscle-invasive bladder cancer (pT2-4): An autopsy study on 367 patients. Urol Int 62(2):69–75
317. Walters L, Martin O, Price J, Sula MM (2018) Expression of receptor tyrosine kinase targets PDGFR-β, VEGFR2 and KIT in canine transitional cell carcinoma. Vet Comp Oncol 16(1):E117–E122
318. Wang X, Ji P, Zhang Y, LaComb JF, Tian X, Li E et al (2016) Aberrant DNA methylation: implications in racial health disparity. PLoS One 11(4):e0153125
319. Watanabe R, Tomita Y, Nishiyama T, Tanikawa T, Sato S (1994) Correlation of p53 protein expression in human urothelial transitional cell cancers with malignant potential and patient survival. Int J Urol 1(1):43–48
320. Wen L, Zhong G, Zhang Y, Zhong M (2022) Risk and prognosis of secondary bladder cancer after post-operative radiotherapy for gynecological cancer. Bosn J Basic Med Sci 22(3):471–480
321. Willeit P, Willeit J, Mayr A, Weger S, Oberhollenzer F, Brandstätter A et al (2010) Telomere length and risk of incident cancer and cancer mortality. JAMA 304(1):69–75
322. Williams JR, Ayscue JM (2023) Colorectal cancer screening: a review of current screening options, timing, and guidelines. J Surg Oncol 127(8):1236–1246
323. Wise CF, Hammel SC, Herkert N, Ma J, Motsinger-Reif A, Stapleton HM et al (2020) Comparative exposure assessment using silicone passive samplers indicates that domestic dogs are sentinels to support human health research. Environ Sci Technol 54(12):7409–7419
324. Wise CF, Hammel SC, Herkert NJ, Ospina M, Calafat AM, Breen M et al (2022) Comparative assessment of pesticide exposures in domestic dogs and their owners using silicone passive samplers and biomonitoring. Environ Sci Technol 56(2):1149–1161
325. Woldemeskel M (2017) Primary urinary bladder osteosarcoma in a dog. J Comp Pathol 157(2–3):141–144
326. Wolfe AJ, Toh E, Shibata N, Rong R, Kenton K, Fitzgerald M et al (2012) Evidence of uncultivated bacteria in the adult female bladder. J Clin Microbiol 50(4):1376–1383
327. Wong K, Abascal F, Ludwig L, Aupperle-Lellbach H, Grassinger J, Wright CW et al (2023) Cross-species oncogenomics offers insight into human muscle-invasive bladder cancer. Genome Biol 24(1):191
328. World Health Organization, International Agency for Research on Cancer (n.d.). https://www.iarc.who.int/cancer-type/bladder-cancer. Accessed 07 25/2023
329. Wu P, Zhang G, Zhao J, Chen J, Chen Y, Huang W et al (2018) Profiling the urinary microbiota in male patients with bladder cancer in china. Front Cell Infect Microbiol 8:167
330. Wülfing C, Machiels JPH, Richel DJ, Grimm MO, Treiber U, De Groot MR et al (2009) A single-arm, multicenter, open-label phase 2 study of lapatinib as the second-line treatment of patients with locally advanced or metastatic transitional cell carcinoma. Cancer 115(13):2881–2890
331. Xiong S, Huang W, Liu X, Chen Q, Ding Y, Huang H et al (2022) Celecoxib synergistically enhances MLN4924-induced cytotoxicity and EMT inhibition via AKT and ERK pathways in human urothelial carcinoma. Cell Transplant 31:9636897221077921
332. Yamasaki H, Uematsu Y, Hayashi Y, Yamashita M, Tei M, Uchida K et al (2022) Coincidence of v-raf murine sarcoma viral oncogene homolog B mutation (V595E) with phosphorylated v-raf murine sarcoma viral oncogene homolog B in urothelial carcinoma in dogs. Can J Vet Res 86(4):286–293
333. Yarchoan M, Hopkins A, Jaffee EM (2017) Tumor mutational burden and response rate to PD-1 inhibition. N Engl J Med 377(25):2500–2501
334. Yi L, Ai K, Li X, Li Z, Li Y (2022) Bone metastasis in bladder cancer. J Pers Med 13(1):54
335. Yoshitake R, Saeki K, Eto S, Shinada M, Nakano R, Sugiya H et al (2020) Aberrant expression of the COX2/PGE2 axis is induced by activation of the RAF/MEK/ERK pathway in BRAFV595E canine urothelial carcinoma. Sci Rep 10(1):7826
336. Yu Y, Sikorski P, Bowman-Gholston C, Cacciabeve N, Nelson KE, Pieper R (2015) Diagnosing inflammation and infection in the urinary system via proteomics. J Transl Med 13:111
337. Zaman A, Bivona TG (2022) Quantitative framework for bench-to-bedside cancer research. Cancers (Basel) 14(21):5254
338. Zeegers MP, Swaen GM, Kant I, Goldbohm RA, van den Brandt PA (2001) Occupational risk factors for male bladder cancer: results from a population based case cohort study in the Netherlands. Occup Environ Med 58(9):590–596
339. Zhang N, Li D, Shao J, Wang X (2015) Animal models for bladder cancer: the model establishment and evaluation (Review). Oncol Lett 9(4):1515–1519
340. Zhi Y, Ji H, Pan J, He P, Zhou X, Zhang H et al (2017) Downregulated XPA promotes carcinogenesis of bladder cancer via impairment of DNA repair. Tumour Biol 39(2):1010428317691679
341. Zhou J, Yang C, Lu Z, Zhang L, Yin Y, Tai S et al (2019) Primary urothelial carcinoma of the prostate: a rare case report. Medicine (Baltimore) 98(3):e14155

Melanoma

Philip J. Bergman and Jedd D. Wolchok

1 Introduction

Melanoma is a common cancer of dogs, especially those with significant amounts of skin pigmentation, but melanoma is relatively rare in cats [1]. The most common location for canine melanoma is the haired skin where they grossly appear to be small brown to black masses, but they can also appear as large, flat, and/or wrinkled masses [2, 3]. Primary melanomas can also occur in the oral cavity, nailbed, footpad, eye, gastrointestinal tract, nasal cavity, anal sac, or mucocutaneous junction [4–8]. Metastatic sites are numerous including lymph nodes (LNs), lungs, liver, meninges, and adrenal glands [1, 4, 9].

Melanoma arises from melanocytes, which are cells that generate pigment through the melanosome using a number of melanosomal glycoproteins. In humans, cutaneous melanoma can arise due to mutations induced by repeated, intense exposure to ultraviolet light (for example, frequent tanning or working outdoors). Melanoma is currently the most rapidly increasing incident human cancer [10, 11]. Significant recent research into the etiology of human melanoma suggests multiple causes independent of the aforementioned UV-associated mutagenesis [12, 13]. Since most breeds of dogs have a significant hair coat which likely affords them protection from sunlight, UV exposure is less likely to be a primary causative agent in the dog. Recent investigations have found differential expression of melanocytic markers in dogs across anatomic sites, suggesting melanocyte subpopulations, which may help better delineate melanoma pathogenetic mechanisms [14]. However, risk factors for canine melanoma are not well established.

The most common canine oral malignancy is melanoma [1–3, 15, 16]. Oral melanoma is most commonly diagnosed in Scottish terriers, golden retrievers, Chow Chows, poodles, and Dachshunds [3, 17–20]. Oral melanoma is more commonly seen in heavily pigmented breeds and is primarily a disease of older dogs without gender predilection, but may also be seen in younger dogs [17, 21, 22]. Differential diagnoses for oral tumors include squamous cell carcinoma, fibrosarcoma, osteosarcoma, acanthomatous ameloblastoma, and peripheral odontogenic fibroma [1–3, 16, 23–25]. Canine oral melanomas are found in the following locations by order of decreasing frequency: gingiva, lips, tongue, and hard palate [2, 3, 14, 15, 17]. Feline melanoma is

P. J. Bergman (✉)
Adjunct Associate Faculty, Memorial Sloan-Kettering Cancer Center, New York, NY, USA

Veterinary Program, Focused Ultrasound Foundation, Charlottesville, VA, USA

J. D. Wolchok
Meyer Director of the Sandra and Edward Meyer Cancer Center, Weill Cornell Medical College, Cornell University, New York, NY, USA

M. W. Nolan et al. (eds.), *Comparative Oncology*, https://doi.org/10.1007/978-3-032-04454-9_12

relatively rare, but appears to be malignant in most cases [1, 4, 26–33].

Melanomas in dogs have extremely diverse biologic behaviors depending on a large variety of factors. A greater understanding of these factors helps the clinician to determine the appropriate staging, treatment options, and prognosis. The primary factors which determine the biologic behavior of an oral melanoma in a dog are site, size, stage, and histologic parameters [1, 17, 21, 22, 34, 35]. Unfortunately, even with a comprehensive understanding of all of these factors, there are melanomas that have an unreliable biologic behavior; hence, the need for additional research into this relatively common, heterogeneous, and frequently aggressive tumor.

2 Pathology and Molecular Biology

Melanomas can at times be difficult to diagnose pathologically, especially anaplastic amelanotic melanomas which can masquerade as soft tissue sarcomas [36–38]. Numerous investigators have attempted to increase the precision of identifying melanomas, predominantly through immunohistochemical (IHC) or other expression means [20, 37, 39–42]. This has been accomplished through the use of multiple IHC assays or through the use of an IHC cocktail of antibodies. The use of PNL2, CD34, CALD1, and tyrosinase beyond the typical use of Melan A and S100 appears to hold particular promise [43–46]. As IHC cocktails are not always definitive and these biomarkers have differential expressions in various anatomic sites [14], these authors hope that genetic signature testing (e.g., through commercial platforms such as those currently offered by Vidium/Anivive, Vetomics, or Fidocure) may improve our abilities to obtain a definitive diagnosis in difficult cases and strongly recommend these be investigated for this unmet clinical need. An additional area of melanoma biomarker investigation that may lead to increased precision of diagnosis is through exosomal cargo identification, such as microRNA and, more specifically, novel small noncoding RNAs [47, 48].

The characterization of canine and feline melanomas by molecular means is significantly limited compared to the more comprehensive evaluation to date of human melanomas [49]. BRAF is a member of the MAPK signaling pathway which is commonly mutated in human cutaneous melanoma, but not in human oral melanoma [50]. Interestingly, BRAF mutations are also uncommon in canine oral malignant melanomas (MMs) [51]. However, downstream constitutive activation of ERK has been identified in both human and canine MMs [52], supporting the idea that certain canine and feline malignancies can have similar molecular signatures to human malignancies, in addition to their already well-known clinical similarities in the context of resistance to chemotherapy and/or radiation therapy (RT) and similar atypical sites of metastasis. A number of other investigators have reported a variety of molecular abnormalities and/or associations in canine and feline melanoma [1, 52–82].

A variety of possible new therapeutic targets in canine melanoma has been recently uncovered through molecular genetics, transcriptome, methylation, and T-cell immune profile analyses [83–107]. The melanoma-associated genes clustered in the areas of focal adhesion and PI3K-Akt (phosphoinositide 3-kinase/protein kinase B) signaling pathways, extracellular matrix-receptor interactions, protein digestion, and absorption, as well as TERT, MDM2, and CDK4. A small subset of dogs with malignant melanoma has *c-kit* gene mutations [62, 108–110], and therefore, the more routine use of *c-kit* mutation analysis by polymerase chain reaction (PCR) or IHC-based expression [111] of canine MMs, and subsequent use of KIT small molecule inhibitors (particularly in dogs with advanced stage disease and/or lack of response to Oncept™), should be considered. In one pilot study, 17 dogs with stage 3 or 4 MM were treated with the KIT inhibitor masitinib; the drug had mild at best effectiveness, with only 2 dogs experiencing a partial response [112]. These dogs did not have Kit status confirmed as an entry criterion, and the impact of advanced and late-stage disease is likely significant and should not deter future studies in this area. Lastly, with somatic mutations in KRAS, NRAS, PTEN, and others being found in canine MM [87, 92, 113, 114], similar to human melanoma hotspot sites, these may represent logical therapeutic targets.

3 Biologic Behavior and Prognostic Factors

The biologic behavior of canine oral melanoma is extremely variable and best characterized based on anatomic site, size, stage, and histologic parameters [1]. On divergent ends of the malignancy spectrum, a low-grade 0.5 cm haired-skin melanocytoma is highly likely to be cured with simple surgical excision, while a 5.0 cm high-grade oral MM has a poor to grave prognosis regardless of treatment options. Similar to the development of a rational staging, prognostic, and therapeutic plan for any tumor, two primary questions must be answered: what is the local invasiveness of the tumor and what is the metastatic potential? These will determine the prognosis and appropriate therapies.

The anatomic site of melanoma is highly, although not completely, predictive of local invasiveness and metastatic propensity. Melanomas involving the haired skin, which are not in proximity to mucosal margins, often, but not always, behave in a benign manner [2, 4, 115]. Surgical excision is often curative, but histopathologic examination is imperative for delineation of margins as well as a description of cytologic features. The use of Ki67 IHC has been reported previously to more reliably predict potential malignant behavior than classical histology for cutaneous melanoma [116].

Oral and mucosal melanoma has been routinely considered an extremely malignant tumor with a high degree of local invasiveness and high metastatic potential [3, 17, 21, 22, 34, 117, 118]. This biologic behavior is similar to human oral and mucosal melanoma [4, 119, 120]. Three studies have called this dogma into question and suggest benign oral melanomas can occur more frequently than previously thought [35, 121, 122]. Extreme caution is necessary when one receives a histopathology report suggesting a benign course with an oral melanoma as this author (PJB) has seen approximately 50 dogs over the last 20 years presenting with florid systemic metastases despite an original histopathology report suggesting benign disease. Similar to cutaneous melanoma, Ki67 appears to hold prognostic importance in canine oral melanoma as well [123].

The anatomic sites that split the opposite ends of the prognostic spectrum of generally benign acting, haired skin versus often malignant and metastatic oral/mucosal melanomas in dogs include melanomas of the digit and foot pad. Dogs with melanoma of the digits without LN or distant metastasis treated with digit amputation have reported median survival times (MSTs) of approximately 12 months, with 1- and 2-year survival rates of 42–57% and 11–13%, respectively [124, 125]. Metastasis at presentation is reported in approximately 30–40% of dogs [125, 126], and the majority of dogs with digit melanoma will develop regional or distant metastatic disease [124–126]. A recent study investigated the breeds involved with various canine digital lesions and as expected found a statistically significant increase in risk for digital MM in Rottweilers and Labrador Retrievers, but even more interestingly a statistically significant decreased risk in Dachshunds and Rhodesian Ridgebacks [87, 127]. This suggests that breed risks may vary depending on the anatomic site of their melanoma, and further studies on this topic are warranted [128].

The prognosis for dogs with melanoma of the foot pad has recently been investigated in 20 dogs and found an overall metastatic rate of 55% with a PFI of 101 days and MST of 240 days [129]. This author (PJB) has found this anatomic site to be anecdotally similar in metastatic potential and prognosis to digit melanoma and is finalizing a manuscript on the efficacy of Oncept in canine foot pad melanoma. Interestingly, human acral lentiginous melanoma (plantar surface of the foot, palms of the hand, and digit) also has an increased potential for metastasis [130].

The most exhaustive consensus reviews of prognostic factors in canine melanocytic neoplasms took a regimented, systematic approach to analyze the studies published to date in order to identify factors which appear to be repeatable, statistical, and therefore likely real, while also identifying areas where additional work is necessary due to incomplete data [131–134]. These studies have found that the most important histopathological prognostic factors include lymphatic invasion, distant metastasis, mitotic count, degree of pigmentation, presence of ulceration, level of nuclear atypia, level of invasion/infiltration, tumor thickness, and Ki67 index. For veterinary clinicians and/or researchers interested in canine melanoma, these publications are strongly recommended, and future histopathological specimens and studies should include an evaluation of these factors. A flurry of recent investigations has given us a much greater understanding of ocular melanoma and iridociliary cysts that are grossly similar to melanoma [7, 8, 135–139]. While Breslow thickness and Clark levels are highly prognostic in human cutaneous melanoma, their use in veterinary medicine is scant; however, a recent paper in canine cutaneous melanoma [140] suggests they may in fact be useful and additional studies in this area are hereby encouraged. The use of all this information by clinicians and pathologists will allow for the best determination of prognosis for a specific patient which then allows for identification of the most logical treatment plans.

4 Size and Stage

For dogs with oral melanoma, primary tumor size has been found to be extremely prognostic. The World Health Organization staging scheme for dogs with oral melanoma is based on local tumor size and regional and distant metastasis, with stage I being a nonmetastatic tumor <2 cm in diameter, stage II being a nonmetastatic tumor 2–4 cm in diameter, stage III being a tumor >4 cm in diameter and/or LN metastasis, and stage IV being a melanoma with distant metastasis (Fig. 1). Unfortunately, this schema works well on the human side with relatively uniform body surface area (BSA), while it may have limitations in veterinary medicine due to the highly various BSAs across different sizes of dogs. To better try to standardize this, some investigators are trying to standardize this based on head volume and other parameters, and these types of studies are further strongly encouraged [141]. The MSTs for dogs with oral melanoma treated with surgery are 511–874 days, 160–818 days, and 168–207 days with stage I, II, and III disease, respectively [21, 142]. More recent reports suggest dogs with stage I oral melanoma treated with standardized therapies, including surgery, RT, and/or chemotherapy, have a MST of approximately 12–14 months, with most dogs dying of distant metastatic disease and not local recurrence [143, 144]. Other investigators have found dogs with stage I oral melanoma have a median progression-free survival time (PFS) of 19 months [145].

5 Diagnostic Workup and Clinical Staging

The diagnosis and clinical staging of dogs with melanoma is relatively straightforward. A minimum database should include a thorough history and physical exam, complete blood count, biochemical profile, and urinalysis. While there are no typical constellation of bloodwork findings suggestive of the diagnosis of melanoma; however, similar to human melanoma, studies confirm that dogs with melanoma have elevations in serum lactate dehydrogenase (LDH) and C-reactive protein (CRP) [146, 147]. Furthermore, there appear to be numerous differences in tumor-associated macrophages and peripheral leukocyte ratios across melanocytomas vs. malignant melanoma [146, 148].

Gross characteristics of melanomas, such as pigmentation of mass, should raise the suspicion for a diagnosis of melanoma. Pigmented melanomas can be easily confirmed via fine needle aspiration (FNA) and cytology. In dogs, small (< 2 cm), mobile, well-circumscribed, slow-growing cutaneous melanomas tend to be benign and easily excisable, whereas large, poorly defined, ulcerated, and rapidly growing tumors can make surgical excision challenging. In the latter

T:	Primary Tumor	
	T1	Tumor ≤ 2 cm in diameter
	T2	Tumor 2–4 cm in diameter
	T3	Tumor > 4 cm in diameter
N:	Regional Lymph Nodes	
	N0	No evidence of regional node involvement
	N1	Histologic/cytologic evidence of regional node involvement
	N2	Fixed nodes
M:	Distant Metastasis	
	M0	No evidence of distant metastasis
	M1	Evidence of distant metastasis

Stage I = T1 N0 M0

Stage II = T2 N0 M0

Stage III = T2 N1 M0 or T3 N0 M0

Stage IV = Any T, Any N and M1

Fig. 1 Traditional World Health Organization TNM-based staging scheme for dogs with oral melanoma. T: Primary tumor. T1. Tumor ≤ 2 cm in diameter. T2. Tumor 2–4 cm in diameter. T3. Tumor >4 cm in diameter. N: Regional lymph nodes. N0. No evidence of regional node involvement. N1. Histologic/cytologic evidence of regional node involvement. N2. Fixed nodes. M: Distant metastasis. M0. No evidence of distant metastasis. M1. Evidence of distant metastasis. Stage I = T1 N0 M0. Stage II = T2 N0 M0. Stage III = T2 N1 M0 or T3 N0 M0. Stage IV = Any T, Any N, and M1

example, incisional biopsy and IHC can be an important part of the diagnostic workup, particularly if the mass is nonpigmented, to allow other tumor types to be ruled out and a diagnosis of melanoma confirmed.

Clinical staging tests routinely include evaluation of the regional LNs and assessment of the thoracic cavity with either three-view thoracic radiographs or thoracic CT scan [134]. The regional LNs should be assessed whether lymphadenomegaly is present or not. LN metastasis is present in approximately 70% of OMM dogs with lymphadenomegaly but, more importantly, in approximately 40% with normal-sized LNs [149]. FNA cytology of the ipsilateral regional LNs has been recommended to assess for nodal metastasis; however, the only generally accessible regional LN is the mandibular LN. This may provide misleading information as the lymphatic drainage of the head is complex and metastases to contralateral LNs have been documented [150, 151]. Furthermore, the mandibular LN can be normal when other LNs, such as the medial retropharyngeal or parotid LN, are metastatic [152]. While earlier studies showed a high concordance of cytology and histopathology in dogs with melanomas, a recent study highlighted discordance between cytology findings and histopathology with a low correlation between the final cytology and histopathology reports in dogs with melanocytic neoplasia [152, 153]. As a result, histologic examination of the LN is recommended either through excision of the major LNs of the head and neck and/or sentinel LN (SLN) mapping [154–156]. Further studies to document best staging practices are highly warranted as the variability across clinicians is significant [134, 157].

Non-discriminate extirpation of the regional LNs of the head and neck has been described in dogs and cats with malignant oral tumors [158, 159]. One approach describes ipsilateral extirpation of the parotid, mandibular, and retropharyngeal LNs, but this requires an extensive dissection and does not investigate the contralateral LNs. A second approach involves extirpation of the left and right mandibular and medial retropharyngeal LNs through a single incision, but does not investigate the parotid LNs [159]. The limitations of both approaches include more extensive dissections and incomplete testing of the regional LNs; hence, there is a risk of postoperative complications and missed metastatic LNs.

SLN mapping allows identification of the direct lymphatic drainage pathway from the tumor to the first draining LN. This LN can then be targeted for selective lymphadenectomy and histopathologic testing. Selective lymphadenectomy avoids the indiscriminate extirpation of multiple LNs because it is a less extensive surgical dissection and reduces the risk of postoperative complications. The use of SLN mapping and lymphadenectomy has been proven to be of diagnostic, prognostic, and clinical benefit in human melanoma [156]. Relatively few investigations have been reported to date for SLN mapping and/or excision for dogs with malignancies [155, 160–162], and the authors strongly encourage additional investigation and clinical adoption in this area.

While not commonly described, abdominal ultrasonography or CT scans should be considered in dogs with melanomas arising from the oral cavity, digits, or pads because of the risk of metastasis to the abdominal LNs, liver, adrenal glands, and other intra-abdominal sites. The use of novel staging modalities, such as gallium citrate scintigraphy, requires further investigation [163].

Cross-sectional imaging (i.e., CT scans or MRI) is critical for surgical planning for oral melanoma, especially melanomas involving the maxilla and caudal mandible. This allows for assessment of the extent of tumor, invasion into soft tissues, bone and the nasal cavity, and assessment of regional LNs, particularly the aforementioned non-palpable medial retropharyngeal, parotid, and buccal LNs [164]. While not routinely available in veterinary medicine, positron emission tomography (PET) scans appear to be more sensitive than CT alone for detection of lymph node metastasis [165].

6 Treatment

6.1 Surgery

Surgery is the most effective local treatment modality for melanoma. Unfortunately, there are relatively few validated and/or objective data available to guide decision making for appropriate surgical margin width for resection of melanomas. Benign cutaneous tumors are typically completely excised with 1 cm skin margins (and ideally one fascial plane for deep margins). Given the invasive nature of MMs, wide margins (2–3 cm) are ideal whenever possible; however, for oral melanomas, wide margins may not be possible due to the limited amount of adjacent normal tissues. In these cases, surgery may need to be combined with RT for adequate local tumor control. Generally, 1–2 cm margins are adequate for complete histologic excision of MMs with well-defined borders. Wider margins are usually possible with cutaneous and digit melanomas [1, 134].

Resection of oral melanomas arising from the gingiva or mucosa in close proximity to the bone often requires partial mandibulectomy or maxillectomy [16]. Resecting a gingival mass without taking underlying bone because bone invasion is not observed is not recommended as this often does not obtain adequate local control (ALC) [1, 134]. Tumors that do occur in mucosal areas that are not adjacent to bone (e.g., buccal mucosa) or originate in the lip or tongue are amenable to excision of the soft tissues only. Complete histologic excision of oral tumors has been shown to significantly impact prognosis in multiple studies [145, 166–168]. Dogs with incomplete histologic excision appear to be approximately four times more likely to die from tumor-related causes compared to dogs with complete histologic excision [168].

Furthermore, dogs with tumors caudal to the third premolar tooth (PM3) were also approximately four times more likely to die from tumor-related causes compared to dogs with tumors located rostral to PM3.

Cross-sectional imaging and increased availability of surgical oncologic training have translated into a greater likelihood of complete histologic excisions. Surgical goals are often driven by clinical stage, tumor location, owner preferences, and the ability of the surgeon to perform a wide resection in locations where surgery is difficult. Poorly planned or limited attempts at excision should not be made whenever possible as these will often leave either residual gross or microscopic disease, result in rapid tumor recurrence, and likely decrease the ability to reach ALC. The first chance to operate with normal anatomy is invariably the best chance to achieve complete histologic excision with ALC. Quality of life is usually very good with mandibulectomy or maxillectomy, and most dogs resume eating within 3–4 days of surgery. Following mandibulectomy and maxillectomy, owner satisfaction with functional and cosmetic results is high [169]. Functional outcomes with single-digit amputation are excellent, and surgeries requiring excision of more than one digit are also tolerated very well and result in a good functional outcome [170, 171].

When tumors are deemed to not be amenable to wide resection, and when resection results in incomplete histologic margins, the combination of surgery with RT or RT alone with or without adjuvant therapies should be considered. Electrochemotherapy [172, 173] also appears to potentially be beneficial in stage 1 or 2 OMM, but strong arguments can be made that these patients are highly likely to have ALC with appropriate surgery. While surgery has not been typically recommended in the presence of loco-regional nodal metastatic disease, the role of adjuvant therapy in conjunction with cytoreductive surgery is being investigated for metastatic melanoma in people and such approaches are now being explored in dogs [174, 175].

6.2 Radiation Therapy

Radiation therapy (RT) plays a crucial role in the management and treatment of many canine and feline oral melanomas [1]. RT is often used for the purpose of achieving locoregional tumor control when surgery is not able to obtain ALC. RT may be utilized as both a primary and adjuvant therapy with hypofractionated and finely fractionated protocols being reported [28, 143, 144, 176–181].

While melanoma has been generally thought to be a relatively radioresistant tumor type necessitating a higher dose in each fraction to achieve local control, this is controversial [182]. Most published protocols in dogs and cats have used relatively high dose per fraction protocols, although the relative radiosensitivity of melanoma in companion animal species has not been determined and the ideal dose per fraction is unknown [1]. Hypofractionated protocols have the advantage of fewer treatments with fewer anesthetic episodes, lower cost, and less time commitment for the owner. These protocols also result in less severe acute effects. The main disadvantage of hypofractionated protocols is that they typically deliver a lower total dose, which may translate to a lower biologically effective dose with lower rates of local control and an increased risk for late side effects. To reduce that risk for dogs with a better prognosis, lower dose per fraction protocols can be considered. Most veterinary radiation oncologists will treat both the primary tumor and the regional LNs, including the mandibular and medial retropharyngeal LNs [1, 134]. These LNs are generally included because, as noted earlier in this chapter, normal-sized LNs do not preclude the possibility of metastasis [149].

The ranges of partial and complete responses with RT in the treatment of canine melanoma are ~20–70%, yielding an overall response rate of ~80–95% [1, 143, 178, 179, 181]. Responses are often rapid with dramatic decreases in tumor volume seen within several weeks of starting therapy for gross melanomas. The PFS has ranged from ~3 to 9 months [143, 177, 183, 184]. The longest reported PFS was from a study where all dogs had surgery in conjunction with RT. [183] Local recurrence rates after RT of ~26–27% have been reported following the treatment of microscopic disease, while local progression was reported in ~45% of dogs following RT of macroscopic disease [143, 177, 184].

The MSTs for dogs treated with RT range from ~5 to 15 months [1, 143, 144, 177–181, 184]. The existing literature describes a variety of RT protocols, equipment, and adjuvant therapies in myriad retrospective scenarios, but an ideal RT regimen has not been identified [1, 134]. Protocols have been published with 12–19 daily fractions of 2–4 Gy each, 4 Gy per fraction three times weekly for 4 weeks, 6 Gy per fraction twice weekly for 2.5–3 weeks, 6 Gy per fraction once weekly for 4 or 6 weeks, 8 Gy per fraction once weekly for three or four fractions, 9 Gy per fraction once weekly for four fractions, and 10 Gy per fraction once weekly for three fractions. Recently, stereotactic body radiotherapy has been introduced as a way to condense these protocols and enable delivery of large fractional doses in a shorter timeframe while limiting morbidity via high conformity; however, as of yet, there are no published reports describing clinical outcomes with such approaches.

Five cats with oral melanoma treated with RT have been reported [28]. There was one complete response and two partial responses with a MST of 146 days. Three cats received adjuvant treatment, one cat with carboplatin, one cat with carboplatin and mitoxantrone, and one cat with a DNA-based vaccine.

Chemotherapy may play a role in the management of dogs and cats with MMs treated with RT, either as a radiation sensitizer and/or to prevent or delay the onset of distant metastatic disease. When dogs with incompletely excised oral melanomas were treated with a radiation protocol consisting of six once-weekly 6 Gy fractions given along with either cisplatin (10–30 mg/m^2 IV) or carboplatin (90 mg/m^2 IV) once weekly approximately 1 hour before receiving RT, the local recurrence rate was 15%, the median time to metastasis was 10 months, and the MST was approximately 12 months [144]. These results were likely favorably biased as the vast majority of dogs had T1 stage melanomas.

Studies have examined using adjuvant chemotherapy with RT, and in general it can be concluded that addition of chemotherapy to RT does not measurably improve outcomes; this recapitulates the lack of efficacy of postoperative adjuvant chemotherapy in this disease [143, 144, 185]. However, other studies suggest that there may be a role for chemotherapy in the treatment of oral melanoma in combination with RT. In 17 dogs with oral melanoma treated with surgery and carboplatin, including 11 dogs also treated with RT, the overall median PFS (259 days) and MST (440 days) for dogs did not significantly change when RT was added to the treatment protocol [183]. Local recurrence rates, however, were lower in the RT group (27%) compared to dogs not treated with RT (67%). In a prospective study of RT +/− adjuvant temozolomide [184], both groups had similar overall response rates of ~80% with median time to progression (TTP) significantly longer in dogs treated with RT and temozolomide (205 days) compared to dogs treated with RT alone (110 days). One pilot study has examined a combination radio-immunotherapy approach which appears safe and feasible for future investigations [186].

Prognostic factors have been identified in dogs with oral melanoma treated with RT. [1] The size of the irradiated oral melanoma is prognostic in several studies. In one study, the overall median PFS was approximately 8 months [177]. T1 lesion dogs had a median PFS of ~11 months, whereas dogs with T2 and T3 lesions had median PFS of only ~6 months. The most common cause of failure in this study was distant metastasis rather than local tumor recurrence. In another study, dogs with oral tumors less than 5 cm^3 were more likely to achieve a complete response and have significantly better MST than dogs with larger tumors [179]. In a retrospective study of the Veterinary Society for Surgical Oncology (VSSO) in which dogs were treated with a variety of different radiation protocols and adjuvant treatments, dogs with stage I disease had a significantly longer MST (758 days) compared to stage II (278 days), stage III (163 days), and stage IV (80 days) dogs. Dogs without radiographic evidence of bone invasion had significantly longer times to first event and overall survival times than dogs with radiographic evidence of bone changes [143]. One plausible explanation for reduced efficacy for RT in melanomas with bony involvement is intra-osseous hypoxia [84, 114, 187]. However, bony involvement has been reported in the majority of dogs with oral melanoma [143, 188]. Studies have examined the genetic and transcriptomic landscape of canine MM RT responses and are likely to bear fruit on new therapeutic targets [189, 190].

7 Chemotherapy and Immunotherapy

Systemic therapy is indicated in dogs with a moderate to high metastatic risk, such as dogs with oral, digit, or pad melanomas, and dogs with cutaneous MM with a high tumor score and/or increased proliferation index through increased Ki-67 expression [1, 134]. Chemotherapy does not seem to have a role in the management of dogs with MM. Overall response rates for dogs with measurable disease are largely disappointing, especially with single-agent dacarbazine, melphalan, vinorelbine, or doxorubicin [191–193], with the highest reported overall response rates being 18% for dogs treated with cisplatin and piroxicam [194] and 28% for dogs treated with carboplatin [195]. Furthermore, the majority of responses are short-lived. More recently and importantly, multiple retrospective studies investigating the role of chemotherapy in the adjuvant setting following either surgery or RT found no significant differences in outcomes with the addition of chemotherapy to the treatment protocol [143–145, 180, 185]. Other non-immunologic antiproliferative and/or pro-differentiation approaches have included lupeol or targeting SET/I2PP2A, proteasomes, and SINE (selective inhibitor of nuclear export) [196–200]. These studies suggest the recently conditionally approved twice-weekly oral product Laverdia-CA1 (for dogs with lymphoma) from Dechra/Anivive may have activity against melanoma if it garners full FDA approval.

While it can be effectively argued that the studies performed to date to evaluate the activity of chemotherapy in an adjuvant setting for canine melanoma have been suboptimal due to a variety of reasons, the human literature is extensive, and this suggests melanoma is an extremely chemotherapy-resistant tumor [183, 201]. It is clear that new approaches to the systemic treatment of this disease are desperately needed.

One potential clinical therapy avenue which has been minimally reported on to date in canine or feline melanoma is the use of cyclooxygenase (COX)-2 inhibitors. A number of authors have investigated the expression of COX-2 and neurokinin-1 (NK-1) in canine melanoma and/or melanoma cell lines and found positive correlations of expression to proliferation and survival [78, 79, 202–208]. Studies investigating the clinical responsiveness of canine melanoma to COX-2 inhibitors (and potential correlation to COX-2 expression) and/or NK-1 antagonists, such as maropitant, are required. Other modalities reported for local tumor control as case reports and/or case series include intralesional cisplatin implants, intralesional bleomycin with electronic pulsing, and many others, but widespread use has not been reported to date [172, 209–214].

Immunotherapy represents one potential systemic therapeutic strategy for the adjuvant treatment of malignant melanoma [1, 134]. A variety of older immunotherapeutic strategies for the treatment of human melanoma have been reported with typically poor outcomes due to a lack of breaking tolerance. Immunotherapy targets and strategies to date in canine melanoma have used autologous tumor cell vaccines (with or without transfection with immunostimulatory cytokines and/or melanosomal differentiation antigens); allogeneic tumor cell vaccines transfected with interleukin 2 or granulocyte macrophage colony-stimulating factor (GM-CSF); liposomal-encapsulated nonspecific immunostimulators (e.g., L-MTP-PE); intralesional Fas ligand DNA; siRNA (small interfering) against the survivin and/or Bcl-2 genes; bacterial superantigen approaches with GM-CSF or interleukin

2 as immune adjuvants; polyethylene glycol (PEG)ylated TNF-α; suicide gene therapy; adenovector CD40 ligand; chondroitin sulfate proteoglycan 4 (CSPG4); IL-12; IFN-β; re-engineered anthrax toxin; GD3; and lastly canine dendritic cell vaccines loaded with melanosomal differentiation antigens [21, 142, 188, 200, 215–242]. Although these approaches have produced some clinical antitumor responses, the methodologies for the generation of these products are often expensive, time-consuming, sometimes dependent on patient tumor samples being established into cell lines, and fraught with the difficulties of consistency, reproducibility, and other quality control issues, and none are currently commercially available [1, 134, 175, 243]. Furthermore, we now more fully understand the native immune dysregulation potentially induced by the malignancy through increased T regulatory (Treg) cells which suppress antitumor responses [105, 244, 245].

The advent of DNA vaccination circumvents many of the previously encountered hurdles in vaccine development. DNA is relatively inexpensive and simple to purify in large quantities. The antigen of interest is cloned into a bacterial expression plasmid with a constitutively active promoter. The plasmid is introduced into the skin or muscle with an intradermal or intramuscular injection. Once in the skin or muscle, professional antigen presenting cells, particularly dendritic cells, are able to present the transcribed and translated antigen in the proper context of major histocompatibility complex and costimulatory molecules. Although DNA vaccines have induced immune responses to viral proteins, vaccinating against tissue-specific self-proteins on cancer cells is clearly a more difficult problem. One way to induce immunity against a tissue-specific differentiation antigen on cancer cells is to vaccinate with xenogeneic antigen or DNA that is homologous to the cancer antigen. Vaccination with DNA encoding cancer differentiation antigens is ineffective when self DNA is used, but tumor immunity can be induced by orthologous DNA from another species [246].

A xenogeneic DNA vaccine program for melanoma was developed in collaboration with human cancer investigators from Memorial Sloan-Kettering Cancer Center [247, 248]. Preclinical and clinical studies showed that xenogeneic DNA vaccination with tyrosinase family members (e.g., tyrosinase, GP100, GP75) produced immune responses resulting in tumor rejection or protection with prolonged survival times, while syngeneic vaccination with orthologous DNA did not induce an immune response [249]. While tyrosinase may not appear to be a preferred target in amelanotic canine melanoma due to poor expression when assessed by IHC [36], more appropriate and/or sensitive PCR-based studies and other IHC-based studies document significant tyrosinase overexpression in melanotic and amelanotic melanomas across species [20, 44, 250–253]. These studies provided the impetus for development of a xenogeneic tyrosinase DNA vaccine program in canine MM. The antibody and T-cell responses in dogs vaccinated biweekly for a total of four vaccinations with human tyrosinase (huTyr) demonstrated antigen-specific IFNγ T cells with 2- to fivefold increases in circulating antibodies to huTyr which can cross-react to canine tyrosinase, suggesting the breaking of tolerance [247, 254]. The clinical results with prolongation in survival have been reported previously [248, 255].

The results of these trials demonstrate that xenogeneic DNA vaccination in canine MM: (1) is safe, (2) leads to the development of anti-tyrosinase antibodies and T cells, (3) is potentially therapeutic, and (4) is an attractive candidate for further evaluation in an adjuvant, minimal residual disease phase II setting for canine MM. Based on these studies, a multi-institutional safety and efficacy trial compared 58 prospectively enrolled dogs with surgically resected stage II and III oral melanomas treated with adjuvant HuTyr-based canine melanoma vaccine (Oncept®, Merial, Inc. and now Boehringer Animal Health, Inc.) to a historical control group of 53 dogs [256]. Dogs treated with Oncept® had a significantly better outcome; the MST for dogs in the historical group was 324 days compared to an MST which was not reached in the vaccinated group because only

26% of vaccinated dogs died as a result of their disease [256]. Ottnod and colleagues performed a single-site retrospective study on 30 dogs with stage II–III oral malignant melanoma (15 each with and without use of Oncept®). They determined that those dogs receiving Oncept® did not achieve a greater progression-free survival, disease-free interval, or median survival time than dogs that did not receive the vaccine [257]. Contrary to the aforementioned prospective USDA 5-site licensure trial [259], this study had <35% of cases treated surgically with margins of 1 mm or more, suggesting a significant lack of ALC. Furthermore, contrary to the aforementioned prospective USDA 5-site licensure trial, the Ottnod et al. study, similar to other noncontrolled retrospective studies, either had a wide variety of other treatments utilized in both the non-vaccinate and vaccinate groups, had small numbers of patients investigated, and/or the cause (in the context of local or distant disease) of death and/or progression of disease was not reported [145, 258–260]. Not surprisingly, the smaller poorly controlled retrospective studies do not appear to mirror the results seen in larger and more highly controlled studies. A large study by Turek and colleagues has confirmed the importance of ALC when using adjuvant Oncept® for treatment of dogs with MM [261].

The concurrent use of RT and Oncept® has been investigated in dogs with oral MM [262]. This pilot study determined that concurrent use was well tolerated with no unexpected toxicities. Oncept® also appears to be safe for use in cats, horses, and penguins [263–265]. Human clinical trials utilizing various xenogeneic melanosomal antigens as DNA (or peptide with adjuvant) vaccination have begun; however, most current studies are utilizing checkpoint inhibitors [249, 266, 267].

Further evidence for the efficacy of immunotherapy for the treatment of canine oral melanoma has been shown in clinical trials with CSPG4 vaccination [188, 231, 234, 268–270]. In a controlled prospective study of dogs with stage II or III oral MM, 19 dogs were treated with surgical resection only and 23 dogs were treated with surgical resection and adjuvant CSPG4 vaccination. The outcomes were significantly better in the vaccinated group. The median disease-free interval, MST, and 1- and 2-year survival rates in the vaccinated group were 477 days, 684 days, and 73.9% and 30.4%, respectively, compared to 180 days, 200 days, and 26.3% and 5.3%, respectively, in the non-vaccinated group [231].

The role of xenogeneic DNA vaccination in the adjuvant management of dogs with digit MM and a penguin with nasal MM has also been investigated [264, 271]. A staging scheme for digit MM was developed based on tumor size, tumor depth, bone involvement, and presence of nodal and distant metastatic disease. A T1 digit melanoma was defined as <2 cm diameter and superficial or exophytic; a T2 tumor was defined as 2–5 cm in diameter with minimal invasion; a T3 digit melanoma was defined as >5 cm or invading the subcutaneous tissue; and a T4 tumor was defined as invading fascia or bone. Stage I was defined as nonmetastatic T1 digit melanoma; stage II as nonmetastatic T2 digit melanoma; stage III as nonmetastatic T3 or T4 digit melanoma and/or LN metastasis; and stage IV was defined as distant metastasis [271]. Treatment of dogs with digit melanoma with digit amputation and adjuvant Oncept® resulted in significantly improved outcomes compared to historical outcomes with digit amputation only [271]. Dogs presenting with metastatic disease had a significantly worse MST (105 days) than dogs without evidence of metastatic disease at presentation (533 days), with a 3-year survival rate of 48% in the latter group. The clinical staging scheme was also prognostic with MSTs of >952 days, > 1093 days, 321 days, and 76 days for dogs with stage I, II, III, and IV disease, respectively [271].

A critical review of the canine oral melanoma treatment literature was recently published [272, 274]. They reviewed 81 studies and found the overall evidence was low, and they recommended future use of prospective, randomized, and double-blinded clinical trials without confounding factors. The author (PJB) completely agrees with these recommendations; however, the reality of veterinary medicine rarely allows this due to myriad factors, especially those financially based.

8 Melanoma Comparative Oncology

Tumor immunology and immunotherapy is one of the most exciting and rapidly expanding fields at present with major advances occurring in patients with melanoma. Significant resources are focused on mechanisms to simultaneously maximally stimulate an antitumor immune response while minimizing the immunosuppressive aspects of the tumor microenvironment [273]. The recent elucidation and blockade of immunosuppressive cytokines (e.g., TGF-β, IL-10, and IL-13) and/or the negative costimulatory molecule CTLA-4 [105, 274–276] and PD-1 (Programmed Cell Death 1 or CD279) [277] along with the functional characterization of myeloid-derived suppressor cells (MDSC) and T regulatory cells [147, 278–281], have dramatically improved cell-mediated immunity to tumors by "taking the brake" off the immune system. Immunotherapy is unlikely to become a sole modality in the treatment of cancer as the traditional modalities of surgery, radiation, and/or chemotherapy are extremely likely to be used in combination with immunotherapy in the future. Like any form of anticancer treatment, immunotherapy appears to work best in a minimal residual disease setting, suggesting its most appropriate use will be in an adjuvant setting with local tumor therapies such as surgery and/or radiation [282]. Similarly, the long-held belief that chemotherapy (non-corticosteroid) attenuates immune responses from cancer vaccines is beginning to be disproven through investigations on a variety of levels [283, 284].

The aforementioned greatly expanded molecular understanding of the immune system has recently translated into human melanoma (and other histologies) immunotherapeutics which confer a survival benefit such as the use of the checkpoint inhibitor anti-CTLA-4 Ab, ipilimumab (Yervoy®, Bristol-Myers Squibb) and the selective BRAF inhibitors, vemurafenib (Zelboraf®, Genetech) and dabrafenib (GSK2118436, GlaxoSmithKline), in patients who are BRAF V600 mutation positive [120]. Currently, FDA-approved antibodies directed against another checkpoint inhibitor known as PD-1 receptor or against human PDL-1 (L = ligand) such as Nivolumab (Opdivo®, Bristol-Myers Squibb) and Pembrolizumab (Keytruda®, Merck) have generated the most excitement due to ~20–30% of human patients having durable objective tumor responses [277, 285]. The highest objective tumor response rates have been seen to date in patients treated with concurrent PD-1 and CTLA-4 checkpoint inhibitors [277, 286–288]. Furthermore, pembrolizumab was given FDA approval for unresectable or metastatic, microsatellite instability-high (MSI-H) or mismatch repair deficient (dMMR) solid tumors that have progressed following prior treatment [289]. This is truly revolutionary as it represents the first cancer-agnostic FDA approval and is one of many recent FDA approvals based on single-arm studies. A recent veterinary study has found as expected a high tumor mutational burden in canine melanoma, osteosarcoma and hemangiosarcoma [290]. Recently, the USDA has granted conditional licensure to Merck for their canine anti-PD1 monoclonal antibody, Gilvetmab; it is labeled for use in canine melanoma and mast cell tumors, and pivotal clinical studies are ongoing.

There are currently over 100 different checkpoint inhibitors in development and the immuno-oncology (IO) "pendulum" has swung from the previous primarily target-dependent approaches to the current checkpoint inhibitor target-independent approach. The IO pendulum over time is likely to come back to the middle with a concurrent target-dependent approach (i.e., vaccine or similar) alongside target-independent checkpoint inhibitors [291, 292]. Unfortunately, very few biomarkers of response with these clinically important agents have been found to date except for changes in the patient gastrointestinal microbiome and tumors which generate numerous neoantigens from tumor-specific mutations [293–296]. This further highlights why pembrolizumab was given FDA approval for MSI-H or dMMR solid tumors as these tumors "throw off" comparatively much higher numbers of neoantigens. A new and highly innovative personalized human cancer vaccine taking advantage of this biomarker-based approach utilizes the neoantigens specific to that individual's cancer, as they are not present in normal tissues and are highly immunogenic [297].

Another area of extreme promise in IO is a form of adoptive cell therapy called CAR-T (Chimeric Antigen Receptor-T cells). T cells are harvested from a patient and then genetically engineered to express a CAR on their cell surface with expansion in vitro before being reinfused back into the patient [300]. This CAR is specifically designed to recognize a specific TAA with a domain responsible for activating the T cell when the CAR-T binds its TAA. The latest generations of CAR-T are engineered to contain important costimulatory domains that further enhance the immune response against the cancer cell containing the TAA. On August 30, 2017, the FDA approved Tisagenlecleucel (Kymriah®, Novartis), a CAR-T therapy utilizing CD19 as its CAR of choice. Many CAR-T studies have found >80–90% objective tumor responses, but side effects, including death, can occur [298]. Furthermore, CAR-Ts are currently difficult to make and carry a high cost of goods to produce, making for a difficult, but not impossible, commercial development path in veterinary medicine [299–301]. Checkpoints, checkpoint inhibitors, and other adoptive cell transfer technologies like CAR-T and others are also starting to be better understood and pursued in veterinary diseases with early signals of clinical benefit [208, 302–322]. Furthermore, the exciting race to develop commercial veterinary-specific IO therapeutics like checkpoint inhibitors, CAR-T, and other adoptive cell approaches is currently ongoing with a handful of animal health companies. One adoptive cell approach was recently approved by USDA-CVB from Elias Animal Health for dogs with osteosarcoma [322]. As these therapeutics reduce immune tolerance and more easily generate specific antitumor immune responses in patients, pathologic autoimmunity was predicted and is now being seen clinically in human patients as a side effect [286, 323, 324].

9 Human Melanoma

The past 15 years have witnessed a significant change in available treatments as well as expected outcomes for human melanoma patients. In general, these advances have come in two distinct categories, immunologic checkpoint blockade and targeted pathway inhibition. Both of these areas of progress represent instances in which years of basic science research have yielded important data that provided a foundation for therapeutic development.

The potential for immune control of melanoma has been the subject of preclinical and clinical research for decades. Indeed, the use of high-dose interleukin-2 (IL-2) resulted in a small subset of patients (~5%) demonstrating long-term survival [325]. Since IL-2's action is not on the tumor cell itself, but rather as a growth and differentiating factor for T cells, this serves as a good initial proof of principle that the immune system could, under some circumstances, control an otherwise fatal malignancy. With a greater understanding of molecular mechanisms controlling T cell activation and immune homeostasis, the CTLA-4 and PD-1 pathways became the subject of therapeutic development. CTLA-4 blockade with ipilimumab, a fully human IgG1 antibody, was the first intervention shown to improve overall survival in metastatic melanoma in humans in a randomized trial [326]. Subsequently, PD-1 blockade with pembrolizumab [327, 328] or nivolumab [328] was shown to have significant clinical activity. Further, the combination of ipilimumab and nivolumab was shown to have a high frequency of clinical responses (53–60%), albeit in the context of a high incidence of immune-related adverse events [285, 329, 330]. All of these agents and combination regimens are now approved by the US FDA for use in treating distantly metastatic or unresectable regionally advanced melanoma. The most recent data indicate that patients initially treated with the combination of ipilimumab and nivolumab in the phase 3 Checkmate-067 trial have a median survival of 72 months [288, 331], a striking change from the 6–7 month median that was routinely observed in the era before checkpoint blockade or targeted therapy. Another major insight which arose from the above studies was the relationship between TMB and response to immunotherapy, based on the idea that mutational neoantigens give rise to a baseline immune response that is non-therapeutic until a checkpoint-blocking antibody allows for supraphysiologic immune function [332]. More recently, The US FDA approved a combination of a monoclonal antibody blocking another immune checkpoint, Lag-3 (relatlimab), in a fixed-dose combination with the PD-1 blocking antibody (nivolumab) in patients with melanoma [333]. The toxicity profile of this combination is more favorable than the ipilimumab + nivolumab combination, but no comparative efficacy data are available.

The feasibility of high throughput next-generation sequencing has given rise to the ability to classify melanomas based on a small number of oncogenic driver mutations. The most frequent of these conserved mutations involve the BRAF kinase gene, and there are now three approved pairs of BRAF and MEK inhibitors that each provides substantial responses with reasonable toxicity profiles. Although the emergence of resistance is common, there is a subset of ~20% of patients who show durable disease control at 5 years with targeted therapy [334]. New approaches are being developed for addressing other oncogenic drivers such as NRAS [335].

References

1. Bergman PK, Kent M, Selmic L (2019) Melanoma. In: Vail DM, Thamm DH, Liptak JM (eds) Withrow & MacEwen's small animal clinical oncology. Elsevier. https://doi.org/10.1016/C2016-0-01939-3
2. Goldschmidt MH (1994) Pigmented lesions of the skin. Clin Dermatol 12:507–514
3. Goldschmidt MH (1985) Benign and malignant melanocytic neoplasms of domestic animals. Am J Dermatopathol 7(Suppl):203–212
4. Smith SH, Goldschmidt MH, McManus PM (2002) A comparative review of melanocytic neoplasms. Vet Pathol 39:651–678
5. Lemetayer J, Al-Dissi A, Tryon K et al (2017) Primary intranasal melanoma with brain invasion in a dog. Can Vet J 58:391–396
6. Vinayak A, Frank CB, Gardiner DW et al (2017) Malignant anal sac melanoma in dogs: eleven cases (2000 to 2015). J Small Anim Pract 58:231–237
7. Wang AL, Kern T (2015) Melanocytic ophthalmic neoplasms of the domestic veterinary species: a review. Top Companion Anim Med 30:148–157
8. Moreira MVL, Langohr IM, Campos MRA et al (2022) Canine and feline uveal melanocytic tumours: histologic and immunohistochemical characteristics of 32 cases. Vet Med Sci 8:1036–1048
9. Razmara AM, Wittenburg LA, Al-Nadaf S et al (2022) Prevalence and clinicopathologic features of canine metastatic melanoma involving the central nervous system: a retrospective analysis and comparative review. Front Oncol 12:868004
10. Leiter U, Garbe C (2008) Epidemiology of melanoma and nonmelanoma skin cancer–the role of sunlight. Adv Exp Med Biol 624:89–103
11. Erdmann F, Lortet-Tieulent J, Schuz J et al (2013) International trends in the incidence of malignant melanoma 1953-2008–are recent generations at higher or lower risk? Int J Cancer 132:385–400
12. Ragnarsson-Olding BK (2011) Spatial density of primary malignant melanoma in sun-shielded body sites: a potential guide to melanoma genesis. Acta Oncol 50:323–328
13. Gillard M, Cadieu E, De BC et al (2014) Naturally occurring melanomas in dogs as models for non-UV pathways of human melanomas. Pigment Cell Melanoma Res 27:90–102
14. Porcellato I, Orlandi M, Lo GA et al (2023) Canine melanocytes: immunohistochemical expression of melanocytic markers in different somatic areas. Vet Dermatol
15. Todoroff RJ, Brodey RS (1979) Oral and pharyngeal neoplasia in the dog: a retrospective survey of 361 cases. J Am Vet Med Assoc 175:567–571
16. Wallace J, Matthiesen DT, Patnaik AK (1992) Hemimaxillectomy for the treatment of oral tumors in 69 dogs. Vet Surg 21:337–341
17. Hahn KA, DeNicola DB, Richardson RC et al (1994) Canine oral malignant melanoma: prognostic utility of an alternative staging system. J Small Anim Pract 35:251–256
18. Dobson JM (2013) Breed-predispositions to cancer in pedigree dogs. ISRN Vet Sci 2013:941275
19. Boerkamp KM, Teske E, Boon LR et al (2014) Estimated incidence rate and distribution of tumours in 4,653 cases of archival submissions derived from the Dutch golden retriever population. BMC Vet Res 10:34
20. Ramos-Vara JA, Beissenherz ME, Miller MA et al (2000) Retrospective study of 338 canine oral melanomas with clinical, histologic, and immunohistochemical review of 129 cases. Vet Pathol 37:597–608
21. MacEwen EG, Patnaik AK, Harvey HJ et al (1986) Canine oral melanoma: comparison of surgery versus surgery plus corynebacterium parvum. Cancer Investig 4(5):397–402

22. Harvey HJ, MacEwen G, Braun D et al (1981) Prognostic criteria for dogs with oral melanoma. JAVMA 178(6):580–582
23. Bradley RL, MacEwen EG, Loar AS (1984) Mandibular resection for removal of oral tumors in 30 dogs and 6 cats. J Am Vet Med Assoc 184:460–463
24. Harvey HJ (1985) Oral tumors. Vet Clin North Am Small Anim Pract 15:493–500
25. Kosovsky JK, Matthiesen DT, Marretta SM et al (1991) Results of partial mandibulectomy for the treatment of oral tumors in 142 dogs. Vet Surg 20:397–401
26. Schobert CS, Labelle P, Dubielzig RR (2010) Feline conjunctival melanoma: histopathological characteristics and clinical outcomes. Vet Ophthalmol 13:43–46
27. Planellas M, Pastor J, Torres MD et al (2010) Unusual presentation of a metastatic uveal melanoma in a cat. Vet Ophthalmol 13:391–394
28. Farrelly J, Denman DL, Hohenhaus AE et al (2004) Hypofractionated radiation therapy of oral melanoma in five cats. Vet Radiol Ultrasound 45:91–93
29. Patnaik AK, Mooney S (1988) Feline melanoma: a comparative study of ocular, oral, and dermal neoplasms. Vet Pathol 25:105–112
30. Luna LD, Higginbotham ML, Henry CJ et al (2000) Feline non-ocular melanoma: a retrospective study of 23 cases (1991-1999). J Feline Med Surg 2:173–181. https://doi.org/10.1053/jfms.2000.0092
31. Munday JS, French AF, Martin SJ (2011) Cutaneous malignant melanoma in an 11-month-old Russian blue cat. NZ Vet J 59:143–146. https://doi.org/10.1080/00480169.2011.561779
32. Morges MA, Zaks K (2011) Malignant melanoma in pleural effusion in a 14-year-old cat. J Feline Med Surg 13:532–535. https://doi.org/10.1016/j.jfms.2011.05.011
33. Grahn BH, Peiffer RL, Cullen CL et al (2006) Classification of feline intraocular neoplasms based on morphology, histochemical staining, and immunohistochemical labeling. Vet Ophthalmol 9:395–403. https://doi.org/10.1111/j.1463-5224.2006.00479.x
34. Bostock DE (1979) Prognosis after surgical excision of canine melanomas. Vet Pathol 16:32–40. https://doi.org/10.1177/030098587901600103
35. Spangler WL, Kass PH (2006) The histologic and epidemiologic bases for prognostic considerations in canine melanocytic neoplasia. Vet Pathol 43:136–149. https://doi.org/10.1354/vp.43-2-136
36. Smedley RC, Lamoureux J, Sledge DG et al (2011) Immunohistochemical diagnosis of canine oral amelanotic melanocytic neoplasms. Vet Pathol 48:32–40. https://doi.org/10.1177/0300985810387447
37. Choi C, Kusewitt DF (2003) Comparison of tyrosinase-related protein-2, S-100, and Melan A immunoreactivity in canine amelanotic melanomas. Vet Pathol 40:713–718. https://doi.org/10.1354/vp.40-6-713
38. Przezdziecki R, Czopowicz M, Sapierzynski R (2015) Accuracy of routine cytology and immunocytochemistry in preoperative diagnosis of oral amelanotic melanomas in dogs. Vet Clin Pathol 44:597–604
39. Koenig A, Wojcieszyn J, Weeks BR et al (2001) Expression of S100a, vimentin, NSE, and melan A/MART-1 in seven canine melanoma cells lines and twenty-nine retrospective cases of canine melanoma. Vet Pathol 38:427–435
40. Ramírez-Hernández C, García-Márquez LJ, Ramírez-Romero R (2022) Primary angiomatoid melanomas in dogs. J Comp Pathol 199:8–11
41. Berrington AJ, Jimbow K, Haines DM (1994) Immunohistochemical detection of melanoma-associated antigens on formalin-fixed, paraffin-embedded canine tumors. Vet Pathol 31:455–461. https://doi.org/10.1177/030098589403100408
42. Sandusky GE Jr, Carlton WW, Wightman KA (1985) Immunohistochemical staining for S100 protein in the diagnosis of canine amelanotic melanoma. Vet Pathol 22:577–581. https://doi.org/10.1177/030098588502200611
43. Giudice C, Ceciliani F, Rondena M et al (2010) Immunohistochemical investigation of PNL2 reactivity of canine melanocytic neoplasms and comparison with Melan A. J Vet Diagn Invest 22:389–394. https://doi.org/10.1177/104063871002200307
44. Ramos-Vara JA, Miller MA (2011) Immunohistochemical identification of canine melanocytic neoplasms with antibodies to melanocytic antigen PNL2 and tyrosinase: comparison with Melan A. Vet Pathol 48:443–450. https://doi.org/10.1177/0300985810382095
45. Grandi F, Rocha RM, Miot HA et al (2014) Immunoexpression of S100A4 in canine skin melanomas and correlation with histopathological parameters. Vet Q 34:98–104
46. Tsoi MF, Thaiwong T, Smedley RC et al (2021) Quantitative expression of TYR, CD34, and CALD1 discriminates between canine oral malignant melanomas and soft tissue sarcomas. Front Vet Sci 8:701457
47. Husna AA, Rahman MM, Chen HW et al (2022) Long non-coding RNA and transfer RNA-derived small fragments in exosomes are potential biomarkers for canine oral melanoma. Vet Comp Oncol 20:653–663
48. Hasan MN, Rahman MM, Husna AA et al (2024) Elevated expression of miR-301a and its functional roles in canine oral melanoma. Vet Comp Oncol 22:78–88. https://doi.org/10.1111/vco.12954
49. Colombino M, Casula M, Paliogiannis P et al (2024) Heterogeneous pathogenesis of melanoma: BRAF mutations and beyond. Crit Rev Oncol Hematol 201:104435. https://doi.org/10.1016/j.critrevonc.2024.104435
50. Bollag G, Hirth P, Tsai J et al (2010) Clinical efficacy of a RAF inhibitor needs broad target blockade in BRAF-mutant melanoma. Nature 467:596–599. https://doi.org/10.1038/nature09454

51. Shelly S, Chien MB, Yip B et al (2005) Exon 15 BRAF mutations are uncommon in canine oral malignant melanomas. Mamm Genome 16:211–217. https://doi.org/10.1007/s00335-004-2441-x
52. Fowles JS, Denton CL, Gustafson DL (2015) Comparative analysis of MAPK and PI3K/AKT pathway activation and inhibition in human and canine melanoma. Vet Comp Oncol 13:288–304
53. Roels S, Tilmant K, Ducatelle R (2001) p53 expression and apoptosis in melanomas of dogs and cats. Res Vet Sci 70:19–25. https://doi.org/10.1053/rvsc.2000.0435
54. Roels SL, Van Daele AJ, Van Marck EA et al (2000) DNA ploidy and nuclear morphometric variables for the evaluation of melanocytic tumors in dogs and cats. Am J Vet Res 61:1074–1079. https://doi.org/10.2460/ajvr.2000.61.1074
55. Modiano JF, Ritt MG, Wojcieszyn J (1999) The molecular basis of canine melanoma: pathogenesis and trends in diagnosis and therapy. J Vet Intern Med 13:163–174. https://doi.org/10.1892/0891-6640(1999)013<0163:tmbocm>2.3.co;2
56. Ritt MG, Mayor J, Wojcieszyn J et al (2000) Sustained nuclear localization of p21/WAF-1 upon growth arrest induced by contact inhibition. Cancer Lett 158:73–84. https://doi.org/10.1016/s0304-3835(00)00507-3
57. Thamm DH, Huelsmeyer MK, Mitzey AM et al (2010) RT-PCR-based tyrosine kinase display profiling of canine melanoma: IGF-1 receptor as a potential therapeutic target. Melanoma Res 20:35–42. https://doi.org/10.1097/CMR.0b013e328331ca86
58. Taylor KH, Smith AN, Higginbotham M et al (2007) Expression of vascular endothelial growth factor in canine oral malignant melanoma. Vet Comp Oncol 5:208–218. https://doi.org/10.1111/j.1476-5829.2007.00130.x
59. Mayr B, Schaffner G, Reifinger M et al (2003) N-ras mutations in canine malignant melanomas. Vet J 165:169–171. https://doi.org/10.1016/s1090-0233(02)00245-9
60. Mayr B, Wilhelm B, Reifinger M et al (2000) Absence of p21 WAF1 and p27 kip1 gene mutations in various feline tumours. Vet Res Commun 24:115–124. https://doi.org/10.1023/a:1006412623142
61. Sulaimon SS, Kitchell BE (2003) The basic biology of malignant melanoma: molecular mechanisms of disease progression and comparative aspects. J Vet Intern Med 17:760–772. https://doi.org/10.1111/j.1939-1676.2003.tb02513.x
62. Murakami A, Mori T, Sakai H et al (2011) Analysis of KIT expression and KIT exon 11 mutations in canine oral malignant melanomas. Vet Comp Oncol 9:219–224. https://doi.org/10.1111/j.1476-5829.2010.00253.x
63. Abou AS (2017) Immunohistochemical expression of MCAM/CD146 in canine melanoma. J Comp Pathol 157:27–33
64. Heishima K, Ichikawa Y, Yoshida K et al (2017) Circulating microRNA-214 and -126 as potential biomarkers for canine neoplastic disease. Sci Rep 7:2301
65. Starkey MP, Compston-Garnett L, Malho P et al (2017) Metastasis-associated microRNA expression in canine uveal melanoma. Vet Comp Oncol
66. Lee BH, Neela PH, Kent MS et al (2017) IQGAP1 is an oncogenic target in canine melanoma. PLoS One 12:e0176370
67. Ogasawara S, Honma R, Kaneko MK et al (2016) Podoplanin expression in canine melanoma. Monoclon Antib Immunodiagn Immunother 35:304–306
68. Finotello R, Monne Rodriguez JM, Vilafranca M et al (2016) Immunohistochemical expression of MDR1-Pgp 170 in canine cutaneous and oral melanomas: pattern of expression and association with tumour location and phenotype. Vet Comp Oncol
69. Zoroquiain P, Mayo-Goldberg E, Alghamdi S et al (2016) Melanocytoma-like melanoma may be the missing link between benign and malignant uveal melanocytic lesions in humans and dogs: a comparative study. Melanoma Res 26:565–571
70. Wei BR, Michael HT, Halsey CH et al (2016) Synergistic targeted inhibition of MEK and dual PI3K/mTOR diminishes viability and inhibits tumor growth of canine melanoma underscoring its utility as a preclinical model for human mucosal melanoma. Pigment Cell Melanoma Res 29:643–655
71. Lin W, Modiano JF, Ito D (2017) Stage-specific embryonic antigen: determining expression in canine glioblastoma, melanoma, and mammary cancer cells. J Vet Sci 18:101–104
72. Abou AS, Anwar S, Yanai T et al (2016) Immunohistochemical analysis of CD146 expression in canine skin tumours. Histol Histopathol 31:453–459
73. Noguchi S, Mori T, Nakagawa T et al (2015) DNA methylation contributes toward silencing of antioncogenic microRNA-203 in human and canine melanoma cells. Melanoma Res 25:390–398
74. Bongiovanni L, D'Andrea A, Porcellato I et al (2015) Canine cutaneous melanocytic tumours: significance of beta-catenin and survivin immunohistochemical expression. Vet Dermatol 26:270–e259
75. Kawabe M, Baba Y, Tamai R et al (2015) Profiling of plasma metabolites in canine oral melanoma using gas chromatography-mass spectrometry. J Vet Med Sci 77:1025–1028
76. Poorman K, Borst L, Moroff S et al (2015) Comparative cytogenetic characterization of primary canine melanocytic lesions using array CGH and fluorescence in situ hybridization. Chromosom Res 23:171–186
77. Guth AM, Deogracias M, Dow SW (2014) Comparison of cancer stem cell antigen expression by tumor cell lines and by tumor biopsies from dogs with melanoma and osteosarcoma. Vet Immunol Immunopathol 161:132–140

78. Borrego JF, Huelsmeyer MK, Pinkerton ME et al (2016) Neurokinin-1 receptor expression and antagonism by the NK-1R antagonist maropitant in canine melanoma cell lines and primary tumour tissues. Vet Comp Oncol 14:210–224
79. Seo KW, Coh YR, Rebhun RB et al (2014) Antitumor effects of celecoxib in COX-2 expressing and non-expressing canine melanoma cell lines. Res Vet Sci 96:482–486
80. Teixeira TF, Gentile LB, da Silva TC et al (2014) Cell proliferation and expression of connexins differ in melanotic and amelanotic canine oral melanomas. Vet Res Commun 38:29–38
81. Campagne C, Jule S, Alleaume C et al (2013) Canine melanoma diagnosis: RACK1 as a potential biological marker. Vet Pathol 50:1083–1090
82. Chon E, Thompson V, Schmid S et al (2013) Activation of the canonical Wnt/beta-catenin signalling pathway is rare in canine malignant melanoma tissue and cell lines. J Comp Pathol 148:178–187
83. Brachelente C, Cappelli K, Capomaccio S et al (2017) Transcriptome analysis of canine cutaneous melanoma and melanocytoma reveals a modulation of genes regulating extracellular matrix metabolism and cell cycle. Sci Rep 7:6386
84. Hasan MN, Rahman MM, Husna AA et al (2024) Hypoxia-related Y RNA fragments as a novel potential biomarker for distinguishing metastatic oral melanoma from non-metastatic oral melanoma in dogs. Vet Q 44:1–8. https://doi.org/10.1080/01652176.2023.2300943
85. Rahman MM, Lai YC, Husna AA et al (2020) Transcriptome analysis of dog oral melanoma and its oncogenic analogy with human melanoma. Oncol Rep 43:16–30
86. Rahman MM, Lai YC, Husna AA et al (2019) Micro RNA transcriptome profile in canine oral melanoma. Int J Mol Sci 20
87. Conrad D, Kehl A, Beitzinger C et al (2022) Molecular genetic investigation of digital melanoma in dogs. Vet Sci 9
88. Prouteau A, Mottier S, Primot A et al (2022) Canine oral melanoma genomic and transcriptomic study defines two molecular subgroups with different therapeutical targets. Cancers (Basel) 14
89. Sparger EE, Chang H, Chin N et al (2021) T Cell immune profiles of blood and tumor in dogs diagnosed with malignant melanoma. Front Vet Sci 8:772932
90. Scattone NV, Epiphanio TMF, Caddrobi KG et al (2021) Quantification of global DNA methylation in canine melanotic and amelanotic oral mucosal melanomas and peripheral blood leukocytes from the same patients with OMM: first study. Front Vet Sci 8:680181
91. Bongiovanni L, Andriessen A, Silvestri S et al (2021) H2AFZ: a novel prognostic marker in canine melanoma and a predictive marker for resistance to CDK4/6 inhibitor treatment. Front Vet Sci 8:705359
92. Dagli MLZ, Nagamine MK, Ikeda TL et al (2024) Identification of mutations in canine oral mucosal melanomas by exome sequencing and comparison with human melanomas. Sci Rep 14:24174. https://doi.org/10.1038/s41598-024-74748-z
93. Yasumaru CC, Xavier JG, Strefezzi RF et al (2021) Intratumoral T-lymphocyte subsets in canine oral melanoma and their association with clinical and histopathological parameters. Vet Pathol 58:491–502
94. Ishizaki T, Yamazaki J, Jelinek J et al (2020) Genome-wide DNA methylation analysis identifies promoter hypermethylation in canine malignant melanoma. Res Vet Sci 132:521–526
95. Liu IL, Chung TF, Huang WH et al (2021) Kynurenine 3-monooxygenase (KMO), and signal transducer and activator of transcription 3 (STAT3) expression is involved in tumour proliferation and predicts poor survival in canine melanoma. Vet Comp Oncol 19:79–91
96. Silvestri S, Porcellato I, Mechelli L et al (2020) E-Cadherin expression in canine melanocytic tumors: histological, immunohistochemical, and survival analysis. Vet Pathol 57:608–619
97. Shinada M, Kato D, Kamoto S et al (2020) PDPN is expressed in various types of canine tumors and its silencing induces apoptosis and cell cycle arrest in canine malignant melanoma. Cells 9
98. Brocca G, Ferraresso S, Zamboni C et al (2019) Array comparative genomic hybridization analysis reveals significantly enriched pathways in canine oral melanoma. Front Oncol 9:1397
99. Vargas THM, Pulz LH, Ferro DG et al (2019) Galectin-3 expression correlates with post-surgical survival in canine oral melanomas. J Comp Pathol 173:49–57
100. Porcellato I, Silvestri S, Menchetti L et al (2020) Tumour-infiltrating lymphocytes in canine melanocytic tumours: An investigation on the prognostic role of CD3(+) and CD20(+) lymphocytic populations. Vet Comp Oncol 18:370–380
101. Zamboni C, Brocca G, Ferraresso S et al (2020) Cyclin D1 immunohistochemical expression and somatic mutations in canine oral melanoma. Vet Comp Oncol 18:231–238
102. Prouteau A, Chocteau F, De BC et al (2020) Prognostic value of somatic focal amplifications on chromosome 30 in canine oral melanoma. Vet Comp Oncol 18:214–223
103. Hitte C, BgC L, Cadieu E et al (2019) Genome-wide analysis of long non-coding RNA profiles in canine oral melanomas. Genes (Basel) 10
104. Bowlt Blacklock KL, Birand Z, Selmic LE et al (2019) Genome-wide analysis of canine oral malignant melanoma metastasis-associated gene expression. Sci Rep 9:6511
105. Porcellato I, Brachelente C, Cappelli K et al (2021) FoxP3, CTLA-4, and IDO in canine melanocytic tumors. Vet Pathol 58:42–52

106. Porcellato I, Brachelente C, De PL et al (2019) FoxP3 and IDO in canine melanocytic tumors. Vet Pathol 56:189–199
107. Hendricks WPD, Zismann V, Sivaprakasam K et al (2018) Somatic inactivating PTPRJ mutations and dysregulated pathways identified in canine malignant melanoma by integrated comparative genomic analysis. PLoS Genet 14:e1007589
108. Tani H, Miyamoto R, Noguchi S et al (2021) A canine case of malignant melanoma carrying a KIT c.1725_1733del mutation treated with toceranib: a case report and in vitro analysis. BMC Vet Res 17:147
109. Brocca G, Poncina B, Sammarco A et al (2020) KIT somatic mutations and immunohistochemical expression in canine oral melanoma. Animals (Basel) 10
110. Chu PY, Pan SL, Liu CH et al (2013) KIT gene exon 11 mutations in canine malignant melanoma. Vet J 196:226–230. https://doi.org/10.1016/j.tvjl.2012.09.005
111. Smedley RC, Thaiwong T, Deeth LE et al (2021) Correlation between KIT expression and c-Kit mutations in 2 subtypes of canine oral melanocytic neoplasms. Vet Pathol 58:683–691
112. Giuliano A, Dobson J (2020) Prospective clinical trial of masitinib mesylate treatment for advanced stage III and IV canine malignant melanoma. J Small Anim Pract 61:190–194
113. Gillardon F, Wickert H, Zimmermann M (1995) Up-regulation of bax and down-regulation of bcl-2 is associated with kainate-induced apoptosis in mouse brain. Neurosci Lett 192:85–88
114. Gola C, Maniscalco L, Iussich S et al (2024) Hypoxia-associated markers in the prognosis of oral canine melanoma. Vet Pathol 61:721–731. https://doi.org/10.1177/03009858241244853
115. Laver T, Feldhaeusser BR, Robat CS et al (2018) Post-surgical outcome and prognostic factors in canine malignant melanomas of the haired skin: 87 cases (2003-2015). Can Vet J 59:981–987
116. Laprie C, Abadie J, Amardeilh MF et al (2001) MIB-1 immunoreactivity correlates with biologic behaviour in canine cutaneous melanoma. Vet Dermatol 12:139–147. https://doi.org/10.1046/j.1365-3164.2001.00236.x
117. Millanta F, Fratini F, Corazza M et al (2002) Proliferation activity in oral and cutaneous canine melanocytic tumours: correlation with histological parameters, location, and clinical behaviour. Res Vet Sci 73:45–51. https://doi.org/10.1016/s0034-5288(02)00041-3
118. Carroll KA, Kuntz CA, Heller J et al (2020) Tumor size as a predictor of lymphatic invasion in oral melanomas of dogs. J Am Vet Med Assoc 256:1123–1128
119. Vail DM, MacEwen EG (2000) Spontaneously occurring tumors of companion animals as models for human cancer. Cancer Investig 18:781–792. https://doi.org/10.3109/07357900009012210
120. Brown LM, Olino K (2025) Non-cutaneous melanoma: biology, clinical management, current therapy, and future directions in treatment. Surg Oncol Clin N Am 34:453–471. https://doi.org/10.1016/j.soc.2024.12.006
121. Esplin DG (2008) Survival of dogs following surgical excision of histologically well-differentiated melanocytic neoplasms of the mucous membranes of the lips and oral cavity. Vet Pathol 45:889–896. https://doi.org/10.1354/vp.45-6-889
122. Kim WS, Vinayak A, Powers B (2021) Comparative review of malignant melanoma and histologically well-differentiated melanocytic neoplasm in the oral cavity of dogs. Vet Sci 8
123. Bergin IL, Smedley RC, Esplin DG et al (2011) Prognostic evaluation of Ki67 threshold value in canine oral melanoma. Vet Pathol 48:41–53. https://doi.org/10.1177/0300985810388947
124. Wobeser BK, Kidney BA, Powers BE et al (2007) Diagnoses and clinical outcomes associated with surgically amputated canine digits submitted to multiple veterinary diagnostic laboratories. Vet Pathol 44:355–361. https://doi.org/10.1354/vp.44-3-355
125. Henry CJ, Brewer WG Jr, Whitley EM et al (2005) Canine digital tumors: a veterinary cooperative oncology group retrospective study of 64 dogs. J Vet Intern Med 19:720–724. https://doi.org/10.1892/0891-6640(2005)19[720:cdtavc]2.0.co;2
126. Marino DJ, Matthiesen DT, Stefanacci D et al (1995) Evaluation of dogs with digit masses: 117 cases (1981-1991). J Am Vet Med Assoc 207:726–728
127. Grassinger JM, Floren A, Mãller T et al (2021) Digital lesions in dogs: a statistical breed analysis of 2912 cases. Vet Sci 8
128. Porcellato I, Orlandi M, Lo Giudice A et al (2023) Canine melanocytes: immunohistochemical expression of melanocytic markers in different somatic areas. Vet Dermatol 34:284–297. https://doi.org/10.1111/vde.13150
129. Jeon MD, Leeper HJ, Cook MR et al (2022) Multi-institutional retrospective study of canine foot pad malignant melanomas: 20 cases. Vet Comp Oncol 20:854–861
130. Dugan MM, Perez MC, Karapetyan L et al (2024) Management of acral lentiginous melanoma: current updates and future directions. Front Oncol 14:1323933. https://doi.org/10.3389/fonc.2024.1323933
131. Smedley RC, Bongiovanni L, Bacmeister C et al (2022) Diagnosis and histopathologic prognostication of canine melanocytic neoplasms: a consensus of the Oncology-Pathology Working Group. Vet Comp Oncol 20:739–751
132. Smedley RC, Sebastian K, Kiupel M (2022) Diagnosis and prognosis of canine melanocytic neoplasms. Vet Sci 9
133. Smedley RC, Spangler WL, Esplin DG et al (2011) Prognostic markers for canine melanocytic neoplasms: a comparative review of the literature and

goals for future investigation. Vet Pathol 48:54–72. https://doi.org/10.1177/0300985810390717
134. Polton G, Borrego JF, Clemente-Vicario F et al (2024) Melanoma of the dog and cat: consensus and guidelines. Front Vet Sci 11:1359426. https://doi.org/10.3389/fvets.2024.1359426
135. Wiggans KT, Reilly CM, Kass PH et al (2016) Histologic and immunohistochemical predictors of clinical behavior for feline diffuse iris melanoma. Vet Ophthalmol 19(Suppl 1):44–55
136. Rushton JG, Ertl R, Klein D et al (2017) Mutation analysis and gene expression profiling of ocular melanomas in cats. Vet Comp Oncol
137. Fragola JA, Dubielzig RR, Bentley E et al (2017) Iridociliary cysts masquerading as neoplasia in cats: a morphologic review of 14 cases. Vet Ophthalmol
138. Chamel G, Abadie J, Albaric O et al (2017) Non-ocular melanomas in cats: a retrospective study of 30 cases. J Feline Med Surg 19:351–357
139. Badanes Z, Espinheira GF, Ledbetter EC (2020) Choroidal melanocytic tumors in dogs: a retrospective study. Vet Ophthalmol 23:987–993
140. Silvestri S, Porcellato I, Mechelli L et al (2019) Tumor thickness and modified clark level in canine cutaneous melanocytic tumors. Vet Pathol 56:180–188
141. Silva ML, Martinho I, Rocha M et al (2024) Relative tumour volume in canine oral melanoma staging and prognosis. Vet Comp Oncol 22:641–650. https://doi.org/10.1111/vco.13018
142. MacEwen EG, Kurzman ID, Vail DM et al (1999) Adjuvant therapy for melanoma in dogs: results of randomized clinical trials using surgery, liposome-encapsulated muramyl tripeptide, and granulocyte macrophage colony-stimulating factor. Clin Cancer Res 5:4249–4258
143. Proulx DR, Ruslander DM, Dodge RK et al (2003) A retrospective analysis of 140 dogs with oral melanoma treated with external beam radiation. Vet Radiol Ultrasound 44:352–359
144. Freeman KP, Hahn KA, Harris FD et al (2003) Treatment of dogs with oral melanoma by hypofractionated radiation therapy and platinum-based chemotherapy (1987-1997). J Vet Intern Med 17:96–101
145. Boston SE, Lu X, Culp WT et al (2014) Efficacy of systemic adjuvant therapies administered to dogs after excision of oral malignant melanomas: 151 cases (2001-2012). J Am Vet Med Assoc 245:401–407
146. Murray B, Blacklock KLB (2022) Pilot study: assessing the expression of serum lactate dehydrogenase and peripheral leukocyte ratios in canine oral malignant melanoma. Vet Sci 9
147. Garcia JS, Nowosh V, Lãpez RVM et al (2022) Association of systemic inflammatory and immune indices with survival in canine patients with oral melanoma, treated with experimental immunotherapy alone or experimental immunotherapy plus metronomic chemotherapy. Front Vet Sci 9:888411
148. Porcellato I, Sforna M, Lo GA et al (2022) Tumor-associated macrophages in canine oral and cutaneous melanomas and melanocytomas: phenotypic and prognostic assessment. Front Vet Sci 9:878949
149. Williams LE, Packer RA (2003) Association between lymph node size and metastasis in dogs with oral malignant melanoma: 100 cases (1987-2001). J Am Vet Med Assoc 222:1234–1236
150. Skinner OT, Boston SE, Souza CHM (2017) Patterns of lymph node metastasis identified following bilateral mandibular and medial retropharyngeal lymphadenectomy in 31 dogs with malignancies of the head. Vet Comp Oncol 15:881–889
151. Herring ES, Smith MM, Robertson JL (2002) Lymph node staging of oral and maxillofacial neoplasms in 31 dogs and cats. J Vet Dent 19:122–126
152. Grimes JA, Matz BM, Christopherson PW et al (2017) Agreement between cytology and histopathology for regional lymph node metastasis in dogs with melanocytic neoplasms. Vet Pathol 54:579–587
153. Fournier Q, Cazzini P, Bavcar S et al (2018) Investigation of the utility of lymph node fine-needle aspiration cytology for the staging of malignant solid tumors in dogs. Vet Clin Pathol 47:489–500
154. Grimes JA, Mestrinho LA, Berg J et al (2019) Histologic evaluation of mandibular and medial retropharyngeal lymph nodes during staging of oral malignant melanoma and squamous cell carcinoma in dogs. J Am Vet Med Assoc 254:938–943
155. Chiti LE, Stefanello D, Manfredi M et al (2021) To map or not to map the cN0 neck: impact of sentinel lymph node biopsy in canine head and neck tumours. Vet Comp Oncol 19:661–670
156. Dumitra T, Faries MB (2024) Melanoma sentinel lymph node biopsy in the modern era. Surg Oncol 57:102162. https://doi.org/10.1016/j.suronc.2024.102162
157. Congiusta M, Lawrence J, Rendahl A et al (2020) Variability in recommendations for cervical lymph node pathology for staging of canine oral neoplasia: a survey study. Front Vet Sci 7:506
158. Smith MM (2002) Surgical approach for lymph node staging of oral and maxillofacial neoplasms in dogs. J Vet Dent 19:170–174
159. Green K, Boston SE (2017) Bilateral removal of the mandibular and medial retropharyngeal lymph nodes through a single ventral midline incision for staging of head and neck cancers in dogs: a description of surgical technique. Vet Comp Oncol 15:208–214
160. Grimes JA, Secrest SA, Wallace ML et al (2020) Use of indirect computed tomography lymphangiography to determine metastatic status of sentinel lymph nodes in dogs with a pre-operative diagnosis of melanoma or mast cell tumour. Vet Comp Oncol 18:818–824
161. Worley DR (2014) Incorporation of sentinel lymph node mapping in dogs with mast cell tumours: 20 consecutive procedures. Vet Comp Oncol 12:215–226

162. Brissot HN, Edery EG (2017) Use of indirect lymphography to identify sentinel lymph node in dogs: a pilot study in 30 tumours. Vet Comp Oncol 15:740–753
163. Liuti T, de Vos J, Bosman T et al (2009) 67Gallium citrate scintigraphy to assess metastatic spread in a dog with an oral melanoma. J Small Anim Pract 50:31–34
164. Cotter B, Zwicker LA, Waldner C et al (2022) Inter- and intraobserver agreement for CT measurement of mandibular and medial retropharyngeal lymph nodes is excellent in dogs with histologically confirmed oral melanoma. Vet Radiol Ultrasound 63:73–81
165. Willcox JL, Spriet M, Zwingenberger AL et al (2021) Evaluation of accuracy for (18) F-FDG positron emission tomography and computed tomography for detection of lymph node metastasis in canine oral malignant melanoma. Vet Comp Oncol 19:463–472
166. Sarowitz BN, Davis GJ, Kim S (2017) Outcome and prognostic factors following curative-intent surgery for oral tumours in dogs: 234 cases (2004 to 2014). J Small Anim Pract 58:146–153
167. Schwarz PD, Withrow SJ, Curtis CR et al (1991) Mandibular resection as a treatment for oral cancer in 81 dogs. J Am Anim Hosp Assoc 27:601–610
168. Schwarz PD, Withrow SJ, Curtis CR et al (1991) Partial maxillary resection as a treatment for oral cancer in 61 dogs. J Am Anim Hosp Assoc 27:617–624
169. Fox LE, Geoghegan SL, Davis LH et al (1997) Owner satisfaction with partial mandibulectomy or maxillectomy for treatment of oral tumors in 27 dogs. J Am Anim Hosp Assoc 33:25–31
170. Liptak JM, Dernell WS, Rizzo SA et al (2005) Partial foot amputation in 11 dogs. J Am Anim Hosp Assoc 41:47–55
171. Kaufman KL, Mann FA (2013) Short- and long-term outcomes after digit amputation in dogs: 33 cases (1999-2011). J Am Vet Med Assoc 242:1249–1254
172. Tellado M, De Robertis M, Montagna D et al (2023) Electrochemotherapy plus IL-2+IL-12 gene electrotransfer in spontaneous inoperable stage III-IV canine oral malignant melanoma. Vaccines (Basel) 11. https://doi.org/10.3390/vaccines11061033
173. Tellado MN, Maglietti FH, Michinski SD et al (2020) Electrochemotherapy in treatment of canine oral malignant melanoma and factors influencing treatment outcome. Radiol Oncol 54:68–78
174. Morton DL (2001) Cytoreductive surgery and adjuvant immunotherapy in the management of metastatic melanoma. Tumori 87:S57–S59
175. Bergman PJ (2019) Cancer immunotherapies. Vet Clin North Am Small Anim Pract 49:881–902
176. Baja AJ, Kelsey KL, Ruslander DM et al (2022) A retrospective study of 101 dogs with oral melanoma treated with a weekly or biweekly 6 Gy ×6 radiotherapy protocol. Vet Comp Oncol 20:623–631. https://doi.org/10.1111/vco.12815
177. Théon AP, Rodriquez C, Madewell BR (1997) Analysis of prognostic factors and patterns of failure in dogs with malignant oral tumors treated with megavoltage irradiation. J Am Vet Med Assoc 210:778–784
178. Bateman KE, Catton PA, Pennock PW et al (1994) 0-7-21 radiation therapy for the treatment of canine oral melanoma. J Vet Intern Med 8:267–272
179. Blackwood L, Dobson JM (1996) Radiotherapy of oral malignant melanomas in dogs. J Am Vet Med Assoc 209:98–102
180. Murphy S, Hayes AM, Blackwood L et al (2005) Oral malignant melanoma – the effect of coarse fractionation radiotherapy alone or with adjuvant carboplatin therapy. Vet Comp Oncol 3:222–229
181. Kawabe M, Mori T, Ito Y et al (2015) Outcomes of dogs undergoing radiotherapy for treatment of oral malignant melanoma: 111 cases (2006-2012). J Am Vet Med Assoc 247:1146–1153
182. Khan N, Khan MK, Almasan A et al (2011) The evolving role of radiation therapy in the management of malignant melanoma. Int J Radiat Oncol Biol Phys 80:645–654
183. Dank G, Rassnick KM, Sokolovsky Y et al (2014) Use of adjuvant carboplatin for treatment of dogs with oral malignant melanoma following surgical excision. Vet Comp Oncol 12:78–84
184. Cancedda S, Rohrer BC, Aresu L et al (2016) Efficacy and side effects of radiation therapy in comparison with radiation therapy and temozolomide in the treatment of measurable canine malignant melanoma. Vet Comp Oncol 14:e146–e157
185. Brockley LK, Cooper MA, Bennett PF (2013) Malignant melanoma in 63 dogs (2001-2011): the effect of carboplatin chemotherapy on survival. N Z Vet J 61:25–31
186. Magee K, Marsh IR, Turek MM et al (2021) Safety and feasibility of an in situ vaccination and immunomodulatory targeted radionuclide combination immuno-radiotherapy approach in a comparative (companion dog) setting. PLoS One 16:e0255798
187. Noguchi S, Yagi K, Okamoto N et al (2022) Prognostic factors for the efficiency of radiation therapy in dogs with oral melanoma: a pilot study of hypoxia in intraosseous lesions. Vet Sci 10
188. Camerino M, Giacobino D, Manassero L et al (2022) Prognostic impact of bone invasion in canine oral malignant melanoma treated by surgery and anti-CSPG4 vaccination: a retrospective study on 68 cases (2010-2020). Vet Comp Oncol 20:189–197
189. Mucignat G, Montanucci L, Elgendy R et al (2024) A whole-transcriptomic analysis of canine oral melanoma: a chance to disclose the radiotherapy effect and outcome-associated gene signature. Genes (Basel) 15. https://doi.org/10.3390/genes15081065
190. Giannuzzi D, Marconato L, Elgendy R et al (2019) Longitudinal transcriptomic and genetic landscape of radiotherapy response in canine melanoma. Vet Comp Oncol 17:308–316
191. Ogilvie GK, Reynolds HA, Richardson RC et al (1989) Phase II evaluation of doxorubicin for treatment of various canine neoplasms. JAVMA 195(11):1580–1583

192. Wouda RM, Miller ME, Chon E et al (2015) Clinical effects of vinorelbine administration in the management of various malignant tumor types in dogs: 58 cases (1997-2012). J Am Vet Med Assoc 246:1230–1237
193. Page RL, Thrall DE, Dewhirst MW et al (1991) Phase I study of melphalan alone and melphalan plus whole body hyperthermia in dogs with malignant melanoma. Int J Hyperth 7:559–566
194. Boria PA, Murry DJ, Bennett PF et al (2004) Evaluation of cisplatin combined with piroxicam for the treatment of oral malignant melanoma and oral squamous cell carcinoma in dogs. J Am Vet Med Assoc 224:388–394
195. Rassnick KM, Ruslander DM, Cotter SM et al (2001) Use of carboplatin for treatment of dogs with malignant melanoma: 27 cases (1989-2000). J Am Vet Med Assoc 218:1444–1448
196. Enjoji S, Yabe R, Fujiwara N et al (2015) The therapeutic effects of SET/I2PP2A inhibitors on canine melanoma. J Vet Med Sci 77:1451–1456
197. Breit MN, Kisseberth WC, Bear MD et al (2014) Biologic activity of the novel orally bioavailable selective inhibitor of nuclear export (SINE) KPT-335 against canine melanoma cell lines. BMC Vet Res 10:160
198. London CA, Bernabe LF, Barnard S et al (2014) Preclinical evaluation of the novel, orally bioavailable Selective Inhibitor of Nuclear Export (SINE) KPT-335 in spontaneous canine cancer: results of a phase I study. PLoS One 9:e87585
199. Ito K, Kobayashi M, Kuroki S et al (2013) The proteasome inhibitor bortezomib inhibits the growth of canine malignant melanoma cells in vitro and in vivo. Vet J 198:577–582
200. Yokoe I, Azuma K, Hata K et al (2015) Clinical systemic lupeol administration for canine oral malignant melanoma. Mol Clin Oncol 3:89–92
201. Jarab AS, Al-Qerem WA, Khdour LM et al (2024) New emerging treatment options for metastatic melanoma: a systematic review and meta-analysis of skin cancer therapies. Arch Dermatol Res 316:735. https://doi.org/10.1007/s00403-024-03467-2
202. Martínez CM, Peñafiel-Verdú C, Vilafranca M et al (2011) Cyclooxygenase-2 expression is related with localization, proliferation, and overall survival in canine melanocytic neoplasms. Vet Pathol 48:1204–1211. https://doi.org/10.1177/0300985810396517
203. Gregorio H, Raposo TP, Queiroga FL et al (2016) Investigating associations of cyclooxygenase-2 expression with angiogenesis, proliferation, macrophage and T-lymphocyte infiltration in canine melanocytic tumours. Melanoma Res 26:338–347
204. Pires I, Garcia A, Prada J et al (2010) COX-1 and COX-2 expression in canine cutaneous, oral and ocular melanocytic tumours. J Comp Pathol 143:142–149. https://doi.org/10.1016/j.jcpa.2010.01.016
205. Paglia D, Dubielzig RR, Kado-Fong HK et al (2009) Expression of cyclooxygenase-2 in canine uveal melanocytic neoplasms. Am J Vet Res 70:1284–1290. https://doi.org/10.2460/ajvr.70.10.1284
206. Yoshitake R, Saeki K, Watanabe M et al (2017) Molecular investigation of the direct anti-tumour effects of nonsteroidal anti-inflammatory drugs in a panel of canine cancer cell lines. Vet J 221:38–47
207. Silveira TL, Pang LY, Di DA et al (2021) COX-2 silencing in canine malignant melanoma inhibits malignant behaviour. Front Vet Sci 8:633170
208. Maekawa N, Konnai S, Asano Y et al (2022) Exploration of serum biomarkers in dogs with malignant melanoma receiving anti-PD-L1 therapy and potential of COX-2 inhibition for combination therapy. Sci Rep 12:9265
209. Kitchell BE, Brown DM, Luck EE et al (1994) Intralesional implant for treatment of primary oral malignant melanoma in dogs. J Am Vet Med Assoc 204:229–236
210. Theon AP, Madewell BR, Moore AS et al (1991) Localized thermo-cisplatin therapy: a pilot study in spontaneous canine and feline tumours. Int J Hyperth 7:881–892
211. Spugnini EP, Dragonetti E, Vincenzi B et al (2006) Pulse-mediated chemotherapy enhances local control and survival in a spontaneous canine model of primary mucosal melanoma. Melanoma Res 16:23–27. https://doi.org/10.1097/01.cmr.0000195702.73192.a0
212. Moretti G, Dentini A, Beccati F et al (2022) Palliative repeated electroporations of oral tumours in dogs: a case series. Front Vet Sci 9:1004811
213. Wei BR, Hoover SB, Peer CJ et al (2020) Efficacy, tolerability, and pharmacokinetics of combined targeted MEK and Dual mTORC1/2 inhibition in a preclinical model of mucosal melanoma. Mol Cancer Ther 19:2308–2318
214. Tunikowska J, Antończyk A, Rembiałkowska N et al (2020) The first application of nanoelectrochemotherapy in feline oral malignant melanoma treatment-case study. Animals (Basel) 10. https://doi.org/10.3390/ani10040556
215. Alexander AN, Huelsmeyer MK, Mitzey A et al (2006) Development of an allogeneic whole-cell tumor vaccine expressing xenogeneic gp100 and its implementation in a phase II clinical trial in canine patients with malignant melanoma. Cancer Immunol Immunother 55:433–442. https://doi.org/10.1007/s00262-005-0025-6
216. Hogge GS, Burkholder JK, Culp J et al (1999) Preclinical development of human granulocyte-macrophage colony-stimulating factor-transfected melanoma cell vaccine using established canine cell lines and normal dogs. Cancer Gene Ther 6:26–36. https://doi.org/10.1038/sj.cgt.7700015
217. Dow SW, Elmslie RE, Willson AP et al (1998) In vivo tumor transfection with superantigen plus cytokine genes induces tumor regression and prolongs

survival in dogs with malignant melanoma. J Clin Invest 101:2406–2414
218. Gyorffy S, Rodriguez-Lecompte JC, Woods JP et al (2005) Bone marrow-derived dendritic cell vaccination of dogs with naturally occurring melanoma by using human gp100 antigen. J Vet Intern Med 19:56–63. https://doi.org/10.1892/0891-6640(2005)19<56:bmdcvo>2.0.co;2
219. Helfand SC, Soergel SA, Donner RL et al (1994) Potential to involve multiple effector cells with human recombinant interleukin-2 and antiganglioside monoclonal antibodies in a canine malignant melanoma immunotherapy model. J Immunother 16:188–197
220. Watanabe Y, Kano R, Maruyama H et al (2010) Small interfering RNA (siRNA) against the Bcl-2 gene increases apoptosis in a canine melanoma cell line. J Vet Med Sci 72:383–386. https://doi.org/10.1292/jvms.09-0159
221. Moriyama M, Kano R, Maruyama H et al (2010) Small interfering RNA (siRNA) against the survivin gene increases apoptosis in a canine melanoma cell line. J Vet Med Sci 72:1643–1646. https://doi.org/10.1292/jvms.10-0119
222. Thamm DH, Kurzman ID, Clark MA et al (2010) Preclinical investigation of PEGylated tumor necrosis factor alpha in dogs with spontaneous tumors: phase I evaluation. Clin Cancer Res 16:1498–1508. https://doi.org/10.1158/1078-0432.Ccr-09-2804
223. Allende JB, Finocchiaro LME, Glikin GC (2022) Therapeutic potential of the cytosine deaminase::uracil phosphoribosyl transferase/5-fluorocytosine suicide system for canine melanoma. Vet Comp Oncol 20:372–380
224. Fondello C, Agnetti L, Glikin GC et al (2020) Proliferation index and pseudoprogression as predictors of the therapeutic efficacy of suicide gene therapy for canine melanoma. Melanoma Res 30:126–135
225. Finocchiaro LME, Agnetti L, Fondello C et al (2019) Combination of cytokine-enhanced vaccine and chemo-gene therapy as surgery adjuvant treatments for spontaneous canine melanoma. Gene Ther 26:418–431
226. Finocchiaro LM, Fondello C, Gil-Cardeza ML et al (2015) Cytokine-enhanced vaccine and interferon-beta plus suicide gene therapy as surgery adjuvant treatments for spontaneous canine melanoma. Hum Gene Ther 26:367–376
227. Finocchiaro LM, Glikin GC (2012) Cytokine-enhanced vaccine and suicide gene therapy as surgery adjuvant treatments for spontaneous canine melanoma: 9 years of follow-up. Cancer Gene Ther 19:852–861
228. Finocchiaro LM, Glikin GC (2008) Cytokine-enhanced vaccine and suicide gene therapy as surgery adjuvant treatments for spontaneous canine melanoma. Gene Ther 15:267–276
229. Finocchiaro LM, Fiszman GL, Karara AL et al (2008) Suicide gene and cytokines combined nonviral gene therapy for spontaneous canine melanoma. Cancer Gene Ther 15:165–172
230. von Euler H, Sadeghi A, Carlsson B et al (2008) Efficient adenovector CD40 ligand immunotherapy of canine malignant melanoma. J Immunother 31:377–384
231. Piras LA, Riccardo F, Iussich S et al (2017) Prolongation of survival of dogs with oral malignant melanoma treated by en bloc surgical resection and adjuvant CSPG4-antigen electrovaccination. Vet Comp Oncol 15:996–1013
232. Paoloni M, Mazcko C, Selting K et al (2015) Defining the pharmacodynamic profile and therapeutic index of NHS-IL12 immunocytokine in dogs with malignant melanoma. PLoS One 10:e0129954
233. Rossi UA, Gil-Cardeza ML, Villaverde MS et al (2015) Interferon-beta gene transfer induces a strong cytotoxic bystander effect on melanoma cells. Biomed Pharmacother 72:44–51
234. Camerino M, Giacobino D, Tarone L et al (2025) Clinical evaluation of HuDo-CSPG4 DNA electroporation as adjuvant treatment for canine oral malignant melanoma: comparison of two vaccination protocols. Vet Q 45:1–16. https://doi.org/10.1080/01652176.2025.2473717
235. Rinaldi V, Bongiovanni L, Crisi PE et al (2024) APAVAC immunotherapy for the adjuvant treatment of a canine mucosal melanoma. Vet Sci 11. https://doi.org/10.3390/vetsci11120628
236. Riccardo F, Tarone L, Camerino M et al (2022) Antigen mimicry as an effective strategy to induce CSPG4-targeted immunity in dogs with oral melanoma: a veterinary trial. J Immunother Cancer 10
237. Westberg S, Sadeghi A, Svensson E et al (2013) Treatment efficacy and immune stimulation by AdCD40L gene therapy of spontaneous canine malignant melanoma. J Immunother 36:350–358
238. Saellstrom S, Sadeghi A, Eriksson E et al (2021) Adenoviral CD40 ligand immunotherapy in 32 canine malignant melanomas-long-term follow up. Front Vet Sci 8:695222
239. Nishiya AT, Nagamine MK, Fonseca IIMD et al (2020) Inhibitory effects of a reengineered anthrax toxin on canine oral mucosal melanomas. Toxins (Basel) 12
240. Hutchison S, Sahay B, de Mello SC et al (2019) Characterization of myeloid-derived suppressor cells and cytokines GM-CSF, IL-10 and MCP-1 in dogs with malignant melanoma receiving a GD3-based immunotherapy. Vet Immunol Immunopathol 216:109912
241. Milner RJ, Salute M, Crawford C et al (2006) The immune response to disialoganglioside GD3 vaccination in normal dogs: a melanoma surface antigen vaccine. Vet Immunol Immunopathol 114:273–284
242. Milevoj N, Tratar UL, Nemec A et al (2019) A combination of electrochemotherapy, gene electrotransfer of plasmid encoding canine IL-12 and

cytoreductive surgery in the treatment of canine oral malignant melanoma. Res Vet Sci 122:40–49
243. Bongiovanni L, Brachelente C, Dow S et al (2022) Editorial: canine melanoma in comparative oncology: Translate research advances to develop new diagnostic and therapeutic options. Front Vet Sci 9:1127527
244. Fortuna L, Relf J, Chang YM et al (2016) Prevalence of FoxP3(+) cells in canine tumours and lymph nodes correlates positively with glucose transporter 1 expression. J Comp Pathol 155:171–180
245. Pinheiro D, Chang YM, Bryant H et al (2014) Dissecting the regulatory microenvironment of a large animal model of non-Hodgkin lymphoma: evidence of a negative prognostic impact of FOXP3+ T cells in canine B cell lymphoma. PLoS One 9:e105027
246. Guevara-Patiño JA, Turk MJ, Wolchok JD et al (2003) Immunity to cancer through immune recognition of altered self: studies with melanoma. Adv Cancer Res 90:157–177. https://doi.org/10.1016/s0065-230x(03)90005-4
247. Liao JC, Gregor P, Wolchok JD et al (2006) Vaccination with human tyrosinase DNA induces antibody responses in dogs with advanced melanoma. Cancer Immun 6:8
248. Bergman PJ, McKnight J, Novosad A et al (2003) Long-term survival of dogs with advanced malignant melanoma after DNA vaccination with xenogeneic human tyrosinase: a phase I trial. Clin Cancer Res 9:1284–1290
249. Wolchok JD, Yuan J, Houghton AN et al (2007) Safety and immunogenicity of tyrosinase DNA vaccines in patients with melanoma. Mol Ther 15:2044–2050
250. Gradilone A, Gazzaniga P, Ribuffo D et al (2012) Prognostic significance of tyrosinase expression in sentinel lymph node biopsy for ultra-thin, thin, and thick melanomas. Eur Rev Med Pharmacol Sci 16:1367–1376
251. Phillips JC, Lembcke LM, Noltenius CE et al (2012) Evaluation of tyrosinase expression in canine and equine melanocytic tumors. Am J Vet Res 73:272–278
252. Cangul IT, van Garderen E, van der Poel HJ et al (1999) Tyrosinase gene expression in clear cell sarcoma indicates a melanocytic origin: insight from the first reported canine case. APMIS 107:982–988. https://doi.org/10.1111/j.1699-0463.1999.tb01500.x
253. de Vries TJ, Smeets M, de Graaf R et al (2001) Expression of gp100, MART-1, tyrosinase, and S100 in paraffin-embedded primary melanomas and locoregional, lymph node, and visceral metastases: implications for diagnosis and immunotherapy. A study conducted by the EORTC Melanoma Cooperative Group. J Pathol 193:13–20. https://doi.org/10.1002/1096-9896(2000)9999:9999<::Aid-path729>3.0.Co;2-d
254. Goubier A, Fuhrmann L, Forest L et al (2008) Superiority of needle-free transdermal plasmid delivery for the induction of antigen-specific IFNgamma T cell responses in the dog. Vaccine 26:2186–2190
255. Bergman PJ, Camps-Palau MA, McKnight JA et al (2006) Development of a xenogeneic DNA vaccine program for canine malignant melanoma at the Animal Medical Center. Vaccine 24:4582–4585
256. Grosenbaugh DA, Leard AT, Bergman PJ et al (2011) Safety and efficacy of a xenogeneic DNA vaccine encoding for human tyrosinase as adjunctive treatment for oral malignant melanoma in dogs following surgical excision of the primary tumor. Am J Vet Res 72:1631–1638
257. Ottnod JM, Smedley RC, Walshaw R et al (2013) A retrospective analysis of the efficacy of Oncept vaccine for the adjunct treatment of canine oral malignant melanoma. Vet Comp Oncol 11:219–229
258. Verganti S, Berlato D, Blackwood L et al (2017) Use of Oncept melanoma vaccine in 69 canine oral malignant melanomas in the UK. J Small Anim Pract 58:10–16
259. Treggiari E, Grant JP, North SM (2016) A retrospective review of outcome and survival following surgery and adjuvant xenogeneic DNA vaccination in 32 dogs with oral malignant melanoma. J Vet Med Sci 78:845–850
260. McLean JL, Lobetti RG (2015) Use of the melanoma vaccine in 38 dogs: The South African experience. J S Afr Vet Assoc 86:1246
261. Turek M, Ladue T, Looper J et al (2020) Multimodality treatment including ONCEPT for canine oral melanoma: a retrospective analysis of 131 dogs. Vet Radiol Ultrasound 61:471–480
262. Herzog A, Buchholz J, Ruess-Melzer K et al (2013) Combined use of irradiation and DNA tumor vaccine to treat canine oral malignant melanoma: a pilot study. Schweiz Arch Tierheilkd 155:135–142
263. Sarbu L, Kitchell BE, Bergman PJ (2015) Safety of administering the canine melanoma DNA vaccine (Oncept) to cats with malignant melanoma - a retrospective study. J Feline Med Surg
264. Mangold BJ, Flower JE, Burgess KE et al (2021) Use of a canine melanoma vaccine in the management of malignant melanoma in an African penguin (Spheniscus demersus). J Am Vet Med Assoc 260:455–460
265. Phillips JCBJ, Lembcke LM, Grosenbaugh DA, Leard AT (2011) Evaluation of needle-free injection devices for intramuscular vaccination in horses. J Eq VetSci 31:738–743
266. Perales MA, Yuan J, Powel S et al (2008) Phase I/II study of GM-CSF DNA as an adjuvant for a multipeptide cancer vaccine in patients with advanced melanoma. Mol Ther 16:2022–2029
267. Yuan J, Ku GY, Gallardo HF et al (2009) Safety and immunogenicity of a human and mouse gp100 DNA vaccine in a phase I trial of patients with melanoma. Cancer Immun 9:5
268. Giacobino D, Camerino M, Riccardo F et al (2021) Difference in outcome between curative intent vs marginal excision as a first treatment in dogs with

oral malignant melanoma and the impact of adjuvant CSPG4-DNA electrovaccination: a retrospective study on 155 cases. Vet Comp Oncol 19:651–660
269. Camerino M, Giacobino D, Iussich S et al (2021) Evaluation of prognostic impact of pre-treatment neutrophil to lymphocyte and lymphocyte to monocyte ratios in dogs with oral malignant melanoma treated with surgery and adjuvant CSPG4-antigen electrovaccination: anÂ explorativeÂ study. Vet Comp Oncol 19:353–361
270. Riccardo F, Iussich S, Maniscalco L et al (2014) CSPG4-specific immunity and survival prolongation in dogs with oral malignant melanoma immunized with human CSPG4 DNA. Clin Cancer Res 20:3753–3762
271. Manley CA, Leibman NF, Wolchok JD et al (2010) Xenogeneic murine tyrosinase DNA vaccine for malignant melanoma of the digit of dogs. J Vet Intern Med
272. Pazzi P, Steenkamp G, Rixon AJ (2022) Treatment of canine oral melanomas: a critical review of the literature. Vet Sci 9
273. Catchpole B, Gould SM, Kellett-Gregory LM et al (2002) Immunosuppressive cytokines in the regional lymph node of a dog suffering from oral malignant melanoma. J Small Anim Pract 43:464–467. https://doi.org/10.1111/j.1748-5827.2002.tb00015.x
274. Peggs KS, Quezada SA, Korman AJ et al (2006) Principles and use of anti-CTLA4 antibody in human cancer immunotherapy. Curr Opin Immunol 18:206–213. https://doi.org/10.1016/j.coi.2006.01.011
275. Graves SS, Stone D, Loretz C et al (2009) Establishment of long-term tolerance to SRBC in dogs by recombinant canine CTLA4-Ig. Transplantation 88:317–322. https://doi.org/10.1097/TP.0b013e3181ae3285
276. Takeuchi H, Konnai S, Maekawa N et al (2021) Canine transforming growth factor-β receptor 2-Ig: a potential candidate biologic for melanoma treatment that reverses transforming growth factor-β1 immunosuppression. Front Vet Sci 8:656715. https://doi.org/10.3389/fvets.2021.656715
277. Callahan MK, Wolchok JD (2013) At the bedside: CTLA-4- and PD-1-blocking antibodies in cancer immunotherapy. J Leukoc Biol 94:41–53
278. Biller BJ, Elmslie RE, Burnett RC et al (2007) Use of FoxP3 expression to identify regulatory T cells in healthy dogs and dogs with cancer. Vet Immunol Immunopathol 116:69–78
279. Itoh H, Horiuchi Y, Nagasaki T et al (2009) Evaluation of immunological status in tumor-bearing dogs. Vet Immunol Immunopathol 132:85–90. https://doi.org/10.1016/j.vetimm.2009.04.020
280. O'Neill K, Guth A, Biller B et al (2009) Changes in regulatory T cells in dogs with cancer and associations with tumor type. J Vet Intern Med 23:875–881. https://doi.org/10.1111/j.1939-1676.2009.0333.x
281. Sherger M, Kisseberth W, London C et al (2012) Identification of myeloid derived suppressor cells in the peripheral blood of tumor bearing dogs. BMC Vet Res 8:209. https://doi.org/10.1186/1746-6148-8-209
282. Thamm DH (2006) Interactions between radiation therapy and immunotherapy: the best of two worlds? Vet Comp Oncol 4:189–197
283. Walter CU, Biller BJ, Lana SE et al (2006) Effects of chemotherapy on immune responses in dogs with cancer. J Vet Intern Med 20:342–347. https://doi.org/10.1892/0891-6640(2006)20[342:eocoir]2.0.co;2
284. Emens LA, Jaffee EM (2005) Leveraging the activity of tumor vaccines with cytotoxic chemotherapy. Cancer Res 65:8059–8064. https://doi.org/10.1158/0008-5472.Can-05-1797
285. Wolchok JD, Kluger H, Callahan MK et al (2013) Nivolumab plus ipilimumab in advanced melanoma. N Engl J Med 369:122–133
286. Ott PA, Hodi FS, Kaufman HL et al (2017) Combination immunotherapy: a road map. J Immunother Cancer 5:16
287. Hellmann MD, Friedman CF, Wolchok JD (2016) Combinatorial cancer immunotherapies. Adv Immunol 130:251–277
288. Wolchok JD, Chiarion-Sileni V, Rutkowski P et al (2025) Final, 10-year outcomes with nivolumab plus ipilimumab in advanced melanoma. N Engl J Med 392:11–22. https://doi.org/10.1056/NEJMoa2407417
289. Le D, Uram J, Wang H et al (2015) PD-1 blockade in tumors with mismatch-repair deficiency. N Engl J Med 372:2509–2520
290. Alsaihati BA, Ho KL, Watson J et al (2021) Canine tumor mutational burden is correlated with TP53 mutation across tumor types and breeds. Nat Commun 12:4670
291. Karaki S, Anson M, Tran T et al (2016) Is there still room for cancer vaccines at the era of checkpoint inhibitors. Vaccines (Basel):4
292. Lai X, Friedman A (2017) Combination therapy of cancer with cancer vaccine and immune checkpoint inhibitors: a mathematical model. PLoS One 12:e0178479
293. Yuasa T, Masuda H, Yamamoto S et al (2017) Biomarkers to predict prognosis and response to checkpoint inhibitors. Int J Clin Oncol 22:629–634
294. Khagi Y, Kurzrock R, Patel SP (2017) Next generation predictive biomarkers for immune checkpoint inhibition. Cancer Metastasis Rev 36:179–190
295. Luksza M, Riaz N, Makarov V et al (2017) A neoantigen fitness model predicts tumour response to checkpoint blockade immunotherapy. Nature 551:517–520
296. Pinto C, Aluai-Cunha C, Santos A (2023) The human and animals' malignant melanoma: comparative tumor models and the role of microbiome in dogs and humans. Melanoma Res 33:87–103
297. Ott PA, Hu Z, Keskin DB et al (2017) An immunogenic personal neoantigen vaccine for patients with melanoma. Nature 547:217–221

298. Jackson HJ, Rafiq S, Brentjens RJ (2016) Driving CAR T-cells forward. Nat Rev Clin Oncol 13:370–383
299. Atherton MJ, Rotolo A, Haran KP et al (2022) Case report: clinical and serological hallmarks of cytokine release syndrome in a canine B Cell lymphoma patient treated with autologous CAR-T cells. Front Vet Sci 9:824982. https://doi.org/10.3389/fvets.2022.824982
300. Panjwani MK, Smith JB, Schutsky K et al (2016) Feasibility and safety of RNA-transfected CD20-specific chimeric antigen receptor T cells in dogs with spontaneous B cell lymphoma. Mol Ther 24:1602–1614
301. Smith JB, Panjwani MK, Schutsky K et al (2015) Feasibility and safety of cCD20 RNA CAR-bearing T cell therapy for the treatment of canine B cell malignancies. J Immunother Cancer 3:123
302. Foiani G, Melchiotti E, Capello K et al (2025) PD-L1, PD-1, and CTLA-4 mRNA in situ expression by canine oral melanoma cells and immune cells of the tumour microenvironment. Vet Comp Oncol. https://doi.org/10.1111/vco.13039
303. Igase M, Inanaga S, Nishibori S et al (2024) Proof-of-concept study of the caninized anti-canine programmed death 1 antibody in dogs with advanced non-oral malignant melanoma solid tumors. J Vet Sci 25:e15. https://doi.org/10.4142/jvs.23144
304. Maekawa N, Konnai S, Asano Y et al (2023) Molecular characterization of feline immune checkpoint molecules and establishment of PD-L1 immunohistochemistry for feline tumors. PLoS One 18:e0281143. https://doi.org/10.1371/journal.pone.0281143
305. Sirivisoot S, Boonkrai C, Wongtangprasert T et al (2023) Development and characterization of mouse anti-canine PD-L1 monoclonal antibodies and their expression in canine tumors by immunohistochemistry in vitro. Vet Q 43:1–9. https://doi.org/10.1080/01652176.2023.2240380
306. Yoshimoto S, Chester N, Xiong A et al (2023) Development and pharmacokinetic assessment of a fully canine anti-PD-1 monoclonal antibody for comparative translational research in dogs with spontaneous tumors. MAbs 15:2287250. https://doi.org/10.1080/19420862.2023.2287250
307. Igase M, Inanaga S, Tani K et al (2022) Long-term survival of dogs with stage 4 oral malignant melanoma treated with anti-canine PD-1 therapeutic antibody: a follow-up case report. Vet Comp Oncol 20:901–905
308. Pantelyushin S, Ranninger E, Guerrera D et al (2021) Cross-reactivity and functionality of approved human immune checkpoint blockers in dogs. Cancers (Basel):13. https://doi.org/10.3390/cancers13040785
309. Stevenson VB, Perry SN, Todd M et al (2021) PD-1, PD-L1, and PD-L2 gene expression and tumor infiltrating lymphocytes in canine melanoma. Vet Pathol 58:692–698
310. Ganbaatar O, Konnai S, Okagawa T et al (2020) PD-L1 expression in equine malignant melanoma and functional effects of PD-L1 blockade. PLoS One 15:e0234218. https://doi.org/10.1371/journal.pone.0234218
311. Igase M, Nemoto Y, Itamoto K et al (2020) A pilot clinical study of the therapeutic antibody against canine PD-1 for advanced spontaneous cancers in dogs. Sci Rep 10:18311
312. Nemoto Y, Shosu K, Okuda M et al (2018) Development and characterization of monoclonal antibodies against canine PD-1 and PD-L1. Vet Immunol Immunopathol 198:19–25
313. Coy J, Caldwell A, Chow L et al (2017) PD-1 expression by canine T cells and functional effects of PD-1 blockade. Vet Comp Oncol
314. Maekawa N, Konnai S, Okagawa T et al (2016) Immunohistochemical analysis of PD-L1 expression in canine malignant cancers and PD-1 expression on lymphocytes in canine oral melanoma. PLoS One 11:e0157176
315. Maekawa N, Konnai S, Hosoya K et al (2023) Safety and clinical efficacy of an anti-PD-L1 antibody (c4G12) in dogs with advanced malignant tumours. PLoS One 18:e0291727. https://doi.org/10.1371/journal.pone.0291727
316. Maekawa N, Konnai S, Takagi S et al (2017) A canine chimeric monoclonal antibody targeting PD-L1 and its clinical efficacy in canine oral malignant melanoma or undifferentiated sarcoma. Sci Rep 7:8951
317. Forsberg EMV, Riise R, Saellström S et al (2023) Treatment with anti-HER2 chimeric antigen receptor tumor-infiltrating lymphocytes (CAR-TILs) is safe and associated with antitumor efficacy in mice and companion dogs. Cancers (Basel) 15. https://doi.org/10.3390/cancers15030648
318. Sakai O, Yamamoto H, Igase M et al (2022) Optimization of culture conditions for the generation of canine CD20-CAR-T cells for adoptive immunotherapy. In Vivo 36:764–772. https://doi.org/10.21873/invivo.12763
319. Cutmore LC, Marshall JF (2021) Current perspectives on the use of off the shelf CAR-T/NK cells for the treatment of cancer. Cancers (Basel) 13. https://doi.org/10.3390/cancers13081926
320. Razmara AM, Farley LE, Harris RM et al (2024) Preclinical evaluation and first-in-dog clinical trials of PBMC-expanded natural killer cells for adoptive immunotherapy in dogs with cancer. J Immunother Cancer 12. https://doi.org/10.1136/jitc-2023-007963
321. Kisseberth WC, Lee DA (2021) Adoptive natural killer cell immunotherapy for canine osteosarcoma. Front Vet Sci 8:672361. https://doi.org/10.3389/fvets.2021.672361
322. Flesner BK, Wood GW, Gayheart-Walsten P et al (2020) Autologous cancer cell vaccination, adoptive T-cell transfer, and interleukin-2 administration results in long-term survival for companion dogs

with osteosarcoma. J Vet Intern Med 34:2056–2067. https://doi.org/10.1111/jvim.15852
323. Heinzerling L, Goldinger SM (2017) A review of serious adverse effects under treatment with checkpoint inhibitors. Curr Opin Oncol 29:136–144
324. Kumar V, Chaudhary N, Garg M et al (2017) Current diagnosis and management of immune related adverse events (irAEs) induced by immune checkpoint inhibitor therapy. Front Pharmacol 8:49
325. Atkins MB, Lotze MT, Dutcher JP et al (1999) High-dose recombinant interleukin 2 therapy for patients with metastatic melanoma: analysis of 270 patients treated between 1985 and 1993. J Clin Oncol 17:2105–2116
326. Hodi FS, O'Day SJ, McDermott DF et al (2010) Improved survival with ipilimumab in patients with metastatic melanoma. N Engl J Med 363:711–723
327. Hamid O, Robert C, Daud A et al (2013) Safety and tumor responses with lambrolizumab (anti-PD-1) in melanoma. N Engl J Med 369:134–144
328. Robert C, Schachter J, Long GV et al (2015) Pembrolizumab versus Ipilimumab in advanced melanoma. N Engl J Med 372:2521–2532
329. Wolchok JD, Chiarion-Sileni V, Gonzalez R et al (2017) Overall survival with combined nivolumab and Ipilimumab in advanced melanoma. N Engl J Med 377:1345–1356
330. Postow MA, Chesney J, Pavlick AC et al (2015) Nivolumab and ipilimumab versus ipilimumab in untreated melanoma. N Engl J Med 372:2006–2017
331. Wolchok JD, Chiarion-Sileni V, Gonzalez R et al (2022) Long-term outcomes with nivolumab plus ipilimumab or nivolumab alone versus ipilimumab in patients with advanced melanoma. J Clin Oncol 40:127–137
332. Snyder A, Makarov V, Merghoub T et al (2014) Genetic basis for clinical response to CTLA-4 blockade in melanoma. N Engl J Med 371:2189–2199
333. Tawbi HA, Schadendorf D, Lipson EJ et al (2022) Relatlimab and nivolumab versus nivolumab in untreated advanced melanoma. N Engl J Med 386:24–34
334. Robert C, Grob JJ, Stroyakovskiy D et al (2019) Five-year outcomes with dabrafenib plus trametinib in metastatic melanoma. N Engl J Med 381:626–636
335. Bai X, Flaherty KT (2025) The rise of new targets in melanoma. Br J Dermatol. https://doi.org/10.1093/bjd/ljaf251

Head and Neck Cancer

Pooja Karukonda, Ashlyn Rickard, Katherine Gonzalez, Yvonne M. Mowery, and Michael. W. Nolan

Abbreviations

HNC	Head and neck cancer
HNSCC	Head and neck squamous cell carcinoma
SCC	Squamous cell carcinoma
HPV	Human papillomavirus
EBV	Epstein-Barr virus
CT	Computed tomography
MRI	Magnetic resonance imaging
PET	Positron emission tomography
FDG	Fluorodeoxyglucose
FNA	Fine needle aspiration
AJCC	American Joint Committee on Cancer
UICC	Union for International Cancer Control
TNM	Tumor, node, metastasis (TNM) system
RT	Radiation therapy
IMRT	Intensity-modulated radiation therapy
CRT	Chemoradiation
SIB	Simultaneous integrated boost
Gy	Gray
EGFR	Epidermal growth factor receptor
PD-1	Programmed cell death protein 1
PD-L1	Programmed death-ligand 1
PFS	Progression-free survival
OS	Overall survival
SBRT	Stereotactic body radiation therapy
WHO	World Health Organization

Authors Mowery and Nolan have equally contributed to this chapter.

P. Karukonda
Department of Radiation Oncology, Duke University, Durham, NC, USA

Duke Cancer Institute, Duke University, Durham, NC, USA

A. Rickard
Department of Radiation Oncology, UPMC Hillman Cancer Center, Pittsburgh, PA, USA

K. Gonzalez
Department of Head and Neck Surgery & Communication Sciences, Duke University, Durham, NC, USA

Y. M. Mowery
Department of Radiation Oncology, Duke University, Durham, NC, USA

Duke Cancer Institute, Duke University, Durham, NC, USA

Department of Radiation Oncology, UPMC Hillman Cancer Center, Pittsburgh, PA, USA

Department of Head and Neck Surgery & Communication Sciences, Duke University, Durham, NC, USA

M. W. Nolan (✉)
Duke Cancer Institute, Duke University, Durham, NC, USA

Department of Clinical Sciences, North Carolina State University, Raleigh, NC, USA
e-mail: mwnolan@ncsu.edu

M. W. Nolan et al. (eds.), *Comparative Oncology*, https://doi.org/10.1007/978-3-032-04454-9_13

ACR	American College of Radiology
TI-RADS	Thyroid Imaging Reporting and Data System
TSH	Thyroid stimulating hormone
RAI	Radioactive iodine
MTC	Medullary thyroid carcinoma
MEN	Multiple endocrine neoplasia
a4NQO	4-Nitroquinoline 1-oxide
TME	Tumor microenvironment
DMBA	7,12-Dimethylbenz[a]anthracene
NOD/SCID	Nonobese diabetic/severe combined immunodeficiency
CDX	Cell-derived xenograft
PDX	Patient-derived xenograft
GEMM	Genetically engineered mouse model
FOSCC	Feline oral and oropharyngeal squamous cell carcinoma

1 Part 1. Introduction: The Current State of Knowledge of Human Head and Neck Cancer

1.1 Overview

Head and neck cancer (HNC) is the seventh most common type of cancer affecting humans worldwide, with around 900,000 new cases and 460,000 deaths annually [183]. In the United States, HNC accounts for approximately 3% of all cancers diagnosed. HNC comprises a heterogeneous group of tumors with regard to epidemiology, pathology, prognosis, and treatment. Despite recent therapeutic advances within surgical oncology, radiation oncology, and medical oncology, survival rates for HNC have remained largely stable over the past few decades, highlighting the need for further novel practice-changing research [70]. The primary focus of this chapter will be head and neck squamous cell carcinomas (HNSCC), as these constitute the majority of HNCs afflicting both humans and companion animals. While nasopharyngeal carcinomas in humans include keratinizing squamous cell carcinoma and basaloid squamous cell carcinoma, the most common histologic subtypes are differentiated nonkeratinizing carcinoma and undifferentiated nonkeratinizing carcinoma. In addition to HNSCC and nasopharyngeal carcinomas, human salivary gland cancers and thyroid carcinomas will be discussed. While sarcomas, melanomas, and lymphomas also occur within the head and neck region, these tumor types will be covered in other chapters.

1.2 Head and Neck Squamous Cell Carcinoma

HNC is typically categorized by the anatomic subsite in which the primary tumor is felt to originate. The principal anatomic subsites are oral cavity, pharynx (including nasopharynx, oropharynx, and hypopharynx), larynx, nasal cavity/paranasal sinuses, and salivary glands. Squamous cell carcinomas (SCC), which arise from the mucosal epithelial cells lining the upper aerodigestive tracts, comprise ~90% of HNC [70]. Perineural invasion commonly occurs in HNC, with prevalence observed on pathologic evaluation varying widely from 5% to 90% depending on histology, anatomic subsite, grade, and location [168].

1.2.1 Epidemiology and Biology

An increasing incidence of HNC has been noted in both developed and developing countries, with a predicted 30% annual increase by 2030 [91, 183]. Men have a two- to fourfold increased risk of developing HNC compared to women. Other risk factors for HNSCC in humans include advanced age, exposure to airborne pollutants/chemicals, tobacco usage, areca nut/betel quid consumption, and alcohol use. The combination of heavy tobacco and alcohol usage has been linked to at least a 35-fold synergistic increase in the risk of developing HNSCC [91]. Within the last few decades, human papillomavirus (HPV) infection has emerged as a major risk factor for developing oropharyngeal cancer. The rising incidence of oropharyngeal cancer has been attributed to the prevalence of anogenital HPV infection (particularly high-risk serotype HPV-

16) subsequently transmitted through oral sex [39]. Patients with HPV-related oropharyngeal cancer tend to be younger than patients with HPV-negative disease, with a median age at diagnosis of 53 versus 66, respectively [91]. The typical latency period from HPV infection to diagnosis of HPV-related oropharyngeal cancer is 10–30 years; thus, the effects of HPV vaccination will not be seen for decades. However, HPV vaccination will likely decrease the prevalence of high-risk oral HPV infections and therefore the incidence of HPV-related oropharyngeal cancer [34]. HPV has also been implicated in nasopharyngeal carcinoma to a lesser extent, with Epstein-Barr virus (EBV) representing the most common etiologic factor, particularly for undifferentiated nonkeratinizing nasopharyngeal carcinoma.

HPV is a double-stranded DNA virus that encodes two key oncogenes, E6 and E7, which drive carcinogenesis largely through inhibition of TP53 and RB, leading to loss of cell-cycle checkpoints [105]. Over 80% of smoking-related, HPV-negative HNC tumors exhibit loss-of-function *TP53* mutations. Inactivating *CDKN2A* and copy number alterations are also common in HPV-negative disease. By contrast, HPV-positive tumors typically have wild type *TP53*, with mutations in oncogene *PIK3CA* being relatively common [32].

1.2.2 Clinical Presentation, Diagnosis, and Staging

No screening strategy has yet proven effective for HNSCC. The primary approach to detection is thus based on physical exam and a thorough history, including assessment of risk factors and suspicious symptoms. SCC of the oral cavity (oral tongue, floor of mouth, retromolar trigone, buccal mucosa, hard palate, gingiva) typically presents as a nonhealing ulcer or mass, often associated with pain or functional deficits such as decreased tongue mobility, difficulty with mastication, or dysarthria [91]. Patients with SCC of the oropharynx (base of tongue, palatine tonsils, soft palate, and posterior pharyngeal wall) often describe dysphagia, odynophagia, globus sensation, trismus, and/or otalgia. However, these patients most commonly present with a painless neck mass and an otherwise asymptomatic or occult primary lesion. Patients with SCC of the larynx (true vocal cords, false vocal cords, epiglottis, arytenoids, aryepiglottic folds) or hypopharynx (pyriform sinuses, postcricoid area, posterior pharyngeal wall) usually present with hoarseness, other voice changes, and/or otalgia; if diagnosis and subsequent treatment are delayed, dyspnea and airway compromise may ensue [34].

Workup for suspected HNC includes fiberoptic nasopharyngolaryngoscopy and radiologic imaging, typically contrast-enhanced computed tomography (CT) extending from skull base to the thoracic inlet to determine the extent of locoregional disease (representative CT images of a human patient with HNC are shown in Fig. 1). Magnetic resonance imaging (MRI) is indicated for nasopharyngeal carcinomas and paranasal sinus tumors, as well as concern for perineural spread, skull base/orbital/intracranial invasion, and sometimes for delineation of oral cavity or laryngeal tumors. Extending the imaging range to the carina may be indicated in select situations, such as low-lying nodal disease, extensive subglottic extension, and/or thyroid malignancies. Chest CT or ^{18}F-fluorodeoxyglucose (FDG) positron emission tomography (PET)/CT to rule out distant metastatic disease is indicated for locally advanced primary tumors and/or nodal disease. ^{18}FDG PET/CT also has higher sensitivity and specificity for detecting cervical lymph node metastases compared to MRI or CT [34].

Diagnosis is ultimately contingent on biopsy, with primary lesion biopsy often requiring exam under anesthesia. Fine needle aspiration (FNA) of cervical lymphadenopathy also has a high sensitivity and specificity; excisional biopsy of a lymph node is not typically indicated unless FNA and/or core needle biopsies have been persistently nondiagnostic. In the case of an occult primary lesion which cannot be detected on imaging or direct laryngoscopy, bilateral palatine tonsillectomy and biopsies of the base of the tongue and nasopharynx are standardly obtained [34]. If nodal biopsy is consistent with HPV-related dis-

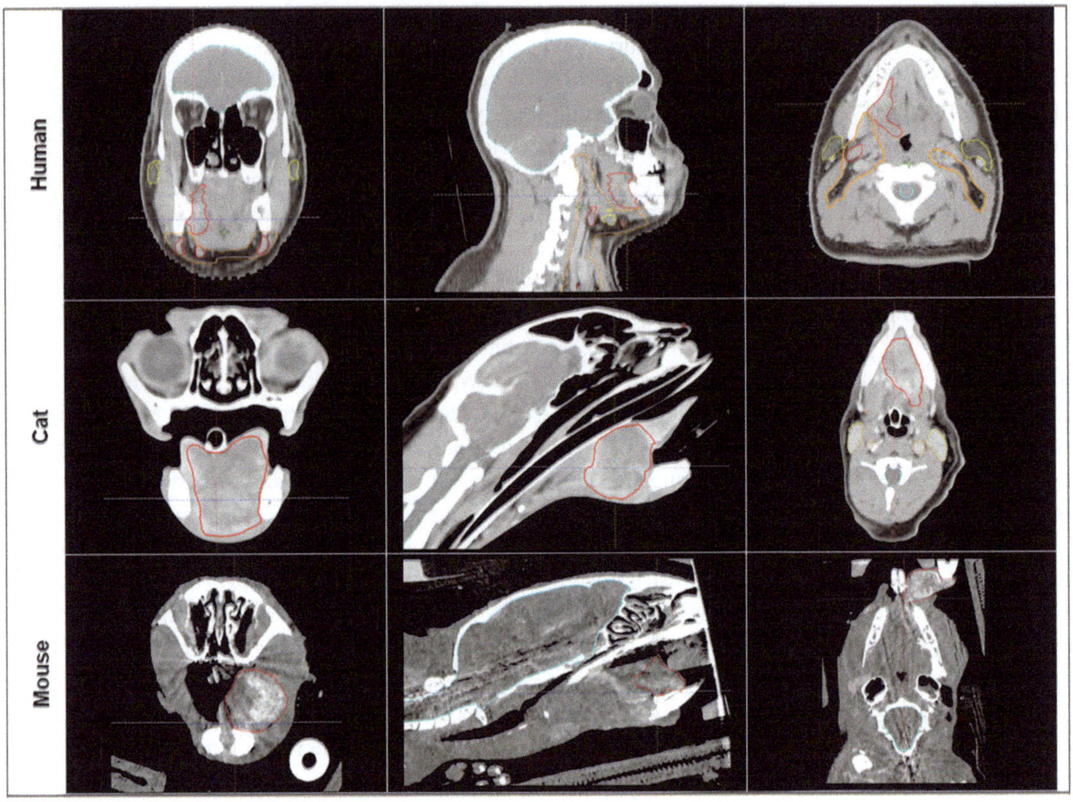

Fig. 1 Comparative anatomy of head and neck cancers. Representative computed tomography (CT) images are shown for a human (top row), pet cat (middle row), and mouse (bottom row), each with head and neck squamous cell carcinoma (SCC). The human has SCC of the lateral oral tongue and floor of mouth, extending posteriorly to include tonsil and inferiorly to base of tongue. The cat has naturally occurring sublingual/lingual SCC. The mouse has an SCC lesion that was induced via injection of MOC2 cells into the tongue. In all three species, the primary tumor is outlined in red with involved lymph nodes also outlined in red for the human case. In the human and cat, cervical lymph nodes that would be targeted for irradiation are outlined in orange; equivalent lymph nodes cannot be reliably visualized on the mouse CT. Likewise, regional salivary glands (a critical organ at risk during radiotherapy) cannot be seen clearly on the mouse CT, but are outlined in yellow on the cat and human CT. In all three species, the brain and spinal cord are outlined in cyan

ease, then nasopharyngeal biopsy is typically excluded, with oropharynx presumed to be the primary site. HPV DNA or RNA can be detected from a tumor sample by in situ hybridization or polymerase chain reaction; however, immunohistochemical staining for the validated surrogate marker p16 is most commonly used.

Disease staging assists with determination of treatment options as well as prognosis. The American Joint Committee on Cancer (AJCC) and Union for International Cancer Control (UICC) have published staging guidelines which incorporate a tumor, node, metastasis (TNM) system, as well as factors such as anatomic subsite. Given the differing biology and prognosis of HPV-positive and HPV-negative oropharyngeal cancers, the AJCC/UICC incorporated separate oropharyngeal cancer staging guidelines based on HPV status in 2018. The revised guidelines resulted in downward stage migration of many patients with HPV-positive oropharyngeal cancer, more accurately reflecting the similar survival rates observed among patients with previously stage I-IVA HPV-positive oropharyngeal cancer [39, 145].

1.2.3 Treatment

Evaluation by a multidisciplinary team including oncologic surgeons, medical oncologists, and radiation oncologists is crucial to formulate and execute an appropriate treatment regimen for any patient with HNC. Furthermore, dietitian, audiologists, dentists, occupational and physical therapists, social workers, psychologists, and speech therapists often play a critical role before, during, and after treatment, particularly in managing acute and chronic treatment-related toxicities. Treatment at high-volume centers with expertise in HNC management has been associated with improved patient outcomes [55]. Counseling patients who are actively using tobacco products regarding cessation and ensuring access to evidence-based interventions is extremely important to improve treatment efficacy, decrease morbidity, and ultimately reduce the risk of developing a second primary malignancy [91]. Dental evaluation and necessary extractions should be completed prior to initiation of definitive radiation therapy (RT) if possible, as long-term RT-related toxicities can complicate wound healing after dental extractions [34].

Approximately 30–40% of patients present with early-stage HNSCC (AJCC stage I–II), which can typically be managed with single-modality surgery or RT. The remaining 60–70% of patients present with more locally advanced disease (AJCC stage III–IV) necessitating multimodality treatment, typically some sequence or combination of RT, chemotherapy, and/or surgery to achieve locoregional tumor control [156]. Treatment plans are tailored to maximize the chance of cure while preserving function and minimizing toxicity. For patients with metastatic disease, treatment typically includes chemotherapy and/or immunotherapy. Palliative surgery may be performed, e.g., tracheostomy for airway maintenance, and palliative RT may be employed to treat specific symptoms.

In recent decades, both surgical and RT techniques have been refined, resulting in optimized locoregional control and decreased treatment-related toxicity. Minimally invasive robotic and/or laser-assisted surgical techniques, as well as advanced reconstructions, have expanded the indications for surgical management of HNSCC [39]. Intensity-modulated radiation therapy (IMRT) with image guidance has become the standard of care for curative-intent conventionally fractionated RT, with the superior conformality afforded by IMRT resulting in reduced long-term treatment-related toxicities compared to two-dimensional or three-dimensional conformal techniques [75].

There are two key components to both surgical resection and RT: management of the primary tumor and the lymphatic drainage basins in the neck. For early-stage disease, upfront surgery and RT result in similar survival outcomes; therefore, the choice between definitive surgery and RT typically involves assessment of the anatomical extent of the tumor, which affects the feasibility and morbidity of surgery versus RT. Primary oral cavity tumors are typically readily accessible via a transoral surgical approach, and thus, surgery is usually the primary treatment recommendation, with favorable survival outcomes and treatment-related toxicity [34]. Importantly, upfront surgery for oral cavity cancer facilitates lower radiation dose to the mandible, which reduces the risk of osteoradionecrosis. Paranasal sinus tumors are similarly most often managed with a primary surgical approach, while nasopharyngeal carcinomas are typically treated nonsurgically regardless of stage. Early-stage oropharyngeal and laryngeal cancers can usually be managed with either definitive surgery or RT alone depending on the individual presentation. While definitive RT for the majority of HNSCC entails 6–7 weeks of conventionally fractionated treatment, a moderately hypofractionated schedule yields improved locoregional control and survival outcomes in early-stage laryngeal cancers (stage I-II), and is therefore standard of care when RT is the primary modality of choice [18].

For patients undergoing upfront surgery, adjuvant RT with or without concurrent chemotherapy may be indicated based on adverse or high-risk pathologic features such as positive/close margins, T3-T4 primary tumor, nodal disease (particularly ≥2 lymph nodes), extranodal extension, lymphovascular invasion, and/or perineural invasion, with the goal of reducing locoregional recurrence rates and improving survival [13]. Importantly, use of multiple treatment modalities is associated with increased late toxicity and non-cancer-related mortality. Neck management is based on primary tumor stage and patterns of lymphatic drainage. In general, even patients with early stage clinically node-negative HNSCC should undergo selective neck dissection or elective nodal RT (ipsilateral or bilateral depending on primary tumor location and depth of invasion). An exception can be made specifically for clinically node-negative oral cavity tumors with depth of invasion <2 mm and for T1-T2 glottic cancers due to low risk of occult nodal disease. When there is concern for bilateral lymphatic drainage based on primary tumor site (such as tumors involving the nasopharynx, soft palate, posterior pharyngeal wall, base of tongue, supraglottic/subglottic larynx, hypopharynx) and/or tumor extent (deep invasion, approaching midline, tonsillar tumor extending >1 cm into the base of tongue), then bilateral selective neck dissection or elective nodal RT should target the nodal levels at highest risk of harboring disease. In the setting of residual or recurrent locoregional disease, salvage treatment with the previously unused modality is typically indicated and can still result in cure [34].

Unfortunately, about 60–70% of patients with HNSCC present with locally advanced disease, characterized by a bulky and/or extensive primary tumor, regional nodal disease, or both. Treatment approaches are frequently multimodal and can entail significant short-term morbidity, requiring complex care coordination and management [25]. Surgical resection of the primary tumor and selective or comprehensive lymph node dissection, followed by RT with or without concurrent chemotherapy, is typically the sequence of choice for resectable locally advanced oral cavity cancers. As discussed above, there are numerous adverse pathologic features for which adjuvant RT is indicated, and concurrent chemotherapy is typically recommended in cases with positive margins and/or extranodal extension, due to demonstrated improvements in locoregional control, progression-free survival, and overall survival [13]. For locally advanced oropharyngeal cancers for which upfront surgery may result in significant loss of function or necessitate adjuvant RT or chemoradiation (CRT), primary concurrent CRT is typically preferred. It is important to attempt to anticipate and limit the number of patients who undergo triple-modality therapy, which can result in significant morbidity [34]. Primary CRT is also typically the treatment of choice for locally advanced laryngeal cancers deemed appropriate for larynx preservation, though extensive tumors will require total laryngectomy/neck dissection followed by adjuvant RT or CRT [59].

Definitive RT for HNSCC is typically delivered once daily, Monday-Friday, for 6–7 weeks. Sequential boost and simultaneous integrated boost (SIB) are two IMRT techniques that can be utilized. Primary sequential boost IMRT typically entails delivering 44–50 Gray (Gy) in 2 Gy daily fractions to a "low-risk" area inclusive of elective nodal basins, followed by a sequential boost of 20–26 Gy to a "high-risk" area inclusive of gross disease. For SIB technique, subclinical disease is typically treated to 44–63 Gy with concurrent boost to 66–72 Gy to gross disease using different fraction sizes. These boost techniques can be used interchangeably based on institutional/physician preference and expertise, as a meta-analysis showed no difference in survival outcomes or toxicity between them [90]. Adjuvant RT is usually similarly fractionated, but the total dose is slightly lower, typically 50 Gy for lower-risk areas and 60–66 Gy for high-risk areas. The preferred interval between surgery and RT is less than six weeks to maximize treatment efficacy.

The primary function of chemotherapy given concurrently with RT for HNSCC is to radiosensitize the tumor. Administration of concurrent chemotherapy with RT in the definitive treatment of HNSCC has been shown in a large meta-analysis to decrease 5-year mortality by 6.5%, though usage should be individually tailored [100, 157]. Single-agent cisplatin is the preferred concurrent chemotherapy for patients with adequate performance status and is typically administered at a bolus dose of 100 mg/m^2 every 3 weeks or 40 mg/m^2 weekly, though there is conflicting evidence regarding the weekly regimen [95, 141]. Many patients are not cisplatin candidates based on comorbid conditions such as pre-existing hearing loss or renal dysfunction. One approach for cisplatin-ineligible patients is to utilize accelerated RT fractionation, typically 6 fractions per week rather than 5 fractions [149]. Alternative agents administered concurrently with RT include carboplatin or the epidermal growth factor receptor (EGFR) inhibitor cetuximab; however, these drugs are regarded as inferior to cisplatin [67, 73, 124]. Thus, further research is needed to define alternative and/or superior concurrent systemic therapy agents with RT in the definitive treatment setting.

De-escalating definitive treatment for HPV-positive oropharyngeal cancer is a major research interest, with the goal of maintaining excellent survival outcomes while decreasing the significant acute and late treatment-related toxicity burden. Clinical trials are investigating several strategies, including de-escalation of chemotherapy regimens, decreasing RT dose and/or the extent of elective nodal RT, and utilizing proton beam therapy, with the intent of maximizing the therapeutic window [39]. At this time, it is not standard practice to de-escalate treatment of patients with HPV-positive oropharyngeal cancer outside of a clinical trial; however, results from ongoing randomized phase III clinical trials are eagerly awaited to guide management in this evolving space.

The role of immunotherapy in the treatment of patients with HNSCC is also an area of active research. Programmed cell death protein 1 (PD-1) is a transmembrane protein that is part of the CD28 family of T cell co-stimulatory receptors. Binding of programmed death-ligand 1 (PD-L1) to PD-1 inhibits T cell activation. Cancer cells have co-opted this immune checkpoint to evade detection and elimination by the host immune system. PD-1/PD-L1 immune checkpoint blockade has emerged as a promising and effective therapeutic strategy for numerous malignancies [111]. Several ongoing trials are evaluating immune checkpoint inhibitors in the definitive treatment setting for HNSCC. NRG-HN003 is investigating the combination of PD-1 inhibitor pembrolizumab and CRT in the adjuvant setting for stage III-IV HNSCC, and NRG-HN005 is evaluating RT with cisplatin versus the PD-1 inhibitor nivolumab. However, the phase III JAVELIN study evaluating PD-L1 inhibitor avelumab with CRT compared to placebo with CRT for locally advanced HNSCC showed no improvement in progression-free survival (PFS) or overall survival (OS) with the addition of avelumab [108]. Similarly NRG-HN004, investigating concurrent PD-L1 inhibitor durvalumab with definitive RT for cisplatin-ineligible patients with HNSCC, was closed to accrual at the first interval analysis due to 2-year locoregional failure in the durvalumab arm of 32% compared to 15% in the cetuximab arm [125]. These disappointing immunotherapy clinical trial results despite promising preclinical data may reflect the limitations of traditional mouse models that typically inform investigational trial designs.

The technique of stereotactic body radiotherapy (SBRT), involving delivery of limited-fraction, high-dose RT typically targeted to gross disease with minimal margin, has increasingly been used to treat many cancers, including metastatic disease. Advantages of the technique include shorter treatment time and often decreased acute toxicity. SBRT is not currently recommended for definitive treatment of HNSCC given insufficient supportive evidence; however, it is an area of active research particularly in the setting of recurrent tumors in previously irradiated areas [34]. While fractionation schedules vary across institutions, typical SBRT reirradiation dose is 30–50 Gy in 5 fractions with improved local control for doses ≥35 Gy [107, 199]. Given that hypofractionated RT in the definitive setting is more feasible and widely adopted in the care of companion animals with HNSCC, this poses a unique comparative research opportunity.

1.2.4 Toxicity

Patients with HNSCC commonly present with debilitating disease-related symptoms such as odynophagia and dysphagia with sequelae including weight loss, dehydration, and aspiration. Treatment can exacerbate these symptoms in the acute setting and can also result in significant long-term toxicity. Among cancer survivors, patients with a history of HNSCC have the second highest rates of suicide, likely reflecting jeopardized quality of life in addition to psychological distress. Extensive supportive care is thus essential to managing this challenging patient population. Oral mucositis is a common morbid acute toxicity of RT that is further worsened by concurrent chemotherapy. Mucositis results in pain that makes eating and drinking challenging, particularly in the setting of treatment-related dysgeusia, another common acute RT-related toxicity. These side effects can lead to significant weight loss and/or dehydration, resulting in treatment breaks, feeding tube placement, and/or hospitalizations [180]. After completion of definitive RT for HNSCC, increased frequency of oral and dental evaluation is recommended due to the potential for RT-induced xerostomia, bone demineralization, and trismus. Referral to physical and/or occupational therapy can be beneficial for other late toxicities such as RT- or surgery-induced neck fibrosis and lymphedema. Swallowing rehabilitation may be necessary to manage chronic dysphagia, which occurs in approximately 45% of HNSCC survivors regardless of the utilized treatment modality. Speech therapy can also help alleviate treatment-related dysarthria and/or voice changes, which can affect up to 68% of HNSCC survivors [91]. Further research is indicated to improve management of acute RT-related toxicities, as well as to evaluate agents that are selectively radioprotective of normal tissues without sparing tumor to reduce the severity and duration of both acute and late treatment-related toxicities.

1.2.5 Prognosis

HNSCC prognosis is largely related to stage at diagnosis, with 70–90% of patients with early-stage disease having high rates of cancer-specific survival [156]. Locally advanced disease is associated with a high risk of locoregional recurrence and/or distant metastasis (up to 40%), with a correspondingly low 5-year OS of <50% [23]. Locoregional tumor progression is the most common cause of death, for example due to asphyxiation, aspiration, catastrophic bleed, or malnutrition secondary to dysphagia and/or pain. Additionally, metastatic disease and treatment-related toxicities contribute to poor survival. The adjusted mortality risk of HPV-positive HNSCC is notably almost 60% lower than HPV-negative HNSCC [9, 70, 203]. Other risk factors, such as tobacco and alcohol usage, also impact prognosis. A greater than 10 pack-year smoking history is associated with worse prognosis, even in individuals with HPV-related oropharyngeal cancers [66]. Other important modifiers of prognosis include performance status, comorbidities, and age [19, 171, 197]. Importantly, second neoplasms are also common, contributing to mortality and warranting long-term follow-up for patients with a history of HNSCC [10, 114].

1.3 Salivary Gland Carcinoma

Primary salivary gland malignancies are rare (~0.5–1% of all cancers) and heterogeneous, with over 20 types described by the 2017 World Health Organization (WHO) classification system. Mucoepidermoid carcinoma and adenoid cystic carcinoma account for approximately half of malignant salivary gland tumors, with other common histologies including carcinoma ex-pleomorphic adenoma, adenocarcinoma and squamous cell carcinoma [213]. These tumors can arise within major salivary glands such as the parotid, submandibular, and sublingual glands, or within minor salivary glands scattered throughout the mucosal surfaces of the head and neck. The majority of malignant salivary gland tumors arise from the parotid gland. Prognosis depends primarily on grade, histology, tumor size, and extent of local invasion. Surgical resection is the preferred frontline treatment. However, adequate resection of tumors within the parotid gland in particular can be challenging, given branching of the facial nerve within the gland. In the setting of close or positive surgical margins, and also in the presence of other adverse features, many malignant salivary gland tumors require adjuvant RT with dose and fractionation similar to that described for HNSCC: typically 60–66 Gy at

2 Gy/fraction. Indications for RT include poorly differentiated and/or high-risk histologic subtype (particularly adenoid cystic carcinoma), extraparenchymal extension, T4 (and select T3) disease, nodal involvement, perineural invasion, and lymphovascular invasion. Definitive RT may be utilized for patients who are not surgical candidates. There is notably insufficient evidence to recommend concurrent systemic therapy in most cases, even when tumors are deemed unresectable [34].

1.4 Thyroid Cancer

The lifetime risk of thyroid cancer in the United States is 1.2% [136], and approximately 586,000 new cases are diagnosed globally each year (NCI Surveillance, Epidemiology, and End Results (SEER) Program). There are several histologic types of thyroid cancer: differentiated (encompassing papillary, follicular and Hurthle cell types), medullary, and anaplastic. Exposure to ionizing radiation is the most common environmental risk factor for the development of thyroid cancer. The vast majority (almost 90%) of thyroid cancers are papillary type, which typically carry an excellent prognosis with 10-year survival rates >90%. Very few prospective randomized trials for thyroid cancer have been performed, though results from large cohort studies help to guide management [16]. Differentiated thyroid cancers typically present as solitary, relatively asymptomatic thyroid nodules. About half of these nodules are discovered incidentally on routine physical exams or on imaging studies. The American College of Radiology (ACR) Thyroid Imaging Reporting and Data System (TI-RADS) categorizes thyroid nodules into five risk levels based on ultrasound features (composition, echogenicity, shape, margin, and echogenic foci), with corresponding management recommendations ranging from no further follow-up to biopsy [185]. Ultrasound-guided FNA for cytopathologic evaluation is the initial diagnostic procedure of choice. The Bethesda system includes six classes for reporting thyroid cytopathology: nondiagnostic (I), benign (II), atypia or follicular lesion of undetermined significance (III), follicular neoplasm or suspicion for follicular neoplasm (IV), suspicious for malignancy (V), and malignant (VI) [42]. Importantly, FNA is not adequate for the diagnosis of follicular and Hurthle cell carcinomas, as diagnostic criteria mandate demonstration of pathological architectural features such as vascular or capsular invasion.

Further workup for thyroid nodules includes thyroid function testing, as well as thyroid scintigraphy to evaluate functional status in patients with low thyroid stimulating hormone (TSH). Patients with benign follicular adenomas often have autonomously functioning “hot” nodules, whereas hypo-functioning “cold” nodules carry a higher suspicion of malignancy. For patients with biopsy-proven thyroid malignancy, cross-sectional contrast-enhanced CT and/or MRI should be performed to evaluate for locally advanced disease. In the setting of voice changes, the vocal cords should also be directly visualized given risk of vocal cord paralysis due to recurrent laryngeal nerve involvement by tumor. Patients with suspicious clinical, imaging, and FNA findings with hypo-functioning nodules should proceed to surgical evaluation, namely diagnostic thyroid lobectomy (in the setting of low-risk disease) or total thyroidectomy. After total thyroidectomy for differentiated thyroid carcinomas, diagnostic whole-body iodine-131 imaging can be indicated to assess for residual disease. Radioactive iodine (RAI) is typically administered to patients at high risk of persistent or recurrent disease, based on risk factors such as large tumor size, extra-thyroid extension, nodal disease burden, and/or high thyroglobulin levels (indicative of residual thyroid tissue or carcinoma). RAI dose is based on the extent of residual disease burden, typically ranging from 30 to 200 millicuries (mCi) [82]. TSH can stimulate tumor growth; thus, TSH suppression through administration of exogenous thyroid hormone (levothyroxine) is typically indicated. Adjuvant external beam RT may be beneficial after RAI in the setting of locally advanced primary tumors, lymph node involvement, and/or positive margins. IMRT is usually delivered in 2 Gy daily fractions to a total dose of 60–70 Gy, depending on the extent of resection. Age is the most important factor for prognosis, with more lethal disease occurring in patients older than 40 years of age. Other factors that affect prognosis include locoregional tumor extent and the presence of distant metastases [16].

Medullary thyroid carcinoma (MTC) arises from neuroendocrine C cells of the thyroid gland. About 20% of cases are associated with inherited tumor syndromes such as multiple endocrine neoplasia (MEN) types 2A and 2B. Patients with these hereditary syndromes can also present with pheochromocytomas, which can result in hypertensive crisis during surgery if not properly managed. It is thus important to perform preoperative genetic screening if there is any suspicion of MTC. Total thyroidectomy and neck dissection are recommended for most patients with MTC. RAI is not indicated for MTC, given that these tumor cells do not concentrate iodine. Adjuvant RT is rarely indicated for MTC given a lack of data indicating benefit, though definitive IMRT (dosing as above) can be indicated in the setting of unresectable disease or incomplete resection [16].

Anaplastic thyroid carcinomas are aggressive, undifferentiated malignancies that are rarely curable. Given their aggressive nature, they are often diagnosed in the setting of symptoms such as a rapidly enlarging neck mass, Horner's syndrome, dyspnea, dysphagia, and/or voice changes. Furthermore, patients commonly present with distant metastases at diagnosis. Surgical resection is the primary treatment option; however, most patients have unresectable and/or metastatic disease at presentation. Total thyroidectomy has only been shown to improve survival in the rare patients who present with small, confined tumors. Similar to MTC, these tumors do not concentrate iodine, so RAI is not used. RT or CRT has been shown to improve local control and short-term survival in certain patients, independent of the extent of resection [16]. Weekly paclitaxel or doxorubicin (sometimes combined with docetaxel or cisplatin) is commonly used in combination with RT for definitive or adjuvant treatment. For patients with *BRAF* V600E mutation, dabrafenib and trametinib may be used in the neoadjuvant setting or for unresectable disease. Given generally poor outcomes for anaplastic thyroid cancer with standard therapies, clinical trials should be considered for patients with adequate functional status.

2 Part 2. Conventional Animal Models

2.1 Overview

Small (mouse, rat, guinea pig, hamster) or large (nonhuman primates) animals are utilized as preclinical models for biomedical research. Mice and rats are used most commonly in oncology research, largely due to the feasibility of large-scale studies given their small size and relatively low expense [208]. In this chapter, we will focus primarily on murine models of HNC. A primary goal of preclinical research is to improve care for patients. Unfortunately, only ~8% of preclinical oncology studies translate successfully to clinical practice, likely due to limited similarities between murine models and human cancer [120]. Often, several types of mouse models are necessary to understand the full scope of disease and potential effects of a treatment. Accounting for both the strengths and limitations of available mouse models is necessary to increase translational probability.

2.2 Transplant Tumor Mouse Models

Transplant tumor models require in vitro cultivation of tumor cells and injecting a bolus of these cells into the mouse; mice can also be injected with small pieces of solid tumor, though the former method is more common. The location for tumor cell injection has proven to be critical for studying patterns of metastasis, as growth, invasion, and interaction with the host immune system can be site-specific [52]. Cells are often injected heterotopically in the hind flank, leading to homogenous tumors that are simple to visualize and measure. This can be a useful site when studying radiation therapy because the acute, normal tissue effects are minimal at therapeutic doses, and the flank can be targeted without an image-guided small animal irradiator. Orthotopic tumor models provide a more clinically relevant tumor microenvironment. For HNSCC, orthotopic models typically entail tumor cell injection into the tongue, floor of mouth, or buccal mucosa (representative CT images of a mouse with an orthotopically grown tongue tumor are provided in Fig. 1).

Transplant models provide a relatively cheap, high-throughput platform for studying novel treatments. They also can be easily genetically modified; for example, utilizing CRISPR/Cas9 technology to mutate genes of interest in tumor cells prior to injection. However, two-dimensional culturing prior to in vivo transplant may lead to genetic instabilities and clonal selection that can affect treatment response and contribute to poor repeatability [167, 190]. Transplant tumors also develop substantially differently than spontaneous tumors such as those that develop in humans and companion animals. Briefly, transplanted tumors grow much more quickly than spontaneous cancers, leading to a tumor microenvironment unique to transplant models: (1) Decreased stromal component in transplant tumors can affect the distribution of immune cells within a tumor, as well as its metastatic potential. Cells that have been cultured often lack the ability to undergo epithelial-mesenchymal transition, significantly altering tumor architecture, though this is somewhat dependent on transplant location [74, 148]. (2) Transplant tumors typically lack functional vasculature, with blood vessels exhibiting fragile, leaky endothelial cell linings and chaotic organization. This can impact response to RT and chemotherapy due to a lack of vascular coverage and leakiness [74, 164]. (3) Immune cell infiltration can be affected by the immune response induced by injecting a large bolus of tumor cells, which starkly contrasts the gradual co-evolution of tumor and host immune system in spontaneous tumors [49, 206].

2.2.1 Syngeneic Mouse Models

Syngeneic mouse models require utilizing cancer cells with the same genetic background as the animal into which they are transplanted to avoid immune-mediated rejection. Particularly when implanted orthotopically, these models can be used to study immune responses, stromal signaling, angiogenesis, and metastasis [74]. Early syngeneic models utilized cells from a spontaneous abdominal wall SCC in C3H/HeJ mice (SCC VII/SF) [35]. It has a Toll-like receptor 4 (TLR4) mutation which regulates inflammatory and immune pathways and is upregulated in ~50% of human HNSCC [92, 166, 184]. While this model is less clinically relevant for human HNSCC because it did not originate in the head and neck region, it was critical to developing orthotopic models that exhibit local invasion and lymph and lung metastases upon injection into the floor of mouth [144]. Several review articles describe similar HNC models, including JC1-2 and 4MOSC in detail [109, 175, 202]. Recent preclinical HNSCC research has focused on models that exhibit clinically relevant mutations and are often categorized based on HPV status.

Studying HPV+ HNSCC in preclinical models is critical for understanding biological mechanisms of progression, novel treatments, and potential causes of treatment resistance. The mEERL cell line is a HPV+ SCC developed by transducing C57BL/6 murine tonsillar epithelial cells to stably express HPV16 E6, HPV16 E7, and hRas [200]. Although *HRAS* is only mutated in ~3–4% of human HNSCC, the HPV-associated oncoproteins E6 and E7 are nearly ubiquitously expressed in HPV16+ human HNSCC [44]. Daughter metastatic cell lines (MLM#1, #3, #5, #10) were generated from lung metastases that developed in a mouse with an mEERL tumor treated with cisplatin and RT. In a recent study, both mEERL and MLM #10 transplant tumors were cured by cisplatin and RT (20 mg/m^2 and 8 Gy, respectively, delivered on days 4, 11, and 18). Conversely, MLM #1, #3, and #5 showed heterogeneous treatment responses [200]. Thus, the parental mEERL and daughter MLM cell lines may facilitate understanding of chemoradiation resistance in HPV+ HNSCC and evaluating potential treatments to overcome therapeutic resistance.

Mouse oral carcinoma (MOC) cell lines developed in C57BL/6 mice exposed to 7,12-dimethylbenz[a]anthracene (DMBA), a carcinogen primarily found in fossil-fuel-contaminated environments, are commonly used in transplant models to study HPV-HNSCC [93]. Three SCC cell lines were developed: MOC1 from a mucosal lip tumor, MOC2 from a floor of mouth tumor, and MOC22 from a buccal tumor [98]. MOC1 and MOC2 exhibit different rates of cancer cell proliferation, immune cell infiltrates, and metastatic potential. MOC1 tumors grow more slowly, have higher CD8+ T cell infiltrates, and are less likely to metastasize to draining lymph nodes. Similarly, MOC22 tumors do not spread regionally or distantly, and they have relatively high infiltration of CD4+ and CD8+ T cells. In contrast, MOC2 tumors enlarge rapidly, exhibit immunosuppressive regulatory T cell infiltrates, and demonstrate a metastatic phenotype [93]. Ongoing studies are investigating MOC tumor sensitivity and resistance to standard therapies like RT and cisplatin, as well as immune checkpoint blockade.

2.2.2 Xenograft Mouse Models

Xenograft tumor models are generated by transplanting human tumors (patient-derived, i.e., PDX) or human cancer cells (CDX) into an immunodeficient mouse [139]. Immunodeficient mice lack a functional immune system and therefore avoid xenograft rejection; however, they cannot be used to study antitumor immune response or efficacy of immunotherapies, which is a significant limitation [1, 109]. Common CDX models include JHU-011 (and its derivative lines like JHU-029), derived from a human laryngeal SCC, and FaDu, established from a hypopharyngeal SCC [160]. Though CDX tumors have higher tumor penetrance and are simpler to utilize, PDX models provide advantages over CDX because they retain the heterogeneity of the original tumor, promoting conditions similar to those observed in the tumor microenvironment in human HNC, including a similar stromal component [190]. Thus, they provide an attractive model to investigate anticancer therapies and potentially provide an opportunity to facilitate personalized treatment selection for the patient from whom the PDX was derived [38, 169]. Humanized mice, in which immunodeficient mice have been engrafted with human CD34+ hematopoietic stem cells or peripheral blood mononuclear cells, provide a platform for studying human tumors in vivo with a relatively functional immune system [190]. However, the high expense of these models makes them impractical for high-throughput, large-scale studies.

2.3 Spontaneous Tumor Mouse Models

There are multiple methods for inducing spontaneous tumors in mice, including carcinogen exposure, utilization of transgenic mice, and introduction of DNA constructs, e.g., through electroporation, lentiviral infection, or Sleeping Beauty transposase. While this chapter discusses a few spontaneous HNC models, several articles provide a comprehensive review of spontaneous murine tumor models, including historical and practical perspectives [81, 94, 190]. Spontaneous tumor models offer numerous strengths: (1) These murine tumors develop similarly to their human counterparts, often beginning with mutation(s) in a single cell leading to a survival advantage, accumulation of additional mutations, and gradual growth to become cancer. The stepwise development and interaction with surrounding nonmalignant cells over a period of weeks to months lead to a tumor microenvironment comparable to human malignancies. Spontaneous tumors exhibit increased stromal components compared to transplant tumors, affecting tumor architecture and interactions with the immune system. The vasculature also grows more slowly, increasing the proportion of mature, functional vasculature relative to chaotic, leaky, and inefficient vessels [74]. (2) The genetic alterations in these models are usually similar to human HNC, including common mutations in *TP53*, *RAS*, *PIK3CA*, etc. Mutational load can be modulated via carcinogenic exposure that mimics tobacco use [175, 190]. Specific mutations have variable effects on tumor behavior and treatment response, which can be studied in a controlled manner using genetically engineered mouse models (GEMMs). (3) Immunotherapy has generated a surge of interest with paradigm-shifting improvements in outcomes for numerous human malignancies. Notably, immunotherapy response depends both on innate properties of the tumor and host immune system, and immunogenic transplant tumor models often demonstrate high rates of immunotherapy response that have not translated well to patients with HNC [41]. In spontaneous models, tumors grow under normal immunosurveillance and co-evolve with the host immune system typically leading to immune profiles more similar to poorly immunogenic human tumors compared to transplant tumors [74].

Major limiting factors that reduce the use of spontaneous tumor models include the high cost and time-consuming nature of these models compared to transplant models. Obtaining the correct genotype for a GEMM may take over a year, and developing new transgenic mice takes several months and thousands of dollars. While carcinogen exposure is less costly, these models often require administering a chemical for several months. Inducing tumors by lentiviral infection or electroporation to introduce DNA containing oncogenes or CRISPR/Cas9 constructs often has low penetrance and a long tumor latency period. GEMMs with constitutive whole-animal mutations, as opposed to inducible tissue-specific conditional mutations, frequently develop off-target tumors requiring euthanasia prior to the planned study endpoint.

2.3.1 Carcinogen-Induced Tumor Models

Exposure to tobacco accounts for ~70% of human HNSCC via formation of carcinogen-DNA adducts that lead to mutations [89]. 4-Nitroquinoline 1-oxide (4NQO) causes similar DNA damage and tumor formation when mice are exposed over the course of weeks, typically in drinking water [87]. This method reliably induces tumors in immunocompetent, wild type mice and can also be combined with transgenic models to study the involvement of specific genes in cancer development and progression. 4NQO-induced oral carcinogenesis recapitulates the gradual HNSCC development that occurs in humans and companion animals, offering an opportunity to study genetic similarities in an immunocompetent model [38, 202]. This model has also been used to investigate how cancer stem cells impact treatment resistance and metastasis [36]. However, notable limitations include a long time to tumor onset (sometimes >40 weeks) and the risk of off-target gastrointestinal tumors due to 4NQO ingestion [190].

2.3.2 Genetically Engineered Mouse Models (GEMMs)

GEMMs fill a unique role in preclinical models because they provide a platform to study specific genetic mutations in a controlled background. They can be established through a multitude of methods (e.g., microinjection of exogenous DNA into mouse embryonic stem cells, Sleepy Beauty transposon system, and CRISPR/Cas9), leading to alterations in the mouse genome, with potential augmentation of mutational burden by additional carcinogen exposure [88, 94]. Recently developed GEMM HNSCC models include an HPV+ model that uses tamoxifen-activated Cre-recombinase under the control of the cytokeratin-14 promoter to express HPV16 oncoproteins E6 and E7, along with mutated Pik3ca, which is altered in ~50% of HPV+ HNSCC cases [33]. Histopathologically, these tumors resemble human oropharyngeal SCC; however, most are exophytic and do not exhibit invasive features. Another model uses the Sleeping Beauty transposon system to introduce HPV16-E6/7 and constitutively active mutant *Nras* (altered in 2% of HNSCC [143]) into the genome of murine oral mucosal epithelial cells [110]. These tumors metastasized to draining lymph nodes and distant sites, with malignant cells demonstrating high mitotic activity, as observed in aggressive HNSCC [110].

2.3.3 Murine Papillomavirus-Induced Tumors

Papillomaviruses are small, species-specific double-stranded DNA viruses [83]. The species specificity posed a challenge in studying the role of HPV in HNSCC development in mouse models. In recent years, infection-based models using murine papillomavirus (MmuPV1) have emerged as preclinical models to investigate infection-mediated carcinogenesis [83, 86]. Mice infected with MmuPV1 in the oral epithelia develop neoplastic lesions that can progress to high-grade dysplasia. Exposure to 4NQO causes progression to invasive SCC [204]. Similar to 4NQO-only models, the MmuPV1 4NQO model provides the benefit of histological stepwise progression from mild dysplasia to carcinoma, comparable to HNSCC development in humans and companion animals. Given the tropism of MmuPV1, which can infect mucosal and cutaneous tissues, viral carcinogenesis can also be evaluated in other anatomic sites where HPV-related tumors develop, including the vaginal canal and anus [43]. Papillomavirus infection activates the adaptive and innate immune systems, so these models provide an opportunity to study the interplay between host immune response and tumor development [83].

3 Part 3. Companion Animal Models and Comparative Oncology

3.1 Overview

Companion dogs and cats are affected by a variety of head and neck tumors, including tumors of the oral cavity, pharynx, larynx, nasal cavity, paranasal sinuses, salivary glands, and thyroid. Tumors are classified by histology and location. Oral tumors are particularly common, accounting for approximately 6–7% of all neoplasms in dogs and 10% in cats. The most common canine oral tumors are malignant melanoma, squamous cell carcinoma, and fibrosarcoma. In cats, a large majority of oral tumors are SCC. Sinonasal and nasopharyngeal tumors account for approximately 1% of all cancers in dogs; carcinomas comprise approximately two thirds of intranasal tumors, and the remainder are largely sarcomas and round cell tumors. Sinonasal cancer is less frequent in cats; in order of decreasing frequency are intranasal lymphomas, carcinomas, and sarcomas. This section will focus on diseases of clinical relevance in human patients, including oral SCC, nasal carcinoma, salivary gland neoplasia, and thyroid cancers. Canine oral melanoma is discussed elsewhere.

3.2 Canine Oral and Oropharyngeal Squamous Cell Carcinoma

3.2.1 Etiology, Epidemiology, and Biological Behavior

In dogs, SCC is the second most common type of tumor occurring in the oral cavity and oropharynx [128], and a distinction is made between tonsillar and nontonsillar forms of SCC due to divergent clinical behavior. Tonsillar SCC is highly metastatic, and prognosis is poor even with intensive treatment. Nontonsillar SCC is locally invasive, but because about three-quarters of tumors are low grade [153] and the metastatic rate is <20% [191], prognosis tends to be good when local control can be achieved with surgery or RT.

The prevalence of canine nontonsillar oral SCC has been estimated in 6.4 to 7.3 cases per 100,000 [127]. Rates are more variable for tonsillar SCC in the dog, with 91 to 120 per 100,000 cases in large cities and essentially none in rural communities [127]. Overall, the occurrence of oral and oropharyngeal SCC in the dog is similar to humans, for whom the average incidence rate for head and neck cancers is estimated to be 8.8 and 5.1 per 100,000 men and women, respectively [159].

Dogs can be infected with canine papillomaviruses (CPV), and CPV DNA has been identified in canine malignancies. In a research colony with X-linked severe combined immunodeficiency, CPV-2 was associated with the development of metastatic SCC of the skin [69]. There are also scattered reports of various CPVs being associated with cutaneous and oral SCC lesions in immunocompetent dogs [115–117, 131, 132]. However, most canine SCC lesions are CPV-negative. Without any known shared environmental risk factors, canine oral and oropharyngeal SCCs may be most like the 10–15% of HPV-negative HNSCC cases that develop in patients who neither use tobacco nor drink alcohol [50, 61].

3.2.2 Biology

Several histologic subtypes of oral nontonsillar SCC have been described. In a study by Nemec and colleagues, 48% of lesions were well-differentiated and 45% were moderately differentiated. Less common subtypes include poorly differentiated, papillary, basaloid, adenosquamous, and spindle cell carcinoma [137]. Moderately to well-differentiated oral SCC tends to occur in older dogs, and while not restricted to any single breed, English springer spaniels and Shetland sheepdogs are overrepresented. More than 70% are associated with the dentate jaws, but well-differentiated lesions are most often associated with the tongue and other mucosal surfaces. Nearly 80% are proliferative, either with or without ulceration. There is evidence for lymphovascular invasion in 6% of cases, and perineural invasion in 10% of cases. Histologically, tumor-associated inflammation is reported to be mild in 30% of cases, moderate in 44%, and severe in 12% [137]. Tumor-associated inflammation, perineural invasion, and lymphovascular invasion are all associated with increased risk of death after surgical excision [64].

A set of 33 canine oral SCC lesions was studied to characterize the microenvironmental immune landscape; the predominating immune infiltrates were CD3+ T cells and CD204+ macrophages [21]. Based upon CD3+ T cell microanatomical distribution, 77% of samples had labeling consistent with a "pre-existing immunity" pattern, which is considered highly inflamed. Only 14% were non-inflamed ("immunologically ignorant" staining pattern), and the remaining 6% were characterized by an immunosuppressive immune landscape ("excluded infiltrates") [21, 79]. Immunologically "hot" tumors had high expression of CXCL2, a chemokine associated with myeloid-derived suppressor cell (MDSC) recruitment and differentiation [21].

Nine spontaneous canine oral nontonsillar lesions have been characterized via genome-wide analyses, including high-density array comparative genomic hybridization and RNA sequencing [112]. Similar to human HNSCC, canine disease is characterized by variations in the extent of genomic copy number abnormalities, with significantly more in buccal and lingual tumors as compared with gingival tumors [112]. Consistent with human tumors, there were generally more amplifications than deletions, and the most enriched genes were associated with protein kinase activity. The canine tumors were also characterized by loss of the cell cycle gene *CDKN2A*, which is commonly mutated in human HNSCC. By contrast, *TP53* mutations appeared less frequently than have been observed in HPV-negative human HNSCC [112].

3.2.3 Treatment

In dogs with tonsillar SCC, the clinical workup ideally includes sedated oral examination, either ultrasound or CT of the neck, FNA and cytology of the draining lymph nodes, and thoracic imaging. The vast majority have unilateral disease; interestingly, the primary tumor is often quite small relative to metastatic medial retropharyngeal lymph nodes. At the time of diagnosis, metastasis to regional lymph nodes and lungs has been reported in 47–82% and 5–15% of cases, respectively [72, 122, 192]. In a study of 123 dogs, median survival was 381 days for dogs presenting without evidence of metastasis, 153 days for dogs with a single affected lymph node, and 88 days for dogs with either multiple metastatic lymph nodes or distant dissemination. On multivariate analysis, performing lymphadenectomy was associated with improved survival (hazard ratio: 0.5; $p = 0.01$) [192]. Adjunctive therapies may further improve prognosis. In dogs treated with surgery and chemotherapy, reported median survival ranges from 212 to 465 days [72, 122]. In a series of dogs treated with chemotherapy and radiotherapy, median survival was 355 days

[122]. Surgery followed by radiotherapy and then chemotherapy has been associated with median survival ranging from 243 to 270 days [29, 133]. There is no standard irradiation protocol; most reported cases have been treated with once-weekly hypofractionated external beam radiotherapy directed at the primary tumor and regional lymph nodes. It is unknown whether radiation dose intensification might improve outcomes. Notably, when dogs receive either carboplatin or toceranib phosphate as their sole treatment, response rates are low; approximately 30% of dogs exhibit stable disease or a partial response [192]. Likewise, in the absence of surgery or radiotherapy, multi-agent injectable chemotherapy appears to be of limited value, with infrequent responses and rapid death [29].

For dogs with locoregionally confined nontonsillar oral SCC, surgery is generally regarded as the treatment of choice. Complete excision often requires either partial mandibulectomy or maxillectomy [99, 201]. While some dogs have trouble eating after such procedures, most pet owners perceive quality of life to be improved postoperatively [60]. When histologic margins are negative, surgery alone is sufficient to yield excellent prognoses. In a study of 25 juvenile dogs with oral nontonsillar SCC undergoing surgery alone, negative margins were achieved in 24 cases. The median follow-up time was >1500 days with no dogs developing evidence of either metastatic disease or locoregional tumor recurrence, and there were no tumor-attributable deaths [170]. In adult dogs, 1-year survival rates range from 84% to 94% [64, 99, 201, 205].

With incomplete excision, postoperative radiotherapy protects against recurrence and has been associated with a median survival of >2000 days [165]. Radiotherapy can also be used as the primary definitive therapy. In a study of 14 dogs treated with 48 to 57 Gy total in 3 to 4 Gy fractions administered daily (Monday through Friday), the median disease-free and overall survival times were 365 and 450 days, respectively [101]. With these types of RT protocols, the incidence of moderate radiodermatitis and oral mucositis is nearly 100%, but only 8% have treatment discontinued due to severe toxicity, and the incidence of severe late toxicities (e.g., bone necrosis, fistula formation) is similar (7.6%) [188]. With RT alone, there is a clear dose-response relationship, with 57% of tumors controlled by 40 Gy and 75% controlled by 45 Gy (given in 10 daily fractions); the dose for 50% tumor control probability at 1 year is 38 Gy (again, in 10 daily fractions). This knowledge can be leveraged to study the impact of experimental radiosensitizers, as has been demonstrated in a study wherein thermal enhancement was studied with the dose for 50% tumor control probability reduced to 33 Gy by the combination of RT and heat [65].

Regardless of whether treatment involves surgery, RT, or a combination thereof, the risk of lymph node metastasis is low for nontonsillar SCC. It is recommended that initial staging include FNA and cytologic evaluation of the regional (mandibular and medial retropharyngeal) lymph nodes. However, treatment of nodes is generally reserved for cases with known metastasis [15, 45]. This is in contrast to humans, where elective nodal irradiation is standard.

For dogs with small oral SCC lesions, electrochemotherapy (electroporation after intravenous administration of bleomycin) appears to be a viable alternative when surgery and/or radiotherapy are opted against. In a study of 11 dogs, the overall response rate was 90.9%; during the follow-up period, 3 dogs experienced recurrence at a median of 50 days [174].

Canine oral papillary SCC is a rare subtype that represents a distinct clinical entity. It is diagnosed at a median age of 4 years [137, 181], and is characterized by an exophytic growth pattern [128] with no known relation to CPV infection [146, 186]. The metastatic potential is low [138], and surgery is the treatment of choice [146, 178, 181]. Radiotherapy can be used postoperatively [146] or as the primary definitive-intent treatment [196]. In a retrospective study of 10 dogs treated with definitive RT (10 to 16 daily fractions of 3.2 Gy), 9 achieved a complete response. Two of those complete responders died of unrelated causes, and the remaining 7 were alive at the time of publication, with a median follow-up time of 961 days. The one remaining dog had a partial response that progressed 228 days after RT [196].

3.3 Feline Oral and Oropharyngeal Squamous Cell Carcinoma

3.3.1 Etiology and Epidemiology

Similar to SCC comprising ~90% of head and neck cancers in people, feline oral and oropharyngeal SCC lesions (FOSCC) account for up to 7% of all feline malignancies and 80% of all oral tumors in domestic cats. As with human HNSCC, tobacco smoke is a known risk factor for FOSCC [176, 214]. Other environmental factors that increase the risk of a cat developing FOSCC include living in a rural environment, outdoor access, being fed pet food containing chemical additives, eating canned food or tuna, and wearing certain flea collars [14, 214].

Nearly 25% of human HNSCC cases are associated with human papillomavirus (HPV) infection, and a similar proportion of FOSCC lesions contain viral DNA for *Felis catus* papillomavirus (FcaPV) [6, 7]. In both species, papillomavirus-induced carcinogenesis is mediated by the E6 and E7 oncogenes [4, 5]. Epstein-Barr virus has been identified in FOSCC lesions, but infrequently [40].

Just as occurs in human HNSCC, FOSCC is characterized by frequent EGFR overexpression and dysregulation of p53 and CK2 [12, 56, 113, 210].

3.3.2 Biologic Behavior, Treatment, and Prognosis

Clinical features of human HNSCC and FOSCC are also similar (representative CT images of a pet cat with spontaneously occurring SCC of the tumor are shown in Fig. 1). In both species there is an approximately 15–20% risk of metastasis (namely to regional lymph nodes, and later to the lungs) [177]. However, the main challenge is a destructive and potentially bone-invasive primary tumor that, in some cases, can be successfully managed with surgery, and in other cases requires (chemo)RT. Cats amenable to surgery are generally restricted to those with small and rostrally located tumors [22, 84, 142]. A 2001 publication by Bregazzi and colleagues described 7 cats treated with 24 Gy in 3 weekly fractions of 8 Gy. Three of the cats failed to complete treatment, and six were euthanized at a median of 60 days. It was concluded that this coarse fractionation protocol did not result in palliation [27]. A subsequent paper described treatment of 11 cats with 20 Gy in 5 consecutive daily fractions of 4 Gy. The overall response rate was 55% with a median overall survival time of 3 months [123]. A paper describing outcomes in 15 cats treated with either stereotactic radiosurgery (20 Gy in a single fraction) or stereotactic radiotherapy (30 Gy total in 3 consecutive daily fractions of 10 Gy) reported an overall response rate of 39% and a median overall survival time of 106 days. There was very little acute toxicity, and responders had rapid tumor volume reduction. However, as with the aforementioned protocols, recurrence led to rapid euthanasia [211]. Somewhat improved outcomes have been reported for cats treated with higher total RT doses. In a group of 21 cats treated with 10 daily fractions of 4.8 Gy, the overall response rate was 71% with a median overall survival time of 174 days [158]. In a group of 31 cats undergoing 14 twice-daily fractions of 3.5 Gy with concurrent carboplatin (100 mg/m^2 IV on days 1 and 4.5 of RT), about half of cats had a complete response to therapy, and the median overall survival time was 163 days [57]. Notably, nearly all cats treated with these more intensive protocols experienced moderate to severe oral mucositis.

3.4 Canine Nasal, Sinonasal, and Nasopharyngeal Tumors

Nasal tumors represent about 1% of all canine malignancies, with two-thirds being carcinomas (either adenocarcinoma, SCC, or undifferentiated) and the rest largely being sarcomas (e.g., fibrosarcoma, chondrosarcoma, osteosarcoma, and undifferentiated sarcoma) [118, 119, 152]. While there are no epidemiological studies to substantiate the claim, it is often proffered that long-nosed (dolicocephalic) breeds are at higher risk due to trapping of inhaled carcinogens [30, 163]. While gross metastatic disease is infrequently identified at initial diagnosis, necropsy studies indicate that up to 40% have regional nodal or distant (e.g., pulmonary) metastases at the time of death [151]. Limited data suggest that the presence of metastatic disease at the time of diagnosis may be associated with poor survival even with treatment [80].

Left untreated, the median survival time for dogs with nasal carcinoma is reported to be 95 days; presence of epistaxis is predictive of early euthanasia [161]. Clinically, canine intranasal tumors recur quickly after surgical debulking, and responses to cytotoxic chemotherapy are short-lived [76, 207]. At present, external beam megavoltage radiotherapy represents the treatment of choice, and various treatment protocols have been reported. While coarsely fractionated radiotherapy (i.e., weekly 8 Gy fractions with a total dose of 32 Gy) alone can improve quality of life, the longest reported survivals are in populations of dogs treated with radiotherapy (42 Gy in 10 daily fractions) followed by exenteration [2], radiotherapy (54 Gy in 18 fractions) along with cisplatin (60 mg/m^2 given once) that slowly elutes from an intramuscular device (sponge) implanted at a distant site [102], or SBRT (30 Gy in 3 daily fractions) [140].

It is possible that oncologic outcomes could be further improved with novel targeted therapies and combinatorial approaches. However, scientific advances in that regard have been limited by the fact that the biology of canine nasal tumors has not been particularly well characterized. Several factors have been identified which may predict outcomes after RT. For example, dogs with intranasal carcinomas are reported to have a 3.3-fold higher risk of relapse after RT as compared with dogs with intranasal sarcomas [187]. Poor survival has also been associated with tumor histology (anaplastic tumors and keratinizing or non-keratinizing SCC), as well as local tumor stage [3, 46]. With regard to their molecular biology, a majority of canine nasal carcinomas express cyclooxygenase isoform 2 [20, 85, 97], but expression level is not known to be predictive of survival after tumor irradiation [11, 62]. Many canine nasal carcinomas express EGFR, and overexpression has been negatively correlated with survival after radiotherapy [62, 173]. Likewise, nasal carcinomas overexpress vascular endothelial growth factor receptor, as well as platelet-derived growth factor receptor [71]; this has been offered as the biological basis for treating nasal carcinomas with the receptor tyrosine kinase inhibitor toceranib phosphate, and indeed nasal carcinomas do seem to respond favorably to that drug when given alone or in combination with radiotherapy [53, 126]. From an immune-oncology perspective, limited data suggest that immune infiltrates in the canine nasal tumor microenvironment differ by carcinoma subtype [198]; all are heavily infiltrated by neutrophils and macrophages, and T cells are particularly prominent in transitional carcinomas (nonkeratinizing SCC).

3.5 Feline Nasal, Sinonasal, and Nasopharyngeal Tumors

Sinonasal tumors account for between 1% and 8.4% of all tumors in cats, though the latter number likely overrepresents the true incidence, as it includes SCCs of the nasal planum rather than the nasal cavity or paranasal sinuses. Of the intranasal tumors that occur in cats, nearly half are carcinomas and the predominant subtype is adenocarcinoma [47]. Feline sinonasal carcinomas develop in older cats, and there is no known association with feline papillomaviruses or retroviruses (e.g., feline immunodeficiency virus and feline leukemia virus). They are locally invasive and slow to metastasize to either regional lymph nodes or distant organs (e.g., lungs) [130]. Radiotherapy is the treatment of choice and a variety of RT protocols have been reported.

In a 2014 retrospective study by Fujiwara-Igarashi and colleagues, 29 cats with lymphomatous and 36 cats with non-lymphomatous nasal tumors were evaluated [63]. Each had been treated with weekly fractions of 6–8.4 Gy to total doses of 16–36 Gy. The gross tumor and an additional 3–5 mm of surrounding tissue were treated with three-dimensional conformal radiotherapy using a 4 MV linear accelerator. Acute radiotoxicity was observed in 58.5% of cases and included alopecia (37%), ocular discharge (23%) and keratoconjunctivitis (19%). Other toxicities (e.g., moist desquamation, oral mucositis) were observed in fewer than 15% of animals. Of the irradiated cats, 39 were observable for late toxicity, the most common of which was cataract formation (21% of cases). Median PFS was 229 days, and the median OS was 432 days with 25% alive at 2 years. In this study, there was no detectable difference in outcome based on tumor type.

In a 2020 retrospective study by Giuliano and Dobson, outcomes were reported for 28 cats with intranasal carcinomas that had been treated with either four once-weekly fractions of 8.5 Gy or six twice-weekly fractions of 6 Gy, planned manually (non-graphic planning) and delivered with a single (fixed SSD) 6 MV photon beam, with an aim of covering 90–99% of the tumor with 2 to 5 mm of margin [68]. Clinical improvement was noted in 92% of cases. Mild radiotoxicity was reported in 10 cases. Median OS was 342 days. The presence of facial deformity from tumor stage IV disease (i.e., cribriform lysis) was associated with short survival.

Stiborova and colleagues reported the outcomes of 27 cats with sinonasal carcinomas that had been treated with 42 Gy total in 10 daily (Monday through Friday) fractions [182]. Complete clinical resolution of nasal signs was observed in 11% of cases, and 63% had partial responses. Progressive disease was noted within 3 months of treatment in 15% of cats. The median time to progression was 269 days, with 24% progression-free at one year. Median OS was 452 days with 27% alive at 2 years. Tumor stage was not statistically associated with outcome. However, cats with epistaxis lived longer than those without (median OS of 828 and 296 days respectively), suggesting that epistaxis may allow early detection and treatment of disease. While Veterinary Radiation Therapy Oncology Group (VRTOG) grade I acute skin toxicity was common (44.4% of cases), moderate to severe acute toxicity was infrequent (grade II ocular and mucosal toxicity recorded for one cat, and grade 3 mucosal toxicity occurred in one cat). Following irradiation, 40.7% of animals did show signs of intermittent or chronic rhinitis; there were no other severe late toxicities.

A 2021 multi-institutional retrospective study compared outcomes of 42 cats having undergone either palliative- or definitive-intent RT [212]. Eighteen cats had been treated with definitive-intent stereotactic radiotherapy, which in most cases consisted of 3 consecutive daily fractions of 10 Gy. Eight cats were treated with definitive-intent conventionally fractionated radiotherapy with total doses of 42 to 54 Gy in 10 to 20 daily fractions. Sixteen animals were treated with daily or weekly palliative-intent RT, with total doses of 16 to 36 Gy. Regardless of treatment intent, most cats had improvement of clinical signs, and treatment was well-tolerated with no cats reported to experience grade III or higher acute radiotoxicity. Median OS was longer with definitive-intent therapy (721 versus 284 days). Seven cats underwent a second course of RT at the time of locoregional disease progression; their outcomes were better than those who only underwent a single course of treatment (median OS of 824 versus 434 days). None were reported to have severe complications of such treatment (whereas in humans, there is concern for carotid blowout, brachial plexopathy, etc.).

3.6 Salivary Cancers in Veterinary Species

As in humans, cancers of the salivary glands are rarely diagnosed in companion animals. The incidence is calculated to be 15.3 per 100,000 dogs and 26.3 per 100,000 cats. Whereas older studies suggested a potential overrepresentation of salivary carcinoma in Siamese cats, more recent data fail to support this [48]. Poodles may have increased risk [48]. In dogs and cats, the most common histologic diagnosis is adenocarcinoma. The parotid gland is most affected in dogs, and the mandibular gland (analogous to submandibular gland in humans) is the predominant site in cats [77, 179].

Until recently, there were very few published data describing outcomes of dogs or cats treated for salivary tumors. In a 2001 retrospective study, median OS times were 550 days for 24 dogs and 516 days for 30 cats treated with surgery with or without adjunctive chemotherapy or radiotherapy [77]. Local control was best achieved with either adjunctive RT or multiple surgeries. Since then, few additional data have been added to the published literature regarding feline salivary tumors. In a series of six cats receiving RT as primary or postoperative therapy, none died of metastasis but at least two developed locoregional progression, and survival ranged from 55 to >776 days [17]. There has been a recent expansion in knowledge regarding management of canine salivary tumors. A 2023 multi-institutional retrospective study of the Veterinary Society of Surgical Oncology reported outcomes of 72 dogs having undergone surgery for salivary gland carcinoma [31]. Overall, 42% of cases experienced local recurrence at a median of 191 days, and 32% developed metastasis at a median of 299 days. This supports the notion that postoperative RT should improve prognosis. Presence of nodal metastasis at the time of surgery was associated with short disease-free survival (98 days) even when lymphadenectomy was performed.

3.7 Thyroid Cancers in Veterinary Species

Hyperthyroidism is the most common endocrine disorder in cats. It is almost always caused by multinodular adenomatous hyperplasia; malignant carcinomas account for no more than 3% of cases, and nonfunctional carcinomas are rare in this species [134]. Treatment for feline hyperthyroidism may include medical management with antithyroid drugs, surgical thyroidectomy, or radioactive iodine therapy. Methimazole is the most commonly used antithyroid drug in North America, and carbimazole predominates in Europe [129, 155]. While these drugs have no direct antitumor effects, they are often used for long-term management of feline hyperthyroidism. Definitive tumor-directed therapy consists of either surgical treatment or RAI, with the latter often being regarded as treatment of choice. In cats with benign thyroid disease, the typical dose is 2 to 6 mCi; with this dose, <5% of cats remain hyperthyroid or relapse [154]. Cats with thyroid carcinomas require higher doses, in the range of 20 to 30 mCi.

Thyroid tumors account for up to 3.8% of all tumors in dogs, and about half are malignant [28, 78, 209]. Whereas papillary thyroid carcinomas predominate in humans, the most common types in dogs are compact (solid) and follicular carcinomas [78]. A majority of canine thyroid carcinomas are nonfunctional, meaning that most dogs will be euthyroid and present with a palpable cervical mass. It has been estimated that 10% of dogs with thyroid tumors are hyperthyroid, and 30% are hypothyroid. Up to 40% have gross metastatic disease at the time of diagnosis, and as many as 80% ultimately develop metastasis. Risk of metastasis increases with tumor size, and is higher for dogs with bilateral tumors (which occurs in as many as 60% of cases) [121, 189]. Freely moveable tumors are generally amenable to surgical resection [96]. Median OS for dogs undergoing surgery for thyroid tumors exceeds 2 years [54, 162], and outcomes can be favorable even in the setting of gross vascular invasion [103] or bilateral carcinomas [194]. Nonresectable tumors can be managed with external beam radiotherapy or RAI.

In a study of 66 dogs undergoing treatment with RAI, the overall response rate was 35% with clinical improvement observed in 76% of dogs. The median progression-free interval was 301 days, and median OS was 564 days. Similarly long survival times were reported in another study, where the median OS was 839 days for dogs with local or regional tumors, and 366 days for dogs with distant metastatic disease at the time of treatment [195]. The primary complication of RAI in dogs is bone marrow suppression. While RAI is generally effective and well-tolerated, the dose is relatively high; in one study, the average dose was 4.1 mCi per kilogram of body weight, and the median dose in a population of 39 dogs was 100 mCi total [195]. There are many logical factors that have historically limited enthusiasm for this treatment: need for building infrastructure to isolate/house dogs while radioactive, cost of licensing, and need to hospitalize and isolate dogs while radioactive, which is a particular challenge in dogs with nonresectable thyroid cancer as they often have large cervical masses with concern for dyspnea from airway compromise and/or esophageal and pharyngeal compression that results in dysphagia and predisposes to aspiration pneumonia.

External beam radiotherapy has also been used successfully to manage canine thyroid carcinomas. Data regarding hypofractionated radiotherapy have been mixed. In an early study of 13 dogs having undergone 4 weekly fractions of 9 Gy, median OS was 672 days [26]. In a more recent study of 20 dogs undergoing four weekly fractions of 6.5 to 8 Gy, 5 dogs had either partial or complete responses to therapy, but three dogs failed to complete RT, and the median OS was only 170 days [193]. In a study of 23 dogs having undergone SBRT (15 to 40 Gy total in 1 to five fractions), the overall response rate was 80%, with 81% experiencing clinical improvement at a median of 16 days. Median PFS was 315 days, and median OS was 362 days. Even with gross metastatic disease present at diagnosis, median OS was 347 days [106]. While there have been no head-to-head comparisons or prospective trials, outcomes may improve with higher total doses of radiation. In a study of 8 dogs receiving 46.8 to 48 Gy in 11 to 12 fractions administered on alternating days, all dogs had complete resolution of their palpable thyroid tumor. The minimum OS was 12 months, and median OS was 24.5 months [150]. In a study of 25 dogs receiving 48 Gy in 4 Gy fractions for nonmetastatic locally advanced thyroid carcinomas, 72% remained progression-free at 3 years. While external beam RT is generally well-tolerated, as many as half of treated patients may ultimately require thyroid supplementation due to post-radiotherapy hypothyroidism [8].

While there is no defined role for cytotoxic chemotherapy as primary therapy or in the postoperative setting for canine thyroid tumors [58, 135, 147], there is recent and growing enthusiasm for the receptor tyrosine kinase inhibitor toceranib phosphate [172].

4 Conclusion

Head and neck cancers occur frequently both in humans (accounting for ~3% of newly diagnosed cancers in the United States) and companion animals (~7% of neoplasms in canines and 10% in felines) [183]. The relatively poor prognosis for HPV-negative HNC and limited treatment options for recurrent disease highlight the importance of research to improve understanding of the biology underlying this challenging disease and to evaluate new therapies. Similarities between HNC in humans and companion animals make the latter an attractive model for studying disease mechanisms and novel therapeutics. Current work in canines includes novel imaging and immune-radio-oncology interventions [24, 51]; there is also considerable interest in investigating methods to overcome normal tissue toxicity [37, 104]. Cats offer additional possibilities; however, translation from both canine and feline models is limited by a lack of in-depth characterization of naturally occurring HNC in these species. Despite this, companion-animal models provide numerous advantages, including the ability to image and treat tumors in a manner that closely recapitulates human treatment protocols, e.g., radiotherapy with image-guided linear accelerators, with the potential for acquisition of serial tissue samples for correlative studies.

Mouse models pose challenges given that expensive, specialized equipment is necessary to treat and image their smaller anatomy. However, preclinical murine models provide opportunities for large-scale studies with in-depth characterization of the tumor microenvironment in a controlled genetic background. Furthermore, transplant models are ideal platforms for high-throughput drug screening studies. The in vivo dynamics of tumor growth, particularly interactions with the immune system, are challenging to recapitulate in transplant models; however, spontaneous tumors often overcome this limitation through gradual development in an immunocompetent host. GEMMs provide the additional benefit of tightly regulating the mutational status of tumor cells and/or stromal tissues, facilitating in-depth mechanistic studies. Like companion-animal studies, these models are often limited by expense, though GEMMs are gradually becoming more widely available. Ultimately, complementary data obtained through studies in mice, companion animals, and humans will improve understanding of HNC pathogenesis and treatment resistance and facilitate development of improved diagnostic and therapeutic approaches.

References

1. Abdolahi S, Ghazvinian Z, Muhammadnejad S, Saleh M, Asadzadeh Aghdaei H, Baghaei K (2022) Patient-derived xenograft (PDX) models, applications and challenges in cancer research. J Transl Med 20:206
2. Adams WM, Bjorling DE, Mcanulty JE, Green EM, Forrest LJ, Vail DM (2005) Outcome of accelerated radiotherapy alone or accelerated radiotherapy followed by exenteration of the nasal cavity in dogs with intranasal neoplasia: 53 cases (1990-2002). J Am Vet Med Assoc 227:936–941
3. Adams WM, Kleiter MM, Thrall DE, Klauer JM, Forrest LJ, La Due TA, Havighurst TC (2009) Prognostic significance of tumor histology and computed tomographic staging for radiation treatment response of canine nasal tumors. Vet Radioliol Ultrasound 50:330–335
4. Altamura G, Corteggio A, Pacini L, Conte A, Pierantoni GM, Tommasino M, Accardi R, Borzacchiello G (2016) Transforming properties of Felis catus papillomavirus type 2 E6 and E7 putative oncogenes in vitro and their transcriptional activity in feline squamous cell carcinoma in vivo. Virology 496:1–8
5. Altamura G, Power K, Martano M, Degli Uberti B, Galiero G, De Luca G, Maiolino P, Borzacchiello G (2018) Felis catus papillomavirus type-2 E6 binds to E6AP, promotes E6AP/p53 binding and enhances p53 proteasomal degradation. Sci Rep 8:17529
6. Altamura G, Cardeti G, Cersini A, Eleni C, Cocumelli C, Bartolomé Del Pino LE, Razzuoli E, Martano M, Maiolino P, Borzacchiello G (2020) Detection of Felis catus papillomavirus type-2 DNA and viral gene expression suggest active infection in feline oral squamous cell carcinoma. Vet Comp Oncol 18:494–501
7. Altamura G, Cuccaro B, Eleni C, Strohmayer C, Brandt S, Borzacchiello G (2022) Investigation of multiple Felis catus papillomavirus types (-1/-2/-3/-4/-5/-6) DNAs in feline oral squamous cell carcinoma: a multicentric study. J Vet Med Sci 84:881–884
8. Amores-Fuster I, Cripps P, Blackwood L (2017) Post-radiotherapy hypothyroidism in dogs treated for thyroid carcinomas. Vet Comp Oncol 15:247–251
9. Ang KK, Harris J, Wheeler R, Weber R, Rosenthal DI, Nguyen-Tan PF, Westra WH, Chung CH, Jordan RC, Lu C, Kim H, Axelrod R, Silverman CC, Redmond KP, Gillison ML (2010) Human papillomavirus and survival of patients with oropharyngeal cancer. N Engl J Med 363:24–35
10. Baxi SS, Pinheiro LC, Patil SM, Pfister DG, Oeffinger KC, Elkin EB (2014) Causes of death in long-term survivors of head and neck cancer. Cancer 120:1507–1513
11. Belshaw Z, Constantio-Casas F, Brearley MJ, Dunning MD, Holmes MA, Dobson JM (2011) COX-2 expression and outcome in canine nasal carcinomas treated with hypofractionated radiotherapy. Vet Comp Oncol 9:141–148
12. Bergkvist GT, Argyle DJ, Morrison L, Macintyre N, Hayes A, Yool DA (2011) Expression of epidermal growth factor receptor (EGFR) and Ki67 in feline oral squamous cell carcinomas (FOSCC). Vet Comp Oncol 9:106–117
13. Bernier J, Cooper JS, Pajak TF, Van Glabbeke M, Bourhis J, Forastiere A, Ozsahin EM, Jacobs JR, Jassem J, Ang KK, Lefebvre JL (2005) Defining risk levels in locally advanced head and neck cancers: a comparative analysis of concurrent postoperative radiation plus chemotherapy trials of the EORTC (#22931) and RTOG (# 9501). Head Neck 27:843–850
14. Bertone ER, Snyder LA, Moore AS (2003) Environmental and lifestyle risk factors for oral squamous cell carcinoma in domestic cats. J Vet Intern Med 17:557–562
15. Biau J, Lapeyre M, Troussier I, Budach W, Giralt J, Grau C, Kazmierska J, Langendijk JA, Ozsahin M, O'sullivan B, Bourhis J, Gregoire V (2019) Selection of lymph node target volumes for definitive head and neck radiation therapy: a 2019 Update. Radiother Oncol 134:1–9
16. Bishop G, Cooney K, Cox S, Downing R, Mitchener K, Shanan A, Soares N, Stevens B, Wynn T (2016) 2016 AAHA/IAAHPC end-of-life care guidelines. J Am Anim Hosp Assoc 52:341–356
17. Blackwood L, Harper A, Elliott J, Gramer I (2019) External beam radiotherapy for the treatment of feline salivary gland carcinoma: six new cases and a review of the literature. J Feline Med Surg 21:186–194
18. Bledsoe TJ, Park HS, Stahl JM, Yarbrough WG, Burtness BA, Decker RH, Husain ZA (2017) Hypofractionated radiotherapy for patients with early-stage glottic cancer: patterns of care and survival. J Natl Cancer Inst 109
19. Boje CR (2014) Impact of comorbidity on treatment outcome in head and neck squamous cell

carcinoma – a systematic review. Radiother Oncol 110:81–90
20. Borzacchiello G, Paciello O, Papparella S (2004) Expression of cyclooxygenase-1 and -2 in canine nasal carcinomas. J Comp Pathol 131:70–76
21. Boss MK, Harrison LG, Gold A, Karam SD, Regan DP (2022) Canine oral squamous cell carcinoma as a spontaneous, translational model for radiation and immunology research. Front Oncol 12:1033704
22. Boston SE, Van Stee LL, Bacon NJ, Szentimrey D, Kirby BM, Van Nimwegen S, Wavreille VA (2020) Outcomes of eight cats with oral neoplasia treated with radical mandibulectomy. Vet Surg 49:222–232
23. Braakhuis BJ, Brakenhoff RH, Leemans CR (2012) Treatment choice for locally advanced head and neck cancers on the basis of risk factors: biological risk factors. Ann Oncol 23(Suppl 10):x173–x177
24. Bradshaw TJ, Bowen SR, Deveau MA, Kubicek L, White P, Bentzen SM, Chappell RJ, Forrest LJ, Jeraj R (2015) Molecular imaging biomarkers of resistance to radiation therapy for spontaneous nasal tumors in canines. Int J Radiat Oncol Biol Phys 91:787–795
25. Brana I, Siu LL (2012) Locally advanced head and neck squamous cell cancer: treatment choice based on risk factors and optimizing drug prescription. Ann Oncol 23(Suppl 10):x178–x185
26. Brearley MJ, Hayes AM, Murphy S (1999) Hypofractionated radiation therapy for invasive thyroid carcinoma in dogs: a retrospective analysis of survival. J Small Anim Pract 40:206–210
27. Bregazzi VS, Larue SM, Powers BE, Fettman MJ, Ogilvie GK, Withrow SJ (2001) Response of feline oral squamous cell carcinoma to palliative radiation therapy. Vet Radiol Ultrasound 42:77–79
28. Brodey RS, Kelly DF (1968) Thyroid neoplasms in the dog. A clinicopathologic study of fifty-seven cases. Cancer 22:406–416
29. Brooks MB, Matus RE, Leifer CE, Alfieri AA, Patnaik AK (1988) Chemotherapy versus chemotherapy plus radiotherapy in the treatment of tonsillar squamous cell carcinoma in the dog. J Vet Intern Med 2:206–211
30. Bukowski JA, Wartenberg D, Goldschmidt M (1998) Environmental causes for sinonasal cancers in pet dogs, and their usefulness as sentinels of indoor cancer risk. J Toxicol Environ Health A 54:579–591
31. Bush KM, Grimes JA, Linden DS, Plavec T, Kessler M, Rossanese M, Bennett B, Chadsey L, Coggeshall WS, Matz BM (2023) Outcomes and clinical features associated with surgically excised canine salivary gland carcinoma: a multi-institutional, retrospective, Veterinary Society of Surgical Oncology study. Vet Surg 52:370–378
32. Cancer Genome Atlas, N (2015) Comprehensive genomic characterization of head and neck squamous cell carcinomas. Nature 517:576–582
33. Carper MB, Troutman S, Wagner BL, Byrd KM, Selitsky SR, Parag-Sharma K, Henry EC, Li W, Parker JS, Montgomery SA, Cleveland JL, Williams SE, Kissil JL, Hayes DN, Amelio AL (2019) An immunocompetent mouse model of HPV16(+) head and neck squamous cell carcinoma. Cell Rep 29:1660–1674. e7
34. Caudell JJ, Gillison ML, Maghami E, Spencer S, Pfister DG, Adkins D, Birkeland AC, Brizel DM, Busse PM, Cmelak AJ, Colevas AD, Eisele DW, Galloway T, Geiger JL, Haddad RI, Hicks WL, Hitchcock YJ, Jimeno A, Leizman D, Mell LK, Mittal BB, Pinto HA, Rocco JW, Rodriguez CP, Savvides PS, Schwartz D, Shah JP, Sher D, St. John M, Weber RS, Weinstein G, Worden F, Yang Bruce J, Yom SS, Zhen W, Burns JL, Darlow SD (2022) NCCN guidelines® insights: head and neck cancers, version 1.2022: featured updates to the NCCN guidelines. J Natl Compr Cancer Netw 20:224–234
35. Chaves P, Garrido M, Oliver J, Perez-Ruiz E, Barragan I, Rueda-Dominguez A (2023) Preclinical models in head and neck squamous cell carcinoma. Br J Cancer 128:1819–1827
36. Chen D, Wu M, Li Y, Chang I, Yuan Q, Ekimyan-Salvo M, Deng P, Yu B, Yu Y, Dong J, Szymanski JM, Ramadoss S, Li J, Wang CY (2017) Targeting BMI1(+) cancer stem cells overcomes chemoresistance and inhibits metastases in squamous cell carcinoma. Cell Stem Cell 20:621–634. e6
37. Ching SV, Gillette SM, Powers BE, Roberts SM, Gillette EL, Withrow SJ (1990) Radiation-induced ocular injury in the dog: a histological study. Int J Radiat Oncol Biol Phys 19:321–328
38. Chiu WC, Ou DL, Tan CT (2022) Mouse models for immune checkpoint blockade therapeutic research in oral cancer. Int J Mol Sci 23
39. Chow LQM (2020) Head and neck cancer. N Engl J Med 382:60–72
40. Chu S, Wylie TN, Wylie KM, Johnson GC, Skidmore ZL, Fleer M, Griffith OL, Bryan JN (2020) A virome sequencing approach to feline oral squamous cell carcinoma to evaluate viral causative factors. Vet Microbiol 240:108491
41. Chulpanova DS, Kitaeva KV, Rutland CS, Rizvanov AA, Solovyeva VV (2020) Mouse tumor models for advanced cancer immunotherapy. Int J Mol Sci 21
42. Cibas ES, Ali SZ (2017) The 2017 Bethesda system for reporting thyroid cytopathology. Thyroid 27:1341–1346
43. Cladel NM, Budgeon LR, Cooper TK, Balogh KK, HU J, Christensen ND (2013) Secondary infections, expanded tissue tropism, and evidence for malignant potential in immunocompromised mice infected with Mus musculus papillomavirus 1 DNA and virus. J Virol 87:9391–9395
44. Coleman N, Marcelo KL, Hopkins JF, Khan NI, Du R, Hong L, Park E, Balsara B, Leoni M, Pickering C, Myers J, Heymach J, Albacker LA, Hong D, Gillison M, Le X (2023) HRAS mutations define a distinct subgroup in head and neck squamous cell carcinoma. JCO Precis Oncol 7:e2200211
45. Congiusta M, Lawrence J, Rendahl A, Goldschmidt S (2020) Variability in recommendations for cervi-

cal lymph node pathology for staging of canine oral neoplasia: a survey study. Front Vet Sci 7:506
46. Correa SS, Mauldin GN, Mauldin GE, Patnaik AK (2003) Efficacy of cobalt-60 radiation therapy for the treatment of nasal cavity nonkeratinizing squamous cell carcinoma in the dog. J Am Anim Hosp Assoc 39:86–89
47. Cox N, Brawner W, Powers R, Wright J (1991) Tumors of the nose and paranasal sinuses in cats: 32 cases with comparison to a national database (1977 through 1987). J Am Anim Hosp Assoc
48. Cray M, Selmic LE, Ruple A (2020) Salivary neoplasia in dogs and cats: 1996-2017. Vet Med Sci 6:259–264
49. Crittenden MR, Zebertavage L, Kramer G, Bambina S, Friedman D, Troesch V, Blair T, Baird JR, Alice A, Gough MJ (2018) Tumor cure by radiation therapy and checkpoint inhibitors depends on pre-existing immunity. Sci Rep 8:7012
50. Dahlstrom KR, Little JA, Zafereo ME, Lung M, Wei Q, Sturgis EM (2008) Squamous cell carcinoma of the head and neck in never smoker-never drinkers: a descriptive epidemiologic study. Head Neck 30:75–84
51. Darragh LB, Gadwa J, Pham TT, Van Court B, Neupert B, Olimpo NA, Nguyen K, Nguyen D, Knitz MW, Hoen M, Corbo S, Joshi M, Zhuang Y, Amann M, Wang XJ, Dow S, Kedl RM, Samedi V, Boss MK, Karam SD (2022) Elective nodal irradiation mitigates local and systemic immunity generated by combination radiation and immunotherapy in head and neck tumors. Nat Commun 13:7015
52. Day CP, Merlino G, Van Dyke T (2015) Preclinical mouse cancer models: a maze of opportunities and challenges. Cell 163:39–53
53. Ehling TJ, Klein MK, Smith L, Prescott D, Haney S, Looper J, Ladue T, Brawner W, Fidel J, Shiomitsu K, Green E, Saba C, Turek M, Farrelly J (2022) A prospective, multi-centre, Veterinary Radiation Therapy Oncology Group study reveals potential efficacy of toceranib phosphate (Palladia) as a primary or adjuvant agent in the treatment of canine nasal carcinoma. Vet Comp Oncol 20:293–303
54. Enache D, Ferro L, Morello EM, Massari F, Romanelli G, Nicoli S, Guazzetti S, Porporato F, Zini E (2023) Thyroidectomy in dogs with thyroid tumors: Survival analysis in 144 cases (1994-2018). J Vet Intern Med 37:635–647
55. Eskander A, Irish J, Groome PA, Freeman J, Gullane P, Gilbert R, Hall SF, Urbach DR, Goldstein DP (2014) Volume-outcome relationships for head and neck cancer surgery in a universal health care system. Laryngoscope 124:2081–2088
56. Faust RA, Gapany M, Tristani P, Davis A, Adams GL, Ahmed K (1996) Elevated protein kinase CK2 activity in chromatin of head and neck tumors: association with malignant transformation. Cancer Lett 101:31–35
57. Fidel J, Lyons J, Tripp C, Houston R, Wheeler B, Ruiz A (2011) Treatment of oral squamous cell carcinoma with accelerated radiation therapy and concomitant carboplatin in cats. J Vet Intern Med 25:504–510
58. Fineman LS, Hamilton TA, De Gortari A, Bonney P (1998) Cisplatin chemotherapy for treatment of thyroid carcinoma in dogs: 13 cases. J Am Anim Hosp Assoc 34:109–112
59. Forastiere AA, Zhang Q, Weber RS, Maor MH, Goepfert H, Pajak TF, Morrison W, Glisson B, Trotti A, Ridge JA, Thorstad W, Wagner H, Ensley JF, Cooper JS (2013) Long-term results of RTOG 91-11: a comparison of three nonsurgical treatment strategies to preserve the larynx in patients with locally advanced larynx cancer. J Clin Oncol 31:845–852
60. Fox LE, Geoghegan SL, Davis LH, Hartzel JS, Kubilis P, Gruber LA (1997) Owner satisfaction with partial mandibulectomy or maxillectomy for treatment of oral tumors in 27 dogs. J Am Anim Hosp Assoc 33:25–31
61. Foy JP, Bertolus C, Michallet MC, Deneuve S, Incitti R, Bendriss-Vermare N, Albaret MA, Ortiz-Cuaran S, Thomas E, Colombe A, Py C, Gadot N, Michot JP, Fayette J, Viari A, Van Den Eynde B, Goudot P, Devouassoux-Shisheboran M, Puisieux A, Caux C, Zrounba P, Lantuejoul S, Saintigny P (2017) The immune microenvironment of HPV-negative oral squamous cell carcinoma from never-smokers and never-drinkers patients suggests higher clinical benefit of IDO1 and PD1/PD-L1 blockade. Ann Oncol 28:1934–1941
62. Fu DR, Kadosawa T (2022) Comparison of epidermal growth factor receptor (EGFR) and cyclooxygenase-2 (COX-2) immunohistochemical expression and outcomes in canine nasal carcinomas treated with radiation therapy. J Vet Med Sci 84:1237–1243
63. Fujiwara-Igarashi A, Fujimori T, Oka M, Nishimura Y, Hamamoto Y, Kazato Y, Sawada H, Yayoshi N, Hasegawa D, Fujita M (2014) Evaluation of outcomes and radiation complications in 65 cats with nasal tumours treated with palliative hypofractionated radiotherapy. Vet J 202:455–461
64. Fulton AJ, Nemec A, Murphy BG, Kass PH, Verstraete FJ (2013) Risk factors associated with survival in dogs with nontonsillar oral squamous cell carcinoma 31 cases (1990-2010). J Am Vet Med Assoc 243:696–702
65. Gillette EL, Mcchesney SL, Dewhirst MW, Scott RJ (1987) Response of canine oral carcinomas to heat and radiation. Int J Radiat Oncol Biol Phys 13:1861–1867
66. Gillison ML, Zhang Q, Jordan R, Xiao W, Westra WH, Trotti A, Spencer S, Harris J, Chung CH, Ang KK (2012) Tobacco smoking and increased risk of death and progression for patients with p16-positive and p16-negative oropharyngeal cancer. J Clin Oncol 30:2102–2111
67. Gillison ML, Trotti AM, Harris J, Eisbruch A, Harari PM, Adelstein DJ, Jordan RCK, Zhao W, Sturgis EM, Burtness B, Ridge JA, Ringash J, Galvin J, Yao M, Koyfman SA, Blakaj DM, Razaq MA, Colevas

AD, Beitler JJ, Jones CU, Dunlap NE, Seaward SA, Spencer S, Galloway TJ, Phan J, Dignam JJ, Le QT (2019) Radiotherapy plus cetuximab or cisplatin in human papillomavirus-positive oropharyngeal cancer (NRG Oncology RTOG 1016): a randomised, multicentre, non-inferiority trial. Lancet 393:40–50
68. Giuliano A, Dobson J (2020) Clinical response and survival time of cats with carcinoma of the nasal cavity treated with palliative coarse fractionated radiotherapy. J Feline Med Surg 22:922–927
69. Goldschmidt MH, Kennedy JS, Kennedy DR, Yuan H, Holt DE, Casal ML, Traas AM, Mauldin EA, Moore PF, Henthorn PS, Hartnett BJ, Weinberg KI, Schlegel R, Felsburg PJ (2006) Severe papillomavirus infection progressing to metastatic squamous cell carcinoma in bone marrow-transplanted X-linked SCID dogs. J Virol 80:6621–6628
70. Gormley M, Creaney G, Schache A, Ingarfield K, Conway DI (2022) Reviewing the epidemiology of head and neck cancer: definitions, trends and risk factors. Br Dent J 233:780–786
71. Gramer I, Killick D, Scase T, Chandry D, Marrington M, Blackwood L (2017) Expression of VEGFR and PDGFR-α/−β in 187 canine nasal carcinomas. Vet Comp Oncol 15:1041–1050
72. Grant J, North S (2016) Evaluation of the factors contributing to long-term survival in canine tonsillar squamous cell carcinoma. Aust Vet J 94:197–202
73. Guan J, Zhang Y, Li Q, Zhang Y, Li L, Chen M, Xiao N, Chen L (2016) A meta-analysis of weekly cisplatin versus three weekly cisplatin chemotherapy plus concurrent radiotherapy (CRT) for advanced head and neck cancer (HNC). Oncotarget 7:70185–70193
74. Guerin MV, Finisguerra V, Van Den Eynde BJ, Bercovici N, Trautmann A (2020) Preclinical murine tumor models: a structural and functional perspective. elife 9
75. Gupta T, Kannan S, Ghosh-Laskar S, Agarwal JP (2018) Systematic review and meta-analyses of intensity-modulated radiation therapy versus conventional two-dimensional and/or or three-dimensional radiotherapy in curative-intent management of head and neck squamous cell carcinoma. PLoS One 13:e0200137
76. Hahn KA, Knapp DW, Richardson RC, Matlock CL (1992) Clinical response of nasal adenocarcinoma to cisplatin chemotherapy in 11 dogs. J Am Vet Med Assoc 200:355–357
77. Hammer A, Getzy D, Ogilvie G, Upton M, Klausner J, Kisseberth WC (2001) Salivary gland neoplasia in the dog and cat: survival times and prognostic factors. J Am Anim Hosp Assoc 37:478–482
78. Harari J, Patterson JS, Rosenthal RC (1986) Clinical and pathologic features of thyroid tumors in 26 dogs. J Am Vet Med Assoc 188:1160–1164
79. Hegde PS, Karanikas V, Evers S (2016) The where, the when, and the how of immune monitoring for cancer immunotherapies in the era of checkpoint inhibition. Clin Cancer Res 22:1865–1874
80. Henry CJ, Brewer WG Jr, Tyler JW, Brawner WR, Henderson RA, Hankes GH, Royer N (1998) Survival in dogs with nasal adenocarcinoma: 64 cases (1981-1995). J Vet Intern Med 12:436–439
81. Heyer J, Kwong LN, Lowe SW, Chin L (2010) Non-germline genetically engineered mouse models for translational cancer research. Nat Rev Cancer 10:470–480
82. Hong CM, Ahn BC (2018) Factors associated with dose determination of radioactive iodine therapy for differentiated thyroid cancer. Nucl Med Mol Imaging 52:247–253
83. Hu J, Cladel N, Budgeon L, Balogh K, Christensen N (2017) The mouse papillomavirus infection model. Viruses 9:246
84. Hutson CA, Willauer CC, Walder EJ, Stone JL, Klein MK (1992) Treatment of mandibular squamous cell carcinoma in cats by use of mandibulectomy and radiotherapy: seven cases (1987-1989). J Am Vet Med Assoc 201:777–781
85. Impellizeri JA, Esplin DG (2008) Expression of cyclooxygenase-2 in canine nasal carcinomas. Vet J 176:408–410
86. Ingle A, Ghim S, Joh J, Chepkoech I, Bennett Jenson A, Sundberg JP (2011) Novel laboratory mouse papillomavirus (MusPV) infection. Vet Pathol 48:500–505
87. Ishida K, Tomita H, Nakashima T, Hirata A, Tanaka T, Shibata T, Hara A (2017) Current mouse models of oral squamous cell carcinoma: genetic and chemically induced models. Oral Oncol 73:16–20
88. Jabbar S, Strati K, Shin MK, Pitot HC, Lambert PF (2010) Human papillomavirus type 16 E6 and E7 oncoproteins act synergistically to cause head and neck cancer in mice. Virology 407:60–67
89. Jethwa AR, Khariwala SS (2017) Tobacco-related carcinogenesis in head and neck cancer. Cancer Metastasis Rev 36:411–423
90. Jiang L, Zhang Y, Yang Z, Liang F, Wu J, Wang R (2019) A comparison of clinical outcomes between simultaneous integrated boost (SIB) versus sequential boost (SEQ) intensity modulated radiation therapy (IMRT) for head and neck cancer: a meta-analysis. Medicine (Baltimore) 98:e16942
91. Johnson DE, Burtness B, Leemans CR, Lui VWY, Bauman JE, Grandis JR (2020) Head and neck squamous cell carcinoma. Nat Rev Dis Primers 6:92
92. Ju H, Hu Z, Lu Y, Wu Y, Zhang L, Wei D, Guo W, Xia W, Liu S, Ren G, Hu J (2020) TLR4 activation leads to anti-EGFR therapy resistance in head and neck squamous cell carcinoma. Am J Cancer Res 10:454–472
93. Judd NP, Allen CT, Winkler AE, Uppaluri R (2012) Comparative analysis of tumor-infiltrating lymphocytes in a syngeneic mouse model of oral cancer. Otolaryngol Head Neck Surg 147:493–500
94. Kersten K, De Visser KE, Van Miltenburg MH, Jonkers J (2017) Genetically engineered mouse models in oncology research and cancer medicine. EMBO Mol Med 9:137–153

95. Kiyota N, Tahara M, Mizusawa J, Kodaira T, Fujii H, Yamazaki T, Mitani H, Iwae S, Fujimoto Y, Onozawa Y, Hanai N, Ogawa T, Hara H, Monden N, Shimura E, Minami S, Fujii T, Tanaka K, Homma A, Yoshimoto S, Oridate N, Omori K, Ueda T, Okami K, Ota I, Shiga K, Sugasawa M, Asakage T, Saito Y, Murono S, Nishimura Y, Nakamura K, Hayashi R, Head & Neck Cancer Study Group of the Japan Clinical Oncology, G (2022) Weekly cisplatin plus radiation for postoperative head and neck cancer (JCOG1008): a multicenter, noninferiority, phase II/III randomized controlled trial. J Clin Oncol 40:1980–1990
96. Klein MK, Powers BE, Withrow SJ, Curtis CR, Straw RC, Ogilvie GK, Dickinson KL, Cooper MF, Baier M (1995) Treatment of thyroid carcinoma in dogs by surgical resection alone: 20 cases (1981-1989). J Am Vet Med Assoc 206:1007–1009
97. Kleiter M, Malarkey DE, Ruslander DE, Thrall DE (2004) Expression of cyclooxygenase-2 in canine epithelial nasal tumors. Vet Radiol Ultrasound 45:255–260
98. Kono M, Saito S, Egloff AM, Allen CT, Uppaluri R (2022) The mouse oral carcinoma (MOC) model: a 10-year retrospective on model development and head and neck cancer investigations. Oral Oncol 132:106012
99. Kosovsky JK, Matthiesen DT, Marretta SM, Patnaik AK (1991) Results of partial mandibulectomy for the treatment of oral tumors in 142 dogs. Vet Surg 20:397–401
100. Lacas B, Carmel A, Landais C, Wong SJ, Licitra L, Tobias JS, Burtness B, Ghi MG, Cohen EEW, Grau C, Wolf G, HITT R, Corvo R, Budach V, Kumar S, Laskar SG, Mazeron JJ, Zhong LP, Dobrowsky W, Ghadjar P, Fallai C, Zakotnik B, Sharma A, Bensadoun RJ, Ruo Redda MG, Racadot S, Fountzilas G, Brizel D, Rovea P, Argiris A, Nagy ZT, Lee JW, Fortpied C, Harris J, Bourhis J, Auperin A, Blanchard P, Pignon JP, Group MNC (2021) Meta-analysis of chemotherapy in head and neck cancer (MACH-NC): An update on 107 randomized trials and 19,805 patients, on behalf of MACH-NC Group. Radiother Oncol 156:281–293
101. Ladue-Miller T, Price GS, Page RL, Thrall DE (1996) Radiotherapy of canine non-tonsillar squamous cell carcinoma. Vet Radiol Ultrasound 37:74–77
102. Lana SE, Dernell WS, Lafferty MH, Withrow SJ, Larue SM (2004) Use of radiation and a slow-release cisplatin formulation for treatment of canine nasal tumors. Vet Radiol Ultrasound 45:577–581
103. Latifi M, Skinner OT, Spoldi E, Ackerman L, Souza CHM, Yoon J, Vinayak A, Tuohy JL, Wallace ML, Dornbusch JA, Selmic LE, Menard J, Sumner JP, Schrock KC, Wustefeld-Janssens BG, Matz BM, Daniel TE, Mickelson MA (2021) Outcome and postoperative complications in 73 dogs with thyroid carcinoma with gross vascular invasion managed with thyroidectomy. Vet Comp Oncol 19:685–696
104. Lawrence JA, Forrest LJ, Turek MM, Miller PE, Mackie TR, Jaradat HA, Vail DM, Dubielzig RR, Chappell R, Mehta MP (2010) Proof of principle of ocular sparing in dogs with sinonasal tumors treated with intensity-modulated radiation therapy. Vet Radiol Ultrasound 51:561–570
105. Lechner M, Liu J, Masterson L, Fenton TR (2022) HPV-associated oropharyngeal cancer: epidemiology, molecular biology and clinical management. Nat Rev Clin Oncol 19:306–327
106. Lee BI, Larue SM, Seguin B, Griffin L, Prebble A, Martin T, Leary D, Boss MK (2020a) Safety and efficacy of stereotactic body radiation therapy (SBRT) for the treatment of canine thyroid carcinoma. Vet Comp Oncol 18:843–853
107. Lee J, Kim WC, Yoon WS, Koom WS, Rim CH (2020b) Reirradiation using stereotactic body radiotherapy in the management of recurrent or second primary head and neck cancer: a meta-analysis and systematic review. Oral Oncol 107:104757
108. Lee NY, Ferris RL, Psyrri A, Haddad RI, Tahara M, Bourhis J, Harrington K, Chang PM, Lin JC, Razaq MA, Teixeira MM, Lovey J, Chamois J, Rueda A, Hu C, Dunn LA, Dvorkin MV, De Beukelaer S, Pavlov D, Thurm H, Cohen E (2021) Avelumab plus standard-of-care chemoradiotherapy versus chemoradiotherapy alone in patients with locally advanced squamous cell carcinoma of the head and neck: a randomised, double-blind, placebo-controlled, multicentre, phase 3 trial. Lancet Oncol 22:450–462
109. Li Q, Dong H, Yang G, Song Y, Mou Y, Ni Y (2020) Mouse tumor-bearing models as preclinical study platforms for oral squamous cell carcinoma. Front Oncol 10:212
110. Lin YH, Yang MC, Tseng SH, Jiang R, Yang A, Farmer E, Peng S, Henkle T, Chang YN, Hung CF, Wu TC (2018) Integration of oncogenes via sleeping beauty as a mouse model of HPV16(+) oral tumors and immunologic control. Cancer Immunol Res 6:305–319
111. Ling DC, Bakkenist CJ, Ferris RL, Clump DA (2018) Role of immunotherapy in head and neck cancer. Semin Radiat Oncol 28:12–16
112. Liu D, Xiong H, Ellis AE, Northrup NC, Dobbin KK, Shin DM, Zhao S (2015) Canine spontaneous head and neck squamous cell carcinomas represent their human counterparts at the molecular level. PLoS Genet 11:e1005277
113. Looper JS, Malarkey DE, Ruslander D, Proulx D, Thrall DE (2006) Epidermal growth factor receptor expression in feline oral squamous cell carcinomas. Vet Comp Oncol 4:33–40
114. Lop J, Venegas MDP, Pujol A, Sauter B, Vasquez R, Casasayas M, Quer M, Leon X (2022) Causes of long-term mortality in patients with head and neck squamous cell carcinomas. Eur Arch Otorrinolaringol 279:3657–3664
115. Luff J, Mader M, Britton M, Fass J, Rowland P, Orr C, Schlegel R, Yuan H (2015) Complete genome

sequence of canine papillomavirus type 16. Genome Announc 3
116. Luff J, Rowland P, Mader M, Orr C, Yuan H (2016) Two canine papillomaviruses associated with metastatic squamous cell carcinoma in two related basenji dogs. Vet Pathol 53:1160–1163
117. Luff J, Mader M, Rowland P, Britton M, Fass J, Yuan H (2019) Viral genome integration of canine papillomavirus 16. Papillomavirus Res 7:88–96
118. Macewen EG, Withrow SJ, Patnaik AK (1977) Nasal tumors in the dog: retrospective evaluation of diagnosis, prognosis, and treatment. J Am Vet Med Assoc 170:45–48
119. Madewell BR, Priester WA, Gillette EL, Snyder SP (1976) Neoplasms of the nasal passages and paranasal sinuses in domesticated animals as reported by 13 veterinary colleges. Am J Vet Res 37:851–856
120. Mak IW, Evaniew N, Ghert M (2014) Lost in translation: animal models and clinical trials in cancer treatment. Am J Transl Res 6:114–118
121. Marks SL, Koblik PD, Hornof WJ, Feldman EC (1994) 99mTc-pertechnetate imaging of thyroid tumors in dogs: 29 cases (1980-1992). J Am Vet Med Assoc 204:756–760
122. Mas A, Blackwood L, Cripps P, Murphy S, De Vos J, Dervisis N, Martano M, Polton GA (2011) Canine tonsillar squamous cell carcinoma – a multi-centre retrospective review of 44 clinical cases. J Small Anim Pract 52:359–364
123. McDonald C, Looper J, Greene S (2012) Response rate and duration associated with a 4Gy 5 fraction palliative radiation protocol. Vet Radiol Ultrasound 53:358–364
124. Mehanna H, Robinson M, Hartley A, Kong A, Foran B, Fulton-Lieuw T, Dalby M, Mistry P, Sen M, O'Toole L, Al Booz H, Dyker K, Moleron R, Whitaker S, Brennan S, Cook A, Griffin M, Aynsley E, Rolles M, De Winton E, Chan A, Srinivasan D, Nixon I, Grumett J, Leemans CR, Buter J, Henderson J, Harrington K, McConkey C, Gray A, Dunn J, De EHPVTG (2019) Radiotherapy plus cisplatin or cetuximab in low-risk human papillomavirus-positive oropharyngeal cancer (De-ESCALaTE HPV): an open-label randomised controlled phase 3 trial. Lancet 393:51–60
125. Mell LK, Torres-Saavedra P, Wong S, Chang S, Kish JA, Minn AJ, Jordan R, Liu T, Truong MT, Winquist E, Wise-Draper T, Rodriguez CP, Musaddiq A, Beadle BM, Henson C, Narayan S, Spencer SA, Harris J, Yom SS (2022) Radiotherapy with durvalumab vs. cetuximab in patients with locoregionally advanced head and neck cancer and a contraindication to cisplatin: phase II results of NRG-HN004. Int J Radiat Oncol Biol Phys 114:1058
126. Merino-Gutierrez V, Borrego JF, Puig J, Hernández A, Clemente-Vicario F (2021) Treatment of advanced-stage canine nasal carcinomas with toceranib phosphate: 23 cases (2015-2020). J Small Anim Pract 62:881–885
127. Meuten D (2002) Tumors in domestic animals. Iowa State University Press, Ames
128. Mikiewicz M, Paździor-Czapula K, Gesek M, Lemishevskyi V, Otrocka-Domagała I (2019) Canine and feline oral cavity tumours and tumour-like lesions: a Retrospective study of 486 cases (2015-2017). J Comp Pathol 172:80–87
129. Mooney CT, Thoday KL, Doxey DL (1992) Carbimazole therapy of feline hyperthyroidism. J Small Anim Pract 33:228–235
130. Mukaratirwa S, Van Der Linde-Sipman JS, Gruys E (2001) Feline nasal and paranasal sinus tumours: clinicopathological study, histomorphological description and diagnostic immunohistochemistry of 123 cases. J Feline Med Surg 3:235–245
131. Munday JS, Tucker RS, Kiupel M, Harvey CJ (2015) Multiple oral carcinomas associated with a novel papillomavirus in a dog. J Vet Diagn Invest 27:221–225
132. Munday JS, Dunowska M, Laurie RE, Hills S (2016) Genomic characterisation of canine papillomavirus type 17, a possible rare cause of canine oral squamous cell carcinoma. Vet Microbiol 182:135–140
133. Murphy S, Hayes A, Adams V, Maglennon G, Neath P, Ladlow J, Brearley MJ (2006) Role of carboplatin in multi-modality treatment of canine tonsillar squamous cell carcinoma–a case series of five dogs. J Small Anim Pract 47:216–220
134. Naan EC, Kirpensteijn J, Kooistra HS, Peeters ME (2006) Results of thyroidectomy in 101 cats with hyperthyroidism. Vet Surg 35:287–293
135. Nadeau ME, Kitchell BE (2011) Evaluation of the use of chemotherapy and other prognostic variables for surgically excised canine thyroid carcinoma with and without metastasis. Can Vet J 52:994–998
136. NCI Surveillance, E., and the End Results Program (n.d.) Cancer stat facts: thyroid cancer. seer.cancer.gov.
137. Nemec A, Murphy B, Kass PH, Verstraete FJ (2012) Histological subtypes of oral non-tonsillar squamous cell carcinoma in dogs. J Comp Pathol 147:111–120
138. Nemec A, Murphy BG, Jordan RC, Kass PH, Verstraete FJ (2014) Oral papillary squamous cell carcinoma in twelve dogs. J Comp Pathol 150:155–161
139. Nitschinsk K, Idris A, McMillan N (2018) Patient derived xenografts as models for head and neck cancer. Cancer Lett 434:114–119
140. Nolan MW, Berman AR, Watson-Skaggs ML, Quinn CN, Marcus KL, Russell K, Yoshikawa H, Olby NJ, Gieger TL (2022) Stereotactic radiotherapy (10 Gy X 3) for canine nonlymphomatous intranasal tumors is associated with prolonged survival and minimal risk of severe radiotoxicity. J Am Vet Med Assoc 260:1496–1506
141. Noronha V, Joshi A, Patil VM, Agarwal J, Ghosh-Laskar S, Budrukkar A, Murthy V, Gupta T, D'Cruz AK, Banavali S, Pai PS, Chaturvedi P, Chaukar D, Pande N, Chandrasekharan A, Talreja V, Vallathol DH, Mathrudev V, Manjrekar A, Maske K, Bhelekar

AS, Nawale K, Kannan S, Gota V, Bhattacharjee A, Kane S, Juvekar SL, Prabhash K (2018) Once-a-week versus once-every-3-weeks cisplatin chemoradiation for locally advanced head and neck cancer: a phase III randomized noninferiority trial. J Clin Oncol 36:1064–1072
142. Northrup NC, Selting KA, Rassnick KM, Kristal O, O'Brien MG, Dank G, Dhaliwal RS, Jagannatha S, Cornell KK, Gieger TL (2006) Outcomes of cats with oral tumors treated with mandibulectomy: 42 cases. J Am Anim Hosp Assoc 42:350–360
143. Novoplansky O, Jagadeeshan S, Regev O, Menashe I, Elkabets M (2022) Worldwide prevalence and clinical characteristics of RAS mutations in head and neck cancer: a systematic review and meta-analysis. Front Oncol 12:838911
144. O'Malley BW Jr, Cope KA, Johnson CS, Schwartz MR (1997) A new immunocompetent murine model for oral cancer. Arch Otolaryngol Head Neck Surg 123:20–24
145. O'Sullivan B, Huang SH, Su J, Garden AS, Sturgis EM, Dahlstrom K, Lee N, Riaz N, Pei X, Koyfman SA, Adelstein D, Burkey BB, Friborg J, Kristensen CA, Gothelf AB, Hoebers F, Kremer B, Speel EJ, Bowles DW, Raben D, Karam SD, Yu E, Xu W (2016) Development and validation of a staging system for HPV-related oropharyngeal cancer by the International Collaboration on Oropharyngeal cancer Network for Staging (ICON-S): a multicentre cohort study. Lancet Oncol 17:440–451
146. Ogilvie GK, Sundberg JP, O'Banion MK, Badertscher RR 2nd, Wheaton LG, Reichmann ME (1988) Papillary squamous cell carcinoma in three young dogs. J Am Vet Med Assoc 192:933–936
147. Ogilvie GK, Reynolds HA, Richardson RC, Withrow SJ, Norris AM, Henderson RA, Klausner JS, Fowler JD, Mccaw D (1989) Phase II evaluation of doxorubicin for treatment of various canine neoplasms. J Am Vet Med Assoc 195:1580–1583
148. Onaciu A, Munteanu R, Munteanu VC, Gulei D, Raduly L, Feder RI, Pirlog R, Atanasov AG, Korban SS, Irimie A, Berindan-Neagoe I (2020) Spontaneous and Induced animal models for cancer research. Diagnostics (Basel) 10
149. Overgaard J, Hansen HS, Specht L, Overgaard M, Grau C, Andersen E, Bentzen J, Bastholt L, Hansen O, Johansen J, Andersen L, Evensen JF (2003) Five compared with six fractions per week of conventional radiotherapy of squamous-cell carcinoma of head and neck: DAHANCA 6 and 7 randomised controlled trial. Lancet 362:933–940
150. Pack L, Roberts RE, Dawson SD, Dookwah HD (2001) Definitive radiation therapy for infiltrative thyroid carcinoma in dogs. Vet Radiol Ultrasound 42:471–474
151. Patnaik AK (1989) Canine sinonasal neoplasms – clinicopathological study of 285 cases. J Am Anim Hosp Assoc 25:103–114
152. Patnaik AK, Lieberman PH, Erlandson RA, Liu SK (1984) Canine sinonasal skeletal neoplasms: chondrosarcomas and osteosarcomas. Vet Pathol 21:475–482
153. Pereira MC, Oliveira DT, Landman G, Kowalski LP (2007) Histologic subtypes of oral squamous cell carcinoma: prognostic relevance. J Can Dent Assoc 73:339–344
154. Peterson ME, Becker DV (1995) Radioiodine treatment of 524 cats with hyperthyroidism. J Am Vet Med Assoc 207:1422–1428
155. Peterson ME, Kintzer PP, Hurvitz AI (1988) Methimazole treatment of 262 cats with hyperthyroidism. J Vet Intern Med 2:150–157
156. Pfister DG, Spencer S, Brizel DM, Burtness B, Busse PM, Caudell JJ, Cmelak AJ, Colevas AD, Dunphy F, Eisele DW, Gilbert J, Gillison ML, Haddad RI, Haughey BH, Hicks WL Jr, Hitchcock YJ, Jimeno A, Kies MS, Lydiatt WM, Maghami E, Martins R, Mccaffrey T, Mell LK, Mittal BB, Pinto HA, Ridge JA, Rodriguez CP, Samant S, Schuller DE, Shah JP, Weber RS, Wolf GT, Worden F, Yom SS, Mcmillian NR, Hughes M, National Comprehensive Cancer, N (2014) Head and neck cancers, Version 2.2014. Clinical practice guidelines in oncology. J Natl Compr Cancer Netw 12:1454–1487
157. Pignon JP, Le Maitre A, Maillard E, Bourhis J, Group MNC (2009) Meta-analysis of chemotherapy in head and neck cancer (MACH-NC): an update on 93 randomised trials and 17,346 patients. Radiother Oncol 92:4–14
158. Poirier VJ, Kaser-Hotz B, Vail DM, Straw RC (2013) Efficacy and toxicity of an accelerated hypofractionated radiation therapy protocol in cats with oral squamous cell carcinoma. Vet Radiol Ultrasound 54:81–88
159. Ragin CC, Modugno F, Gollin SM (2007) The epidemiology and risk factors of head and neck cancer: a focus on human papillomavirus. J Dent Res 86:104–114
160. Rangan SR (1972) A new human cell line (FaDu) from a hypopharyngeal carcinoma. Cancer 29:117–121
161. Rassnick KM, Goldkamp CE, Erb HN, Scrivani PV, Njaa BL, Gieger TL, Turek MM, Mcniel EA, Proulx DR, Chun R, Mauldin GE, Phillips BS, Kristal O (2006) Evaluation of factors associated with survival in dogs with untreated nasal carcinomas: 139 cases (1993-2003). J Am Vet Med Assoc 229:401–406
162. Reagan JK, Selmic LE, Fallon C, Sutton B, Lafferty M, Ben-Aderet D, Culp WTN, Liptak JM, Duffy D, Simons M, Boston S, Lana S (2019) Complications and outcomes associated with unilateral thyroidectomy in dogs with naturally occurring thyroid tumors: 156 cases (2003-2015). J Am Vet Med Assoc 255:926–932
163. Reif JS, Cohen D (1971) The environmental distribution of canine respiratory tract neoplasms. Arch Environ Health 22:136–140
164. Rickard AG, Palmer GM, Dewhirst MW (2019) Clinical and pre-clinical methods for quantifying tumor hypoxia. Adv Exp Med Biol 1136:19–41
165. Riggs J, Adams VJ, Hermer JV, Dobson JM, Murphy S, Ladlow JF (2018) Outcomes following surgical excision or surgical excision combined with adjunctive, hypofractionated radiotherapy in dogs with oral

squamous cell carcinoma or fibrosarcoma. J Am Vet Med Assoc 253:73–83
166. Rossa C Jr, D'Silva NJ (2019) Immune-relevant aspects of murine models of head and neck cancer. Oncogene 38:3973–3988
167. Sajjad H, Imtiaz S, Noor T, Siddiqui YH, Sajjad A, Zia M (2021) Cancer models in preclinical research: a chronicle review of advancement in effective cancer research. Anim Model Exp Med 4:87–103
168. Schmitd LB, Scanlon CS, D'Silva NJ (2018) Perineural invasion in head and neck cancer. J Dent Res 97:742–750
169. Schuch LF, Silveira FM, Wagner VP, Borgato GB, Rocha GZ, Castilho RM, Vargas PA, Martins MD (2020) Head and neck cancer patient-derived xenograft models - a systematic review. Crit Rev Oncol Hematol 155:103087
170. Sharma S, Boston SE, Skinner OT, Perry JA, Verstraete FJM, Lee DB, Van Stee LLL, Thompson C, Boylan M, Mckee T, Bergman PJ (2021) Survival time of juvenile dogs with oral squamous cell carcinoma treated with surgery alone: a Veterinary Society of Surgical Oncology retrospective study. Vet Surg 50:740–747
171. Shen W, Sakamoto N, Yang L (2015) Cancer-specific mortality and competing mortality in patients with head and neck squamous cell carcinoma: a competing risk analysis. Ann Surg Oncol 22:264–271
172. Sheppard-Olivares S, Bello NM, Wood E, Szivek A, Biller B, Hocker S, Wouda RM (2020) Toceranib phosphate in the treatment of canine thyroid carcinoma: 42 cases (2009-2018). Vet Comp Oncol 18:519–527
173. Shiomitsu K, Johnson CL, Malarkey DE, Pruitt AF, Thrall DE (2009) Expression of epidermal growth factor receptor and vascular endothelial growth factor in malignant canine epithelial nasal tumours. Vet Comp Oncol 7:106–114
174. Simčič P, Lowe R, Granziera V, Pierini A, Torrigiani F, Lubas G (2020) Electrochemotherapy in treatment of canine oral non-tonsillar squamous cell carcinoma. A case series report. Vet Comp Oncol 18:428–432
175. Smith LP, Thomas GR (2006) Animal models for the study of squamous cell carcinoma of the upper aerodigestive tract: a historical perspective with review of their utility and limitations. Part A. Chemically-induced de novo cancer, syngeneic animal models of HNSCC, animal models of transplanted xenogeneic human tumors. Int J Cancer 118:2111–2122
176. Snyder LA, Bertone ER, Jakowski RM, Dooner MS, Jennings-Ritchie J, Moore AS (2004) p53 expression and environmental tobacco smoke exposure in feline oral squamous cell carcinoma. Vet Pathol 41:209–214
177. Soltero-Rivera MM, Krick EL, Reiter AM, Brown DC, Lewis JR (2014) Prevalence of regional and distant metastasis in cats with advanced oral squamous cell carcinoma: 49 cases (2005-2011). J Feline Med Surg 16:164–169
178. Soukup JW, Snyder CJ, Simmons BT, Pinkerton ME, Chun R (2013) Clinical, histologic, and computed tomographic features of oral papillary squamous cell carcinoma in dogs: 9 cases (2008-2011). J Vet Dent 30:18–24
179. Spangler WL, Culbertson MR (1991) Salivary gland disease in dogs and cats: 245 cases (1985-1988). J Am Vet Med Assoc 198:465–469
180. Sroussi HY, Epstein JB, Bensadoun RJ, Saunders DP, Lalla RV, Migliorati CA, Heaivilin N, Zumsteg ZS (2017) Common oral complications of head and neck cancer radiation therapy: mucositis, infections, saliva change, fibrosis, sensory dysfunctions, dental caries, periodontal disease, and osteoradionecrosis. Cancer Med 6:2918–2931
181. Stapleton BL, Barrus JM (1996) Papillary squamous cell carcinoma in a young dog. J Vet Dent 13:65–68
182. Stiborova K, Meier VS, Takada M, Turek M, Poirier VJ, Laliberte S, Rohrer Bley C (2020) Definitive-intent radiotherapy for sinonasal carcinoma in cats: A multicenter retrospective assessment. Vet Comp Oncol 18:626–633
183. Sung H, Ferlay J, Siegel RL, Laversanne M, Soerjomataram I, Jemal A, Bray F (2021) Global cancer statistics 2020: globocan estimates of incidence and mortality worldwide for 36 cancers in 185 countries. CA Cancer J Clin 71:209–249
184. Szczepanski MJ, Czystowska M, Szajnik M, Harasymczuk M, Boyiadzis M, Kruk-Zagajewska A, Szyfter W, Zeromski J, Whiteside TL (2009) Triggering of toll-like receptor 4 expressed on human head and neck squamous cell carcinoma promotes tumor development and protects the tumor from immune attack. Cancer Res 69:3105–3113
185. Tessler FN, Middleton WD, Grant EG (2018) Thyroid imaging reporting and data system (TI-RADS): a user's guide. Radiology 287:1082
186. Thaiwong T, Sledge DG, Collins-Webb A, Kiupel M (2018) Immunohistochemical characterization of canine oral papillary squamous cell carcinoma. Vet Pathol 55:224–232
187. Théon AP, Madewell BR, Harb MF, Dungworth DL (1993) Megavoltage irradiation of neoplasms of the nasal and paranasal cavities in 77 dogs. J Am Vet Med Assoc 202:1469–1475
188. Théon AP, Rodriguez C, Madewell BR (1997) Analysis of prognostic factors and patterns of failure in dogs with malignant oral tumors treated with megavoltage irradiation. J Am Vet Med Assoc 210:778–784
189. Théon AP, Marks SL, Feldman ES, Griffey S (2000) Prognostic factors and patterns of treatment failure in dogs with unresectable differentiated thyroid carcinomas treated with megavoltage irradiation. J Am Vet Med Assoc 216:1775–1779
190. Tinhofer I, Braunholz D, Klinghammer K (2020) Preclinical models of head and neck squamous cell carcinoma for a basic understanding of cancer biology and its translation into efficient therapies. Cancers Head Neck 5:9

191. Todoroff RJ, Brodey RS (1979) Oral and pharyngeal neoplasia in the dog: a retrospective survey of 361 cases. J Am Vet Med Assoc 175:567–571
192. Treggiari E, Pellin MA, Romanelli G, Maresca G, Gramer I, Yale AD, Pecceu E, Pignanelli M, Borrego J, Purzycka K, Berlato D (2023) Tonsillar carcinoma in dogs: treatment outcome and potential prognostic factors in 123 cases. J Vet Intern Med 37:247–257
193. Tsimbas K, Turek M, Christensen N, Vail DM, Forrest L (2019) Short survival time following palliative-intent hypofractionated radiotherapy for non-resectable canine thyroid carcinoma: a retrospective analysis of 20 dogs. Vet Radiol Ultrasound 60:93–99
194. Tuohy JL, Worley DR, Withrow SJ (2012) Outcome following simultaneous bilateral thyroid lobectomy for treatment of thyroid gland carcinoma in dogs: 15 cases (1994-2010). J Am Vet Med Assoc 241:95–103
195. Turrel JM, Mcentee MC, Burke BP, Page RL (2006) Sodium iodide I 131 treatment of dogs with nonresectable thyroid tumors: 39 cases (1990-2003). J Am Vet Med Assoc 229:542–548
196. Van Der Steen F, Zandvliet M (2021) Treatment of canine oral papillary squamous cell carcinoma using definitive-intent radiation as a monotherapy-a case series. Vet Comp Oncol 19:152–159
197. Van Nieuwenhuizen AJ, Buffart LM, Brug J, Leemans CR, Verdonck-De Leeuw IM (2015) The association between health related quality of life and survival in patients with head and neck cancer: a systematic review. Oral Oncol 51:1–11
198. Vanherberghen M, Day MJ, Delvaux F, Gabriel A, Clercx C, Peeters D (2009) An immunohistochemical study of the inflammatory infiltrate associated with nasal carcinoma in dogs and cats. J Comp Pathol 141:17–26
199. Vargo JA, Moiseenko V, Grimm J, Caudell J, Clump DA, Yorke E, Xue J, Vinogradskiy Y, Moros EG, Mavroidis P, Jain S, El Naqa I, Marks LB, Heron DE (2021) Head and neck tumor control probability: radiation dose-volume effects in stereotactic body radiation therapy for locally recurrent previously-irradiated head and neck cancer: report of the AAPM Working Group. Int J Radiat Oncol Biol Phys 110:137–146
200. Vermeer DW, Coppock JD, Zeng E, Lee KM, Spanos WC, Onken MD, Uppaluri R, Lee JH, Vermeer PD (2016) Metastatic model of HPV+ oropharyngeal squamous cell carcinoma demonstrates heterogeneity in tumor metastasis. Oncotarget 7:24194–24207
201. Wallace J, Matthiesen DT, Patnaik AK (1992) Hemimaxillectomy for the treatment of oral tumors in 69 dogs. Vet Surg 21:337–341
202. Wang Z, Wu VH, Allevato MM, Gilardi M, He Y, Luis Callejas-Valera J, Vitale-Cross L, Martin D, Amornphimoltham P, Mcdermott J, Yung BS, Goto Y, Molinolo AA, Sharabi AB, Cohen EEW, Chen Q, Lyons JG, Alexandrov LB, Gutkind JS (2019) Syngeneic animal models of tobacco-associated oral cancer reveal the activity of in situ anti-CTLA-4. Nat Commun 10:5546
203. Warnakulasuriya S (2009) Global epidemiology of oral and oropharyngeal cancer. Oral Oncol 45:309–316
204. Wei T, Buehler D, Ward-Shaw E, Lambert PF (2020) An infection-based murine model for papillomavirus-associated head and neck cancer. MBio 11
205. White RAS (1991) Mandibulectomy and maxillectomy in the dog: long term survival in 100 cases. J Small Anim Pract 32:69–74
206. Wisdom AJ, Mowery YM, Hong CS, Himes JE, Nabet BY, Qin X, Zhang D, Chen L, Fradin H, Patel R, Bassil AM, Muise ES, King DA, Xu ES, Carpenter DJ, Kent CL, Smythe KS, Williams NT, Luo L, Ma Y, Alizadeh AA, Owzar K, Diehn M, Bradley T, Kirsch DG (2020) Single cell analysis reveals distinct immune landscapes in transplant and primary sarcomas that determine response or resistance to immunotherapy. Nat Commun 11:6410
207. Woodruff MJ, Heading KL, Bennett P (2019) Canine intranasal tumours treated with alternating carboplatin and doxorubin in conjunction with oral piroxicam: 29 cases. Vet Comp Oncol 17:42–48
208. Workman P, Aboagye EO, Balkwill F, Balmain A, Bruder G, Chaplin DJ, Double JA, Everitt J, Farningham DA, Glennie MJ, Kelland LR, Robinson V, Stratford IJ, Tozer GM, Watson S, Wedge SR, Eccles SA, Committee of the National Cancer Research, I (2010) Guidelines for the welfare and use of animals in cancer research. Br J Cancer 102:1555–1577
209. Wucherer KL, Wilke V (2010) Thyroid cancer in dogs: an update based on 638 cases (1995-2005). J Am Anim Hosp Assoc 46:249–254
210. Yoshikawa H, Ehrhart EJ, Charles JB, Thamm DH, Larue SM (2012) Immunohistochemical characterization of feline oral squamous cell carcinoma. Am J Vet Res 73:1801–1806
211. Yoshikawa H, Ehrhart EJ, Charles JB, Custis JT, Larue SM (2016) Assessment of predictive molecular variables in feline oral squamous cell carcinoma treated with stereotactic radiation therapy. Vet Comp Oncol 14:39–57
212. Yoshikawa H, Gieger TL, Saba CF, Fredrickson K, Kubicek L, Haney S, Ruslander D, Kelsey KL, Mcentee MC, Nolan MW (2021) Retrospective evaluation of intranasal carcinomas in cats treated with external-beam radiotherapy: 42 cases. J Vet Intern Med 35:1018–1030
213. Young A, Okuyemi OT (2023) Malignant salivary gland tumors. StatPearls. Treasure Island (FL) ineligible companies. Disclosure: Oluwafunmilola Okuyemi declares no relevant financial relationships with ineligible companies
214. Zaccone R, Renzi A, Chalfon C, Lenzi J, Bellei E, Marconato L, Ros E, Rigillo A, Bettini G, Faroni E, Guerra D, Sabattini S (2022) Environmental risk factors for the development of oral squamous cell carcinoma in cats. J Vet Intern Med 36:1398–1408

Central Nervous System Malignancies

Christopher L. Mariani, Lucas P. Wachsmuth, and Peter Fecci

1 Part 1. Human CNS Malignancies

1.1 Overview of Human CNS Tumors

Tumors of the central nervous system (CNS) arise from a variety of cell types comprising the brain, spinal cord, and their respective connective tissues [1, 2]. Such tumors are the most common solid malignancies and leading cause of death in the human pediatric population [3]. Although they comprise only approximately 2% of all adult malignancies, CNS tumors represent a significant burden of disease, as they are extremely difficult to successfully treat; the most common malignant primary CNS tumor in humans, glioblastoma, portends a 2-year survival rate of less than 30% [2, 4].

CNS tumors may be primary (i.e., derived from glial cells, meningeal cells, or neurons), or metastatic, of which lung, breast, and melanoma are the most common origins [2, 5, 6]. Primary brain tumors are further subdivided into benign or malignant etiologies based on their aggressiveness and natural history [1, 7]. Because primary brain tumors do not typically metastasize, specialized grading according to the World Health Organization Classification of Tumors of the Central Nervous System (WHO CNS) is used for definitive diagnosis and prognostication [7, 8]. While earlier versions of this classification scheme largely utilized histology as the basis for tumor grading, these features are frequently heterogeneous within brain tumors and subject to sampling bias. The advent of multi-omic technologies has enabled increased understanding of the molecular markers and drivers in individual CNS tumor types, and molecular alterations are typically more uniform within a given tumor, yielding a more accurate diagnosis and nuanced prognosis. Thus, the modernized diagnosis scheme in the updated 2021 (5th) edition of the WHO CNS integrates both histopathologic and molecular features to classify tumors [8]. Tumor grade describes the microscopic appearance of the tumor, incorporating features such as cellular and nuclear atypia, mitoses, microvascular proliferation, and necrosis, with the grade increasing as the tumor histology exhibits more atypical and aggressive features. According to the updated 2021 WHO CNS classification scheme, CNS tumors are now graded within tumor type rather than across types.

C. L. Mariani (✉)
Department of Small Animal Clinical Sciences, North Carolina State University, Raleigh, NC, USA
e-mail: clmarian@ncsu.edu

L. P. Wachsmuth
Duke Medical Scientist Training Program, Duke University, Durham, NC, USA

P. Fecci
Department of Neurosurgery, University of Colorado Anschutz Medical Campus, Aurora, CO, USA

M. W. Nolan et al. (eds.), *Comparative Oncology*, https://doi.org/10.1007/978-3-032-04454-9_14

Glioblastoma, an adult-type diffuse glioma, represents the most common malignant primary CNS tumor in humans, comprising 14.2% of all CNS tumors, with approximately 13,000 cases diagnosed in the United States each year [4]. Meningiomas, derived from the meninges, comprise 39.7% of all human CNS tumors, with an annual average of approximately 35,000 diagnoses [4]. Despite their benign designation, the location and long disease course of meningiomas can cause significant morbidity to patients [9]. In addition to these primary tumor types, the neuro-oncology community has begun to focus increased efforts on the treatment of brain metastases [5]. With improvements in systemic cancer therapies, the incidence of late brain metastasis is expected to increase, with such tumors comprising approximately half of the burden of CNS disease in humans [5].

Given the varied functional specializations of brain regions, intracranial disease may present with focal neurological deficits dependent on tumor location. Roughly 50% of patients with newly diagnosed brain tumors present with headaches [2]. Additional signs may include seizures (present in up to 74% of lower-grade gliomas), as well as nausea, vomiting, and other symptoms of increased intracranial pressure [2]. Given the limited specificity of clinical signs and symptoms, magnetic resonance imaging (MRI) is the preferred modality for imaging of suspected brain tumors, with imaging characteristics of specific tumor types discussed below [2, 10]. However, the appearance of many CNS malignancies is similar to several non-neoplastic disease processes, including intracranial abscess and variants of multiple sclerosis [11]. As a result, tissue diagnosis via stereotactic biopsy or surgical resection is the gold standard, allowing for molecular characterization and assignment of a WHO CNS diagnosis.

In several tumor types, decades of neurosurgical literature have illustrated the importance of surgical cytoreduction in prolonging survival or freedom from progression [6, 12, 13]. More recent research has focused on the role of so-called "supramaximal" or "supratotal" resections in which large regions of MRI-FLAIR abnormality without a contrasted T1 correlate are removed with the goal of excising invading tumor cells [14]. On the whole, modern neurosurgical practice has focused on the idea of "onco-functional balance," that is, balancing maximal resection with patient debility and lesion proximity to eloquent cortex [15]. Fractionated, involved-field radiotherapy (FRT) is an essential adjunctive therapy to resection, including both the surgical cavity and a margin of approximately 2–3 cm to aid in local control [1, 2, 10, 16]. Delivery of drug therapies to the CNS is limited by the blood-brain barrier (BBB) and is a critical barrier to drug development in neuro-oncology, with the alkylating agent temozolomide (TMZ) remaining an important tool for treatment of a variety of glioma subtypes [1, 17, 18]. Additionally, immunotherapy has failed to yield the same success in brain tumors as it has in many extracranial malignancies [17, 19–21]. While interest in developing efficacious immunotherapeutic platforms to treat CNS tumors remains strong, we are only in the early stages of understanding how tumor-intrinsic, BBB-related, and immune factors have limited the successful application of immunotherapy in brain tumors.

1.2 Adult-Type Diffuse Gliomas

The first of the six families of glial, glioneuronal, or neuronal tumors in the 2021 WHO CNS comprises adult-type diffuse gliomas, which make up the majority of primary brain tumors in adults [2, 10]. This family is further divided into three tumor types on the basis of the presence of mutations in isocitrate dehydrogenase (*IDH*) and codeletion of chromosomes 1p and 19q: astrocytoma, *IDH*-mutant; oligodendroglioma, *IDH*-mutant and 1p/19q-codeleted; and glioblastoma, *IDH*-wildtype [7, 10]. These tumors rarely occur in the pediatric population; however, this specific family designation recognizes the particular molecular drivers that are most common in adults.

1.2.1 Astrocytoma, IDH-Mutant

Up to 80% of gliomas with low-grade histology are *IDH*-mutant [10]. The defining criteria for astrocytomas are the presence of *IDH* mutations without codeletion of chromosome 1p/19q [7]. The IDH gene is responsible for the conversion of isocitrate to α-ketoglutarate as part of normal metabolism, with gain-of-function mutations leading to the accumulation of the oncometabolite 2-hydroxyglutarate, resulting in global aberrations in chromatin modification [10, 22]. Common additional markers in astrocytomas include tumor protein 53 (*TP53*) and α-thalassemia/mental retardation, X-linked (*ATRX*) loss of function mutations. Such tumors are most common in the fourth to fifth decades of life, and patients often present with seizures [1, 8, 10].

As stated above, MR imaging is the first step in evaluation for a suspected astrocytoma, with lower-grade astrocytomas (e.g., Grade 2) lesions typically displaying no contrast enhancement on T1-weighted sequences with increased signal on T2-weighted or fluid-attenuated inversion recovery (FLAIR) sequences [10]. Following upfront treatment with maximal safe resection or biopsy, tumors may be assigned grades 2–4 on the basis of cellularity, mitoses, and overall differentiation [23]. Presence of microvascular proliferation, necrosis, or homozygous deletions of *CDKN2A/B* are sufficient for assignment of grade 4. Such tumors were previously considered *IDH*-mutant glioblastomas, but the prolonged survival of these patients relative to *IDH*-wildtype GBM has led to recognition of grade 4 astrocytoma as an altogether different entity [1, 2, 10].

1.2.2 Oligodendroglioma, *IDH*-Mutant, and 1p/19q Co-deleted

Oligodendrogliomas are diffuse gliomas characterized by the presence of both *IDH* mutations and loss of chromosome arms 1p and 19q (1p/19q codeletion) [1, 8, 10]. Approximately 1000 such tumors are diagnosed in the United States each year, with a peak incidence in the fifth decade of life [4]. Such tumors are thought to arise from oligodendroglial precursors, although tumors with a primarily astrocytic or a mixed cellular appearance (previously termed oligoastrocytomas) on histology and presence of 1p/19q codeletion are still considered oligodendrogliomas [1]. Mutations in *ATRX* and *TP53* are infrequent in oligodendroglioma and tend to be mutually exclusive with 1p/19q codeletion overall [10].

MRI typically reveals no to minimal enhancement with calcifications, though higher-grade oligodendrogliomas may eventually develop a gliomatosis cerebri-like growth pattern (i.e., diffuse widespread growth involving three or more cerebral lobes) [10, 23]. Patients may present with seizures. Following resection or biopsy, tumors are graded 2 or 3, a retained system from previous editions of the WHO CNS classification [2, 23]. Under the current WHO classification, grade 2 and 3 oligodendrogliomas are purely histologically differentiated and have a similar prognosis for survival of 12–15 years [10].

1.2.3 Glioblastoma, *IDH*-Wildtype

Glioblastoma is the most common malignant primary brain tumor, with a median age at diagnosis of 65 and median survival of approximately 15 months. The advent of molecular screening has played a key role in diagnosis, treatment, and prognostication of glioblastoma over the past two decades. Previously, a subset of *IDH*-mutant astrocytomas with histological features consistent with glioblastoma (necrosis, microvascular proliferation) was considered to be "secondary" glioblastomas, often arising from a previously diagnosed, lower-grade-appearing tumor. However, these patients are often younger and have a different mutational profile, affording improved prognosis. As of the 2021 WHO CNS, only *IDH*-wildtype tumors are classifiable as glioblastomas, with grade 4 *IDH*-mutant tumors reclassified as astrocytoma, *IDH*-mutated, WHO grade 4 (see above) [1, 2, 8, 10, 23].

On MRI, glioblastomas classically demonstrate a "ring-enhancing" contrast enhancement pattern, with invasive tumor surrounded by central necrosis [10]. *IDH*-wildtype, molecularly defined glioblastomas may have a more diffuse or non-contrast-enhancing pattern, but be highly invasive, with features of gliomatosis cerebri [24, 25]. Tumors may spread across the corpus callosum, with significant FLAIR abnormality due to peritumoral edema [2, 10]. As a result, patients may variably present with headaches, altered mental status, changes in cognition or behavior, seizures, or focal neurological deficits [10]. Diagnosis is established by the presence of necrosis and microvascular proliferation in *IDH*-wildtype tumors, or, for lower-grade-appearing tumors, by the presence of *EGFR* amplification, *TERT* promoter mutations, or gain of chromosome 7 with loss of chromosome 10 [1, 23]. The inclusion of previously classed *IDH*-wildtype grade 2 or 3 astrocytomas with these "molecular features of glioblastoma" is a key change in the 2021 WHO CNS; histologic astrocytomas that do not have these molecular features should be evaluated for histone H3 mutations and may in fact be pediatric-type tumors [26]. A further key biomarker is methylation status of the O^6--methylguanine-DNA-methyltransferase (*MGMT*) promoter, which encodes an enzyme capable of repairing the toxic DNA adducts induced by TMZ treatment; *MGMT* promoter methylation is associated with a significant survival advantage [10, 23].

1.3 Pediatric-Type Diffuse High-Grade Gliomas

The first of two new families of tumors added to the 2021 WHO CNS consists of pediatric-type diffuse high-grade gliomas. Four tumor types make up this family of tumors, which most commonly occur in children [7]. In the 2016 WHO CNS, the clinical entity diffuse intrinsic pontine glioma (DIPG) was incorporated as diffuse midline glioma (DMG), H3 K27M-mutant, in recognition of gain-of-function histone mutations that drive this devastating childhood tumor. In the years since, understanding of DMG has increased such that thalamic and spinal cord variants have been documented in young adults, with the discovery of mutations in non-histone genes (*EZHIP* and *ACVR1*) sufficient to cause loss of H3 K27 methylation [1, 8, 23]. These changes have resulted in such tumors being classified as diffuse midline glioma, H3 K27M-altered in the 2021 WHO CNS [7]. For 2018, the first year with available data, 197 pediatric DMG cases were diagnosed in the United States [3]. Patients typically present with headaches and cranial nerve deficits, prompting imaging. DMG is typically only responsive to radiation, with their diffuse spread and location precluding resection [1, 23]. Therapy for this disease is an active area of investigation, with investigations focusing on proteasomal inhibition and engineered chimeric antigen receptor (CAR)-T cells [27, 28].

Three additional tumor types are incorporated into this family: diffuse hemispheric glioma, H3 G34-mutant; diffuse pediatric-type high-grade glioma, H3-wildtype and IDH-wildtype; and infant-type hemispheric glioma. Diffuse hemispheric glioma, H3 G34-mutant, shares loss of histone trimethylation with DMG, but appears to have a predilection for the hemispheres rather than the midline. Such tumors may also display *MGMT* promoter methylation. High-grade gliomas without characteristic driver mutations in histone H3 or IDH are classed separately, and may resemble glioblastomas histologically and molecularly, with methylation patterns that are different from adult-type tumors. Infant-type hemispheric gliomas may be driven by a number of receptor tyrosine kinase fusion genes, including *ROS1*, *ALK*, or *MET*, and may be responsive to small molecule inhibitors targeting these mutations. Prognosis is poor for all tumor types, with infant-type hemispheric gliomas having an approximate 5-year survival of 25–50% [1, 8, 23].

1.4 Pediatric-Type Diffuse Low-Grade Gliomas

Diffuse low-grade gliomas comprise the second family of pediatric-type gliomas included in the 2021 WHO CNS. The four tumor types in this family—diffuse astrocytoma, *MYB*- or *MYBL1*-*altered*; angiocentric glioma; polymorphous low-grade neuroepithelial tumor of the young (PLNTY) and diffuse low-grade glioma, *MAPK* pathway-altered—may invade the brain parenchyma, but generally are associated with long-term survival following resection [7]. There is further a degree of histological and molecular overlap in this family, with angiocentric gliomas often displaying *MYB* fusion, and both PLNTY and diffuse low-grade glioma, *MAPK* pathway-altered may have *MAPK*-activating mutations, an important therapeutic target. This family does not display the IDH or histone mutations mentioned in the previously discussed tumor families. Deletion of *CDKN2A/B* is a poor prognostic factor associated with tumor transformation and shortened time to recurrence [1, 8, 23].

On MRI, these tumors often display similar features to other low-grade glial tumors, including no to minimal contrast enhancement. They most frequently occur in teenagers or young adults, and may present with seizures. The role of chemotherapy, radiation, and targeted *MAPK*-pathway inhibition using approved therapies (i.e., BRAF or MEK inhibitors) is still being explored for these newly defined tumor types [1].

1.5 Circumscribed Astrocytic

The above families of diffuse gliomas are distinguished in the 2021 WHO CNS from tumors in which the border between tumor tissue and normal brain structures is more distinct, termed circumscribed astrocytic gliomas [1, 7, 8]. Several of these diagnoses are well-established and were previously referred to as "other astrocytic tumors." [23] Pilocytic astrocytomas are the most common tumor type, comprising 15.3% of CNS tumors in children aged 0–19 years, and are grade 1 tumors associated with *BRAF* mutations and a predilection for the posterior fossa [3, 8, 29]. Other tumor types include pleomorphic xanthoastrocytoma (PXA), subependymal giant cell astrocytoma (SEGA), chordoid glioma, astroblastoma, *MN1*-altered, and high-grade astrocytoma with piloid features. These tumors similarly tend to cluster in children and young adults, with some specific associations. For example, SEGAs are associated with *TSC1* or *TSC2* mutations causing tuberous sclerosis complex (TSC) and are slow-growing tumors that may progress to cause hydrocephalus. Multiple tumors in this family may have overlapping features (mitoses, necrosis) with diffuse gliomas that are associated with higher grade and worsened overall survival. In particular, high-grade astrocytomas with piloid features were recently defined by methylation profiling and may mirror outcomes in *IDH*-mutant astrocytoma, grade 4 [1, 8, 23].

1.6 Glioneuronal Tumors

The family of rare glial tumors for which a neuronal cellular component exists in tandem is termed glioneuronal or neuronal tumors. This category has a large number of entities, with three added (one provisional) as of the 2021 WHO CNS: myxoid glioneuronal tumor, multinodular and vacuolating neuronal tumor, and diffuse glioneuronal tumor with oligodendroglioma-like features and nuclear clusters. Gangliogliomas or neurocytomas are typically graded 1 or 2 but may occasionally have more anaplastic features [7, 8].

1.7 Ependymomas

Ependymomas comprise the sixth and final family of glial tumors in the 2021 WHO CNS [7]. Such tumors are thought to arise from ependymal linings of the brain's CSF spaces, and were historically classified based on histology alone, though differences in disease phenotype had been noted based on patient age and location [7]. Key advances in methylation profiling have led to integration of molecular features, location data, and histopathology to define ependymomas [1]. Supratentorial ependymomas are defined by fusions involving *ZFTA* or *YAP1*, with *ZFTA* fusion being the more common (25–58% of adult and 66–84% of pediatric cases) and aggressive tumor type [1, 23]. The *RELA* gene is the most common fusion partner, and tumors may also have *CDKN2A/B* mutations, portending a worsened prognosis [23]. Posterior fossa A (PFA) ependymomas are defined based on loss of H3K27 trimethylation (H3K27me3) driven by EZHIP overexpression, a shared mechanism with rare subsets of non-histone mutated diffuse midline glioma [8]. Posterior fossa B tumors (PFB) are associated with older age of onset relative to PFA tumors and typically have whole chromosome abnormalities. Spinal ependymomas may share chromosome 22q loss with PFB ependymomas, and typically present as indolent intramedullary cervicothoracic tumors. *MYCN* amplification in spinal ependymomas is associated with CSF dissemination [8, 23]. Anatomic features on imaging guide clinical suspicion for ependymoma, and tumors may be graded 2 or 3 based on histological features [29].

2 Part 2. Conventional Murine Models of CNS Malignancy

Conventional mouse models of primary CNS malignancies can be divided into three major groups: 1. transplant models, including syngeneic and xenograft models, 2. genetically engineered mouse models (GEMMs), and 3. humanized mouse models (Fig. 1) [30–32]. Syngeneic transplant models consist of tumor cell lines that are derived from primary malignancies from a specific mouse strain. These tumor lines most commonly were either generated via chemical induction or isolated from a spontaneously arising tumor. After being cultured in vitro, these cells can then be injected into syngeneic mice that share the same genetic background as the originating tumor-bearing animal, where they will continue to grow. Xenograft models include immortalized human glioma lines and patient-derived xenografts (PDXs). PDX models involve implanting cells derived from patient tumors into mice to study the development of clinically relevant tumors, but require immunocompromised mice, as immunocompetent strains would reject the xenograft as non-self. GEMMs describe models in which the mouse line has been engineered to either lack tumor suppressors and/or activate oncogenes that are important for tumorigenesis. Specific gene combinations can be used to drive development of specific tumor types. Lastly, humanized mouse models are emerging tools that can bridge some of the gaps between murine and human disease. These models consist of immunocompromised mouse lines that possess some element of human biology (Figs. 2 and 3).

Transplant, i.e., injection, models are the most ubiquitous and oldest mouse models of primary CNS malignancies. Syngeneic models consist of tumor lines that were generated on a specific mouse strain and therefore are genetically matched; immunocompetent recipient mice can be implanted with tumor and will not recognize the tumor cells as non-self, thereby allowing for tumor engraftment. Regarding glioma specifically, the most common models were generated either via chemical induction on the C57BL/6 background (GL261 and CT-2A) or isolated from a spontaneously arising astrocytoma (SMA-560, on the VM/Dk background). GL261 was generated by implanting 3-methylcholantrene in the brain of a C57BL/6 mouse and then serially transplanting tumor cells into C57BL/6 mice to isolate the final line [33]. Similarly, CT-2A was generated via intracranial injection of 20-methylcholantrene in C57BL/6 mice with subsequent serial subcutaneous transplantation to isolate the final line [34]. SMA-560 was isolated from a spontaneous astrocytoma in a VM/Dk mouse, an incredibly rare event, making it a valuable injection model [35].

A more recently developed cell line that is gaining increasing attention as a transplant model that better recapitulates the immunosuppressive microenvironment of human glioma is SB28 [36, 37]. SB28 was generated on the C57BL/6 background using sleeping beauty transposons to target the p53, RAS, and PDGF pathways [38]. This line is less immunogenic than the more well-established models and does not respond to immune checkpoint inhibitor therapy, paralleling human disease [36, 37]. All of these syngeneic tumor cell lines are typically injected intracranially to model orthotopic disease, but will also grow when injected subcutaneously, allowing researchers to study tumor growth, microenvironment, and treatment response both within the brain and in the absence of brain-specific microenvironment features. Overall advantages to these models include the high degree of control

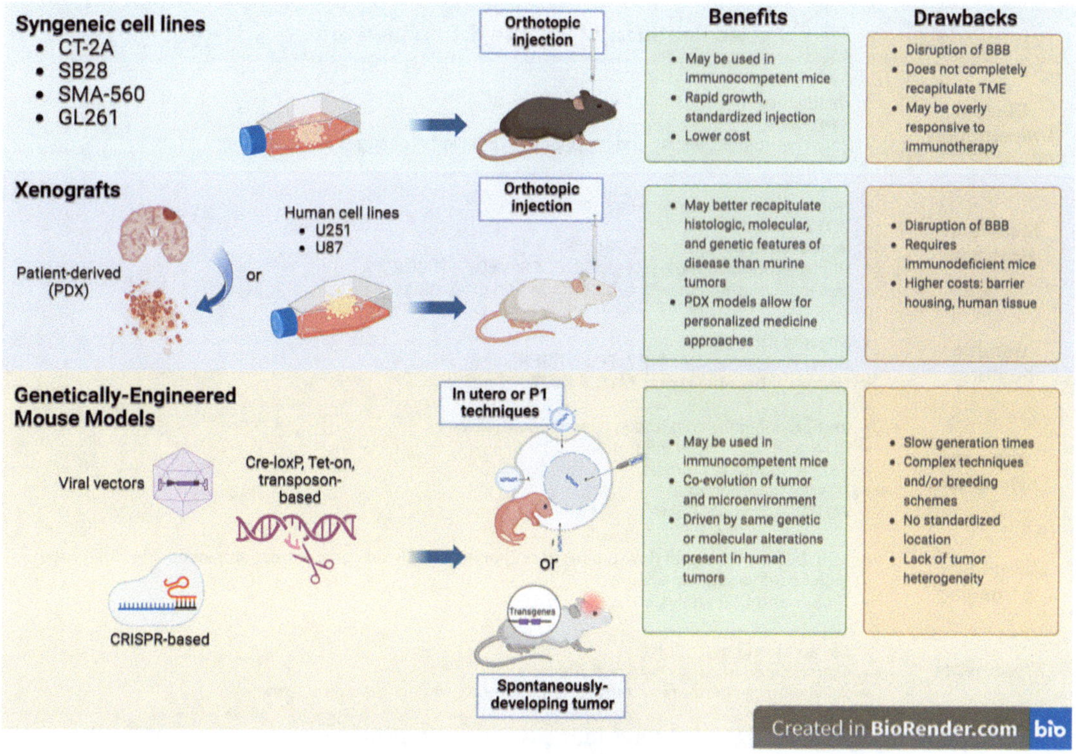

Fig. 1 Mouse models of glioma. Mouse models of glioma may be syngeneic, consisting of previously derived murine cell lines grown in culture prior to orthotopic implantation into the brain of immunocompetent mice. Alternatively, xenograft models from patient-derived (PDX) tissue or stable, immortalized human cell lines may be similarly orthotopically implanted in immunocompromised mice. In genetically engineered mouse models (GEMMs), a variety of molecular techniques, including viral vectors, transgenes, or CRISPR-Cas9, among others, may be used to generate mice that develop spontaneous gliomas via breeding or in utero/P1 injection. Abbreviations: *BBB* blood-brain barrier

they afford with regard to cell dose and tumor location, the experimental efficiency they provide (larger experiments can be conducted relatively quickly), and that they allow for study of immune responses and immunotherapy as mice are immunocompetent.

CT-2A results in an angiogenic, aggressive tumor with 100% penetrance in C57BL/6 mice [39]. Histologically, it is consistent with poorly differentiated malignant astrocytoma, and it exhibits features of high-grade astrocytoma, including a high mitotic index, microvascular proliferation, central necrosis, and glial marker expression [39]. SMA-560, which similarly demonstrates 100% penetrance in VM/Dks, has been shown to better recapitulate immunosuppressive aspects of the tumor microenvironment found in humans and is TMZ resistant, paralleling human disease [40–42]. The drawbacks of syngeneic injection models are primarily related to their reduced capacity to recapitulate key facets of human disease. First, the act of injecting tumor cells in and of itself is a significant contrast with spontaneously arising tumors, as the tumor does not co-evolve with the tumor microenvironment over time, and implantation necessitates tissue trauma and disruption of normal anatomy, including the dura and blood vessels. Second, these tumor lines exhibit a higher mutational burden than that observed in human glioma, rendering them more responsive to various therapies, especially immunotherapy [36, 37]. As a homogenous population of cells, the tumors formed from injection models lack intra-tumoral heterogeneity,

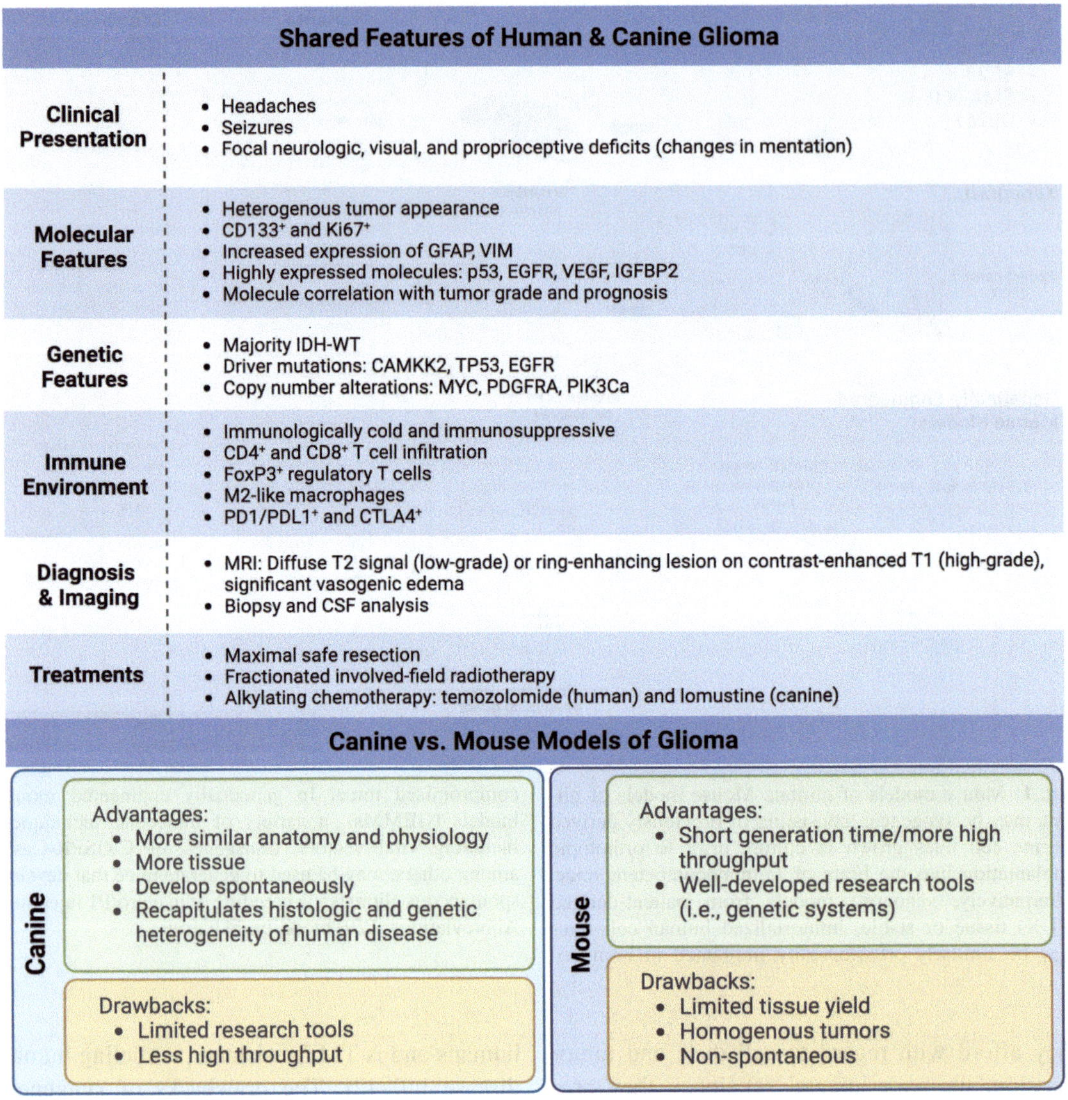

Fig. 2 Shared features of gliomas across species

a critical facet of human disease underlying treatment failure and recurrence [43]. Additionally, they are typically not highly infiltrative and form more discrete tumor masses than observed in humans [44]. GL261 in particular has increasingly been recognized as a sub-optimal model, as it lacks expression of key glial markers, is highly immunogenic and overly responsive to immunotherapy, and is relatively radiosensitive [33, 45].

The other major category of transplant models, xenografts, is similar to syngeneic models in that they involve injection or implantation of tumor cells into recipient mice. The most commonly used xenografts in glioma research are immortalized human cell lines, namely U87 and U251 [46, 47]. Importantly, in any xenograft model, immunocompromised mice must be used to ensure that tumors are not rejected as non-self foreign tissue, given that these cell lines are of human origin. Accordingly, these models have minimal utility for studying the anti-tumor immune response and immunotherapeutic platforms, although the addition of human immune cells into these systems can provide some limited

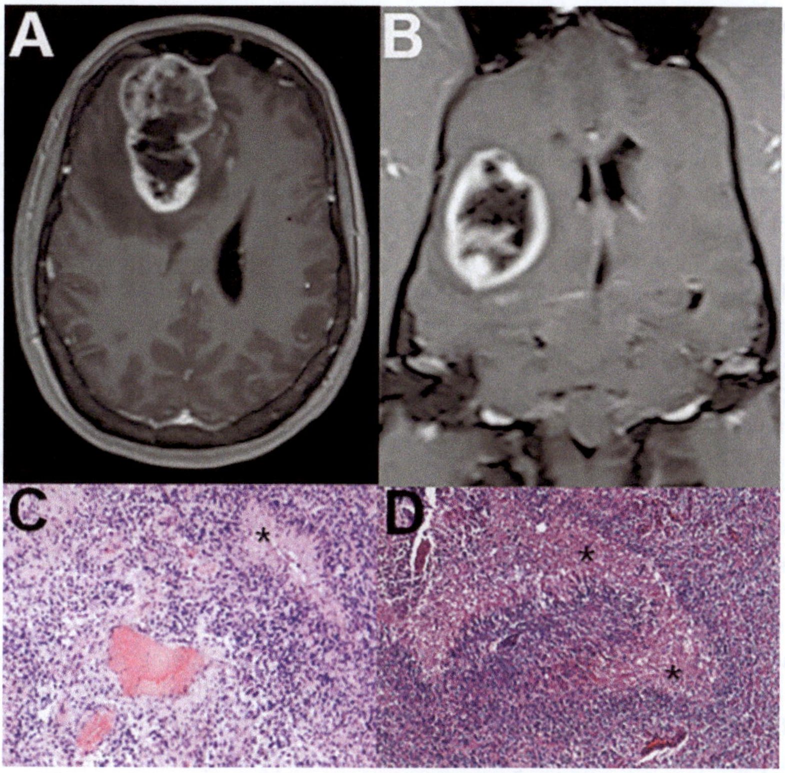

Fig. 3 Magnetic resonance imaging and histopathology of human and canine gliomas. Human and canine high-grade gliomas have similar appearances on both magnetic resonance imaging and histopathological studies. (**a**) Post-contrast, T1-weighted image of a glioblastoma in a human patient. Note the ring-like enhancement of the tumor. (**b**) Post-contrast, T1-weighted image of a high-grade oligodendroglioma in a canine patient with a similar enhancement pattern. (**c**) Histopathological section of a glioblastoma in a human patient including a region of pseudopalisading necrosis (asterisk). (**d**) Histopathological section of a high-grade astrocytoma in a canine patient, showing a similar region of pseudopalisading necrosis (asterisks). (Image courtesy of Dr. Gregory Krane)

insights [31, 48]. In general, human xenograft models exhibit more translationally relevant histologic, molecular, and genetic features of disease than murine tumor lines [49–51]. Non-immortalized PDXs, while difficult to establish, best recapitulate human disease as compared to the transplanted human cell lines and syngeneic models, as these tumors are directly derived from human tumors and undergo minimal in vitro manipulation [52]. As with the syngeneic injection models, drawbacks of the xenograft models include the traumatic tissue disruption inherent in tumor implantation, lack of co-evolution of the tumor and microenvironment, tumor formation of discrete masses exhibiting minimal invasion, and less tumor heterogeneity than observed in human disease [31, 46, 47, 53].

GEMMs utilize genetic tools, such as the Cre-loxP and Tet-on systems, to modulate the expression of genes and drive tumor development [54, 55]. These genetic manipulations typically involve abrogating the activity of tumor suppressors, such as PTEN, TP53, and CDKN2A, and/or upregulating oncogenic pathways, such as EGFR, PI3K, and p21-RAS, that have been implicated in human disease [56–59]. GEMMs can be created via a variety of approaches, including conventional knockout/knockin, conditional knockout, CRISPR Cas9, transgenic, and viral techniques [54, 55, 60–63]. These models allow for the study of the genetic and molecular drivers underlying gliomagenesis and progression, as well as relevant targeted therapies [64–66]. Compared to injection models, GEMMs more closely recapitulate human disease in that they develop over time in an intact microenvironment and avoid the inflammation and blood-brain barrier disruption inherent in injection [31, 46, 67]. Additionally, they allow for the study of these processes in immune-intact mice, which PDX models cannot [67]. However, GEMMs present multiple logistical challenges: tumors typically take time to develop, complex breeding schemes are usually required, and tumors can develop anywhere in the brain, limiting their utility for studies requiring easily accessible and reproducibly located tumors [67, 68]. The major biological drawback of GEMMs is that the driver genes utilized predominate the resultant tumor biology, and they therefore largely do not recapitulate the tumor heterogeneity observed in human disease [47, 68, 69].

Humanized mouse models are relatively new and understudied but offer unique advantages over traditional mouse models [70, 71]. By introducing specific aspects of human biology, e.g., human hematopoietic stem cells that give rise to a competent human immune system, into the murine system, these models allow researchers to conduct controlled in vivo studies that more closely mirror human disease [70–72]. However, in order to tolerate the "humanized" state, humanized mice must be generated from immunocompromised mouse lines. While a step toward improving the translational potential of mouse models, these models are in the early stages of study, and much remains to be learned about their performance in the context of CNS malignancies.

3 Part 3. Companion Animal Models and Comparative Oncology

3.1 Overview of Canine CNS Tumors

The incidence of CNS tumors in companion animals is relatively understudied, and estimates vary widely across species. Interestingly, current research on the incidence of CNS tumors in non-human mammalian species suggests that such neoplasms are rare. Even in non-human primates, intracranial malignancies are observed at a much lower frequency than in humans [73, 74]. Dogs are the only mammalian species aside from humans in which tumors arise frequently in the CNS [75–78]. The estimated total incidence of intracranial tumors in dogs ranges from 14.5 per 100,000 in one study [79] up to 2–4.5% on postmortem examination [75, 78, 80]. One postmortem study found that approximately 50% of intracranial neoplasms in dogs are primary tumors arising from CNS tissue [78], although other studies and clinical experience would suggest that this proportion is substantially higher [81]. Dogs develop a range of primary CNS tumors, but the precise distribution of tumor types varies widely across studies [75–79]. Meningiomas (~40–50%), glial tumors (~35–40%; including oligodendroglioma, astrocytoma, and glioblastoma), and choroid plexus tumors (~7%) together comprise approximately 90% of primary brain tumors observed in dogs, with other types (ependymomas, lymphoma, germ cell tumors, and embryonal tumors) presenting only rarely [75, 77, 78]. However, histiocytic sarcoma is an increasingly recognized CNS neoplasm in dogs easily mistaken for meningioma on imaging [81–83]. While canine primary CNS malignancies can occur at any age in any breed, incidence increases with age, and most intracranial neoplasms occur in dogs middle-aged and older [77, 78]. The majority of cases reported are in dogs older than 5 years of age, and there are no consistent sex predispositions, although this may be complicated by the frequency of neutering in these populations [84, 85]. While rare, cases of synchronous distinct primary brain tumors with different primary histology or simultaneous primary and secondary neoplasms have been reported [86–88].

Certain breeds are at markedly increased risk of developing specific types of primary CNS tumors, suggesting strong genetic components to disease etiology, which is unsurprising given the extensive selective pressure applied over centuries of canine breeding [75, 77, 78]. Consistent with this notion, a number of driver mutations have been implicated in certain types of CNS neoplasms in breeds at increased risk [89–91]. Considering other companion animal species, domestic cats also develop CNS neoplasms, although seemingly at much lower rates. While the incidence of these diseases in cats has been less clearly established, estimates range from 2.2 to 3.5 out of 100,000, and the vast majority described are meningiomas and lymphomas [79, 92]. As research on CNS tumors in companion animals has expanded, the many advantages they offer as translational models of human disease have become increasingly clear; canine primary intracranial neoplasms represent an especially valuable opportunity given their relatively high incidence.

3.2 Canine Glial Tumors

3.2.1 Tumor Biology

Glial tumors, or gliomas, are the second most common primary CNS malignancy in dogs, comprising 35–40% of all canine primary CNS tumors [75–78]. As in humans, the term "glioma" encompasses a diverse group of brain tumors which are derived from support cells in the brain known as glial cells; gliomas are divided into types based on their presumed cellular origin and grade. The most common glial cell tumors found in dogs are oligodendrogliomas (~50–60%) and astrocytomas (~20–40) [75, 77, 78]. The distribution of tumors across types and grades in dogs is quite different from that observed in humans; glioblastoma is the most common glial tumor overall in humans, and oligodendrogliomas comprise only ~5% of human glial tumors [93]. Dogs develop oligodendrogliomas (usually high grade) at higher rates than astrocytomas and exhibit a relatively even distribution of astrocytomas across grades II–IV, contrasting with the predilection toward high-grade astrocytoma in humans [77, 78, 93]. Brachycephalic breeds (those with short skulls and condensed snouts) develop gliomas at relatively high rates, with over half of canine glioma cases occurring in these breeds [75, 78, 94].

3.2.1.1 Pathologic Features

As it has not been updated since its original development in 1999, the WHO classification scheme for canine gliomas has been superseded by a more recently proposed histopathological system [95, 96]. This updated classification scheme divides gliomas into oligodendrogliomas, astrocytomas (including tumors previously classified as grade IV or glioblastoma), and undefined gliomas. Within each subtype, tumors are divided into high- and low-grade based on the presence of high-grade features, including microvascular proliferation, areas of necrosis with or without surrounding pseudopalisading architecture, increased mitotic activity, or features of malignancy (anisocytosis, anisokaryosis, or atypia) [96]. As in humans, these features have been found to correlate with decreased survival and worse prognosis in dogs, confirming their utility in identifying more aggressive glial neoplasms across species [97, 98].

Oligodendroglioma

Grossly, canine oligodendrogliomas span a spectrum from fleshy, soft, well-demarcated masses to infiltrative, poorly defined tumors [99]. They often have a gelatinous consistency due to their high mucin content [99]. Generally, oligodendrogliomas consist of sheets and linear cords of round to polygonal cells with variable amounts of cytoplasm, round nuclei, and a finely stippled chromatin pattern [99]. The vasculature in low-grade malignancies tends to be more delicate and branching, while high-grade tumors demonstrate a high degree of vascular proliferation with a glomeruloid appearance [96].

Astrocytoma

Unlike oligodendrogliomas, astrocytomas tend to form tumors that are not obvious masses and blend into the surrounding brain tissue [99]. Higher-grade tumors tend to be more invasive than low-grade neoplasms, and share the same high-grade features of high-grade oligodendroglioma [96]. While the highest grade of astrocytoma has classically been referred to as glioblastoma, the most recent classification has replaced that nomenclature with the more general classifier of high-grade astrocytoma [96]. Cellular features include variable amounts of eosinophilic cytoplasm, elongate to ovoid nuclei, and an open chromatin pattern [100].

Undefined Glioma

To be classified as an oligodendroglioma or astrocytoma, >80% of the tumor should feature the respective histologic criteria described above. Tumors with mixed histologies occurring at lower frequencies (i.e., 30–40% of each subtype) or those with undifferentiated cellular morphologies are classified as undefined gliomas [96]. Grades are determined as with other glioma subtypes.

3.2.1.2 Molecular Features

Canine gliomas share many molecular features with their human counterparts. Higher-grade tumors, regardless of subtype, demonstrate increased expression of the neural stem cell markers nestin and CD133 [101]. $CD133^{+}nestin^{+}$ cells are putative cancer stem cells and have also been identified in human gliomas. In humans, an increased proportion of $CD133^{+}$ cells has been linked to poorer prognosis and is associated with increased tumor grade [101–105]. Higher-grade canine tumors have also been found to have increased Antigen Kiel 67 (Ki-67) expression, mirroring findings in human glioma [101, 106]. S100 has been found to be expressed across tumor subtypes in both dogs and humans [101]. Regarding glioma subtypes, there are general molecular feature patterns that can be used to aid in distinguishing between canine oligodendrogliomas and astrocytomas. Oligodendrocyte transcription factor 2 (OLIG2), a transcription factor normally expressed in cells of the oligodendrocyte lineage, has also been found to be expressed across human glioma subtypes [103, 107, 108]. Canine oligodendrogliomas tend to demonstrate robust and diffuse, predominantly nuclear immunoreactivity for OLIG2, while astrocytoma OLIG2 expression is mixed, with studies reporting similar or decreased staining compared to oligodendrogliomas [96, 101]. 2′,3′-cyclic-nucleotide 3′-phosphodiesterase (CNPase) is another available immunohistochemical marker that has been used to identify oligodendrogliomas [96]. Additionally, canine astrocytomas tend to show increased expression of both glial fibrillary acidic protein (GFAP) and vimentin (VIM); canine oligodendrogliomas may demonstrate some VIM expression but are largely not immunoreactive for GFAP [96, 101]. These trends mirror human disease [109]. Notably, one study found that canine gliomas are not immunoreactive for neuronal nuclei (NeuN) or βIII-tubulin, markers of neuronal differentiation that have been found in high-grade human tumors [101, 103, 110]. This might suggest that canine gliomas are less differentiated than their human counterparts.

Other important protein markers in human disease include p53, epidermal growth factor receptor (EGFR), vascular endothelial growth factor (VEGF) and its receptor (VEGFR), and insulin-like growth factor-binding protein 2 (IGFBP2). P53 is a potent tumor suppressor protein known as the "guardian of the genome." Interestingly, at the protein level, p53 overexpression is found in ~35% of canine and ~ 60% of human astrocytomas [100, 111, 112]. EGFR amplification and overexpression have been implicated in a number of human malignancies, including gliomas, and impact a number of cellular pathways in glioma, including angiogenesis, apoptosis, and proliferation [113, 114]. A specific EGFR isoform expressed in human glioma, EGFR variant III (EGFRvIII), leads to constitutive signaling and has been extensively studied as both a molecular driver and therapeutic target in human disease. Approximately 30% of human gliomas demonstrate overexpression of both EGFR and EGFRvIII [115]. In canine astrocytomas, EGFR overexpression is also found, with higher-grade tumors more commonly demonstrating overexpression (grade IV 57%, grade III 40%) than lower-grade (grade II 28%) tumors [116]. However, a canine equivalent of EGFRvIII has not yet been identified. In both humans and dogs, VEGF levels have been found to increase with astrocytoma tumor grade [117–119]. VEGFR levels are increased in high-grade astrocytomas in humans, and expression of both receptor isoforms has been confirmed in canine tumors, although expression has not been found to correlate with tumor grade in dogs [117, 120]. Overexpression of IGFBP2 in human high-grade astrocytomas has been associated with worse prognosis, as it is correlated with matrix metalloproteinase 2 expression, which in turn is related to increased invasiveness [121]. Similarly, overexpression of IGFBP2 has been found in canine astrocytomas, and more commonly in higher-grade tumors [116].

3.2.1.3 Genetic Features

As mentioned previously, certain brachycephalic breeds, including Boxers, Boston Terriers, Bullmastiffs, and English and French Bulldogs, have a higher incidence of glioma compared to other breeds [75, 77, 78]. Approximately half of all canine gliomas occur in these breeds; the reported relative risk for Boxers is ~23, and ~ 5 for Boston Terriers and Bulldogs [75, 78]. One study conducting a genome-wide association study of brachycephalic dog breeds at increased risk of developing glial tumors revealed three candidate driver genes implicated in canine glioma: *DENR*, *CAMKK2*, and *P2RX7*, with a single nucleotide variant in *CAMKK2* being most strongly associated [89]. Notably, decreased levels of *CAMKK2*, which is involved in cerebellar precursor cell migration and differentiation during normal development, are found in both human and canine gliomas [89, 122]. Furthermore, increased expression of *CAMKK2* leads to increased differentiation in glioblastoma stem cells [89]; decreased expression may therefore increase the stem-ness of tumor cells and contribute to increased malignancy.

Studies of the genetic alterations present in canine glial tumors have revealed similarities to human disease. In human glial tumors, copy number alterations are more highly associated with tumor grade rather than histologic subtype [123]. Copy number alterations, specifically in CFA 20 and 35, are also significantly associated with glioma grade in dogs, suggesting that the accumulation of copy number variations and changes in the cytogenetic profile may be more closely associated with grade rather than subtype in dogs as well [124]. Specifically, gain of CFA 16, which has areas of synteny with HSA 7, gain of which is a hallmark event early in glioma development, is one of the most common copy number alterations in canine gliomas (63%) [124]. HSA 7p gain, which drives *EGFR* amplification, is a characteristic of high-grade astrocytoma in humans and is mirrored in canine tumors as increased copy number of CFA 18, which includes the canine *EGFR* ortholog, particularly in grade IV astrocytomas [124]. Human gliomas commonly demonstrate gain of HSA 8q, including the *MYC* oncogene, consistent with gain of CFA 13 found in 63% of canine gliomas [124]. Notably, genomic losses of regions corresponding to HSA 1p, which serves as a prognostic marker in both oligodendroglioma and astrocytoma in humans, have not been detected in dogs [124].

Recently, Amin et al. conducted the most comprehensive study of the genetic landscape of canine glioma to date, which involved whole-genome, exome, transcriptome, and methylation sequencing of 83 tumors and 67 germline canine samples, with subsequent comparison to pediatric and adult glioma sequencing libraries [91]. Overall, canine glioma showed a lower mutation rate than high-grade adult human gliomas, but a similar mutation rate to pediatric gliomas. This study detected mutations in *TP53*, *PDGFRA*, *PIK3CA*, and *EGFR* in canine gliomas, all of which are genes implicated in human disease, although there was considerable variation in the percentage of canine tumors with mutations in these genes (4–21%). Consistent with their analysis, a prior study had found *TP53* mutations in canine glioma, but at a lower rate than in humans [125]. They also detected mutations in *IDH1*, a defining characteristic of low-grade adult human gliomas, although only in a very small portion of canine tumors (4%). Interestingly, *TERT* promoter mutations are notably absent in canine gliomas [126]. Their analysis indicated that mutations in some of these genes (*PIK3CA*, *PDGFRA*, and *IDH1*) are driver mutations in canine glioma. Notably, mutation-based pathway alteration analysis indicated that canine gliomas are most similar to pediatric gliomas, specifically the histone 3 (H3) wildtype subtype, and that canine gliomas also show alterations in pathways that allow for immune evasion, mirroring the immune-cold phenotype observed in human tumors. Copy number analysis confirmed previously reported alterations in *MYC*, *PDGFRA*, *TP53*, *PIK3CA*, and *PTEN*, as well as other known human glioma driver genes (*KIT*, *CDKN2A/B*, *RB1*, and *HIST1*); 83% of canine gliomas demonstrated somatic mutations and/or copy number alterations in known human glioma drivers.

Aneuploidy analysis revealed that canine gliomas demonstrate relatively similar levels of aneuploidy to H3-mutant pediatric gliomas (25% vs. 26%, respectively), higher than that observed in adult IDH-mutant (8–9%), adult IDH wildtype (18%), or pediatric H3 wildtype (19%) tumors. The three aneuploidy clusters found in canine glioma correspond to human 1p/19q (common in adult IDH-mutant glioma, present in 20–36% of canine tumors), human 7p (*EGFR*) and 10q (*PTEN*) (common in adult IDH wildtype and pediatric H3 wildtype tumors, present in 5% and 14% of canine tumors, respectively), and human 4p/8q (*PDGFRA* and *MYC*, amplified in 78% of canine gliomas). This study found a bi-modal distribution of canine gliomas in terms of intratumoral heterogeneity, with 25% of tumors being very heterogeneous and 75% demonstrating a proportion of genomic variants consistent with clonal dominance. Canine gliomas were found to be comparably heterogeneous compared to adult human tumors, and more heterogeneous than pediatric human tumors. Similar to human disease, mutations in DNA damage repair pathways were enriched in canine tumors with heavy mutational burden. Despite the age of diagnosis of canine patients in this cohort exceeding the age of canine sexual maturity, DNA methylation pattern analysis revealed that 78% of canine gliomas classify as pediatric glioma, with only 13% and 9% classifying as adult IDH wildtype and IDH-mutant glioma, respectively. O6-Methylguanine-DNA Methyltransferase (MGMT) promoter methylation status is an important prognostic factor in human glioma, but data in canine glioma are lacking. The only study to date reporting on MGMT promoter methylation in immortalized canine glioma cell lines found high levels of MGMT promoter methylation in all three lines examined [127]; further research in this area is needed to understand the role played by MGMT promoter methylation status in canine glioma and degree of overlap with human disease.

3.2.1.4 Immune Environment in Canine Gliomas

The immune environment within canine gliomas has been sparsely studied compared to their human and experimental rodent counterparts. However, findings from several reports suggest that parallels in the immune response to glial tumors exist across species. Tumor-infiltrating lymphocytes (TILs) vary among canine tumors but show a predominance of T cells in most gliomas with sparse B cell infiltration [128–130]. T cells can be found diffusely throughout tumors or clustered in perivascular regions, while B cells are generally confined to perivascular areas. Some studies have shown higher numbers of T cells in higher-grade tumors [130], although overall TIL densities are relatively low, suggesting that canine gliomas are relatively immunologically "cold" tumors, as in humans [91, 131]. Subtyping of TILs has been limited by the availability of reagents suitable for immunohistochemistry in dogs, but in situ hybridization and flow cytometry work have shown the presence of both CD4+ and CD8+ T cells in one study [132]. Additionally, infiltration of FoxP3+ (presumed) regulatory T cells has been shown, with robust numbers seen in a subset of canine gliomas [130, 132, 133], and higher-grade tumors have shown greater numbers of FoxP3+ cells in several studies [130, 133].

Microglial and macrophage populations within canine gliomas have also been investigated. Robust numbers of cells positive for the microglial/macrophage marker Iba-1+ are typically seen in both oligodendrogliomas and astrocytomas, although this is variable both between and within individual tumors [129, 131, 133–135]. Many of these cells also express MHC II [129]. Although macrophage functionality has not been well defined in dogs relative to immunohistochemical markers, large numbers of CD163+

cells, suggestive of an immune-suppressive M2 phenotype, have been documented in canine tumors, are found in increased numbers in higher-grade tumors, and predominate relative to macrophages expressing the putative M1 marker Mac387 [91, 133].

The exploration of several immune-modulating molecules has also been undertaken in select studies. In situ hybridization revealed robust expression of PD-L1 within canine gliomas, with documentation of CTLA-4+ and PD-1+ cells within tumors [132]. Indoleamine 2,3 dioxygenase (IDO) expression was found to be limited to a small subset of canine gliomas in another study [133]. The expression of CCL2 within astrocytomas and in the CSF of tumor-bearing dogs suggests a key role in macrophage recruitment to canine gliomas [134, 136]. Finally, robust expression of the immunosuppressive molecule galectin-3 (GAL-3) has been documented in both astrocytomas and oligodendrogliomas [134, 135].

The systemic (peripheral) immune compartment has been even less studied in the context of canine gliomas, but greater proportions of circulating CD4 + FoxP3+ regulatory T cells have been observed in dogs with gliomas relative to clinically normal controls in one study [132]. This same study noted an increase in circulating plasmacytoid dendritic cells DC compared to controls.

3.2.2 Clinical Presentation

Although gliomas can arise in any dog, as mentioned above, many brachycephalic breeds are at increased risk for the development of glial tumors, and Boxers, English and French Bulldogs, and Boston Terriers comprise the majority of cases seen [77, 81, 89, 137–139]. As in humans, risk increases with age, and the median age at diagnosis in dogs is 8.6 years [77]. No consistent sex predilections have been reported.

Gliomas originate from the brain parenchyma and are therefore intra-axial tumors. As they arise from cells within the brain, they infiltrate and displace healthy brain tissue. In dogs, these tumors most frequently develop in the fronto-olfactory, piriform, temporal, and parietal lobes, and much less commonly arise in the brainstem or spinal cord [75, 96, 100, 138]. Certain gliomas have a propensity for infiltration and invasion across hemispheres or diffuse meningeal involvement [140–144]. Focal, progressive, and lateralized neurologic deficits corresponding to the neuroanatomical location of the tumor may be present depending on tumor size and the affected brain region. However, dogs can present with neurological deficits consistent with multifocal intracranial disease, reflecting the finding that up to 50% of solitary tumor cases involve multiple brain regions [77]. Tumors can impact multiple brain regions either via direct tumor invasion or through secondary effects, such as hemorrhage, ischemia, necrosis, peritumoral edema, obstructive hydrocephalus, and brain herniation [145].

Seizures are the most common clinical sign at presentation, with changes in mentation, circling, proprioceptive deficits, and visual deficits also being common findings [77, 98, 138, 139, 145–148]. Vestibular or cerebellar dysfunction, ataxia, and paresis can be seen, and other non-specific clinical signs including lethargy, inappetence, and weight loss may also be observed [77, 138].

3.2.3 Diagnosis of Gliomas

Similar to humans, the cornerstone of the diagnosis of glial tumors in dogs is diagnostic imaging, which is ideally followed by histopathologic confirmation via biopsy or resected tissue. However, antemortem acquisition of tissue is still not standard practice in many veterinary settings, and dogs are frequently managed presumptively based on imaging features and often using cerebrospinal fluid (CSF) analysis as a (poor) surrogate for histopathology and a tool to rule out meningoencephalitides.

3.2.3.1 Imaging Features

Computed tomography and conventional MRI sequences are not capable of reliably distinguishing between the different types of glioma or determining tumor grade, although there are trends toward specific features in different types and grades [149]. While the addition of diffusion-weighted, spectroscopic, and perfusion-weighted imaging to conventional MRI has improved the ability to assess tumor features, the ability of these sequences to enhance the diagnostic accuracy of MRI in dogs has not been rigorously assessed [150]. Findings on CT or conventional MRI vary considerably even within tumor subtype, and the various subsets share many common imaging characteristics due to their intra-axial and infiltrative nature [151–154]. In general, gliomas can appear either poorly or well-defined and demonstrate variable degrees of contrast enhancement [151, 152, 155]. Considering findings from a number of studies of imaging features of canine glioma, approximately 85% show evidence of mass effect, 55% are well-defined, and 60% demonstrate evidence of peritumoral edema [149–153, 155–158]. As a group, canine gliomas demonstrate variable T1W and T2W intensities and contrast enhancement patterns, although most are T2-hyperintense and T1-hypointense [77, 138, 149–151, 153, 155–158]. Most canine gliomas do not show uniform enhancement [153]. A "ring enhancing" pattern of contrast enhancement has been associated with gliomas but is not specific to glial tumors [158, 159]. As in humans, contrast enhancement that is minimal or absent is associated with lower-grade tumors, while more robust enhancement, including ring enhancement, is characteristic of high-grade tumors [153, 154, 160]. Other imaging characteristics reported to be associated with higher-grade canine gliomas have included heterogeneous signal intensities, signal voids on gradient echo imaging indicative of hemorrhage, cystic structures, and location (thalamocapsular region) within the brain [154, 160].

When considering specific tumor types, some trends in imaging findings can be identified. Oligodendrogliomas can be globular or irregularly shaped and commonly have a central mucinous region that results in signal hyperintensity on water-sensitive MRI sequences [77, 153, 161]. Heterogeneity in microvascular proliferation and resultant blood-brain barrier disruption results in varying degrees of peripheral or non-uniform contrast enhancement [153, 161]. In general, oligodendrogliomas are moderately hypointense on T1W images and T2W hyperintense in mucinous tumor areas [153, 161]. As in humans, a mismatch between signal intensities on T2-weighted and FLAIR images has been documented in a subset of canine oligodendrogliomas and appears specific to this tumor subtype [162]. Astrocytomas, which can be spherical or irregularly shaped, generally appear moderately T1W hypointense and moderately T2W hyperintense [151, 153, 155, 157, 161]. They may demonstrate evidence of necrosis or hemorrhage, and their degree of contrast enhancement tends to increase with grade, tracking with increased microvascular proliferation and tissue disorganization in advanced tumors [151, 153, 155, 157, 161]. However, exceptions to these general patterns are frequent, necessitating tissue-based diagnosis in these cases. While most intracranial gliomas are located within the cerebral cortex and underlying white matter tracts, diencephalic involvement has been suggested to be more likely with astrocytomas [77, 153], although this was not confirmed in other studies [138]. Other imaging factors that have been suggested to differentiate tumor type but that have been inconsistent across studies include the degree of tumor contact with the surface of the brain, ventricular distortion, and degree of peritumoral edema [153, 154].

3.2.3.2 Cerebrospinal Fluid Analysis and Biopsy

Cerebrospinal fluid analysis in dogs with gliomas is usually nonspecific, often showing a mild mononuclear or mixed cell pleocytosis or albuminocytologic dissociation, although analysis can also be normal [77, 138]. However, CSF analysis can be helpful in establishing a diagnosis of meningoencephalitis or infectious granuloma, an important differential diagnosis in this setting [159, 163–165].

Although still relatively uncommon, biopsy of intracranial lesions to better establish an antemortem diagnosis of glioma is becoming more frequent in dogs, and a number of biopsy systems have been described [166–170]. Interpretation of the small samples obtained requires a degree of comfort and experience on the part of the pathologist, and it would behoove clinicians to understand that pathological assessment of tissue is not uniform [128]. Further refinement of biopsy systems and interpretation should continue to make antemortem biopsy procedures in dogs quicker, safer, and more reliable.

3.2.4 Treatment of Canine Gliomas

3.2.4.1 Conventional Therapies

As in humans, conventional treatment options for canine gliomas include surgical resection, chemotherapy, and radiation therapy in addition to palliative therapy. Outcomes in pet dogs, particularly the interpretation of survival, are challenging, as they are heavily influenced by owners' decisions on therapy and euthanasia [171]. Administration of glucocorticoids to alleviate peritumoral edema is frequently used and anticonvulsant therapy is also common due to the prevalence of seizures in these dogs. Palliative therapy with glucocorticoids and anticonvulsants can be effective in alleviating clinical signs associated with the tumor but typically results in survival times of only 1–2 months [139, 171–173].

Reports of surgical resection of gliomas have been relatively infrequent in canine patients due to a variety of factors, including a relative lack of clinician training and skill in intra-axial surgery and the treatment preferences and financial limitations of pet owners. However, such interventions are increasing in frequency. As in the majority of human gliomas, resection of glial tumors is not a curative intervention, but serves to reduce tumor burden, ideally down to microscopic disease after gross total resection. Median survival times in dogs after resection of intracranial gliomas have been reported, although these data are complicated by the administration of concurrent therapies in most cases. Suñol et al. reported a median survival time of 66 days in 14 dogs undergoing surgical resection alone [174]. Hubbard et al. reported median survival times of 200 days for grade IV, 301 days for grade III, and 723 days for grade II gliomas in dogs treated with resection and a variety of adjuvant therapies [98]. Tumor size was not associated with outcome after resection in another study by the same group [175]. Thus, the efficacy of glioma resection in dogs is unclear but is likely to be beneficial in reducing tumor burden when used in combination with other therapies, as in humans.

Chemotherapeutic interventions for canine gliomas have also been sparsely studied, and the studies available suffer from a lack of a histologic diagnosis in most cases; diagnosis is often presumptive based on imaging features [172, 173]. The most frequently reported intervention is lomustine, traditionally chosen based on its favorable CNS penetration and relatively low cost. Retrospective studies of lomustine have reported survival times in most presumptive cases of 2–5 months [172, 173, 176]. More recently, as temozolomide has been removed from patent protection and has become more cost-effective for veterinary use, it has also been investigated for canine glial tumors in several reports, typically in combination with other interventions [177, 178]. Crespo et al. reported a median survival of 240 days in dogs treated with temozolomide and surgical debulking [178]. A phase I study of 8 dogs receiving metronomic chlorambucil combined with surgical resection showed an acceptable safety profile and variable accumulation of the drug within glioma tissue. Dogs also received lomustine post-operatively, and the median survival in this small cohort was 257 days [179].

Due to its non-invasive nature and driven by owner preferences, the most frequently utilized intervention for canine gliomas has been radiation therapy. However, as with studies of chemotherapy, veterinary radiotherapy studies are also plagued by the general lack of a histologic diagnosis, which pet owners often opt against due to cost, accessibility of a properly trained neurosurgeon, and perceived risk of the procedure. Nonetheless, various radiotherapeutic protocols have been described in dogs, including conventionally fractionated protocols [180–189], and hypofractionated protocols [190], as well as protocols that incorporate conformal techniques (IMRT) [191], and combinations of conformal RT with extreme hypofractionation: stereotactic radiotherapy [192–194], and stereotactic radiosurgery [82]. As canine patients must be anesthetized for radiation therapy and the limited availability of specialty centers often necessitates long-distance travel, hypofractionated or single-fraction treatments are particularly attractive for both dog owners and clinicians and are being increasingly utilized [192]. However, highly conformal treatment plans may be suboptimal in the setting of glioma due to failure to provide an adequate dose to neoplastic cells at the invasive margin of the tumor and beyond. Overall, regardless of the protocol utilized, radiotherapy appears to increase survival in dogs with intracranial gliomas compared with palliative treatments, resulting in median survival times typically ranging from 6 to 18 months [82, 138, 177, 180, 182–186, 190, 191, 195–197] and even longer in some studies [187, 193].

The effects of combining surgery or chemotherapies with radiation have been poorly studied in dogs, and the addition of a variety of treatments confounds many of the studies mentioned above. Moirano et al. suggest that adding a chemotherapeutic to SRT extends MST (>659 days vs. 230 days) although this study suffers from very small treatment groups and use of a variety of chemotherapeutics [193]. Another study suggested an improved response rate (91% vs. 63%) and median survival (420 days vs. 383 days) with the addition of temozolomide to SRT, but these results didn't reach statistical significance [177].

Despite the limitations of the studies described above, several studies have now shown a correlation of glioma grade with outcome after conventional therapies [97, 98]. Bley et al. found worse outcomes after radiotherapy in presumed (image-diagnosed) gliomas if the tumor was in proximity to the subventricular zone and/or showed ventricular invasion [186]. Tumors frequently recurred at CNS sites distant to the original tumor, and similar patterns of recurrence have been noted by other authors [144]. As in humans, glial tumors have remained incurable in dogs and remain almost uniformly fatal.

3.2.4.2 Experimental Therapies

A variety of studies investigating experimental therapeutic interventions have been performed in dogs with spontaneous intracranial gliomas. These include minimally invasive tumor ablation using electroporation [168] or laser interstitial thermal therapy [198], intratumoral infusion of chemotherapeutics [199–202], or targeted toxins [203], and a variety of immune therapies. Studies in the latter category have included vaccination with tumor lysate [204], checkpoint inhibition [204], delivery of oncolytic viruses [131, 205] and attempts to modulate macrophage immunosuppression in the tumor microenvironment [206].

3.3 Canine Gliomas as Models of Human Disease

Canine gliomas present numerous technical and biological advantages compared to traditional rodent models of CNS malignancies and understanding of the value of the dog as a model system for the study of glial tumors is becoming more widespread [96, 202, 207–214]. Gliomas in dogs develop spontaneously, occur later in life, are of similar relative size to their human counterpart, develop in the setting of an intact immune system and in a similar environment, and share overlapping histopathologic and molecular features with human gliomas [91, 96, 117, 124, 207, 215–219]. From a logistical standpoint, the amount of tissue that can be obtained from canine patients is orders of magnitude greater than that yielded from mice. The small intracranial tumors that can be generated in murine models limit downstream analyses, especially those geared at deep examination of rarer cell populations or *in vivo* imaging-based studies. Perhaps more importantly, the biology of canine neoplasms addresses all of the major drawbacks of murine tumor models. As spontaneously arising, unmanipulated tumors that develop in genetically unique organisms, they recapitulate human disease that is more translationally relevant. Although genetic bottlenecks likely underlie the breed-specific predilections for primary CNS tumor development [89], the amount of genetic diversity between dogs of the same breed is still far greater than that between substrains of research mice. Whereas murine tumor models require external initiation or implantation, yield relatively homogenous, less infiltrative tumors, and utilize genetically inbred animals, canine studies present none of those drawbacks. Furthermore, canine vascular physiology and brain anatomy are more similar to humans, a valuable asset, especially in therapeutic investigations. In the age of immunotherapy specifically, canine tumors represent an incredibly valuable opportunity to study immune-tumor interactions in a native tumor microenvironment, and the genetic diversity in companion dogs compared to research animals means that immune responses are not as artificially skewed by extensive inbreeding.

The noteworthy drawbacks to canine companion animal tumors as models of human disease center on limited ability to power studies as compared to the high-throughput potential of murine models and the lack of research "tools" available in dogs. Production of commercial reagents and therapies for research in dogs significantly lags behind the massive scale at which murine- and human-compatible reagents are produced. Additionally, while genetic manipulation of mice presents biological disadvantages in terms of translational potential, murine genetic systems allow for targeted investigations not possible in companion dogs. While canine gliomas recapitulate most of the variable glioma histologies found in humans, the molecular and genetic underpinnings of these neoplasms are not identical [91, 216, 220, 221]. Researchers must be cognizant of these differences and tailor research questions that will be appropriate to answer in this species.

As detailed above, the conventional options for glioma therapy in both humans and dogs are similar. However, one distinct benefit of canine studies is the potential for earlier novel interventions in treatment-naïve patients, as dogs are not obligated to receive the therapeutic standard of care. Such strategies might remove some of the confounding factors present in human studies, where novel treatments are delivered in the face of standard therapies, or more commonly, at the time of tumor recurrence. Ultimately, utilization of traditional cellular and rodent models, canine studies, and clinical trials in humans will likely all be necessary to develop more effective strategies for the management of glial tumors in both canine and human patients.

4 Part 4: Conclusion

Increased understanding of the molecular drivers of primary and metastatic brain tumors in humans has led to a shift from a purely histologically based diagnostic paradigm to one informed by molecular features. Simultaneously, therapies that inhibit specific molecular targets or activate an anti-tumor immune response have gained traction in extracranial solid malignancies, but lack efficacy in primary brain tumors. Unfortunately, these same investigations have revealed the significant role of glial tumor heterogeneity and tumor-induced immunosuppression in preventing treatment response. This pathobiology is incompletely captured by current murine model systems, which variably rely on genetically homogenous tumors and/or mice without intact immune systems. There is a significant burden of spontaneously developing glioma in brachycephalic canine breeds, with overlap in clinically significant driver mutations as well as populations of tumor-infiltrating immune cells, though both areas remain incompletely characterized. Unlike mice, canine patients may regularly undergo some or all of the standard-of-care interventions performed on humans—radiotherapy, alkylating chemotherapy, and in some cases, surgical resection. Therefore, canine glioma represent an opportunity for both exploration of basic immune and molecular features as well as improved therapeutic translation in a model that better recapitulates the features of human disease.

References

1. Horbinski C, Berger T, Packer RJ, Wen PY (2022) Clinical implications of the 2021 edition of the WHO classification of central nervous system tumours. Nat Rev Neurol 18:515–529
2. Schaff LR, Mellinghoff IK (2023) Glioblastoma and other primary brain malignancies in adults: a review. JAMA 329:574–587

3. Ostrom QT, Price M, Ryan K et al (2022) CBTRUS statistical report: pediatric brain tumor foundation childhood and adolescent primary brain and other central nervous system tumors diagnosed in the United States in 2014–2018. Neuro-Oncology 24:iii1–iii38
4. Ostrom QT, Price M, Neff C et al (2022) CBTRUS statistical report: primary brain and other central nervous system tumors diagnosed in the United States in 2015–2019. Neuro-Oncology 24:v1–v95
5. Nieblas-Bedolla E, Zuccato J, Kluger H et al (2022) Central nervous system metastases. Hematol Oncol Clin North Am 36:161–188
6. Rogers L, Barani I, Chamberlain M et al (2015) Meningiomas: knowledge base, treatment outcomes, and uncertainties. A RANO review. J Neurosurg 122:4–23
7. Louis DN, Perry A, Wesseling P et al (2021) The 2021 WHO classification of tumors of the central nervous system: a summary. Neuro-Oncology 23:1231–1251
8. Torp SH, Solheim O, Skjulsvik AJ (2022) The WHO 2021 classification of central nervous system tumours: a practical update on what neurosurgeons need to know—a minireview. Acta Neurochir 164:2453–2464
9. Brastianos PK, Galanis E, Butowski N et al (2019) Advances in multidisciplinary therapy for meningiomas. Neuro-Oncology 21:i18–i31
10. Berger TR, Wen PY, Lang-Orsini M, Chukwueke UN (2022) World Health Organization 2021 classification of central nervous system tumors and implications for therapy for adult-type gliomas: a review. JAMA Oncol 8:1493–1501
11. Horvath-Rizea D, Surov A, Hoffmann KT et al (2018) The value of whole lesion ADC histogram profiling to differentiate between morphologically indistinguishable ring enhancing lesions-comparison of glioblastomas and brain abscesses. Oncotarget 9:18148–18159
12. Sanai N, Polley MY, McDermott MW et al (2011) An extent of resection threshold for newly diagnosed glioblastomas. J Neurosurg 115:3–8
13. Jakola AS, Myrmel KS, Kloster R et al (2012) Comparison of a strategy favoring early surgical resection vs a strategy favoring watchful waiting in low-grade gliomas. JAMA 308:1881–1888
14. Molinaro AM, Hervey-Jumper S, Morshed RA et al (2020) Association of maximal extent of resection of contrast-enhanced and non–contrast-enhanced tumor with survival within molecular subgroups of patients with newly diagnosed glioblastoma. JAMA Oncol 6:495–503
15. Dadario NB, Brahimaj B, Yeung J, Sughrue ME (2021) Reducing the cognitive footprint of brain tumor surgery. Front Neurol 12:711646
16. Gilbert MR, Wang M, Aldape KD et al (2013) Dose-dense temozolomide for newly diagnosed glioblastoma: a randomized phase III clinical trial. J Clin Oncol 31:4085–4091
17. Aldape K, Brindle KM, Chesler L et al (2019) Challenges to curing primary brain tumours. Nat Rev Clin Oncol 16:509–520
18. Stupp R, Mason WP, van den Bent MJ et al (2005) Radiotherapy plus concomitant and adjuvant temozolomide for glioblastoma. N Engl J Med 352:987–996
19. Lim M, Weller M, Idbaih A et al (2022) Phase III trial of chemoradiotherapy with temozolomide plus nivolumab or placebo for newly diagnosed glioblastoma with methylated MGMT promoter. Neuro-Oncology
20. Omuro A, Brandes AA, Carpentier AF et al (2022) Radiotherapy combined with nivolumab or temozolomide for newly diagnosed glioblastoma with unmethylated MGMT promoter: an international randomized phase III trial. Neuro-Oncology
21. Weller M, Butowski N, Tran DD et al (2017) Rindopepimut with temozolomide for patients with newly diagnosed, EGFRvIII-expressing glioblastoma (ACT IV): a randomised, double-blind, international phase 3 trial. Lancet Oncol 18:1373–1385
22. Mohan AA, Tomaszewski WH, Haskell-Mendoza AP et al (2021) Targeting immunometabolism in glioblastoma. Front Oncol 11:696402
23. Smith HL, Wadhwani N, Horbinski C (2022) Major features of the 2021 WHO classification of CNS tumors. Neurotherapeutics 19:1691–1704
24. Tesileanu CMS, Dirven L, Wijnenga MMJ et al (2020) Survival of diffuse astrocytic glioma, IDH1/2 wildtype, with molecular features of glioblastoma, WHO grade IV: a confirmation of the cIMPACT-NOW criteria. Neuro-Oncology 22:515–523
25. Lee D, Riestenberg RA, Haskell-Mendoza A, Bloch O (2021) Diffuse astrocytic glioma, IDH-Wildtype, with molecular features of glioblastoma, WHO grade IV: a single-institution case series and review. J Neuro-Oncol 152:89–98
26. Komori T (2022) Grading of adult diffuse gliomas according to the 2021 WHO classification of tumors of the central nervous system. Lab Investig 102:126–133
27. Majzner RG, Ramakrishna S, Yeom KW et al (2022) GD2-CAR T cell therapy for H3K27M-mutated diffuse midline gliomas. Nature 603:934–941
28. Lin GL, Wilson KM, Ceribelli M et al (2019) Therapeutic strategies for diffuse midline glioma from high-throughput combination drug screening. Sci Transl Med 11
29. Osborn AG, Louis DN, Poussaint TY et al (2022) The 2021 World Health Organization classification of tumors of the central nervous system: what neuroradiologists need to know. Am J Neuroradiol
30. Haddad AF, Young JS, Amara D et al (2021) Mouse models of glioblastoma for the evaluation of novel therapeutic strategies. Neurooncol Adv 3:vdab100
31. Miyai M, Tomita H, Soeda A et al (2017) Current trends in mouse models of glioblastoma. J Neuro-Oncol 135:423–432

32. Hicks WH, Bird CE, Traylor JI et al (2021) Contemporary mouse models in glioma research. Cells 10
33. Ausman JI, Shapiro WR, Rall DP (1970) Studies on the chemotherapy of experimental brain tumors: development of an experimental model. Cancer Res 30:2394–2400
34. Seyfried TN, el-Abbadi M, Roy ML (1992) Ganglioside distribution in murine neural tumors. Mol Chem Neuropathol 17:147–167
35. Serano RD, Pegram CN, Bigner DD (1980) Tumorigenic cell culture lines from a spontaneous VM/Dk murine astrocytoma (SMA). Acta Neuropathol 51:53–64
36. Genoud V, Marinari E, Nikolaev SI et al (2018) Responsiveness to anti-PD-1 and anti-CTLA-4 immune checkpoint blockade in SB28 and GL261 mouse glioma models. Onco Targets Ther 7:e1501137
37. Johanns TM, Ward JP, Miller CA et al (2016) Endogenous neoantigen-specific CD8 T cells identified in two glioblastoma models using a cancer immunogenomics approach. Cancer Immunol Res 4:1007–1015
38. Wiesner SM, Decker SA, Larson JD et al (2009) De novo induction of genetically engineered brain tumors in mice using plasmid DNA. Cancer Res 69:431–439
39. Martinez-Murillo R, Martinez A (2007) Standardization of an orthotopic mouse brain tumor model following transplantation of CT-2A astrocytoma cells. Histol Histopathol 22:1309–1326
40. Learn CA, Grossi PM, Schmittling RJ et al (2007) Genetic analysis of intracranial tumors in a murine model of glioma demonstrate a shift in gene expression in response to host immunity. J Neuroimmunol 182:63–72
41. Tran TT, Uhl M, Ma JY et al (2007) Inhibiting TGF-beta signaling restores immune surveillance in the SMA-560 glioma model. Neuro-Oncology 9:259–270
42. Weiss T, Schneider H, Silginer M et al (2018) NKG2D-dependent antitumor effects of chemotherapy and radiotherapy against glioblastoma. Clin Cancer Res 24:882–895
43. Becker AP, Sells BE, Haque SJ, Chakravarti A (2021) Tumor heterogeneity in glioblastomas: from light microscopy to molecular pathology. Cancers (Basel) 13
44. Shelton LM, Mukherjee P, Huysentruyt LC et al (2010) A novel pre-clinical in vivo mouse model for malignant brain tumor growth and invasion. J Neuro-Oncol 99:165–176
45. Szatmari T, Lumniczky K, Desaknai S et al (2006) Detailed characterization of the mouse glioma 261 tumor model for experimental glioblastoma therapy. Cancer Sci 97:546–553
46. Akter F, Simon B, de Boer NL et al (2021) Pre-clinical tumor models of primary brain tumors: challenges and opportunities. Biochim Biophys Acta Rev Cancer 1875:188458
47. Lenting K, Verhaak R, Ter Laan M et al (2017) Glioma: experimental models and reality. Acta Neuropathol 133:263–282
48. da Hora CC, Schweiger MW, Wurdinger T, Tannous BA (2019) Patient-derived glioma models: from patients to dish to animals. Cells 8
49. Joo KM, Kim J, Jin J et al (2013) Patient-specific orthotopic glioblastoma xenograft models recapitulate the histopathology and biology of human glioblastomas in situ. Cell Rep 3:260–273
50. Wainwright DA, Horbinski CM, Hashizume R, James CD (2017) Therapeutic hypothesis testing with rodent brain tumor models. Neurotherapeutics 14:385–392
51. Soeda A, Hara A, Kunisada T et al (2015) The evidence of glioblastoma heterogeneity. Sci Rep 5:7979
52. Frese KK, Tuveson DA (2007) Maximizing mouse cancer models. Nat Rev Cancer 7:645–658
53. Teng J, da Hora CC, Kantar RS et al (2017) Dissecting inherent intratumor heterogeneity in patient-derived glioblastoma culture models. Neuro-Oncology 19:820–832
54. Smith HW, Muller WJ (2013) Transgenic mouse models–a seminal breakthrough in oncogene research. Cold Spring Harb Protoc 2013:1099–1108
55. Hanahan D, Wagner EF, Palmiter RD (2007) The origins of oncomice: a history of the first transgenic mice genetically engineered to develop cancer. Genes Dev 21:2258–2270
56. Furnari FB, Fenton T, Bachoo RM et al (2007) Malignant astrocytic glioma: genetics, biology, and paths to treatment. Genes Dev 21:2683–2710
57. Parsons DW, Jones S, Zhang X et al (2008) An integrated genomic analysis of human glioblastoma multiforme. Science 321:1807–1812
58. Ding H, Shannon P, Lau N et al (2003) Oligodendrogliomas result from the expression of an activated mutant epidermal growth factor receptor in a RAS transgenic mouse astrocytoma model. Cancer Res 63:1106–1113
59. Zhu Y, Guignard F, Zhao D et al (2005) Early inactivation of p53 tumor suppressor gene cooperating with NF1 loss induces malignant astrocytoma. Cancer Cell 8:119–130
60. Brinster RL, Chen HY, Messing A et al (1984) Transgenic mice harboring SV40 T-antigen genes develop characteristic brain tumors. Cell 37:367–379
61. Stewart TA, Pattengale PK, Leder P (1984) Spontaneous mammary adenocarcinomas in transgenic mice that carry and express MTV/myc fusion genes. Cell 38:627–637
62. Gu H, Zou YR, Rajewsky K (1993) Independent control of immunoglobulin switch recombination at individual switch regions evidenced through Cre-loxP-mediated gene targeting. Cell 73:1155–1164
63. Jung S, Rajewsky K, Radbruch A (1993) Shutdown of class switch recombination by deletion of a switch region control element. Science 259:984–987

64. Zhu H, Woolfenden S, Bronson RT et al (2010) The novel Hsp90 inhibitor NXD30001 induces tumor regression in a genetically engineered mouse model of glioblastoma multiforme. Mol Cancer Ther 9:2618–2626
65. Lin F, de Gooijer MC, Roig EM et al (2014) ABCB1, ABCG2, and PTEN determine the response of glioblastoma to temozolomide and ABT-888 therapy. Clin Cancer Res 20:2703–2713
66. McConville P, Hambardzumyan D, Moody JB et al (2007) Magnetic resonance imaging determination of tumor grade and early response to temozolomide in a genetically engineered mouse model of glioma. Clin Cancer Res 13:2897–2904
67. Richmond A, Su Y (2008) Mouse xenograft models vs GEM models for human cancer therapeutics. Dis Model Mech 1:78–82
68. McNeill RS, Vitucci M, Wu J, Miller CR (2015) Contemporary murine models in preclinical astrocytoma drug development. Neuro-Oncology 17:12–28
69. Hambardzumyan D, Parada LF, Holland EC, Charest A (2011) Genetic modeling of gliomas in mice: new tools to tackle old problems. Glia 59:1155–1168
70. Buque A, Galluzzi L (2018) Modeling tumor immunology and immunotherapy in mice. Trends Cancer 4:599–601
71. Choi Y, Lee S, Kim K et al (2018) Studying cancer immunotherapy using patient-derived xenografts (PDXs) in humanized mice. Exp Mol Med 50:1–9
72. Ashizawa T, Iizuka A, Nonomura C et al (2017) Antitumor effect of programmed death-1 (PD-1) blockade in humanized the NOG-MHC double knockout mouse. Clin Cancer Res 23:149–158
73. Brown SL, Anderson DC, Dick EJ Jr et al (2009) Neoplasia in the chimpanzee (Pan spp.). J Med Primatol 38:137–144
74. McClure HM (1973) Tumors in nonhuman primates: observations during a six-year period in the Yerkes primate center colony. Am J Phys Anthropol 38:425–429
75. Hayes HM, Priester WA Jr, Pendergrass TW (1975) Occurrence of nervous-tissue tumors in cattle, horses, cats and dogs. Int J Cancer 15:39–47
76. Priester WA, Mantel N (1971) Occurrence of tumors in domestic animals. Data from 12 United States and Canadian colleges of veterinary medicine. J Natl Cancer Inst 47:1333–1344
77. Snyder JM, Shofer FS, Van Winkle TJ, Massicotte C (2006) Canine intracranial primary neoplasia: 173 cases (1986-2003). J Vet Int Med 20:669–675
78. Song RB, Vite CH, Bradley CW, Cross JR (2013) Postmortem evaluation of 435 cases of intracranial neoplasia in dogs and relationship of neoplasm with breed, age, and body weight. J Vet Int Med 27:1143–1152
79. Dorn CR, Taylor DO, Schneider R et al (1968) Survey of animal neoplasms in Alameda and Contra Costa Counties, California. II. Cancer morbidity in dogs and cats from Alameda County. J Natl Cancer Inst 40:307–318
80. Dobson JM, Samuel S, Milstein H et al (2002) Canine neoplasia in the UK: estimates of incidence rates from a population of insured dogs. J Small Anim Pract 43:240–246
81. Kishimoto TE, Uchida K, Chambers JK et al (2020) A retrospective survey on canine intracranial tumors between 2007 and 2017. J Vet Med Sci 82:77–83
82. Mariani CL, Schubert TA, House RA et al (2015) Frameless stereotactic radiosurgery for the treatment of primary intracranial tumours in dogs. Vet Comp Oncol 13:409–423
83. Mai W, Burke EE, Reetz JA et al (2022) High-field MRI using standard pulse sequences has moderate to substantial interobserver agreement and good accuracy for differentiation between intracranial extra-axial histiocytic sarcoma and meningioma in dogs. Vet Radiol Ultrasound 63:176–184
84. Sturges BK, Dickinson PJ, Bollen AW et al (2008) Magnetic resonance imaging and histological classification of intracranial meningiomas in 112 dogs. J Vet Intern Med 22:586–595
85. Westworth DR, Dickinson PJ, Vernau W et al (2008) Choroid plexus tumors in 56 dogs (1985-2007). J Vete Int Med 22:1157–1165
86. Stacy BA, Stevenson TL, Lipsitz D, Higgins RJ (2003) Simultaneously occurring oligodendroglioma and meningioma in a dog. J Vet Intern Med 17:357–359
87. Alves A, Prada J, Almeida JM et al (2006) Primary and secondary tumours occurring simultaneously in the brain of a dog. J Small Anim Pract 47:607–610
88. MacKillop E, Thrall DE, Ranck RS et al (2007) Imaging diagnosis–synchronous primary brain tumors in a dog. Vet Radiol Ultrasound 48:550–553
89. Truve K, Dickinson P, Xiong A et al (2016) Utilizing the dog genome in the search for novel candidate genes involved in glioma development-genome wide association mapping followed by targeted massive parallel sequencing identifies a strongly associated locus. PLoS Genet 12:e1006000
90. Wu K, Rodrigues L, Post G et al (2023) Analyses of canine cancer mutations and treatment outcomes using real-world clinico-genomics data of 2119 dogs. NPJ Precis Oncol 7:8
91. Amin SB, Anderson KJ, Boudreau CE et al (2020) Comparative molecular life history of spontaneous canine and human gliomas. Cancer Cell 37(243–257):e247
92. Zaki FA, Hurvitz AI (1976) Spontaneous neoplasms of the central nervous system of the cat. J Small Anim Pract 17:773–782
93. Ohgaki H, Kleihues P (2005) Population-based studies on incidence, survival rates, and genetic alterations in astrocytic and oligodendroglial gliomas. J Neuropathol Exp Neurol 64:479–489
94. Snyder JM, Lipitz L, Skorupski KA et al (2008) Secondary intracranial neoplasia in the dog: 177 cases (1986-2003). J Vet Intern Med 22:172–177
95. Koestner ABT, Fatzer R, Schulman FY, Summers BA, Van Winkle TJ (1999) Histological classification

of tumors of the nervous system of domestic animals. Armed Forces Institute of Pathology, Washington, DC
96. Koehler JW, Miller AD, Miller CR et al (2018) A revised diagnostic classification of canine glioma: towards validation of the canine glioma patient as a naturally occurring preclinical model for human glioma. J Neuropathol Exp Neurol 77:1039–1054
97. Merickel JL, Pluhar GE, Rendahl A, O'Sullivan MG (2021) Prognostic histopathologic features of canine glial tumors. Vet Pathol 58:945–951
98. Hubbard ME, Arnold S, Bin Zahid A et al (2018) Naturally occurring canine glioma as a model for novel therapeutics. Cancer Investig 36:415–423
99. Miller AD, Miller CR, Rossmeisl JH (2019) Canine primary intracranial cancer: a clinicopathologic and comparative review of glioma, meningioma, and choroid plexus tumors. Front Oncol 9:1151
100. Stoica G, Kim HT, Hall DG, Coates JR (2004) Morphology, immunohistochemistry, and genetic alterations in dog astrocytomas. Vet Pathol 41:10–19
101. Fernandez F, Deviers A, Dally C et al (2016) Presence of neural progenitors in spontaneous canine gliomas: a histopathological and immunohistochemical study of 20 cases. Vet J 209:125–132
102. Beier D, Hau P, Proescholdt M et al (2007) CD133(+) and CD133(−) glioblastoma-derived cancer stem cells show differential growth characteristics and molecular profiles. Cancer Res 67:4010–4015
103. Rebetz J, Tian D, Persson A et al (2008) Glial progenitor-like phenotype in low-grade glioma and enhanced CD133-expression and neuronal lineage differentiation potential in high-grade glioma. PLoS One 3:e1936
104. Zeppernick F, Ahmadi R, Campos B et al (2008) Stem cell marker CD133 affects clinical outcome in glioma patients. Clin Cancer Res 14:123–129
105. Zhang M, Song T, Yang L et al (2008) Nestin and CD133: valuable stem cell-specific markers for determining clinical outcome of glioma patients. J Exp Clin Cancer Res 27:85
106. Hu X, Miao W, Zou Y et al (2013) Expression of p53, epidermal growth factor receptor, Ki-67 and O(6)-methylguanine-DNA methyltransferase in human gliomas. Oncol Lett 6:130–134
107. Ligon KL, Alberta JA, Kho AT et al (2004) The oligodendroglial lineage marker OLIG2 is universally expressed in diffuse gliomas. J Neuropathol Exp Neurol 63:499–509
108. Rhee W, Ray S, Yokoo H et al (2009) Quantitative analysis of mitotic Olig2 cells in adult human brain and gliomas: implications for glioma histogenesis and biology. Glia 57:510–523
109. Schiffer D, Giordana MT, Mauro A et al (1986) Immunohistochemical demonstration of vimentin in human cerebral tumors. Acta Neuropathol 70:209–219
110. Katsetos CD, Draberova E, Smejkalova B et al (2007) Class III beta-tubulin and gamma-tubulin are co-expressed and form complexes in human glioblastoma cells. Neurochem Res 32:1387–1398
111. Hwang SL, Hong YR, Sy WD et al (1999) Expression and mutation analysis of the p53 gene in astrocytoma. J Formos Med Assoc 98:31–38
112. Lang FF, Miller DC, Koslow M, Newcomb EW (1994) Pathways leading to glioblastoma multiforme: a molecular analysis of genetic alterations in 65 astrocytic tumors. J Neurosurg 81:427–436
113. Gullick WJ (1991) Prevalence of aberrant expression of the epidermal growth factor receptor in human cancers. Br Med Bull 47:87–98
114. Louis DN (2006) Molecular pathology of malignant gliomas. Annu Rev Pathol 1:97–117
115. Heimberger AB, Hlatky R, Suki D et al (2005) Prognostic effect of epidermal growth factor receptor and EGFRvIII in glioblastoma multiforme patients. Clin Cancer Res 11:1462–1466
116. Higgins RJ, Dickinson PJ, LeCouteur RA et al (2010) Spontaneous canine gliomas: overexpression of EGFR, PDGFRalpha and IGFBP2 demonstrated by tissue microarray immunophenotyping. J Neuro-Oncol 98:49–55
117. Dickinson PJ, Roberts BN, Higgins RJ et al (2006) Expression of receptor tyrosine kinases VEGFR-1 (FLT-1), VEGFR-2 (KDR), EGFR-1, PDGFRa and c-Met in canine primary brain tumours. Vet Comp Oncol 4:132–140
118. Korkolopoulou P, Patsouris E, Konstantinidou AE et al (2004) Hypoxia-inducible factor 1alpha/vascular endothelial growth factor axis in astrocytomas. Associations with microvessel morphometry, proliferation and prognosis. Neuropathol Appl Neurobiol 30:267–278
119. Pietsch T, Valter MM, Wolf HK et al (1997) Expression and distribution of vascular endothelial growth factor protein in human brain tumors. Acta Neuropathol 93:109–117
120. Huang H, Held-Feindt J, Buhl R et al (2005) Expression of VEGF and its receptors in different brain tumors. Neurol Res 27:371–377
121. Kalya M, Kel A, Wlochowitz D et al (2021) IGFBP2 is a potential master regulator driving the dysregulated gene network responsible for short survival in glioblastoma multiforme. Front Genet 12:670240
122. Kokubo M, Nishio M, Ribar TJ et al (2009) BDNF-mediated cerebellar granule cell development is impaired in mice null for CaMKK2 or CaMKIV. J Neurosci 29:8901–8913
123. Trost D, Ehrler M, Fimmers R et al (2007) Identification of genomic aberrations associated with shorter overall survival in patients with oligodendroglial tumors. Int J Cancer 120:2368–2376
124. Thomas R, Duke SE, Wang HJ et al (2009) 'Putting our heads together': insights into genomic conservation between human and canine intracranial tumors. J Neuro-Oncol 94:333–349
125. York D, Higgins RJ, LeCouteur RA et al (2012) TP53 mutations in canine brain tumors. Vet Pathol 49:796–801

126. Amin S, Boudreau B, Martinez-Ledesma JE et al (2018) COMP-07. Comparative molecular life history of spontaneous canine and human glioma. Neuro-Oncology 20:vi64–vi65
127. Tresch NS, Fuchs D, Morandi L et al (2021) Temozolomide is additive with cytotoxic effect of irradiation in canine glioma cell lines. Vet Med Sci 7:2124–2134
128. Krane GA, Shockley KR, Malarkey DE et al (2022) Inter-pathologist agreement on diagnosis, classification and grading of canine glioma. Vet Comp Oncol
129. Sloma EA, Creneti CT, Erb HN, Miller AD (2015) Characterization of inflammatory changes associated with canine oligodendroglioma. J Comp Pathol 153:92–100
130. Pi Castro D, Jose-Lopez R, Fernandez Flores F et al (2020) Expression of FOXP3 in canine gliomas: immunohistochemical study of tumor-infiltrating regulatory lymphocytes. J Neuropathol Exp Neurol 79:184–193
131. Chambers MR, Foote JB, Bentley RT et al (2021) Evaluation of immunologic parameters in canine glioma patients treated with an oncolytic herpes virus. J Transl Genet Genom 5:423–442
132. Filley A, Henriquez M, Bhowmik T et al (2018) Immunologic and gene expression profiles of spontaneous canine oligodendrogliomas. J Neuro-Oncol 137:469–479
133. Krane GA, O'Dea CA, Malarkey DE et al (2021) Immunohistochemical evaluation of immune cell infiltration in canine gliomas. Vet Pathol 58:952–963
134. Toedebusch R, Grodzki AC, Dickinson PJ et al (2021) Glioma-associated microglia/macrophages augment tumorigenicity in canine astrocytoma, a naturally occurring model of human glioma. Neurooncol Adv 3:vdab062
135. Toedebusch RG, Wei NW, Simafranca KT et al (2023) Intra- and intertumoral microglia/macrophage infiltration and their associated molecular signature is highly variable in canine oligodendroglioma: a preliminary evaluation. Vet Sci 10
136. Boozer LB, Davis TW, Borst LB et al (2012) Characterization of immune cell infiltration into canine intracranial meningiomas. Vet Pathol 49:784–795
137. Dobson JM (2013) Breed-predispositions to cancer in pedigree dogs. ISRN Vet Sci 2013:941275
138. Jose-Lopez R, Gutierrez-Quintana R, de la Fuente C et al (2021) Clinical features, diagnosis, and survival analysis of dogs with glioma. J Vet Intern Med 35:1902–1917
139. Pons-Sorolla M, Dominguez E, Czopowicz M et al (2022) Clinical and Magnetic Resonance Imaging (MRI) features, tumour localisation, and survival of dogs with presumptive brain gliomas. Vet Sci 9
140. Rossmeisl JH, Clapp K, Pancotto TE et al (2016) Canine butterfly glioblastomas: a neuroradiological review. Front Vet Sci 3:40
141. Koch MW, Sanchez MD, Long S (2011) Multifocal oligodendroglioma in three dogs. J Am Anim Hosp Assoc 47:e77–e85
142. Lobacz MA, Serra F, Hammond G et al (2018) Imaging diagnosis-magnetic resonance imaging of diffuse leptomeningeal oligodendrogliomatosis in a dog with "dural tail sign". Vet Radiol Ultrasound 59:E1–E6
143. Bentley RT, Burcham GN, Heng HG et al (2016) A comparison of clinical, magnetic resonance imaging and pathological findings in dogs with gliomatosis cerebri, focusing on cases with minimal magnetic resonance imaging changes (double dagger). Vet Comp Oncol 14:318–330
144. Bentley RT, Yanke AB, Miller MA et al (2021) Cerebrospinal fluid drop metastases of canine glioma: magnetic resonance imaging classification. Front Vet Sci 8:650320
145. Palmer AC, Malinowski W, Barnett KC (1974) Clinical signs including papilloedema associated with brain tumours in twenty-one dogs. J Small Anim Pract 15:359–386
146. Bagley RS, Gavin PR, Moore MP et al (1999) Clinical signs associated with brain tumors in dogs: 97 cases (1992-1997). J Am Vet Med Assoc 215:818–819
147. Bagley RS, Gavin PR (1998) Seizures as a complication of brain tumors in dogs. Clin Tech Small Anim Pract 13:179–184
148. Foster ES, Carrillo JM, Patnaik AK (1988) Clinical signs of tumors affecting the rostral cerebrum in 43 dogs. J Vet Intern Med 2:71–74
149. Stadler KL, Ruth JD, Pancotto TE et al (2017) Computed tomography and magnetic resonance imaging are equivalent in mensuration and similarly inaccurate in grade and type predictability of canine intracranial gliomas. Front Vet Sci 4:157
150. Bentley RT (2015) Magnetic resonance imaging diagnosis of brain tumors in dogs. Vet J 205:204–216
151. Rodenas S, Pumarola M, Gaitero L et al (2011) Magnetic resonance imaging findings in 40 dogs with histologically confirmed intracranial tumours. Vet J 187:85–91
152. Turrel JM, Fike JR, LeCouteur RA, Higgins RJ (1986) Computed tomographic characteristics of primary brain tumors in 50 dogs. J Am Vet Med Assoc 188:851–856
153. Young BD, Levine JM, Porter BF et al (2011) Magnetic resonance imaging features of intracranial astrocytomas and oligodendrogliomas in dogs. Vet Radiol Ultrasound 52:132–141
154. Bentley RT, Ober CP, Anderson KL et al (2013) Canine intracranial gliomas: relationship between magnetic resonance imaging criteria and tumor type and grade. Vet J 198:463–471
155. Wisner ER, Dickinson PJ, Higgins RJ (2011) Magnetic resonance imaging features of canine intracranial neoplasia. Vet Radiol Ultrasound 52:S52–S61

156. Thomas WBWS, Kramer R, Kornegay JN (1996) Magnetic resonance imaging features of primary brain tumors in dogs. Vet Radiol Ultrasound 37:20–27
157. Polizopoulou ZS, Koutinas AF, Souftas VD et al (2004) Diagnostic correlation of CT-MRI and histopathology in 10 dogs with brain neoplasms. J Vet Med A Physiol Pathol Clin Med 51:226–231
158. Wolff CA, Holmes SP, Young BD et al (2012) Magnetic resonance imaging for the differentiation of neoplastic, inflammatory, and cerebrovascular brain disease in dogs. J Vet Intern Med 26:589–597
159. Flegel T (2017) Breed-specific magnetic resonance imaging characteristics of necrotizing encephalitis in dogs. Front Vet Sci 4:203
160. Amphimaque B, Durand A, Oevermann A et al (2022) Grading of oligodendroglioma in dogs based on magnetic resonance imaging. J Vet Intern Med 36:2104–2112
161. Kraft SL, Gavin PR, DeHaan C et al (1997) Retrospective review of 50 canine intracranial tumors evaluated by magnetic resonance imaging. J Vet Intern Med 11:218–225
162. Garcia-Mora J, Parker RL, Cecere T et al (2023) The T2-FLAIR mismatch sign as an imaging biomarker for oligodendrogliomas in dogs. J Vet Intern Med 37:1447–1454
163. Young BD, Fosgate GT, Holmes SP et al (2014) Evaluation of standard magnetic resonance characteristics used to differentiate neoplastic, inflammatory, and vascular brain lesions in dogs. Vet Radiol Ultrasound 55:399–406
164. Diangelo L, Cohen-Gadol A, Heng HG et al (2019) Glioma mimics: magnetic resonance imaging characteristics of granulomas in dogs. Front Vet Sci 6:286
165. Bentley RT, Heng HG, Thompson C et al (2015) Magnetic resonance imaging features and outcome for solitary central nervous system Coccidioides granulomas in 11 dogs and cats. Vet Radiol Ultrasound 56:520–530
166. Koblik PD, LeCouteur RA, Higgins RJ et al (1999) CT-guided brain biopsy using a modified Pelorus MARK III stereotactic system: experience with 50 dogs. Vet Radiol Ultrasound 40:434–440
167. Moissonnier P, Blot S, Devauchelle P et al (2002) Stereotactic CT-guided brain biopsy in the dog. J Small Anim Pract 43:115–123
168. Rossmeisl JH, Andriani RT, Cecere TE et al (2015) Frame-based stereotactic biopsy of canine brain masses: technique and clinical results in 26 cases. Front Vet Sci 2:20
169. James MD, Bova FJ, Rajon DA et al (2017) Novel MRI and CT compatible stereotactic brain biopsy system in dogs using patient-specific facemasks. J Small Anim Pract 58:615–621
170. Gutmann S, Winkler D, Muller M et al (2020) Accuracy of a magnetic resonance imaging-based 3D printed stereotactic brain biopsy device in dogs. J Vet Intern Med 34:844–851
171. Rossmeisl JH Jr, Jones JC, Zimmerman KL, Robertson JL (2013) Survival time following hospital discharge in dogs with palliatively treated primary brain tumors. J Am Vet Med Assoc 242:193–198
172. Van Meervenne S, Verhoeven PS, de Vos J et al (2014) Comparison between symptomatic treatment and lomustine supplementation in 71 dogs with intracranial, space-occupying lesions. Vet Comp Oncol 12:67–77
173. Moirano SJ, Dewey CW, Wright KZ, Cohen PW (2018) Survival times in dogs with presumptive intracranial gliomas treated with oral lomustine: a comparative retrospective study (2008-2017). Vet Comp Oncol 16:459–466
174. Sunol A, Mascort J, Font C et al (2017) Long-term follow-up of surgical resection alone for primary intracranial rostrotentorial tumors in dogs: 29 cases (2002-2013). Open Vet J 7:375–383
175. MacLellan JD, Arnold SA, Dave AC et al (2018) Association of magnetic resonance imaging-based preoperative tumor volume with postsurgical survival time in dogs with primary intracranial glioma. J Am Vet Med Assoc 252:98–102
176. Fulton LM, Steinberg HS (1990) Preliminary study of lomustine in the treatment of intracranial masses in dogs following localization by imaging techniques. Semin Vet Med Surg Small Anim 5:241–245
177. Dolera M, Malfassi L, Bianchi C et al (2018) Frameless stereotactic radiotherapy alone and combined with temozolomide for presumed canine gliomas. Vet Comp Oncol 16:90–101
178. Hidalgo Crespo E, Farré Mariné A, Pumarola IBM et al (2022) Survival time after surgical debulking and temozolomide adjuvant chemotherapy in canine intracranial gliomas. Vet Sci 9
179. Bentley RT, Thomovsky SA, Miller MA et al (2018) Canine (pet dog) tumor microsurgery and Intratumoral concentration and safety of metronomic Chlorambucil for spontaneous glioma: a phase I clinical trial. World Neurosurg 116:e534–e542
180. Heidner GL, Kornegay JN, Page RL et al (1991) Analysis of survival in a retrospective study of 86 dogs with brain tumors. J Vet Intern Med 5:219–226
181. Evans SM, Dayrell-Hart B, Powlis W et al (1993) Radiation therapy of canine brain masses. J Vet Intern Med 7:216–219
182. Norman A, Ingram M, Skillen RG et al (1997) X-ray phototherapy for canine brain masses. Radiat Oncol Investig 5:8–14
183. Brearley MJ, Jeffery ND, Phillips SM, Dennis R (1999) Hypofractionated radiation therapy of brain masses in dogs: a retrospective analysis of survival of 83 cases (1991-1996). J Vet Intern Med 13:408–412
184. Spugnini EP, Thrall DE, Price GS et al (2000) Primary irradiation of canine intracranial masses. Vet Radiol Ultrasound 41:377–380
185. Bley CR, Sumova A, Roos M, Kaser-Hotz B (2005) Irradiation of brain tumors in dogs with neurologic disease. J Vet Intern Med 19:849–854

186. Rohrer Bley C, Staudinger C, Bley T et al (2022) Canine presumed glial brain tumours treated with radiotherapy: Is there an inferior outcome in tumours contacting the subventricular zone? Vet Comp Oncol 20:29–37
187. Debreuque M, De Fornel P, David I et al (2020) Definitive-intent uniform megavoltage fractioned radiotherapy protocol for presumed canine intracranial gliomas: retrospective analysis of survival and prognostic factors in 38 cases (2013-2019). BMC Vet Res 16:412
188. LeCouteur RA, Gillette EL, Powers BE et al (1989) Peripheral neuropathies following experimental intraoperative radiation therapy (IORT). Int J Radiat Oncol Biol Phys 17:583–590
189. Thrall DE, Withrow SJ, Powers BE et al (1990) Radiotherapy prior to cortical allograft limb sparing in dogs with osteosarcoma: a dose response assay. Int J Radiat Oncol Biol Phys 18:1351–1357
190. Schwarz P, Meier V, Soukup A et al (2018) Comparative evaluation of a novel, moderately hypofractionated radiation protocol in 56 dogs with symptomatic intracranial neoplasia. J Vet Intern Med 32:2013–2020
191. Van Asselt N, Christensen N, Meier V et al (2020) Definitive-intent intensity-modulated radiation therapy provides similar outcomes to those previously published for definitive-intent three-dimensional conformal radiation therapy in dogs with primary brain tumors: a multi-institutional retrospective study. Vet Radiol Ultrasound 61:481–489
192. Nolan MW, Gieger TL (2019) Update in veterinary radiation oncology: focus on stereotactic radiation therapy. Vet Clin North Am Small Anim Pract 49:933–947
193. Moirano SJ, Dewey CW, Haney S, Yang J (2020) Efficacy of frameless stereotactic radiotherapy for the treatment of presumptive canine intracranial gliomas: a retrospective analysis (2014-2017). Vet Comp Oncol 18:528–537
194. Dunfield EM, Turek MM, Buhr KA, Christensen NI (2018) A survey of stereotactic radiation therapy in veterinary medicine. Vet Radiol Ultrasound 59:786–795
195. MagalhAes TR, BenoIt J, NECova S et al (2021) Outcome after radiation therapy in canine intracranial meningiomas or gliomas. In Vivo 35:1117–1123
196. Staudinger C, Meier V, Beckmann K et al (2022) Treatment of intracranial neoplasia in dogs using higher doses: a randomized controlled trial comparing a boosted to a conventional radiation protocol. J Vet Intern Med 36:1353–1364
197. Trageser E, Martin T, Burdekin B et al (2023) Efficacy of stereotactic radiation therapy for the treatment of confirmed or presumed canine glioma. Vet Comp Oncol
198. Hicks J, Platt S, Stewart G et al (2019) Intratumoral temozolomide in spontaneous canine gliomas: feasibility of a novel therapy using implanted microcylinders. Vet Med Sci 5:5–18
199. Freeman AC, Platt SR, Holmes S et al (2018) Convection-enhanced delivery of cetuximab conjugated iron-oxide nanoparticles for treatment of spontaneous canine intracranial gliomas. J Neuro-Oncol 137:653–663
200. Young JS, Bernal G, Polster SP et al (2018) Convection-enhanced delivery of polymeric nanoparticles encapsulating chemotherapy in canines with spontaneous supratentorial tumors. World Neurosurg 117:e698–e704
201. Dickinson PJ, LeCouteur RA, Higgins RJ et al (2010) Canine spontaneous glioma: a translational model system for convection-enhanced delivery. Neuro-Oncology 12:928–940
202. Rossmeisl JH, Herpai D, Quigley M et al (2021) Phase I trial of convection-enhanced delivery of IL13RA2 and EPHA2 receptor targeted cytotoxins in dogs with spontaneous intracranial gliomas. Neuro-Oncology 23:422–434
203. Olin MR, Ampudia-Mesias E, Pennell CA et al (2019) Treatment combining CD200 immune checkpoint inhibitor and tumor-lysate vaccination after surgery for pet dogs with high-grade glioma. Cancers (Basel) 11
204. Cloquell A, Mateo I, Gambera S et al (2022) Systemic cellular viroimmunotherapy for canine high-grade gliomas. J Immunother Cancer 10
205. Ammons DT, Guth A, Rozental AJ et al (2022) Reprogramming the canine glioma microenvironment with tumor vaccination plus oral losartan and propranolol induces objective responses. Cancer Res Commun 2:1657–1667
206. Candolfi M, Curtin JF, Nichols WS et al (2007) Intracranial glioblastoma models in preclinical neuro-oncology: neuropathological characterization and tumor progression. J Neuro-Oncol 85:133–148
207. Kimmelman J, Nalbantoglu J (2007) Faithful companions: a proposal for neurooncology trials in pet dogs. Cancer Res 67:4541–4544
208. Olin MR, Pluhar GE, Andersen BM et al (2014) Victory and defeat in the induction of a therapeutic response through vaccine therapy for human and canine brain tumors: a review of the state of the art. Crit Rev Immunol 34:399–432
209. Hicks J, Platt S, Kent M, Haley A (2017) Canine brain tumours: a model for the human disease? Vet Comp Oncol 15:252–272
210. LeBlanc AK, Mazcko C, Brown DE et al (2016) Creation of an NCI comparative brain tumor consortium: informing the translation of new knowledge from canine to human brain tumor patients. Neuro-Oncology 18:1209–1218
211. LeBlanc AK, Mazcko CN (2020) Improving human cancer therapy through the evaluation of pet dogs. Nat Rev Cancer 20:727–742
212. Bentley RT, Ahmed AU, Yanke AB et al (2017) Dogs are man's best friend: in sickness and in health. Neuro-Oncology 19:312–322
213. Schiffman JD, Breen M (2015) Comparative oncology: what dogs and other species can teach us about

humans with cancer. Philos Trans R Soc Lond Ser B Biol Sci 370
214. Boudreau CE, York D, Higgins RJ et al (2017) Molecular signalling pathways in canine gliomas. Vet Comp Oncol 15:133–150
215. Connolly NP, Shetty AC, Stokum JA et al (2018) Cross-species transcriptional analysis reveals conserved and host-specific neoplastic processes in mammalian glioma. Sci Rep 8:1180
216. Dickinson PJ, York D, Higgins RJ et al (2016) Chromosomal aberrations in canine gliomas define candidate genes and common pathways in dogs and humans. J Neuropathol Exp Neurol 75:700–710
217. Stoica G, Levine J, Wolff J, Murphy K (2011) Canine astrocytic tumors: a comparative review. Vet Pathol 48:266–275
218. York D, Sproul CD, Chikere N et al (2018) Expression and targeting of transcription factor ATF5 in dog gliomas. Vet Comp Oncol 16:102–107
219. Reitman ZJ, Olby NJ, Mariani CL et al (2010) IDH1 and IDH2 hotspot mutations are not found in canine glioma. Int J Cancer 127:245–246
220. Fraser AR, Bacci B, le Chevoir MA, Long SN (2018) Isocitrate dehydrogenase 1 expression in canine gliomas. J Comp Pathol 165:33–39

Soft Tissue Sarcoma

Laura E. Selmic, William C. Kisseberth, and John Alexander

1 Overview of Human and Canine Soft Tissue Sarcoma

1.1 Introduction

Soft tissue sarcomas are mesenchymal neoplasms that arise from connective tissues. As such these tumors can arise from anywhere in the body. In humans, STS are a rare group of malignancies (<1% of all adult malignancies) comprised of more than 50 subtypes, of which liposarcoma, leiomyosarcoma, and undifferentiated pleomorphic sarcoma are the most common subtypes. Most sarcomas are diagnosed based on pathologic analysis of tissue biopsies with the subtypes being determined based on morphology, immunohistochemistry (IHC), and molecular genetics. Histologic subtype is critical for predicting clinical behavior and guiding therapy. Histology-tailored staging tests are then performed to determine the extent of disease and ultimately guide treatment. Soft tissue sarcoma patients are typically managed by a multidisciplinary team including medical oncologists, radiation oncologists, surgical oncologists, radiologists, and experienced pathologists. The treatment recommended is often based on subtype and may include surgery, radiation therapy, and systemic therapy including cytotoxic therapy, targeted therapy, and, more recently, immunotherapy.

In dogs, sarcomas represent approximately 10–15% of malignant tumors with about 80% of these occurring as STS and the remaining 20% being bone sarcomas [1]. In this chapter, we will focus on sarcomas arising from soft tissues, i.e., STS. As in humans, STSs are a heterogeneous group of mesenchymal tumors that can be further categorized based on the histologic phenotype or tissue of origin. The more common histologic subtypes of STS seen in dogs include hemangiosarcoma, gastrointestinal stromal tumor (GIST), fibrosarcoma, malignant peripheral nerve sheath tumor (MPNST), histocytic sarcoma, myxosarcoma, liposarcoma, leiomyosarcoma, synovial cell sarcoma, and lymphangiosarcoma [1]. One of the most common sites for STS to arise in the dog is the skin and subcutaneous tissues. Historically, in dogs, STSs of different tissues of origin have been grouped together based on similar morphologic appearance [2, 3]. Furthermore, these tumors share common biological behavior of local invasion and moderate metastatic potential, both at diagnosis and subsequently in surveillance. Generally, metastases occur at higher

L. E. Selmic (✉) · W. C. Kisseberth
Department of Veterinary Clinical Sciences, College of Veterinary Medicine, The Ohio State University, Columbus, OH, USA
e-mail: Selmic.1@osu.edu

J. Alexander
Division of Musculoskeletal Oncology, Department of Orthopaedics, The Ohio State University Wexner Medical Center, Columbus, OH, USA

M. W. Nolan et al. (eds.), *Comparative Oncology*, https://doi.org/10.1007/978-3-032-04454-9_15

rates (22–44%) in high-grade STSs [4–6]. Different histologic subtypes of sarcoma demonstrate different biological behavior, and these can be diagnosed with a combination of morphology and IHC. Following diagnosis, dogs are often staged with three-view thoracic radiographs and abdominal ultrasound or CT imaging to assess for evidence of metastatic spread. If disease is localized, surgical resection of STS is often performed. If the tumor is incompletely excised or is high grade, then other treatments may be recommended including radiation and/or chemotherapy. The benefit of chemotherapy for high-grade skin and subcutaneous STSs in dogs is unclear, but in some STSs, including hemangiosarcoma, a survival benefit has been established.

1.2 Clinical Epidemiology and Risk Factors for Soft Tissue Sarcoma

1.2.1 Human Soft Tissue Sarcoma

In humans, STSs are rare, with only 12,390 cases of STS diagnosed in the United States in 2017. Half the cases diagnosed arise in the limbs, 30% intra-abdominally (including in the retroperitoneum), and 15% occur on the trunk or head and neck region [7]. While certain histologic subtypes are more common in young patients such as rhabdomyosarcoma, synovial sarcoma, and myxoid liposarcoma, the incidence of STS generally increases with increasing age [8, 9]. The pathogenesis of most STSs is unknown, with most tumors arising spontaneously without any apparent cause. There are some rare examples in which genetic or environmental factors have been associated with the development of sarcoma. Radiation and chronic lymphedema can result in secondary angiosarcoma of the breast [10]. Viral infections with HHV8 have been associated with Kaposi sarcoma. Exposure to chemicals, including vinyl chloride, has been associated with hepatic angiosarcoma, and EBV infection in immunodeficient subjects results in the development of smooth muscle tumors. A minority of sarcomas may arise in patients with genetic syndromes such as neurofibromatosis type 1, hereditary retinoblastoma, and Li-Fraumeni syndromes. In neurofibromatosis type 1, up to 10% of affected individuals will develop MPNST and multiple GIST. With Li-Fraumeni syndrome, germline mutations in *TP53*, predispose patients to the development of malignant tumors, one third of which are bone and STSs. About half of sarcoma patients have been shown to have pathogenic monogenic and polygenic variation in both known and novel cancer genes, such as *TP53, ATM, ATR, BRCA2, and ERCC2* [11]. Additionally, in patients with hereditary retinoblastoma, the risk for non-head and neck STS is 45.7-fold compared to the general population [12]. Advances in molecular genetics over the last 20 years have led to a greater understanding of the molecular mechanisms associated with sarcomagenesis [13–15]. Chromosome translocations have been found in several subtypes of STSs. However, the majority of STSs have variably complex karyotypes; one example would be the occurrence of copy number alterations seen in well-differentiated/dedifferentiated liposarcoma, where amplification of MDM2, CDK4, and HMGA2 genes has been found to be the genetic driver of pathogenesis.

1.2.2 Canine Soft Tissue Sarcoma

Most canine sarcomas are diagnosed in older dogs [16]. Sarcomas are proportionally more common in dogs than in humans [17]. In dogs, STS is one of the most common skin malignancies. The total number of canine sarcomas occurring in the United States annually is estimated at 7700–31,800 based on an overall cancer incidence of 99.3–272.1 per 100,000 dogs [18] and a canine population of 78 million in the United States [1].

Dogs have undergone selective breeding to create distinct breeds, and there are known genetic susceptibilities in some dog breeds including susceptibility to the development of cancer [19]. There are rare cancers, including some sarcomas that occur more commonly in specific breeds. One example is histiocytic sarcoma, which is seen more commonly in Bernese Mountain Dogs, Flat Coat Retrievers, and

Rottweilers. Genome-wide association studies (GWAS) in dogs have shown that complex traits (including cancer susceptibility) are influenced strongly by a small set of loci compared to humans, explaining breed-associated differences in cancer risk [20]. These breed-specific tumors in dogs provide excellent spontaneous tumor models for studying the genetics of tumors like sarcoma that exist in both dogs and humans.

1.3 Clinical Presentation and Diagnostic Workup

1.3.1 Human Soft Tissue Sarcoma

The diagnosis of STS relies heavily upon tissue biopsy for directing staging work-up and treatment planning for patients with STS. Soft tissue sarcomas are currently classified based on the 2020 WHO classification of soft tissue tumors, which classifies different tumors based on differences in histomorphometry, immunophenotype, and molecular genetics [21]. The pathologist assesses the microscopic features of the lesion through evaluation of hematoxylin- and eosin-stained slides. The microscopic diagnosis of sarcoma involves assessment of four main features to help determine the choice of ancillary immunohistochemistry and molecular tests. These features are (1) the predominant shape of the neoplastic cells; (2) the pattern of growth; (3) the quality of the background; (4) the architecture of the vascular network. The shape of the neoplastic cells is classified as either: spindle, epithelioid, round, or pleomorphic. The pattern of growth is particularly important for refinement of the differential diagnosis. The main patterns are fascicular, herringbone, storiform, alveolar, solid, and biphasic. The quality of the background refers to characteristics of the stroma surrounding the neoplastic cells. The categories are considered as fibrous, sclerotic, myxoid, myxochondroid, and osteogenic. Finally, the blood vessels in sarcomas can be arranged in different configurations and are described as one of the following architectures: plexiform, archiform, or hemangiopericytoma-like. The assessment of these four features can help narrow the differential diagnosis; however, it is possible that additional testing may be necessary to further subtype/classify the diagnosis. This is critical when the differential diagnosis includes sarcomatoid variants of other cancers including carcinomas and melanoma.

Immunohistochemistry plays a pivotal role in the diagnosis of STS [22, 23]. The chosen panel of immunostains is guided by the morphology, with most of the classic markers having good sensitivity, but lower specificity [22, 23]. The classic myogenic markers are smooth muscle actin, muscle-specific actin, desmin, and h-caldesmon. Differentiation between smooth and striated muscle is important to confirm adult myogenic sarcomas, differentiate pediatric rhabdomyosarcoma from other soft tissue tumors, and identify myogenic differentiation in MPNST and dedifferentiated liposarcoma. S100 can be utilized to differentiate neural or schwannian origin tumors, as S100 positivity can occur in 30% of neoplastic cells in MPNST and is seen in most neoplastic cells with epithelioid MPNST.

The expansion of molecular diagnostics use in combination with histopathology has led to more accurate diagnoses, clarified disease definitions, provided validation of classification schemes, and has allowed the identification of prognostic markers and potential molecular therapeutic targets in STS. Many STSs are known to have relatively specific recurrent point mutations, gene amplifications, and chromosome translocations that can be readily assessed with molecular diagnostic techniques. Gene fusions are particularly frequent in soft tissue tumors. FISH and/or PCR techniques can be used to identify these specific molecular features to confirm specific histologic subtype diagnoses, in particular when supporting the diagnosis in patients with noncanonical clinical presentations or distinguishing sarcoma from benign mimics or metastatic pleomorphic malignancies of non-sarcoma origin. For example, differentiation between subtypes is important for round cell sarcomas which include Ewing sarcoma, desmoplastic small round cell tumor, alveolar rhabdomyosarcoma, poorly differentiated round cell synovial sarcoma, CIC-rearranged, and

BCOR-rearranged undifferentiated round cell sarcomas, and a minority of cases of high-grade liposarcoma featuring a round cell morphology. All these sarcomas are aggressive; however, the therapeutic approach can differ significantly, in particular when considering systemic therapy options/regimens. In these subtypes, there is overlap in the morphologic appearance, and IHC characterization cannot always provide a definitive diagnosis (e.g., keratin-positive Ewing sarcoma vs. poorly differentiated round cell synovial sarcoma), and thus, molecular genetics play a crucial role in their diagnosis. Using FISH to identify translocations involving *EWSR1*, *SS18*, and *FOXO1*, these rearrangements will be found in Ewing's sarcoma, rhabdomyosarcoma, and poorly differentiated synovial sarcoma, respectively. Alternatively, demonstration of specific chimerical transcripts can be performed using PCR-based techniques or using a new generation sequencing-based approach. This identification of gene copy number variations using both techniques has proven useful for certain STSs. For example, amplification of *MDM2* by FISH or quantitative RT-PCR can be used to confirm the diagnosis of dedifferentiated liposarcoma on core needle biopsies where there may not be tissue available/biopsied from the well-differentiated component or when the well-differentiated component is absent. Molecular diagnostics can also provide value when confirming the diagnosis of sarcoma subtypes when they occur in rare anatomical locations, for example primary Ewing sarcoma of the skin or kidney or synovial sarcoma involving the viscera. Molecular genetics can also be helpful to distinguish benign mesenchymal neoplasms from STSs which can be challenging on morphology alone. For example, the differential diagnoses for low-grade fibromyxoid sarcoma include benign soft tissue tumors including perineurioma, neurofibroma, cellular myxoma, nodular fasciitis, and even locally aggressive tumors like desmoid fibromatosis. MUC4 expression is key for diagnosis, but the finding of a *FUS* rearrangement via FISH or the identification of FUS-CREB3L2 or FUS-CREB3L2 transcripts can be very helpful for diagnosis [24].

Although the histologic subtype of STS is prognostic, it does not provide enough information for predicting the clinical course of disease, so grading systems are used to estimate aggressiveness of STSs. There are many different grading schemes reported; however, the two most successful and commonly utilized have been the three-tiered systems of the National Cancer Institute (NCI) and the French Federation of Cancer Centers Sarcoma Group (FNCLCC) scheme. The FNCLCC grading system is based on evaluation of differentiation, mitotic count, and presence of necrosis. This system has shown better discrimination between the low- and high-grade tumors, and results in a smaller group of tumors in the intermediate grade [25, 26].

After a histologic diagnosis is determined, STS patients undergo staging which includes imaging studies to determine the local and systemic extent of disease to assign a clinical stage prior to the initiation of therapy. This generally includes a CT scan of the thorax and other histologic-specific imaging studies [27]. The American Joint Committee on Cancer (AJCC) Cancer Staging System (also called TNM staging system) is commonly used to assign a stage based on the anatomic location given the different biological behavior and clinical course of tumors of the extremities and trunk, retroperitoneum or abdominopelvic cavities, or the head and neck [28]. The T component designates the size and invasion of the primary tumor. The N component designates whether the regional lymph nodes are normal or have tumor present. The M component designates if there are distant metastases present or not. The most recent version applicable for STS is the eighth edition of the AJCC cancer staging manual (Table 1) [29].

1.3.2 Canine Soft Tissue Sarcoma

In dogs, the diagnosis of STS or spindle cell sarcoma may be made presumptively based on fine needle aspirate and cytology; however, cells may not exfoliate, or necrosis can make the sample nondiagnostic. Cytologic samples are submitted to a cytopathologist for diagnosis. The accuracy of cytology for diagnosis of STS is 63–97% [30, 31]. For definitive diagnosis in dogs, histopathol-

Table 1 AJCC staging system (eighth edition) for soft tissue sarcomas [28]

Primary tumor (T)				
T1	Tumor ≤5 cm in greatest dimension			
T2	Tumor >5 cm and ≤ 10 cm in greatest dimension			
T3	Tumor >10 cm and ≤ 15 cm in greatest dimension			
T4	Tumor >15 cm in greatest dimension			
Regional lymph nodes (N)				
N0	No regional lymph node metastasis or unknown lymph node status			
N1	Regional lymph node metastasis			
Distant metastasis (M)				
M0	No distant metastasis			
M1	Distant metastasis			
Stage groups	Tumor (T)	Nodes (N)	Metastasis (M)	Grade
IA	T1	N0	M0	G1
IB	T2, T3, T4	N0	M0	G1
II	T1	N0	M0	G2/3
IIIA	T2	N0	M0	G2/3
IIIB	T3, T4	N0	M0	G2/3
IV	Any T	N1	M0	Any G
	Any T	Any N	M1	Any G

Table 2 Grading system for canine skin and subcutaneous soft tissue sarcomas [32]

Differentiation score	
1	Sarcomas most closely resembling normal adult mesenchymal tissue
2	Sarcomas for which histologic type can be determined, although differentiation is poor
3	Undifferentiated sarcomas, sarcomas of unknown type
Mitotic score: mitoses per 10 high-power fields (400x)	
1	0–9
2	10–19
3	>19
Tumor necrosis score	
0	No necrosis
1	≤50% necrosis
2	>50% necrosis
Histologic grade: total score[a]	
1	≤ 3
2	4–5
3	≥ 6

[a]Combined score from differentiation score, mitotic score, and tumor necrosis scores

ogy is considered the gold standard. A core needle biopsy or an incisional biopsy can be performed under sedation and using local anesthetic. When STSs arise in abdominal visceral organs, clinicians may forego a preoperative biopsy and perform celiotomy and tumor resection instead as the histopathologic diagnosis does not always alter the surgical plan. Core needle biopsy and incisional biopsy yield small tissue samples, so multiple samples must be taken to try to improve the diagnostic yield. Pathologists will assess the tissue to provide a histologic diagnosis and tumor grade for STSs. The canine STS grading scheme was modified from an international human grading scheme [4, 32–34]. The pathologist assesses tumor differentiation, mitotic index (or more accurately a mitotic count), and percent necrosis, and provides a score for each, with the total score determining the tumor grade (Table 2). Most skin and subcutaneous tumors are classified as grade 1 by pathologists [4, 34–37]. This grading system has not been rigorously validated in dogs, but in general, grade 1 tumors have a low rate (7–13%) of metastasis and local recurrence (7% with close margins in one study). When biopsies are performed, due to the small sample size, there can be discordance in the grading of the biopsy sample and the final grade at the time of resection [38].

In dogs, STSs arising in skin and subcutaneous soft tissues were found to display a common biological behavior of local invasion and only moderate metastatic potential, so for simplification many histologic subtypes are considered within the nomenclature of STS. There are a few sarcomas that have historically been excluded from this group due to more malignant biological behavior. These can be identified and differentiated from STS through distinct morphologic characteristics and/or anatomic locations. These excluded sarcomas include hemangiosarcoma, histiocytic sarcoma, lymphangiosarcoma, synovial cell sarcoma, leiomyosarcoma, rhabdomyosarcoma, fibrosarcoma of the oral cavity, and brachial plexus peripheral nerve sheath tumors (PNST). As such in dogs, STS of the skin and subcutaneous tissues is a diagnosis of exclusion which is not the case in humans.

Canine skin and subcutaneous STSs have common features of spindle cells forming bundles, streams and whorls and intercellular collagenous matrix. It can be challenging to identify areas within the tumors that resemble mature tissue or that express cellular markers to diagnose the phenotype. Sometimes these tumors display more than one histologic pattern, or the histologic pattern and immunohistochemistry patterns are not exclusive to a single cell of origin [39–41].

The combination of tests used for the work up and clinical staging may depend on the tumor location (skin or subcutaneous STS) or specific histologic type such as hemangiosarcoma, but generally it includes hematology and biochemistry blood tests, three-view thoracic radiographs or thoracic computed tomography (CT) scan, abdominal ultrasound or abdominal CT scan, and sometimes local imaging of the STS. Local imaging of the primary site may be necessary for surgical or radiation therapy planning. CT or magnetic resonance imaging can provide valuable information regarding the depth of tumor invasion or the extent of gross disease in the subcutaneous tissues. Fine needle aspirates can be performed on any abnormal lesions found on imaging and regional lymph nodes. With skin and subcutaneous STSs, lymph node metastasis is rare, but some STSs have a higher rate of lymph node metastases like hemangiosarcoma, histiocytic sarcoma, lymphangiosarcoma, synovial cell sarcoma, leiomyosarcoma, and rhabdomyosarcoma [42–47].

The canine staging system used has been modified from the original AJCC staging system for human STS. Subsequently, the AJCC staging system has been modified to categorize localized disease with more emphasis on depth of invasion and less on tumor size [48]. The updated modified staging system for animals is summarized in Table 3. This grouping accounts for clinical staging (TMN) and the histologic grade, but this has not been investigated with respect to having prognostic significance in canine STS.

Table 3 Modified staging system for canine soft tissue sarcomas [255]

Primary tumor (T)				
T1	Tumor ≤5 cm in diameter at greatest dimension			
T1a	Superficial tumor			
T1b	Deep tumor			
T2	Tumor >5 cm in diameter at greatest dimension			
T2a	Superficial tumor			
T2b	Deep tumor			
Regional lymph nodes (N)				
N0	No regional lymph node metastasis			
N1	Regional lymph node metastasis			
Distant metastasis (M)				
M0	No distant metastasis			
M1	Distant metastasis			
Stage grouping	Tumor (T)	Nodes (N)	Metastasis (M)	Grade
I	Any T	N0	M0	I–II
II	T1a-1b, T2a	N0	M0	III
III	T2b	N0	M0	III
IV	Any T	N1	Any M	I–III
	Any T	Any N	M1	I–III

1.4 Tumor Subtypes

1.4.1 Human and Canine Leiomyosarcoma and Gastrointestinal Stromal Tumors

Leiomyosarcoma is a malignant mesenchymal tumor of smooth muscle origin. Most commonly leiomyosarcoma in the dog arises from viscera including the gastrointestinal tract, urogenital tract, the liver, and the spleen [43, 49–55]. There are fewer reports about non-visceral locations including the oral cavity, skin, and large blood vessels [56–60]. GISTs develop from the interstitial cells of Cajal, which are important in the coordination of peristalsis [61]. In humans, GIST occurs most commonly in the stomach, then small intestine, colon, and rectum, and rarely in the esophagus or other non-gastrointestinal organs [62]. There is evidence in humans [63, 64] and dogs [43, 53, 58, 65] that leiomyosarcomas show differing biological behavior based on anatomic site.

Pathology

Leiomyosarcoma can be challenging to differentiate from other mesenchymal tumors including fibrosarcoma, myofibroblastic neoplasms, and GIST as these tumors look similar morphologically. There is no gold standard for morphologic diagnosis; however, IHC can be utilized to aid in the diagnosis. Leiomyosarcomas are frequently desmin and smooth muscle actin (SMA) positive, but there are no established cutoffs for the percentage of positive cells. In addition, some of the other tumors like GIST, myofibroblastic tumors, and perivascular wall tumors (PWT) can be positive for SMA. In contrast, GISTs have KIT immunoreactivity regardless of their reactivity to desmin and SMA [66–68]. Antibodies for other markers used in humans like calponin and heavy-caldesmon, both parts of smooth muscle thin filament, are not available for dogs. Performing IHC to distinguish between the two tumor types is as important in dogs as in humans, as a subset of canine GIST has activating mutations in exon 11 of the *c-kit* gene, making these tumors susceptible to treatment with tyrosine kinase inhibitors [69, 70]. An early study identified 6/17 canine GIST cases that had *c-KIT* mutations in the juxtamembrane domain of exon 11, but none of the 17 canine GIST cases had mutations identified in exons 8, 9, 13, and 17 of *c-KIT* nor mutations in *PDGFRA* [69]. The location and nature of the c-KIT mutations of exon 11 are like those seen in humans, making the dog a relevant model for human GIST. Another more recent study demonstrated 47% of the 17 canine GIST cases had mutations of c-KIT (exon 11) and 1 dog also had a *PDGFRA* mutation [61].

1.4.2 Human and Canine Liposarcoma

This is a rare STS subtype in dogs with a different anatomic distribution compared to humans. In dogs, liposarcomas predominantly occur in the subcutaneous tissues but have been reported in the abdominal organs and elsewhere [2, 71, 72] versus in humans they occur more frequently in the deeper soft tissues and muscles of the extremities and the retroperitoneal space [73, 74]. There is no known breed or sex predilection, and these tumors tend to occur in older dogs [71, 75]. Liposarcomas are locally invasive, but the true incidence of metastases in dogs is unknown. CT assessment of lipomatous tumors can provide helpful information to differentiate the mass from other similar tumors (lipoma and infiltrative lipoma) or for staging or treatment planning. On CT, liposarcomas are generally heterogeneous lesions with soft tissue-attenuating components with a multinodular appearance and may be associated with regional lymphadenopathy and amorphous mineralized areas [76].

Pathology

In dogs there are three histological types of liposarcoma that have been suggested based on the World Health Organization panel: well-differentiated, pleomorphic, and myxoid. Two additional histopathologic types have been suggested by others as atypical lipoma and dedifferentiated liposarcoma [77, 78]. Well-differentiated liposarcoma is the most common histopathologic subtype where the majority of cells resemble adipocytes containing a single fat droplet and a peripheral nucleus. Dedifferentiated liposarcoma is a tumor characterized by areas of well-differentiated liposarcoma with adjacent areas of sarcoma resembling fibrosarcoma or undifferentiated pleomorphic sarcoma [79]. Pleomorphic liposarcoma has severe neoplastic cell pleomorphism, multinucleated neoplastic cells, and minimal to no intracellular lipid. Myxoid liposarcoma is characterized by lipoblasts, lipocytes, and spindle cells with a background of mucin. Atypical lipoma has minimal criteria of malignancy and has histological features similar to lipoma with some scattered atypical lipoblasts [80].

A comparative pathology study with veterinary and human pathologists comparing the morphology and IHC of canine STSs to human STSs concluded the five canine liposarcoma subtypes could not completely fit into defined categories due to a mixture of adipocyte and epithelioid cells (some positive for desmin) which is not seen in human liposarcoma cases [73, 81]. Another study sought to evaluate IHC expression of muscle markers including desmin, myogenin, and α-smooth muscle actin (α-SMA) and the brown fat marker, uncoupling protein I (UCPI), in 25 canine liposarcoma cases (15 well-differentiated, 5 pleomorphic, 3 myxoid, and 2 dedifferentiated) [82]. The use of these IHC markers might be needed for differentiation of liposarcoma from hibernoma and rhabdomyosarcomas. IHC results indicated that 23/25 cases expressed UCPI, 7/25 expressed SMA, 7/25 expressed desmin and 3/25 expressed myogenin. These results indicate similar IHC profiles for liposarcoma and rhabdomyosarcoma and could lead to misdiagnosis of liposarcoma subtypes with similar morphology to rhabdomyosarcoma in dogs. In addition, well-differentiated liposarcoma could be challenging to distinguish from hibernoma if only based on UCPI IHC.

Molecular Characteristics

Avallone et al. demonstrated MDM2 and CDK4 expression in canine liposarcomas [78]. Fifty-three liposarcomas were retrospectively evaluated with IHC, 24 were well differentiated (16 expressed MDM2 and 21 CDK4); 7 were myxoid liposarcomas (1 expressed MDM2 and 5 CDK4), and 18 were pleomorphic liposarcomas (all were MDM2 negative and 12 expressed CDK4). Four tumors were classified as dedifferentiated liposarcoma (3 expressed MDM2 and 4 expressed CDK4) for the first time in dogs based on morphology. MDM2 expression was correlated with histopathologic subtype (high expression was seen in well-differentiated and de-differentiated liposarcoma) and grade (highly expressed in grade I tumors). CDK4 expression was less specifically able to differentiate between the liposarcoma subtypes in the Avallone study [78], which contrasts with liposarcoma in humans where in 90% of cases express MDM2 and CDK4 and co-amplification of the respective genes is seen, and this is specific for well- and de-differentiated liposarcoma [73].

Tyrosine kinase receptor expression (fibroblast growth factor receptor I, platelet-derived growth factor receptor β and c-kit) has been reported in canine liposarcoma [79]. The study population was derived from an earlier study [78] and consisted of 14 cases of well-differentiated liposarcoma, 7 myxoid liposarcoma, 25 pleomorphic liposarcoma and 4 dedifferentiated liposarcoma cases. High expression of fibroblast growth factor receptor I, platelet-derived growth factor receptor β, and c-kit was seen in 68%, 71%, and 13%, respectively, of all liposarcomas. A correlation was demonstrated between high expression of FDF2 and low mitotic index suggesting this pathway might be less efficient in inducing proliferation of canine liposarcoma cells. In addition, this would indicate that the FGF2-FGFR1 pathway is not relevant in the pathogenesis of canine liposarcoma. The low rate of expression of c-kit within this canine liposarcoma population does not support c-kit having a primary role in cellular proliferation in canine liposarcoma. The PDGFB-PDGFRB pathway could have a central role in canine liposarcoma progression given there is high expression in greater than 70% of cases. Further research is needed but these could be potential therapeutic targets.

P53 expression determined through IHC has been found to correlate with the myxoid variant and higher proliferative activity in canine liposarcoma. Five of 47 canine liposarcoma cases were p53-positive: 4/7 myxoid and 1/13 well-differentiated liposarcomas. The de-differentiated cases and the pleomorphic liposarcomas were consistently negative. P53 expression correlated with higher Ki67 labeling index and higher mitotic count. The p53 expression by canine myxoid liposarcoma differs from human myxoid liposarcoma which may mean that although these are morphologically similar the genetic alterations of the tumors are different in canine liposarcoma also.

1.4.3 Human and Canine Malignant Peripheral Nerve Sheath Tumor

MPNSTs are classified based on whether they are peripheral (located away from the spine or brain), root (directly adjacent to the brain or spine) or plexus (adjacent to the brachial or lumbosacral plexus). There are no strong breed predilections that have been identified, although German shepherds and females were more common in one study [83].

Pathology

This subtype in dogs is included in the large all-inclusive cutaneous and subcutaneous STS group. This tumor has historically also been referred to as neurofibrosarcoma, and malignant Schwannoma, but these are currently regarded as having a nerve sheath origin so are classified as MPNST [40, 84, 85]. Canine hemangiopericytoma (another subtype in the STS group) is a differential diagnosis for MPNST; however, there is significant overlap in histomorphological and IHC features between them [39, 40, 86, 87]. Differing IHC results for the expression of S100, CD34, and SMA have been reported for canine hemangiopericytoma, this supports the theory that the hemangiopericytoma category in dogs likely encompasses neoplasms of varying histology [39, 84, 85, 87]. These findings and the assessment of ultrastructure led to classification of hemangiopericytoma to canine perivascular wall tumors arising from endothelial mural cells of blood vessels, this parallels the subtypes recognized in humans, which includes myopericytoma, angioleiomyoma/sarcoma, hemangiopericytoma, and angiofibroma [88, 89].

Molecular Characteristics

Very limited genomic assessment of canine MPNST has been performed. *TP53* mutations and *MDM2* amplification were identified in 3 of 7 primary MPNST (and one metastatic lesion showed the same TP53 mutation as the primary), and 2 of 7 primary MPNST [90]. *BRAFV450E* mutation was found in 2/9 PNST [91]. In humans, many of the malignant PNST (87.5%) arise in the setting of neurofibromatosis type 1 (NF1) syndrome. Whole-exome sequencing of 12 malignant PNST revealed recurrent mutations in *NF1* in patients (8/10 with neurofibromatosis 1, and 1 of 2 with spontaneous tumors) [92]. Other recurrent mutations identified included *CDKN2A* (58%), *TP53* (50%), *SUZ12* (42%), and *EED* (33%). In addition, this study identified other RAS pathway activating somatic mutations outside of recurrently mutated genes, overall suggesting a complex genomic landscape.

1.4.4 Human Angiosarcoma and Canine Hemangiosarcoma

Canine hemangiosarcoma is similar to angiosarcoma in humans. There is some similarity to sites of occurrence in both species as these tumors can be seen in cutaneous, subcutaneous, and visceral sites. In humans, the most common site of angiosarcoma is cutaneous, arising in the head and neck [93, 94]. Cutaneous hemangiosarcoma arises particularly in dogs with shorter coats and lightly pigmented skin (most commonly affecting the ventral abdominal skin) leading to the suggestion of development due to exposure to UV radiation [95]. In contrast to humans, in dogs visceral hemangiosarcoma is seen more commonly [96]. Certain dog breeds are affected at higher rates, including boxer and German shepherd dogs, but also Labrador and golden retrievers. Hemangiosarcoma is highly metastatic; dogs may present with vague signs secondary to hemorrhage [1]. Initially hemangiosarcoma was thought to arise from transformed vascular endothelial cells given the histopathologic tumor appearance. More recent genomic evaluation in dogs and humans suggests the cell of origin is a hematopoietic endothelial progenitor cell [97].

Pathology

On histopathology, the neoplastic cells for canine hemangiosarcoma are pleomorphic, polygonal to spindle-shaped cells similar to other canine sarcomas, but these cells form and line irregular, anastomosing spaces [98, 99]. Histological grading of hemangiosarcoma in dogs is based on differentiation, cellular pleomorphism, and necrosis [100]. The prognostic significance of hemangiosarcoma grading has not been extensively evaluated, and in humans the prognostic utility of angiosarcoma grading is debatable [101]. Immunohistochemistry for vascular endothelial markers (CD31, factor VIII-related antigen, and CD34) is often used to differentiate hemangiosarcoma from other canine sarcomas; these markers are also found in human angiosarcoma [102–104]. Tumors of lymphatic origin can be distinguished from canine hemangiosarcoma of vascular origin through the expression of lymphatic markers: lymphatic vessel endothelial receptor-1 (LYVE-1) and prospero-related homeobox gene 1 (PROX-1) [105]. Canine hemangiosarcoma can be differentiated from tumors of lymphatic origin through the lack of expression of lymphatic markers, and other studies have shown expression of other signal transduction proteins including CD117 (c-KIT), VEGFR1, VEGFR2, VEGFR3, and FGFR1 [103, 106].

Molecular Characteristics

The assessment of the molecular characteristics of canine hemangiosarcoma has been through studies of gene expression, comparative genomic hybridization studies to assess copy number aberrations, and GWAS.

Genome-wide association studies have been feasible in golden retrievers, as this breed has been shown to have an increased (20%) lifetime risk of developing hemangiosarcoma [107]. In a cohort of 356 golden retrievers, two loci were identified on chromosome 5 that contributed to around 20% of the risk of developing hemangiosarcoma and B-cell lymphoma [108]. Germline mutations in these two tumor types were found to be associated with the T-cell-mediated immune response. GWAS has not been performed in human angiosarcoma given the rarity of the tumor.

Transcriptional profiling studies have been performed in both canine hemangiosarcoma and human angiosarcoma. In a study by Tamburini et al. in golden retrievers, hemangiosarcoma cells had a robust gene expression signature that distinguished hemangiosarcoma cells from nonmalignant proliferating endothelial cells (from splenic hematoma lesions) and bone marrow-derived tumor cells (lymphoma, leukemia, and osteosarcoma). This gene expression signature included genes involved in inflammation, angiogenesis, adhesion, invasion, metabolism, cell cycle, signaling, and patterning [10]. Genes that were expressed at higher levels in hemangiosarcoma versus non-hemangiosarcoma tumors (lymphoma, leukemia and osteosarcoma) and hemangiosarcoma versus splenic hematomas included *VEGFA*, *TIMP-1*, *FN-1*, *ADAM9*, *PDGFC*, *MMP14*, *TNF*, and acid ceramidase. The origin of hemangiosarcoma from vascular endothelial cells has been questioned through the findings of the Tamburini et al. study and others [10, 109, 110]. A gene expression profiling study of primary tumor samples identified three molecular genotypes of hemangiosarcoma characterized by enrichment of genes associated with blood vessel development, angio- and vasculogenesis, endothelial cell development and migration (group 1, angiogenesis; immune cell differentiation, homeostasis, development, and migration (group 2, inflammation); and lipid and cholesterol transport and metabolism of fatty acids, cholesterol and steroid (group 3, adipogenesis, or lipogenesis). This study supported the idea that hemangiosarcoma cells may arise from cells with multipotency, but it is still possible that these tumors could arise from a mix of progenitor cells that can each differentiate lineage specific differentiation and contribute to tumor progression [97].

There is some overlap between the genes expressed in canine hemangiosarcoma and human angiosarcoma. A gene expression study differentiated angiosarcoma from other sarcomas based on overexpression of genes associated with the different stages of angiogenesis (*TIE1*, *KDR*, *SNRK*, *TEK*, endothelial (*TIE2*), and *FLT1*) and genes known as endothelial markers or associated with endothelial function (*PECAM1*, *EPHA2*, *ANGPT2*, *ENDRB*, *PGF*, *FLI1*, and *VWF*). Growth factor genes, such as KIT ligand and VEGFB, were downregulated in hemangiosarcoma versus other sarcomas [111]. The downregulation of VEGF in this study contrasted with the enriched expression found in golden retriever hemangiosarcoma cells in the Tamburini et al. study.

Comparative genomic hybridization array analysis on 75 primary intra-abdominal hemangiosarcoma tumors from 5 breeds (including golden retrievers) identified the most frequent recurrent copy number aberrations as copy number gains of dog chromosomes 13, 24, and 31, and loss of chromosome 16 [112]. This study identified copy number aberrations involving

CDKN2A, *VEGFA*, and the *SKI* oncogene as potential driver aberrations for the development of hemangiosarcoma [113].

Candidate driver mutations were identified from whole-exome sequencing of hemangiosarcoma and normal tissue samples from 20 dogs [114]. There were somatic mutations in *PIK3CA* (9 cases), *TP53* (7 cases), *PTEN* (2 cases), and phospholipase C gamma (*PLCG1*) (1 case), which are known tumor drivers in human cancer. In 8/9 *PIK3CA*-mutant cases, there was a missense mutation affecting amino acid 1047, which is the same position commonly mutated in human cancers [115, 116]. Activating mutations of *PLCG1* and *PIK3CA* have been reported in human angiosarcomas (3/34 cases and 1/39 cases, respectively) [117]. The most common gene mutation in the study (seen in 10/39 human angiosarcoma cases) was inactivating mutations of *PTPRB*, which is a tyrosine phosphatase specific to vascular endothelium [117]. Targeted panel sequencing of cancer-associated genes in tumor-germline (matched normal tissue) pairs of 15 canine visceral hemangiosarcoma cases revealed the most commonly mutated gene was *TP53* (14/15 cases), with most (13/14) of these mutations occurring in the DNA-binding domain which is also the most commonly mutated domain in TP53 in human cancers [118, 119]. PIK3CA was mutated in 9/15 cases with the majority (6/9) at H1047R in the kinase domain. The next most commonly mutated genes were the tumor suppressor genes *ATRX* and LRP1B (4/15 cases) followed by *GRIN2A* and *NFATC2* (3/15 cases).

MiRNA-sequencing has been performed on samples from splenic and cutaneous hemangiosarcoma, splenic nodular hyperplasia and normal spleen [120]. Twenty-two miRNAs were differentially expressed in the hemangiosarcoma samples (four between hemangiosarcoma and both nodular hyperplasia and normal spleen and 18 between hemangiosarcoma and normal spleen only). For the four miRNAs specific to hemangiosarcoma, two were significantly overexpressed (mir-126 and mir-452) and two were significantly underexpressed (mir-150, mir-203) compared to nodular hyperplasia and normal spleen samples. Mir-126, mir-150, and mir-203 have a role in angiogenesis, and mir-452 although not associated with angiogenesis has been shown to target cyclin-dependent kinase inhibitor 1B, which inhibits the cell cycle checkpoint from G1 to S.

Elevated expression of KIT has been confirmed in canine splenic hemangiosarcomas compared to splenic hematomas, and in patient-derived cell hemangiosarcoma lines [121]. Kit expression has also been found in human angiosarcomas compared to epithelioid hemangioendotheliomas and hemangiomas [122].

Most detailed genetic analyses of canine hemangiosarcoma have focused on visceral sites. Wong et al. performed a targeted panel sequencing on 13 canine cutaneous samples [118]. The most commonly mutated gene was identified as TP53 (9/13 cases), but after exclusion of samples with a UV signature, the only other recurrently mutated gene was the protein kinase PRKDC (2/13 cases). In three canine cutaneous HSAs, there was an elevated mutation rate and the COSMIC mutational signatures SBS7a and SBS7b were found, which is a UV mutational signature found mostly in skin cancers with proposed etiology due to UV exposure [123]. These tumors were from the hindlimb and ventral abdomen of the dogs which are sites exposed to sun, supporting a potential role for UV light exposure in the development of some canine cutaneous hemangiosarcoma like human face and scalp angiosarcoma [124, 125].

1.4.5 Human and Canine Synovial Sarcoma

While this is a common extremity tumor in humans, in dogs synovial cell sarcoma is rare. In humans, less than 10% of synovial sarcomas are intra-articular, and more than 80% originate from the deep soft tissues around the joints or tendons [126], or other sites include the kidney, lungs, mediastinum, and the neck [127]. The cell of origin once thought to be the synoviocyte is now thought to be a pluripotent mesenchymal stem cell; hence, why the terminology of synovial sarcoma is preferred over synovial cell sarcoma in humans [128]. This tumor was originally thought to be the most common joint tumor in dogs; however, later with the use of immunohistochemistry, it was determined that histiocytic sarcoma accounted for the majority of canine joint sarcomas [129].

Pathology

In humans, diagnosis is made through identification of the (t(X;18)(p11;q11)) translocation which is specific for synovial sarcoma [130, 131]. This translocation fuses the *SYT* gene from chromosome 18 to either one of two highly homologous genes at *Xp11*, *SSX1*, or *SSX2* and is detectable through RT-PCR, FISH, or traditional karyotyping [132]. The TLE-1 IHC marker has been shown to be sensitive and specific, and strongly correlated with the translocation in human synovial sarcoma [133].

In dogs, synovial cell sarcoma typically demonstrates immunohistochemical vimentin and pan-cytokeratin co-expression in a low proportion of the cells. This co-expression might not be represented or seen so CD18 (pan-leukocyte marker) is often used to help with the differentiation between synovial cell sarcoma and histiocytic sarcoma. A histologic grading scheme was proposed by Vail et al., but this grading scheme failed to predict survival in a subsequent study [42, 134]. The reason for this could be misdiagnosis, as unfortunately in this study CD18 or IBA1 were not used and only 6/20 cases were positive for both vimentin and cytokeratin. Further molecular characterization of synovial cell sarcomas has not been performed in dogs.

1.4.6 Human and Canine Fibrosarcoma

Fibrosarcoma arises from transformed fibroblasts, occurring primarily in the skin, subcutaneous tissues, and the oral cavity. Although this tumor subtype is recognized, this is one of the subtypes included in the umbrella term of STS and grading scheme in dogs. The clinical importance of distinguishing between fibrosarcoma and other subtypes is unknown in the dog, although it has been noted to potentially be more prevalent in Doberman Pinscher, Rottweilers, and setters [135]. This tumor behaves in a locally invasive manner with metastasis identified at diagnosis in 20% of dogs [136].

Pathology

The diagnosis of fibrosarcoma in dogs is made based on identification of characteristic morphologic features on histopathology. A key characteristic of fibrosarcoma is spindle-shaped cells forming interwoven bundles distributed in a herringbone pattern with underlying collagen stroma. Clearly, the characteristic morphologic features may not be present in undifferentiated tumors, making the diagnosis challenging and necessitating the use of molecular methods. There are no highly specific immunohistochemistry markers to distinguish fibrosarcoma from histomorphologically similar subtypes using histomorphology alone, including MPNST and perivascular wall tumors. S100 expression is found in both MPNST and fibrosarcoma [137–139]. Additionally, PGP9.5, a marker for human MPNST, is expressed in both MPNST and fibrosarcoma [140]. α-SMA is reported in both perivascular wall tumors and fibrosarcoma [85, 87, 139]. Gene expression analysis using RT-PCR revealed that the combination of GLI1 and GLEC3B gene expression had a high sensitivity and specificity for differentiating fibrosarcoma from MPNST [140]. There has been only limited molecular analyses of canine fibrosarcoma to date. In contrast in humans, specific subtypes of fibrosarcoma can be identified based on the presence of specific molecular aberrations, for example: translocations between chromosomes 7 and 16 are seen in low-grade fibromyxoid sarcoma and sclerosing epithelioid fibrosarcoma [141]. One group performed cytogenetic analyses on two poorly differentiated fibrosarcomas (in Labrador retrievers) and identified alterations in chromosomes 11 and 30 [142]. This group also published results from bacterial artificial chromosome mapping in these cases and found more complex chromosome rearrangements on chromosome 11 than they had appreciated with chromosome paint alone in the prior study [143]. These alterations reflected the loss of sequences corresponding to *CDKN2A/2B* genes. Another study utilized differential gene expression to distinguish between canine fibrosarcoma and MPNST [139]. No *TP53* mutations were identified in four dogs with fibrosarcoma [90].

1.5 Treatment and Prognosis

1.5.1 Human Soft Tissue Sarcoma

Human STSs are typically treated in tertiary referral centers with improved outcomes demonstrated with centralized care. A multidisciplinary approach is often necessary for these cancers, with patients frequently receiving both radiation therapy and surgery, the latter of which often includes complex resections and at times soft tissue reconstructions necessitating the involvement of a plastic surgeon. While not universally employed in localized disease, systemic therapy has a more established role in patients with metastatic disease [144].

The overall treatment approach to STSs is dependent upon histology, grade, size, patient age, and anatomic location. With respect to assessing oncologic outcomes, there are three primary outcomes of significance including local recurrence, distant metastatic disease, and overall survival. The impact of distant metastatic disease on overall survival is well-documented; however, in the extremity, the impact of local recurrence on survival has not been established [145–150]. This uncertainty drives significant debate in balancing local control benefit and morbidity when considering the extent of surgery and use of adjuvant therapy. In contrast, local recurrence in retroperitoneal STS is associated with increased mortality [151].

Given the differences in survival and treatment approaches between retroperitoneal and extremity STS, these will be considered separately. In the extremity, STSs can be treated with limb-salvage surgery in the majority of cases. There are no strict contraindications to limb-salvage; however, the surgical morbidity and expected functional outcome must be balanced when considering the complex reconstructions. Leveraging the capabilities of plastic and vascular surgery teams, composite soft tissue defects may be reconstructed, including skin, muscle, bone, nerves, and arteries and veins. In certain cases, the expected functional outcomes and morbidity of an amputation will be superior to limb-salvage. This decision should be made after thoughtful consideration by the patient. Generally, low-grade STSs can be treated with surgery alone, with local recurrence rates of <5% and excellent overall survival (>90%), although radiation therapy may be utilized in scenarios in which a close or potentially positive margin is anticipated [152, 153]. The role of radiation therapy in the treatment of large, high-grade STSs is well established; however, in high-grade tumors measuring less than 5 cm in which negative surgical margins can be anticipated, a negative margin resection alone without radiation therapy has been shown to be associated with acceptable local recurrence rates and overall survival. There is, however, evidence that in superficial STSs, radiation therapy may decrease the risk of local recurrence in high-grade tumors with <5 mm margins, regardless of size. As mentioned previously, the morbidity of radiation therapy must be balanced with its potential benefit as this benefit did not lead to an improvement in overall survival [154–158].

In high-grade extremity (grade 2 and 3) STS, higher rates of local recurrence are observed, and thus, the potential benefit of radiotherapy is more apparent and has allowed for function-preserving surgery [153, 159, 160]. Tumor cells have been identified up to 4 cm beyond the tumor within the peritumoral edema; thus, a marginal resection through the reactive zone may leave behind residual disease and increase the risk for local recurrence [161]. Radiation therapy planning strategies have been developed to account for these satellite lesions and generally include an expansion of the gross tumor volume by 3 cm in the longitudinal direction and 1.5 cm radially [162].

There are several strategies for the delivery of radiation therapy for STSs with variations in the timing, fractionation, delivery method, and type of particle. Radiation therapy may be delivered via external beam radiation therapy (EBRT) with photons which includes image-guided intensity-modulated radiotherapy (IMRT), brachytherapy, or intraoperatively. External beam radiation therapy has evolved since its inception and currently involves the use of three-dimensional planning and conformal radiotherapy which allows radiation to be delivered through multiple trajectories. This technique allows dosing to the tumor to be maximized while minimizing the dose to the surrounding healthy tissue, including critical structures. An expansion upon this is the use of intensity-modulated radiation therapy which allows for additional modification to the intensity of the radiation beam allowing for more reliable sparing of normal tissues and appropriate radiation dosing for three-dimensionally complex tumors. This has been associated with lower local recurrence rates compared to conventional EBRT, 7.6% and 15.1%, respectively [163]. IMRT has also been associated with lower rates of radiation-associated fractures [164, 165]. The dosing of external beam radiation therapy varies depending on the timing of its use. Preoperative radiation therapy is typically 50 Gy delivered in 25 fractions over 5 weeks while postoperative adjuvant radiation therapy is generally between 60 and 66 Gy and delivered over 6–7 weeks. In the setting of unresectable or gross residual disease after a tumor debulking patients are treated with higher doses of radiation therapy which is associated with acceptable rates of local control [166]. It was hoped that a postoperative radiation therapy boost (16 Gy) after preoperative radiation therapy to a total dose of 66 Gy would be associated with improved local recurrence rates in the setting of a positive margin; unfortunately, this did not improve local control at the cost of additional morbidity [167].

The timing of radiation therapy and surgery is of critical importance. A multi-institutional randomized controlled study by O'Sullivan demonstrated similar rates of local control regardless of sequence, but with higher rates of wound healing complications for preoperative radiation therapy (35% versus 17%). In particular, the upper leg anatomic location is associated with a 45% wound complication rate with preoperative radiation therapy compared to 28% with postoperative radiation [168]. However, preoperative radiation therapy is associated with smaller treatment volumes and a lower total dose and lower late complications including fibrosis, edema, and fractures. A final consideration in external beam radiation therapy is timing of surgery after preoperative radiation therapy. In general, a 4-to-6-week delay between completion of radiation therapy and surgery has been employed in order to allow for resolution of the acute toxicities associated with radiation therapy, in particular dermatitis.

Alternative strategies in the timing and dosing of external beam radiation therapy have been employed. Specifically, hypofractionated regimens have been developed for the treatment of STS in an effort to deliver radiobiologicalalally equivalent doses over shorter treatment durations. Uniformity does not exist with respect to total dose, fractionation, and timing of surgery between institutional protocols; however, in general, this treatment approach has been associated with acceptable wound complication profiles and local control [169–174].

An alternative to external beam radiation therapy is brachytherapy. This involves the delivery of radiation to a postoperative wound bed. In STS, this is achieved with the placement of catheters which are secured in the wound bed at the time of surgery. The catheters are then loaded with [192] iridium over 4 to 6 days for a dose of 42 to 45 Gy. The catheters are then removed and the wound, if not previously closed primarily, is closed in a delayed fashion. It is particularly useful for the treatment of in-field local recurrences [175, 176]. Brachytherapy is not universally available creating theoretical issues with accessibility.

Accessibility to proton beam therapy is improving, although there remain significant challenges to the widespread adoption of this advanced radiotherapy technique [177]. Proton therapy provides a few advantages over standard photon therapy, in particular with its ability to spare surrounding normal tissue. There is evidence supporting its use in axial bone sarcomas; however, there is limited experience with proton beam therapy and extremity STS although early results demonstrate an acceptable safety profile [178].

From a surgical perspective, the goal of surgery is to achieve a wide resection of the sarcoma with a cuff of normal tissue between the sarcoma and the resection plane. The definition of what width constitutes an adequate margin is frequently debated without consensus. In addition, the context and qualitative aspects of the margin are critical. Gundle et al. reviewed the experience at Princess Margaret Cancer Centre; they found that an R + 1 mm classification provided no additional benefit with respect to local recurrence risk stratification compared to the R classification. They found that the 5-year local recurrence risk with an R0 margin was 6%, 17% with R1, and 38% with R2. More importantly however, they found that the context of the margin was critical, specifically the risk of local recurrence was not significantly increased for a planned close, but ultimately positive margin when compared to a negative margin resection (10% and 6% 5-year local recurrence rate respectively). In contrast, an inadvertent positive margin was associated with a local recurrence risk for 28% [179]. This finding is supported by prior evidence [180]; however, it is not universally accepted and others advocate for wider margins [149, 181].

In contrast to extremity and chest wall STSs, abdominal and retroperitoneal STSs are associated with higher rates of local recurrence [182–184] which is felt to be due in part to anatomic constraints which limit the ability of surgeons to achieve wide margins. Given the proximity of critical organs to these often large tumors, resection of these normal structures is often necessary contributing to significant surgical morbidity [185]. Furthermore, local recurrence can be associated with morbidity and mortality even in the absence of metastatic disease. Radiation therapy has been used to improve local control rates in retroperitoneal STS, with improved local control with perioperative radiotherapy. Unfortunately, the results of a large, randomized phase 3 study (STRASS) in North America and Europe failed to demonstrate a benefit to preoperative radiotherapy while contributing to increased complication rates [186–188]. Additional studies are ongoing, investigating alternative radiation strategies and histology-specific approaches [189, 190].

The role of systemic therapy in STS is not clearly defined, and there remains significant institutional variation in practice. In the metastatic setting, palliative systemic therapy should balance toxicity and patient-specific goals [191, 192]. Frequently targeted therapies with more tolerable side-effect profiles are utilized albeit with limited success [193–196].

In the localized disease setting, there is evidence to suggest a benefit with doxorubicin and ifosfamide-based adjuvant chemotherapy [197–200]. This marginal benefit must be balanced with the toxicity of cytotoxic chemotherapy. Careful patient selection is required and should be determined by a multi-disciplinary team. Patient and sarcoma factors that influence the decision to administer systemic chemotherapy include age (young versus old), size of the tumor (> 10 cm), grade (high-grade), and histology. Certain STSs have demonstrated response rates to histology-specific chemotherapy regimens. This prompted a multicenter, randomized-controlled, phase 3 trial comparing the oncologic outcomes of high-risk STSs treated with histology-tailored versus standard (epirubicin plus ifosfamide) neoadjuvant chemotherapy regimens. Interestingly, this study demonstrated no benefit of a histology-specific regimen over the standard regimen [201].

In conclusion, human STS is a heterogeneous disease which presents in a wide range of anatomic locations and at various times of life. This along with the variability in histology and clinical behavior makes STS a challenging diagnosis to treat.

1.5.2 Canine Soft Tissue Sarcoma

STSs are a common tumor type in dogs and as a result dogs receive care at primary care clinics, private referral clinics, and academic teaching hospitals. Access to referral care including specialist surgeons and radiation therapy facilities has increased over the last few decades. The challenge to treatment of STSs is generally local tumor control. Surgery is often the treatment of choice, but the definitive treatment options possible differ by location of the tumor, clinical stage, grade, and completeness of surgical resection. In the event a STS is incompletely excised, there are multiple options depending on the client's goals: active surveillance (monitoring for local tumor recurrence), wide excision of the surgical scar, radiation therapy, metronomic chemotherapy, and electrochemotherapy.

Surgery is the most accessible treatment and the treatment of choice for most canine STSs. Sarcomas can be marginally, widely, or radically excised, with the ideal approach needing to be personalized to the individual patient and tumor and will depend on the tumor size, its location, the grade, extent of local invasion, the histologic grade, and the client's goals for outcome. Wide excision of STSs is considered the treatment of choice. This involves planning to remove a 3 cm cuff of normal tissue (lateral surgical margin) around the tumor, and one fascial plane beneath (deep surgical margin), to remove both the gross and microscopic tumor extension [202]. This is a fairly arbitrary recommendation regardless of patient size, tumor size, tumor location, or any knowledge of the tumor biology. Radical excision utilizing surgeries such as amputation or hemipelvectomy may be required when tumors are fixed and invading into deeper structures. When tumors arise on the distal extremities, a more marginal resection approach is sometimes taken when tumors are small and discrete, given there is low skin elasticity and limited tissue availability for reconstruction. STS tumors appear to have a pseudo capsule, which is a layer of compressed tissue that can contain tumor cells, giving the illusion of an encapsulated tumor during surgical excision [2]. Dissection around the tumor pseudocapsule in marginal excision leaves behind microscopic disease, but this might be planned to be treated later with radiation or other therapies. Active surveillance might be utilized in dogs with grade I or grade II tumors (with lower recurrence rates) [37] and if the tumors are located in areas where reoperation would be possible if recurrence occurred.

Fractionated radiation therapy protocols are routinely used for dogs with residual microscopic disease after surgery. In humans, radiation therapy has a well-documented role in improving local control of STSs. Radiation is known to result in long-term local control, but the benefit of radiation above surgery alone in canines with STS is more uncertain than in humans, as all the studies are retrospective and lack a control group receiving surgery alone. Radiation therapy is often used in the adjuvant setting in dogs, either after a planned marginal tumor excision leaving behind microscopic disease or occasionally following unplanned incomplete tumor excision. Distal extremity STS cases may be prescribed adjuvant radiation after surgery to save the limb versus limb amputation. Normally, radiation therapy is started following initial healing from surgery. A full course definitive protocol is recommended normally. This involves the dogs receiving 3 to 4 Gy fractions from Monday to Friday for a total dose of 42–63 Gy [35, 36, 203, 204]. Radiation therapy is generally well tolerated in dogs but involves general anesthesia for each radiation treatment to ensure patient immobilization. Side effects of radiation like moist desquamation are often only mild and resolve quickly. Local recurrence is reported in 16.7–36.8% of cases and the local control rates at 1, 2, 3, and 4 years are 71–84%, 60–81%, 57–81%, and up to 81%, respectively [35, 36, 203, 204].

Adjuvant chemotherapy is often recommended by medical oncologists for dogs that have been diagnosed with high-grade skin and subcutaneous STS or dogs with metastatic disease. The benefit of chemotherapy in this patient population is unclear. A retrospective study looking at 39 dogs with grade III STSs treated with surgery alone (n = 18) or surgery and doxorubicin chemotherapy (n = 21) did not identify a survival benefit with the use of doxorubicin [6]. An alternating protocol with ifosfamide and doxorubicin was reported in 12 dogs that had STSs surgically removed, but this study did not assess survival outcomes [205].

Metronomic chemotherapy has been assessed in dogs to see if this could help with local tumor control through inhibition of tumor angiogenesis and suppression of regulatory T cells. In a clinical study of 30 dogs, oral piroxicam and low-dose cyclophosphamide were administered following incomplete excision of STSs. These dogs had a significantly longer disease-free interval compared to a historical control group of 55 dogs that had incompletely excised STSs but no metronomic chemotherapy [206]. These results should be interpreted cautiously as historical control groups often can lead to bias and inflated type I error. Additional studies are needed to assess the benefits and risks of this treatment.

Tyrosine kinase inhibitors have not been utilized in any large clinical studies for skin and subcutaneous STS, but there may be a role given that increased vascular endothelial growth factor (VEGF) and VEGF receptor expression has been shown to occur in canine STSs [207–210].

Some studies have been performed assessing local release chemotherapy following marginal excision of STS. Studies have reported on tolerability and outcome of implantation of cisplatin-impregnated biodegradable polymer or calcium sulfate and dextran sulfate beads into the surgical wound bed, and injections of 5-fluorouracil into the surgical wound bed weekly for five to six injections [211–213]. The most common complications after treatment were wound complications (47–84% dogs) [211, 212, 214, 215]. The use of electrochemotherapy for local control of incompletely excised high-grade tumors has been reported in 22 dogs [216]. In this study, the local tumor bed was treated with bleomycin and then biphasic electric pulses, following this treatment only 36% of dogs had local recurrence with a mean time to local recurrence of 730 days. Wound healing complications occurred in 14% of dogs.

Local tumor control is crucial for STS treatment. Many factors have been reported to affect the risk of local recurrence in skin and subcutaneous STS, including tumor location, tumor size and characteristics like local invasion, histopathologic grade, completeness of excision, and treatment methods used. Overall, the prognosis for dogs with skin or subcutaneous STS is very good with dogs often dying of other causes. In general, local recurrence rates are 0–5% after wide excision [217, 218], 11–29% after marginal excision [37, 88, 217, 219–221], and 17–37% after incomplete excision and fractionated radiation therapy [35, 36, 203, 204]. For dogs receiving surgery alone, the median disease-free interval is 368 days to 637 days to not reached and the disease-free rates at 1, 2, 3, and 4 years are 71–84%, 60–81%, 57–81%, and up to 81% [4, 30, 218–220]. For dogs that had tumors incompletely excised then had fractionated radiation therapy, the median disease-free interval is 412 days to more than 798 days and the disease-free rates at 1, 2, and 3 years are 81%, 73%, and 73% [35, 36, 203].

Mixed relationships have been reported between completeness of surgical excision of STS and prognosis. The conflicting findings for recurrence rates and risk of recurrence between publications could be complicated by several factors. Excised tumors are formalin fixed and submitted to pathology for tumor diagnosis and surgical margin assessment. Often radial trimming methods are used for surgical margin assessment which results in only a small sample (<1%) of the surgical margins being assessed [222]. Many of the studies are retrospective and the long term follow up can be weak. Wide excision has been associated with an increased likelihood of complete margins [30] and a lower risk of local recurrence [4]. In one study, no tumors recurred which were completely excised, and only 7% of grade 1 and 34% of grade 2 tumors recurred when incompletely excised [218]. Other studies have reported similar low recurrence rates (18–21%) despite the majority of tumors being incompletely excised [88, 220]. Low rates of recurrence (7–30%) have been reported using marginal excision of STSs of the distal extremities below the elbow and stifle [221].

High tumor grade has been associated with a higher risk of local recurrence and metastasis [219]. In one study with 236 dogs with subcutaneous STS treated by excisional biopsy, complete histologic margins resulted in no local recurrence; however, incomplete margins had an overall 19% local recurrence rate. The local recurrence rate was highest for high-grade tumors (grade I: 7%, grade II: 34%, and grade III: 75%). In addition, the metastatic rates are higher for high-grade tumors (grade I: 0–13%, II: 7–27%, and

III: 22–44%) [4–6]. Other factors have been found that increase the risk of metastatic disease; these include more pleomorphic and undifferentiated compared to well differentiated tumors, high mitotic count, percent tumor necrosis, and local tumor recurrence [4, 219].

Reported median survival times for dogs with skin and subcutaneous STS are prolonged (1013–1796 days with surgery only and up to 2270 days with surgery and adjuvant radiation therapy) [4, 36, 203, 217, 219]. Many studies cannot calculate the median survival as only low proportions (9–33%) of dogs die from disease [4, 5, 30, 36, 37, 217–219, 221, 223]. Some of the retrospective studies identified different clinical features that were associated with decreased survival time in the study populations. Two studies identified lower survival times in dogs with invasive and fixed STSs, which were postulated to be due to difficulty with complete excision leading to challenges with local control [217, 219]. Wide surgical excision was associated with a longer median survival time than non-curative intent surgeries (1306 days vs. 164 days) [5]. In addition, dogs with incompletely excised tumors had shorter median survival than dogs with completely excised tumors (657 days vs. 1306 days) [5]. Local recurrence has been found to be associated with increased risk of death due to disease [219]. In addition, some associations have been identified between survival times and histologic and immunohistochemistry features including tumor necrosis, mitotic count, histologic grade, argyrophilic nucleolar organizer region (AgNOR) score, and Ki67 score [4, 5, 219].

Leiomyosarcoma

Differing biological behavior has been reported based on anatomic site [43, 53, 58, 65]. Esophageal leiomyosarcomas are mainly low grade and have more benign behavior as are most smooth muscle tumors of the skin (angioleiomyosarcoma and piloleiomyosarcoma) [58, 65]. In contrast, splenic and hepatic leiomyosarcoma are mostly malignant [43, 53].

Liposarcoma

Baez et al. described outcomes following surgical treatment in 56 dogs diagnosed with liposarcoma: 3 dogs with well-differentiated liposarcoma, 7 with myxoid liposarcoma and 34 with pleomorphic liposarcoma. Local recurrence occurred in 12/56 dogs (28%), but only 3 dogs had suspected metastasis (not confirmed on histopathology) on abdominal ultrasound [71]. The median survival time for all dogs was 694 days (1–1782 days). There were no differences in survival based on histopathologic subtype.

Hemangiosarcoma

The prognosis for canine hemangiosarcoma depends on anatomic site, clinical stage and treatment. The treatment typically needs to involve surgical removal and cytotoxic chemotherapy [224]. Surgical resection alone yields very short survival times (19–86 days) for splenic hemangiosarcoma [224]. The benefit of cytotoxic chemotherapy has been questioned, doxorubicin protocols have been favored, but the majority of dogs experience short survival (141–179 days) and die of metastatic disease [224]. Cutaneous hemangiosarcoma has a better prognosis with surgery alone leading to survival times over 2 years, and dogs dying through other causes [47]. Recurrent local disease is common (up to 77%) with suspected UV-related lesions [225].

Given the poor overall patient outcomes, immunotherapy approaches for the treatment of canine hemangiosarcoma are currently being investigated. Earlier studies showed feasibility of immunotherapy approaches with chemotherapy and also humoral responses to vaccination in dogs with hemangiosarcoma [226–228]. A phase 2, single arm, open-label trial testing a peptide-based anticancer vaccine in addition to standard of care surgery and cytotoxic chemotherapy in 28 dogs reported improvements in time to progressive disease and overall survival compared to historic controls (TTP: 195 vs. 160 days and OS: 276 vs. 175 days) [214]. The peptide-based vaccine was generated from the tumor cell secretome from infection of hemangiosarcoma cells with Salmonella typhi Ty21a to release immunogenic endoplasmic reticulum stress-related peptides.

Fibrosarcoma

Some studies have suggested that fibrosarcoma compared to other histopathologic subtypes might have a worse prognosis [3, 4, 30, 203, 219, 223]. These studies providing prognostic information should be interpreted with care. Many of these studies were performed many years ago using morphology for diagnosis. These studies need to be reevaluated with more robust molecular methods to confirm diagnosis and larger case numbers.

2 Unique Opportunities in Canine Studies

Given STSs are rare in humans, it is challenging to perform clinical trials in some subtypes. Soft tissue sarcoma arises spontaneously more commonly in dogs. Currently there is under-utilization of canine spontaneous sarcomas for clinical trials for diagnostics and therapeutics like immunotherapy despite the advantages of the canine model. Canines are larger in size than rodents, relatively outbred, live in the same environment, and have many physiologic similarities to humans. Canines have an intact immune system, and the STSs that occur display tumor heterogeneity. Due to early domestication and the recent creation of breeds of dogs, GWAS studies in dogs can be performed with 10x fewer SNPs than humans due to the fact purebred dogs have kilobase-sized haplotypes and megabase-sized linkage disequilibrium blocks (within breeds) [229, 230]. Some human sarcomas like angiosarcoma have been too rare for GWAS to be performed to date. The spontaneous development of tumors in canines means these tumors occur naturally and develop therapy resistance and metastasis. Serial sampling of tumors can be performed in dogs that is often challenging to justify in human clinical trials. Furthermore, since STS is often a surface tumor, it is easily accessible for repeated biopsy. This opens the possibility to evaluate intratumoral drug concentrations and assess therapy-induced changes in antitumor immune responses. In addition, there is a lack of an evidence-based standard of care for many canine sarcomas which facilitates evaluation of novel therapies in treatment-naïve patients early in the drug development timeline and permits investigation of novel combinations with other treatment modalities. The costs of care are lower in canines than humans making clinical trials in dogs less expensive to execute and providing the potential to help the participating canine and inform parallel or future human clinical trials.

Immunotherapy The canine model could be very valuable for cancer immunotherapy development specifically given the tumors develop spontaneously, manifest heterogeneity, and dogs have an intact immune system. Dogs could help with both the understanding of immunobiology and treatment development. Soft tissue sarcoma has been considered immunologically barren or cold due to lack of tumor infiltrating T cells on histopathology. However, more work is needed in the form of next-generation sequencing, more extensive IHC assessment to characterize the mutational burden and the immune landscape of molecular subtypes of STS in the dog.

Oncolytic virotherapy involves the therapeutic virus selectively entering, replicating, and then lysing tumor cells. Rodent models have not been reliable predictors of the efficacy of oncolytic virus therapy in humans, so there have been several studies evaluating this therapy in cancer-bearing dogs [231, 232]. Many studies have shown oncolytic virus treatment (adenoviruses, herpesviruses, poxviruses, avipoxviruses, vesicular stomatitis virus, and myxoma virus) is safe in dogs [232–242], and so the canine model could represent a more accurate model to predict response to therapy in humans [243]. A recent review summarized the promise of targeted type I interferon pathway inhibitor and oncolytic viruses to treat sarcomas in dogs and cats [244].

Radiation Therapy FLASH radiotherapy (FLASH-RT) is an emerging radiation treatment modality where an ultrahigh dose of radiation is delivered in less than a second. This treatment is reported to have decreased normal tissue toxicity in mice compared to conventional radiation but performed equally in effectively killing cancer cells [245]. Further in vivo studies confirmed these effects in different cancers [246–251], including two veterinary clinical trials [252, 253]. One clinical trial performed on ten dogs (included three STSs) used a modified clinical linear accelerator for administration of a single fraction of FLASH-RT. [253] The canine patients helped to develop a safe and efficient workflow for FLASH-RT which could inform human clinical trials [253]. Canine patients could help inform radiobiology studies, especially given that the mechanisms behind FLASH sparing normal tissues are not yet fully understood but are thought to potentially involve oxygen depletion. Canine tumors are thought to have similar oxygen profiles to human tumors so they represent a great opportunity to study promising novel treatments like FLASH-RT. [254]

3 Conclusions

In humans, soft tissue sarcomas are rare cancers with many unique histologic subtypes. Therapeutic clinical trials evaluating novel treatments are limited by small sample sizes and disease heterogeneity, limiting opportunities to improve patient outcomes. Canines spontaneously develop soft tissue sarcoma (STS) more commonly than humans, importantly while living in the same environment as their human owners. Molecular characterization of some canine soft tissue sarcoma histologic subtypes has led to recognition of similarities to the corresponding human histologic subtype, but further research is needed in this area. As such, canines with STS provide the opportunity to study cancer genetics and perform clinical trials in real-world conditions. The spontaneous dog STS model provides a unique opportunity to advance device or drug development including immunotherapy. Canine clinical trials allow for the screening of more candidate drugs to streamline and inform human trials, or canine clinical trials can be run in parallel with human clinical trials allowing for improved power due to larger patient populations.

References

1. Gustafson DL, Duval DL, Regan DP et al (2018) Canine sarcomas as a surrogate for the human disease. Pharmacol Ther 188:80–96
2. Dennis MM, McSporran KD, Bacon NJ et al (2011) Prognostic factors for cutaneous and subcutaneous soft tissue sarcomas in dogs. Vet Pathol 48:73–84
3. Bostock DE, Dye MT (1980) Prognosis after surgical excision of canine fibrous connective tissue sarcomas. Vet Pathol 17:581–588
4. Kuntz CA, Dernell WS, Powers BE et al (1997) Prognostic factors for surgical treatment of soft-tissue sarcomas in dogs: 75 cases (1986-1996). J Am Vet Med Assoc 211:1147–1151
5. Ettinger SN, Scase TJ, Oberthaler KT et al (2006) Association of argyrophilic nucleolar organizing regions, Ki-67, and proliferating cell nuclear antigen scores with histologic grade and survival in dogs with soft tissue sarcomas: 60 cases (1996-2002). J Am Vet Med Assoc 228:1053–1062
6. Selting KA, Powers BE, Thompson LJ et al (2005) Outcome of dogs with high-grade soft tissue sarcomas treated with and without adjuvant doxorubicin chemotherapy: 39 cases (1996-2004). J Am Vet Med Assoc 227:1442–1448
7. Sbaraglia M, Dei Tos AP (2019) The pathology of soft tissue sarcomas. Radiol Med 124:266–281
8. Corey RM, Swett K, Ward WG (2014) Epidemiology and survivorship of soft tissue sarcomas in adults: a national cancer database report. Cancer Med 3:1404–1415
9. Weiss AR, Harrison DJ (2024) Soft tissue sarcomas in adolescents and young adults. J Clin Oncol 42:675–685
10. Tamburini BA, Phang TL, Fosmire SP et al (2010) Gene expression profiling identifies inflammation and angiogenesis as distinguishing features of canine hemangiosarcoma. BMC Cancer 10:619
11. Ballinger ML, Goode DL, Ray-Coquard I et al (2016) Monogenic and polygenic determinants of sarcoma risk: an international genetic study. Lancet Oncol 17:1261–1271
12. Kleinerman RA, Schonfeld SJ, Sigel BS et al (2019) Bone and soft-tissue sarcoma risk in long-term survivors of hereditary retinoblastoma treated with radiation. J Clin Oncol 37:3436–3445
13. Barretina J, Taylor BS, Banerji S et al (2010) Subtype-specific genomic alterations define new targets for soft-tissue sarcoma therapy. Nat Genet 42:715–721

14. Brenca M, Maestro R (2015) Massive parallel sequencing in sarcoma pathobiology: state of the art and perspectives. Expert Rev Anticancer Ther 15:1473–1488
15. Cancer Genome Atlas Research Network. Electronic address edsc, Cancer Genome Atlas Research N (2017) Comprehensive and integrated genomic characterization of adult soft tissue sarcomas. Cell 171:950–965. e928
16. Davis BW, Ostrander EA (2014) Domestic dogs and cancer research: a breed-based genomics approach. ILAR J 55:59–68
17. Dobson JM, Samuel S, Milstein H et al (2002) Canine neoplasia in the UK: estimates of incidence rates from a population of insured dogs. J Small Anim Pract 43:240–246
18. Merlo DF, Rossi L, Pellegrino C et al (2008) Cancer incidence in pet dogs: findings of the Animal Tumor Registry of Genoa, Italy. J Vet Intern Med 22:976–984
19. Ostrander EA, Dreger DL, Evans JM (2019) Canine cancer genomics: lessons for canine and human health. Annu Rev Anim Biosci 7:449–472
20. Hedan B, Cadieu E, Rimbault M et al (2021) Identification of common predisposing loci to hematopoietic cancers in four dog breeds. PLoS Genet 17:e1009395
21. The WHO Classification of Tumours Editorial Board (2020) WHO classification of tumours soft tissue and bone tumours, 5th edn. IARC Press, Lyon
22. Hornick JL (2014) Novel uses of immunohistochemistry in the diagnosis and classification of soft tissue tumors. Mod Pathol 27(Suppl 1):S47–S63
23. Miettinen M (2014) Immunohistochemistry of soft tissue tumours – review with emphasis on 10 markers. Histopathology 64:101–118
24. Mertens F, Fletcher CD, Antonescu CR et al (2005) Clinicopathologic and molecular genetic characterization of low-grade fibromyxoid sarcoma, and cloning of a novel FUS/CREB3L1 fusion gene. Lab Investig 85:408–415
25. Coindre JM, Terrier P, Guillou L et al (2001) Predictive value of grade for metastasis development in the main histologic types of adult soft tissue sarcomas: a study of 1240 patients from the French Federation of Cancer Centers Sarcoma Group. Cancer 91:1914–1926
26. Guillou L, Coindre JM, Bonichon F et al (1997) Comparative study of the National Cancer Institute and French Federation of Cancer Centers Sarcoma Group grading systems in a population of 410 adult patients with soft tissue sarcoma. J Clin Oncol 15:350–362
27. von Mehren M, Kane JM, Agulnik M et al (2022) Soft tissue sarcoma, Version 2.2022, NCCN clinical practice guidelines in oncology. J Natl Compr Cancer Netw 20:815–833
28. Amin MB, Edge SB, Greene FL et al (2018) AJCC cancer staging manual. Springer
29. Cates JMM (2018) The AJCC 8th edition staging system for soft tissue sarcoma of the extremities or trunk: a cohort study of the SEER database. J Natl Compr Cancer Netw 16:144–152
30. Baker-Gabb M, Hunt GB, France MP (2003) Soft tissue sarcomas and mast cell tumours in dogs; clinical behaviour and response to surgery. Aust Vet J 81:732–738
31. Ghisleni G, Roccabianca P, Ceruti R et al (2006) Correlation between fine-needle aspiration cytology and histopathology in the evaluation of cutaneous and subcutaneous masses from dogs and cats. Vet Clin Pathol 35:24–30
32. Trojani M, Contesso G, Coindre JM et al (1984) Soft-tissue sarcomas of adults; study of pathological prognostic variables and definition of a histopathological grading system. Int J Cancer 33:37–42
33. McChesney SL, Withrow SJ, Gillette EL et al (1989) Radiotherapy of soft tissue sarcomas in dogs. J Am Vet Med Assoc 194:60–63
34. Gillette SM, Dewhirst MW, Gillette EL et al (1992) Response of canine soft tissue sarcomas to radiation or radiation plus hyperthermia: a randomized phase II study. Int J Hyperth 8:309–320
35. Simon D, Ruslander DM, Rassnick KM et al (2007) Orthovoltage radiation and weekly low dose of doxorubicin for the treatment of incompletely excised soft-tissue sarcomas in 39 dogs. Vet Rec 160:321–326
36. McKnight JA, Mauldin GN, McEntee MC et al (2000) Radiation treatment for incompletely resected soft-tissue sarcomas in dogs. J Am Vet Med Assoc 217:205–210
37. McSporran KD (2009) Histologic grade predicts recurrence for marginally excised canine subcutaneous soft tissue sarcomas. Vet Pathol 46:928–933
38. Perry JA, Culp WT, Dailey DD et al (2014) Diagnostic accuracy of pre-treatment biopsy for grading soft tissue sarcomas in dogs. Vet Comp Oncol 12:106–113
39. Avallone G, Helmbold P, Caniatti M et al (2007) The spectrum of canine cutaneous perivascular wall tumors: morphologic, phenotypic and clinical characterization. Vet Pathol 44:607–620
40. Chijiwa K, Uchida K, Tateyama S (2004) Immunohistochemical evaluation of canine peripheral nerve sheath tumors and other soft tissue sarcomas. Vet Pathol 41:307–318
41. Williamson MM, Middleton DJ (1998) Cutaneous soft tissue tumours in dogs: classification, differentiation, and histogenesis. Vet Dermatol 9:43–48
42. Vail DM, Powers BE, Getzy DM et al (1994) Evaluation of prognostic factors for dogs with synovial sarcoma: 36 cases (1986-1991). J Am Vet Med Assoc 205:1300–1307
43. Kapatkin AS, Mullen HS, Matthiesen DT et al (1992) Leiomyosarcoma in dogs: 44 cases (1983-1988). J Am Vet Med Assoc 201:1077–1079

44. Cohen M, Post GS, Wright JC (2003) Gastrointestinal leiomyosarcoma in 14 dogs. J Vet Intern Med 17:107–110
45. Frost D, Lasota J, Miettinen M (2003) Gastrointestinal stromal tumors and leiomyomas in the dog: a histopathologic, immunohistochemical, and molecular genetic study of 50 cases. Vet Pathol 40:42–54
46. Crawshaw J, Berg J, Sardinas JC et al (1998) Prognosis for dogs with nonlymphomatous, small intestinal tumors treated by surgical excision. J Am Anim Hosp Assoc 34:451–456
47. Ward H, Fox LE, Calderwood-Mays MB et al (1994) Cutaneous hemangiosarcoma in 25 dogs: a retrospective study. J Vet Intern Med 8:345–348
48. Greene FL, Page DL, Fleming ID et al (2002) AJCC cancer staging manual, 6th edn. Springer, New York
49. Day MJ, Lucke VM, Pearson H (1995) A review of pathological diagnoses made from 87 canine splenic biopsies. J Small Anim Pract 36:426–433
50. Heng HG, Lowry JE, Boston S et al (2006) Smooth muscle neoplasia of the urinary bladder wall in three dogs. Vet Radiol Ultrasound 47:83–86
51. Johnson GC, Miller MA, Ramos-Vara JA (1995) Comparison of argyrophilic nucleolar organizer regions (AgNORs) and mitotic index in distinguishing benign from malignant canine smooth muscle tumors and in separating inflammatory hyperplasia from neoplastic lesions of the urinary bladder mucosa. J Vet Diagn Invest 7:127–136
52. Ogden JA, Selmic LE, Liptak JM et al (2020) Outcomes associated with vaginectomy and vulvovaginectomy in 21 dogs. Vet Surg 49:1132–1143
53. Spangler WL, Culbertson MR, Kass PH (1994) Primary mesenchymal (nonangiomatous/nonlymphomatous) neoplasms occurring in the canine spleen: anatomic classification, immunohistochemistry, and mitotic activity correlated with patient survival. Vet Pathol 31:37–47
54. Thacher C, Bradley RL (1983) Vulvar and vaginal tumors in the dog: a retrospective study. J Am Vet Med Assoc 183:690–692
55. Weinstein MJ, Carpenter JL, Schunk CJ (1989) Nonangiogenic and nonlymphomatous sarcomas of the canine spleen: 57 cases (1975-1987). J Am Vet Med Assoc 195:784–788
56. Boy SC, Van Heerden WF, Steenkamp G (2005) Diagnosis and treatment of primary intraoral leiomyosarcomas in four dogs. Vet Rec 156:510–513
57. Callanan JJ, McCarthy GM, McAllister H (2000) Primary pulmonary artery leiomyosarcoma in an adult dog. Vet Pathol 37:663–666
58. Liu SM, Mikaelian I (2003) Cutaneous smooth muscle tumors in the dog and cat. Vet Pathol 40:685–692
59. Pierini A, Cinti F, Binanti D et al (2017) Primary leiomyosarcoma of the jugular vein in a dog. Open Vet J 7:61–64
60. Rabanal RH, Fondevila DM, Montane V et al (1989) Immunocytochemical diagnosis of skin tumours of the dog with special reference to undifferentiated types. Res Vet Sci 47:129–133
61. Morini M, Gentilini F, Turba ME et al (2022) Mutational analysis of c-KIT and PDGFRA in canine gastrointestinal stromal tumors (GISTs). Vet Sci:9
62. Soreide K, Sandvik OM, Soreide JA et al (2016) Global epidemiology of gastrointestinal stromal tumours (GIST): a systematic review of population-based cohort studies. Cancer Epidemiol 40:39–46
63. Carvalho JC, Thomas DG, Lucas DR (2009) Cluster analysis of immunohistochemical markers in leiomyosarcoma delineates specific anatomic and gender subgroups. Cancer 115:4186–4195
64. Grossmann AH, Layfield LJ, Randall RL (2012) Classification, molecular characterization, and the significance of pten alteration in leiomyosarcoma. Sarcoma 2012:380896
65. Farese JP, Bacon NJ, Ehrhart NP et al (2008) Oesophageal leiomyosarcoma in dogs: surgical management and clinical outcome of four cases. Vet Comp Oncol 6:31–38
66. Dailey DD, Ehrhart EJ, Duval DL et al (2015) DOG1 is a sensitive and specific immunohistochemical marker for diagnosis of canine gastrointestinal stromal tumors. J Vet Diagn Invest 27:268–277
67. Hayes S, Yuzbasiyan-Gurkan V, Gregory-Bryson E et al (2013) Classification of canine nonangiogenic, nonlymphogenic, gastrointestinal sarcomas based on microscopic, immunohistochemical, and molecular characteristics. Vet Pathol 50:779–788
68. Russell KN, Mehler SJ, Skorupski KA et al (2007) Clinical and immunohistochemical differentiation of gastrointestinal stromal tumors from leiomyosarcomas in dogs: 42 cases (1990-2003). J Am Vet Med Assoc 230:1329–1333
69. Gregory-Bryson E, Bartlett E, Kiupel M et al (2010) Canine and human gastrointestinal stromal tumors display similar mutations in c-KIT exon 11. BMC Cancer 10:559
70. Berger EP, Johannes CM, Jergens AE et al (2018) Retrospective evaluation of toceranib phosphate (Palladia(R)) use in the treatment of gastrointestinal stromal tumors of dogs. J Vet Intern Med 32:2045–2053
71. Baez JL, Hendrick MJ, Shofer FS et al (2004) Liposarcomas in dogs: 56 cases (1989-2000). J Am Vet Med Assoc 224:887–891
72. Gower KL, Liptak JM, Culp WT et al (2015) Splenic liposarcoma in dogs: 13 cases (2002-2012). J Am Vet Med Assoc 247:1404–1407
73. Goldblum JR, Folpe AL, Weiss SW (2014) Liposarcoma. In: Goldblum JR, Folpe AL, Weiss SW (eds) Enzinger and Weiss's soft tissue tumors, 6th edn. Philadelphia, Elsevier, Saunders, pp 484–522
74. Fletcher CDM, Bridge JA, Hogendoorn PCW et al (2013) Classification of soft tissue and bone. pathology of genetics of tumours of soft tissue and bone, 5th edn. IARC Press, Lyon

75. Strafuss AC, Bozarth AJ (1973) Liposarcomas in dogs. J Am Anim Hosp Assoc:183–187
76. Spoldi E, Schwarz T, Sabattini S et al (2017) Comparisons among computed tomographic features of adipose masses in dogs and cats. Vet Radiol Ultrasound 58:29–37
77. Hendrick MJ, Mahaffey EA, Moore FM et al (1998) Histological classification of mesenchymal tumors of skin and soft tissues of domestic animals. Armed Forces Institute of Pathology, Washington, DC
78. Avallone G, Roccabianca P, Crippa L et al (2016) Histological classification and immunohistochemical evaluation of MDM2 and CDK4 expression in canine Liposarcoma. Vet Pathol 53:773–780
79. Avallone G, Pellegrino V, Roccabianca P et al (2017) Tyrosine kinase receptor expression in canine Liposarcoma. Vet Pathol 54:212–217
80. Gross TL, Ihrke PJ, Walder EJ et al (2005) Lipocytic tumors. In: Gross TL, Ihrke PJ, Walder EJ et al (eds) Skin diseases of the dog and cat clinical and histopathologic diagnosis. Blackwell Science, Oxford, pp 766–777
81. Milovancev M, Hauck M, Keller C et al (2015) Comparative pathology of canine soft tissue sarcomas: possible models of human non-rhabdomyosarcoma soft tissue sarcomas. J Comp Pathol 152:22–27
82. LaDouceur EEB, Stevens SE, Wood J et al (2017) Immunoreactivity of canine liposarcoma to muscle and brown adipose antigens. Vet Pathol 54:885–891
83. Boos GS, Bassunio DM, Wurster F et al (2015) Retrospective canine skin peripheral nerve sheath tumors data with emphasis on histologic, immunohistochemical and prognostic factors. Pesq Vet Bras 35:965–974
84. Mazzei M, Millanta F, Citi S et al (2002) Haemangiopericytoma: histological spectrum, immunohistochemical characterization and prognosis. Vet Dermatol 13:15–21
85. Perez J, Bautista MJ, Rollon E et al (1996) Immunohistochemical characterization of hemangiopericytomas and other spindle cell tumors in the dog. Vet Pathol 33:391–397
86. Goldschmidt MH, Hendrick MJ (2008) Tumors of the skin and soft tissues. In: Tumors in domestic animals. Iowa State Press, pp 45–117
87. Suzuki S, Uchida K, Nakayama H (2014) The effects of tumor location on diagnostic criteria for canine malignant peripheral nerve sheath tumors (MPNSTs) and the markers for distinction between canine MPNSTs and canine perivascular wall tumors. Vet Pathol 51:722–736
88. Avallone G, Boracchi P, Stefanello D et al (2014) Canine perivascular wall tumors: high prognostic impact of site, depth, and completeness of margins. Vet Pathol 51:713–721
89. Palmieri C, Avallone G, Cimini M et al (2013) Use of electron microscopy to classify canine perivascular wall tumors. Vet Pathol 50:226–233
90. Nasir L, Rutteman GR, Reid SW et al (2001) Analysis of p53 mutational events and MDM2 amplification in canine soft-tissue sarcomas. Cancer Lett 174:83–89
91. Mochizuki H, Kennedy K, Shapiro SG et al (2015) BRAF mutations in canine cancers. PLoS One 10:e0129534
92. Brohl AS, Kahen E, Yoder SJ et al (2017) The genomic landscape of malignant peripheral nerve sheath tumors: diverse drivers of Ras pathway activation. Sci Rep 7:14992
93. Antonescu C (2014) Malignant vascular tumors–an update. Mod Pathol 27(Suppl 1):S30–S38
94. Fury MG, Antonescu CR, Van Zee KJ et al (2005) A 14-year retrospective review of angiosarcoma: clinical characteristics, prognostic factors, and treatment outcomes with surgery and chemotherapy. Cancer J 11:241–247
95. Hargis AM, Ihrke PJ, Spangler WL et al (1992) A retrospective clinicopathologic study of 212 dogs with cutaneous hemangiomas and hemangiosarcomas. Vet Pathol 29:316–328
96. Schultheiss PC (2004) A retrospective study of visceral and nonvisceral hemangiosarcoma and hemangiomas in domestic animals. J Vet Diagn Invest 16:522–526
97. Gorden BH, Kim JH, Sarver AL et al (2014) Identification of three molecular and functional subtypes in canine hemangiosarcoma through gene expression profiling and progenitor cell characterization. Am J Pathol 184:985–995
98. Kim JH, Graef AJ, Dickerson EB et al (2015) Pathobiology of hemangiosarcoma in dogs: research advances and future perspectives. Vet Sci 2:388–405
99. Prymak C, McKee LJ, Goldschmidt MH et al (1988) Epidemiologic, clinical, pathologic, and prognostic characteristics of splenic hemangiosarcoma and splenic hematoma in dogs: 217 cases (1985). J Am Vet Med Assoc 193:706–712
100. Ogilvie GK, Powers BE, Mallinckrodt CH et al (1996) Surgery and doxorubicin in dogs with hemangiosarcoma. J Vet Intern Med 10:379–384
101. Dettenborn T, Wermker K, Schulze HJ et al (2014) Prognostic features in angiosarcoma of the head and neck: a retrospective monocenter study. J Craniomaxillofac Surg 42:1623–1628
102. Ferrer L, Fondevila D, Rabanal RM et al (1995) Immunohistochemical detection of CD31 antigen in normal and neoplastic canine endothelial cells. J Comp Pathol 112:319–326
103. Sabattini S, Bettini G (2009) An immunohistochemical analysis of canine haemangioma and haemangiosarcoma. J Comp Pathol 140:158–168
104. von Beust BR, Suter MM, Summers BA (1988) Factor VIII-related antigen in canine endothelial neoplasms: an immunohistochemical study. Vet Pathol 25:251–255
105. Halsey CH, Worley DR, Curran K et al (2016) The use of novel lymphatic endothelial cell-specific immunohistochemical markers to differentiate cuta-

neous angiosarcomas in dogs. Vet Comp Oncol 14:236–244
106. Yonemaru K, Sakai H, Murakami M et al (2006) Expression of vascular endothelial growth factor, basic fibroblast growth factor, and their receptors (flt-1, flk-1, and flg-1) in canine vascular tumors. Vet Pathol 43:971–980
107. Glickman LG, Glickman N, Thorpe R The Golden Retriever Club of America National Health Survey 1998-1999, 2000
108. Tonomura N, Elvers I, Thomas R et al (2015) Genome-wide association study identifies shared risk loci common to two malignancies in golden retrievers. PLoS Genet 11:e1004922
109. Cohen D, Reif JS, Brodey RS et al (1974) Epidemiological analysis of the most prevalent sites and types of canine neoplasia observed in a veterinary hospital. Cancer Res 34:2859–2868
110. Lamerato-Kozicki AR, Helm KM, Jubala CM et al (2006) Canine hemangiosarcoma originates from hematopoietic precursors with potential for endothelial differentiation. Exp Hematol 34:870–878
111. Antonescu CR, Yoshida A, Guo T et al (2009) KDR activating mutations in human angiosarcomas are sensitive to specific kinase inhibitors. Cancer Res 69:7175–7179
112. Thomas R, Borst L, Rotroff D et al (2014) Genomic profiling reveals extensive heterogeneity in somatic DNA copy number aberrations of canine hemangiosarcoma. Chromosom Res 22:305–319
113. Anderson DD, Thomas TP, Campos Marin A et al (2014) Computational techniques for the assessment of fracture repair. Injury 45(Suppl 2):S23–S31
114. Wang G, Wu M, Maloneyhuss MA et al (2017) Actionable mutations in canine hemangiosarcoma. PLoS One 12:e0188667
115. Bader AG, Kang S, Vogt PK (2006) Cancer-specific mutations in PIK3CA are oncogenic in vivo. Proc Natl Acad Sci USA 103:1475–1479
116. Gkeka P, Evangelidis T, Pavlaki M et al (2014) Investigating the structure and dynamics of the PIK3CA wild-type and H1047R oncogenic mutant. PLoS Comput Biol 10:e1003895
117. Behjati S, Tarpey PS, Sheldon H et al (2014) Recurrent PTPRB and PLCG1 mutations in angiosarcoma. Nat Genet 46:376–379
118. Wong K, Ludwig L, Krijgsman O et al (2021) Comparison of the oncogenomic landscape of canine and feline hemangiosarcoma shows novel parallels with human angiosarcoma. Dis Model Mech 14
119. Laptenko O, Prives C (2006) Transcriptional regulation by p53: one protein, many possibilities. Cell Death Differ 13:951–961
120. Grimes JA, Prasad N, Levy S et al (2016) A comparison of microRNA expression profiles from splenic hemangiosarcoma, splenic nodular hyperplasia, and normal spleens of dogs. BMC Vet Res 12:272
121. Chen YC, Liao JW, Hsu WL et al (2016) Identification of the two KIT isoforms and their expression status in canine hemangiosarcomas. BMC Vet Res 12:142
122. Fosmire SP, Dickerson EB, Scott AM et al (2004) Canine malignant hemangiosarcoma as a model of primitive angiogenic endothelium. Lab Investig 84:562–572
123. Alexandrov LB, Kim J, Haradhvala NJ et al (2020) The repertoire of mutational signatures in human cancer. Nature 578:94–101
124. Boichard A, Wagner MJ, Kurzrock R (2020) Angiosarcoma heterogeneity and potential therapeutic vulnerability to immune checkpoint blockade: insights from genomic sequencing. Genome Med 12:61
125. Painter CA, Jain E, Tomson BN et al (2020) The Angiosarcoma Project: enabling genomic and clinical discoveries in a rare cancer through patient-partnered research. Nat Med 26:181–187
126. Changchien YC, Katalin U, Fillinger J et al (2012) A challenging case of metastatic intra-abdominal synovial sarcoma with unusual immunophenotype and its differential diagnosis. Case Rep Pathol 2012:786083
127. Kritsaneepaiboon S, Sangkhathat S, Mitarnun W (2015) Primary synovial sarcoma of the abdominal wall: a case report and literature review. J Radiol Case Rep 9:47–52
128. Craig LE, Dittmer KE, Thompson KG (2016) Tumours and tumour-like lesions of joints. In: Grant Maxie M (ed) Jubb, Kennedy, Palmer's pathology of domestic animals, 6th edn. Elsevier, Missouri, pp 159–163
129. Craig LE, Julian ME, Ferracone JD (2002) The diagnosis and prognosis of synovial tumors in dogs: 35 cases. Vet Pathol 39:66–73
130. Terry J, Saito T, Subramanian S et al (2007) TLE1 as a diagnostic immunohistochemical marker for synovial sarcoma emerging from gene expression profiling studies. Am J Surg Pathol 31:240–246
131. Jagdis A, Rubin BP, Tubbs RR et al (2009) Prospective evaluation of TLE1 as a diagnostic immunohistochemical marker in synovial sarcoma. Am J Surg Pathol 33:1743–1751
132. Kawai A, Woodruff J, Healey JH et al (1998) SYT-SSX gene fusion as a determinant of morphology and prognosis in synovial sarcoma. N Engl J Med 338:153–160
133. Knosel T, Heretsch S, Altendorf-Hofmann A et al (2010) TLE1 is a robust diagnostic biomarker for synovial sarcomas and correlates with t(X;18): analysis of 319 cases. Eur J Cancer 46:1170–1176
134. Fox DB, Cook JL, Kreeger JM et al (2002) Canine synovial sarcoma: a retrospective assessment of described prognostic criteria in 16 cases (1994-1999). J Am Anim Hosp Assoc 38:347–355
135. Gruntzig K, Graf R, Boo G et al (2016) Swiss canine cancer registry 1955-2008: occurrence of the most common tumour diagnoses and influence of age, breed, body size, sex and neutering status on tumour development. J Comp Pathol 155:156–170

136. Ciekot PA, Powers BE, Withrow SJ et al (1994) Histologically low-grade, yet biologicalally high-grade, fibrosarcomas of the mandible and maxilla in dogs: 25 cases (1982-1991). J Am Vet Med Assoc 204:610–615
137. Choi C, Kusewitt DF (2003) Comparison of tyrosinase-related protein-2, S-100, and Melan A immunoreactivity in canine amelanotic melanomas. Vet Pathol 40:713–718
138. Gaitero L, Anor S, Fondevila D et al (2008) Canine cutaneous spindle cell tumours with features of peripheral nerve sheath tumours: a histopathological and immunohistochemical study. J Comp Pathol 139:16–23
139. Klopfleisch R, Meyer A, Lenze D et al (2013) Canine cutaneous peripheral nerve sheath tumours versus fibrosarcomas can be differentiated by neuroectodermal marker genes in their transcriptome. J Comp Pathol 148:197–205
140. Meyer A, Klopfleisch R (2014) Multiple polymerase chain reaction markers for the differentiation of canine cutaneous peripheral nerve sheath tumours versus canine fibrosarcomas. J Comp Pathol 150:198–203
141. Guillou L, Benhattar J, Gengler C et al (2007) Translocation-positive low-grade fibromyxoid sarcoma: clinicopathologic and molecular analysis of a series expanding the morphologic spectrum and suggesting potential relationship to sclerosing epithelioid fibrosarcoma: a study from the French Sarcoma Group. Am J Surg Pathol 31:1387–1402
142. Sargan DR, Milne BS, Hernandez JA et al (2005) Chromosome rearrangements in canine fibrosarcomas. J Hered 96:766–773
143. Aguirre-Hernandez J, Milne BS, Queen C et al (2009) Disruption of chromosome 11 in canine fibrosarcomas highlights an unusual variability of CDKN2B in dogs. BMC Vet Res 5:27
144. Napolitano A, Thway K, Huang P et al (2024) Centralisation of care improves overall survival for sarcoma patients. Ann Oncol
145. Bonvalot S, Levy A, Terrier P et al (2017) Primary extremity soft tissue sarcomas: does local control impact survival? Ann Surg Oncol 24:194–201
146. Brennan MF, Antonescu CR, Moraco N et al (2014) Lessons learned from the study of 10,000 patients with soft tissue sarcoma. Ann Surg 260:416–421. discussion 421-412
147. Abatzoglou S, Turcotte RE, Adoubali A et al (2010) Local recurrence after initial multidisciplinary management of soft tissue sarcoma: is there a way out? Clin Orthop Relat Res 468:3012–3018
148. Gronchi A, Miceli R, Fiore M et al (2007) Extremity soft tissue sarcoma: adding to the prognostic meaning of local failure. Ann Surg Oncol 14:1583–1590
149. Novais EN, Demiralp B, Alderete J et al (2010) Do surgical margin and local recurrence influence survival in soft tissue sarcomas? Clin Orthop Relat Res 468:3003–3011
150. Hasan O, Nasir M, Jessar M et al (2021) Is local recurrence in bone and soft tissue sarcomas just a local recurrence or does it impact the overall survival, retrospective cohort from a sarcoma referral center. J Surg Oncol 124:1536–1543
151. Gronchi A, Colombo C, Raut CP (2014) Surgical management of localized soft tissue tumors. Cancer 120:2638–2648
152. Mollabashy A, Virkus WW, Zlotecki RA et al (2002) Radiation therapy for low-grade soft tissue sarcoma. Clin Orthop Relat Res:190–195
153. Yang JC, Chang AE, Baker AR et al (1998) Randomized prospective study of the benefit of adjuvant radiation therapy in the treatment of soft tissue sarcomas of the extremity. J Clin Oncol 16:197–203
154. Alektiar KM, Leung D, Zelefsky MJ et al (2002) Adjuvant radiation for stage II-B soft tissue sarcoma of the extremity. J Clin Oncol 20:1643–1650
155. Pisters PW, Pollock RE, Lewis VO et al (2007) Long-term results of prospective trial of surgery alone with selective use of radiation for patients with T1 extremity and trunk soft tissue sarcomas. Ann Surg 246:675–681. discussion 681-672
156. Fleming JB, Berman RS, Cheng SC et al (1999) Long-term outcome of patients with American Joint Committee on Cancer stage IIB extremity soft tissue sarcomas. J Clin Oncol 17:2772–2780
157. Baldini EH, Goldberg J, Jenner C et al (1999) Long-term outcomes after function-sparing surgery without radiotherapy for soft tissue sarcoma of the extremities and trunk. J Clin Oncol 17:3252–3259
158. Fujiwara T, Tsuda Y, Le Nail LR et al (2020) The role of radiotherapy in the treatment of superficial soft-tissue sarcomas. Bone Joint J 102-B:1088–1094
159. Fabrizio PL, Stafford SL, Pritchard DJ (2000) Extremity soft-tissue sarcomas selectively treated with surgery alone. Int J Radiat Oncol Biol Phys 48:227–232
160. Rosenberg SA, Tepper J, Glatstein E et al (1982) The treatment of soft-tissue sarcomas of the extremities: prospective randomized evaluations of (1) limb-sparing surgery plus radiation therapy compared with amputation and (2) the role of adjuvant chemotherapy. Ann Surg 196:305–315
161. White LM, Wunder JS, Bell RS et al (2005) Histologic assessment of peritumoral edema in soft tissue sarcoma. Int J Radiat Oncol Biol Phys 61:1439–1445
162. Wang D, Zhang Q, Eisenberg BL et al (2015) Significant reduction of late toxicities in patients with extremity sarcoma treated with image-guided radiation therapy to a reduced target volume: results of Radiation Therapy Oncology Group RTOG-0630 trial. J Clin Oncol 33:2231–2238
163. Folkert MR, Singer S, Brennan MF et al (2014) Comparison of local recurrence with conventional and intensity-modulated radiation therapy for primary soft-tissue sarcomas of the extremity. J Clin Oncol 32:3236–3241

164. Casey DL, Berry SL, Crago A et al (2021) Femoral fracture in primary soft tissue sarcoma treated with intensity-modulated radiation therapy with and without dose constraints. Ann Surg Oncol 28:2700–2704
165. Folkert MR, Casey DL, Berry SL et al (2019) Femoral fracture in primary soft-tissue sarcoma of the thigh and groin treated with intensity-modulated radiation therapy: observed versus expected risk. Ann Surg Oncol 26:1326–1331
166. Allignet B, Waissi W, Geets X et al (2022) Long-term outcomes after definitive radiotherapy with modern techniques for unresectable soft tissue sarcoma. Radiother Oncol 173:55–61
167. Al Yami A, Griffin AM, Ferguson PC et al (2010) Positive surgical margins in soft tissue sarcoma treated with preoperative radiation: is a postoperative boost necessary? Int J Radiat Oncol Biol Phys 77:1191–1197
168. O'Sullivan B, Davis AM, Turcotte R et al (2002) Preoperative versus postoperative radiotherapy in soft-tissue sarcoma of the limbs: a randomised trial. Lancet 359:2235–2241
169. Guadagnolo BA, Bassett RL, Mitra D et al (2022) Hypofractionated, 3-week, preoperative radiotherapy for patients with soft tissue sarcomas (HYPORT-STS): a single-centre, open-label, single-arm, phase 2 trial. Lancet Oncol 23:1547–1557
170. Mayo ZS, Parsai S, Asha W et al (2023) Early outcomes of ultra-hypofractionated preoperative radiation therapy for soft tissue sarcoma followed by immediate surgical resection. Radiother Oncol 180:109439
171. Bedi M, Singh R, Charlson JA et al (2022) Is 5 the new 25? long-term oncologic outcomes from a phase II, prospective, 5-fraction preoperative radiation therapy trial in patients with localized soft tissue sarcoma. Adv Radiat Oncol 7:100850
172. Pennington JD, Eilber FC, Eilber FR et al (2018) Long-term outcomes With Ifosfamide-based hypofractionated preoperative chemoradiotherapy for extremity soft tissue sarcomas. Am J Clin Oncol 41:1154–1161
173. Kalbasi A, Kamrava M, Chu FI et al (2020) A phase II trial of 5-day neoadjuvant radiotherapy for patients with high-risk primary soft tissue sarcoma. Clin Cancer Res 26:1829–1836
174. Valle LF, Bernthal N, Eilber FC et al (2021) Evaluating thresholds to adopt hypofractionated preoperative radiotherapy as standard of care in sarcoma. Sarcoma 2021:3735874
175. Naghavi AO, Gonzalez RJ, Scott JG et al (2016) Implications of staged reconstruction and adjuvant brachytherapy in the treatment of recurrent soft tissue sarcoma. Brachytherapy 15:495–503
176. Campbell SR, Shah C, Scott JG et al (2021) American Brachytherapy Society (ABS) consensus statement for soft-tissue sarcoma brachytherapy. Brachytherapy 20:1200–1218
177. Gaito S, Aznar MC, Burnet NG et al (2023) Assessing equity of access to proton beam therapy: a literature review. Clin Oncol (R Coll Radiol) 35:e528–e536
178. Laughlin BS, Golafshar MA, Ahmed S et al (2022) Early experience using proton beam therapy for extremity soft tissue sarcoma: a multicenter study. Int J Part Ther 9:1–11
179. Gundle KR, Kafchinski L, Gupta S et al (2018) Analysis of margin classification systems for assessing the risk of local recurrence after soft tissue sarcoma resection. J Clin Oncol 36:704–709
180. King DM, Hackbarth DA, Kirkpatrick A (2012) Extremity soft tissue sarcoma resections: how wide do you need to be? Clin Orthop Relat Res 470:692–699
181. McKee MD, Liu DF, Brooks JJ et al (2004) The prognostic significance of margin width for extremity and trunk sarcoma. J Surg Oncol 85:68–76
182. Tan MC, Brennan MF, Kuk D et al (2016) Histology-based classification predicts pattern of recurrence and improves risk stratification in primary retroperitoneal sarcoma. Ann Surg 263:593–600
183. Gronchi A, Strauss DC, Miceli R et al (2016) Variability in patterns of recurrence after resection of primary retroperitoneal sarcoma (RPS): a report on 1007 patients from the multi-institutional collaborative RPS working group. Ann Surg 263:1002–1009
184. Dominguez DA, Sampath S, Agulnik M et al (2023) Surgical management of retroperitoneal sarcoma. Curr Oncol 30:4618–4631
185. MacNeill AJ, Fiore M (2018) Surgical morbidity in retroperitoneal sarcoma resection. J Surg Oncol 117:56–61
186. Kelly KJ, Yoon SS, Kuk D et al (2015) Comparison of perioperative radiation therapy and surgery versus surgery alone in 204 patients with primary retroperitoneal sarcoma: a retrospective 2-institution study. Ann Surg 262:156–162
187. Lane WO, Cramer CK, Nussbaum DP et al (2015) Analysis of perioperative radiation therapy in the surgical treatment of primary and recurrent retroperitoneal sarcoma. J Surg Oncol 112:352–358
188. Bonvalot S, Gronchi A, Le Pechoux C et al (2020) Preoperative radiotherapy plus surgery versus surgery alone for patients with primary retroperitoneal sarcoma (EORTC-62092: STRASS): a multicentre, open-label, randomised, phase 3 trial. Lancet Oncol 21:1366–1377
189. Callegaro D, Raut CP, Ajayi T et al (2023) Preoperative radiotherapy in patients with primary retroperitoneal sarcoma: EORTC-62092 trial (STRASS) versus off-trial (STREXIT) results. Ann Surg 278:127–134
190. Haas RLM, Bonvalot S, Miceli R et al (2019) Radiotherapy for retroperitoneal liposarcoma: a report from the transatlantic retroperitoneal sarcoma working group. Cancer 125:1290–1300
191. Judson I, Verweij J, Gelderblom H et al (2014) Doxorubicin alone versus intensified doxorubicin plus ifosfamide for first-line treatment of advanced or metastatic soft-tissue sarcoma: a randomised controlled phase 3 trial. Lancet Oncol 15:415–423
192. Seddon B, Strauss SJ, Whelan J et al (2017) Gemcitabine and docetaxel versus doxorubicin as

first-line treatment in previously untreated advanced unresectable or metastatic soft-tissue sarcomas (GeDDiS): a randomised controlled phase 3 trial. Lancet Oncol 18:1397–1410

193. Tawbi HA, Burgess M, Bolejack V et al (2017) Pembrolizumab in advanced soft-tissue sarcoma and bone sarcoma (SARC028): a multicentre, two-cohort, single-arm, open-label, phase 2 trial. Lancet Oncol 18:1493–1501
194. Grunwald V, Karch A, Schuler M et al (2020) Randomized comparison of Pazopanib and Doxorubicin as first-line treatment in patients with metastatic soft tissue sarcoma age 60 years or older: results of a German intergroup study. J Clin Oncol 38:3555–3564
195. D'Angelo SP, Mahoney MR, Van Tine BA et al (2018) Nivolumab with or without ipilimumab treatment for metastatic sarcoma (Alliance A091401): two open-label, non-comparative, randomised, phase 2 trials. Lancet Oncol 19:416–426
196. van der Graaf WT, Blay JY, Chawla SP et al (2012) Pazopanib for metastatic soft-tissue sarcoma (PALETTE): a randomised, double-blind, placebo-controlled phase 3 trial. Lancet 379:1879–1886
197. Adjuvant chemotherapy for localised resectable soft tissue sarcoma in adults. Sarcoma Meta-analysis Collaboration (SMAC). Cochrane Database Syst Rev 2000:CD001419
198. Kraybill WG, Harris J, Spiro IJ et al (2010) Long-term results of a phase 2 study of neoadjuvant chemotherapy and radiotherapy in the management of high-risk, high-grade, soft tissue sarcomas of the extremities and body wall: Radiation Therapy Oncology Group Trial 9514. Cancer 116:4613–4621
199. Spunt SL, Million L, Chi YY et al (2020) A risk-based treatment strategy for non-rhabdomyosarcoma soft-tissue sarcomas in patients younger than 30 years (ARST0332): a Children's Oncology Group prospective study. Lancet Oncol 21:145–161
200. Pervaiz N, Colterjohn N, Farrokhyar F et al (2008) A systematic meta-analysis of randomized controlled trials of adjuvant chemotherapy for localized resectable soft-tissue sarcoma. Cancer 113:573–581
201. Gronchi A, Ferrari S, Quagliuolo V et al (2017) Histotype-tailored neoadjuvant chemotherapy versus standard chemotherapy in patients with high-risk soft-tissue sarcomas (ISG-STS 1001): an international, open-label, randomised, controlled, phase 3, multicentre trial. Lancet Oncol 18:812–822
202. Bray JP (2017) Soft tissue sarcoma in the dog - Part 2: surgical margins, controversies and a comparative review. J Small Anim Pract 58:63–72
203. Forrest LJ, Chun R, Adams WM et al (2000) Postoperative radiotherapy for canine soft tissue sarcoma. J Vet Intern Med 14:578–582
204. Heller D, Stebbins ME, Reynolds T et al (2005) A retrospective study of 87 cases of canine soft tissue sarcomas, 1986-2001. Int J Appl Res Vet Med 3:81–87
205. Payne SE, Rassnick KM, Northrup NC et al (2003) Treatment of vascular and soft-tissue sarcomas in dogs using an alternating protocol of ifosfamide and doxorubicin. Vet Comp Oncol 1:171–179
206. Elmslie RE, Glawe P, Dow SW (2008) Metronomic therapy with cyclophosphamide and piroxicam effectively delays tumor recurrence in dogs with incompletely resected soft tissue sarcomas. J Vet Intern Med 22:1373–1379
207. de Queiroz GF, Dagli ML, Fukumasu H et al (2010) Vascular endothelial growth factor expression and microvascular density in soft tissue sarcomas in dogs. J Vet Diagn Invest 22:105–108
208. de Queiroz GF, Dagli ML, Meira SA et al (2013) Serum vascular endothelial growth factor in dogs with soft tissue sarcomas. Vet Comp Oncol 11:230–235
209. Al-Dissi AN, Haines DM, Singh B et al (2009) Immunohistochemical expression of vascular endothelial growth factor and vascular endothelial growth factor receptor in canine cutaneous fibrosarcomas. J Comp Pathol 141:229–236
210. Avallone G, Stefanello D, Boracchi P et al (2015) Growth factors and COX2 expression in canine perivascular wall tumors. Vet Pathol 52:1034–1040
211. Havlicek M, Straw RS, Langova V et al (2009) Intra-operative cisplatin for the treatment of canine extremity soft tissue sarcomas. Vet Comp Oncol 7:122–129
212. Bergman NS, Urie BK, Pardo AD et al (2016) Evaluation of local toxic effects and outcomes for dogs undergoing marginal tumor excision with intralesional cisplatin-impregnated bead placement for treatment of soft tissue sarcomas: 62 cases (2009-2012). J Am Vet Med Assoc 248:1148–1156
213. Marconato L, Comastri S, Lorenzo MR et al (2007) Postsurgical intra-incisional 5-fluorouracil in dogs with incompletely resected, extremity malignant spindle cell tumours: a pilot study. Vet Comp Oncol 5:239–249
214. Marconato L, Albanese F, Viacava P et al (2007) Paraneoplastic alopecia associated with hepatocellular carcinoma in a cat. Vet Dermatol 18:267–271
215. Dernell WS, Withrow SJ, Straw RC et al (1997) Intracavitary treatment of soft tissue sarcomas in dogs using cisplatin in a biodegradable polymer. Anticancer Res 17:4499–4505
216. Spugnini EP, Vincenzi B, Citro G et al (2007) Adjuvant electrochemotherapy for the treatment of incompletely excised spontaneous canine sarcomas. In Vivo 21:819–822
217. Chase D, Bray J, Ide A et al (2009) Outcome following removal of canine spindle cell tumours in first opinion practice: 104 cases. J Small Anim Pract 50:568–574
218. Banks T, Straw R, Thomson M et al (2004) Soft tissue sarcomas in dogs: a study correlating optimal surgical margin with tumour grade. Aust Vet Pract 34:158–163

219. Bray JP, Polton GA, McSporran KD et al (2014) Canine soft tissue sarcoma managed in first opinion practice: outcome in 350 cases. Vet Surg 43:774–782
220. Stefanello D, Avallone G, Ferrari R et al (2011) Canine cutaneous perivascular wall tumors at first presentation: clinical behavior and prognostic factors in 55 cases. J Vet Intern Med 25:1398–1405
221. Stefanello D, Morello E, Roccabianca P et al (2008) Marginal excision of low-grade spindle cell sarcoma of canine extremities: 35 dogs (1996-2006). Vet Surg 37:461–465
222. Stromberg PC, Meuten DJ (2017) Trimming tumors for diagnosis and prognosis. In: Meuten DJ (ed) Tumors in domestic animals, 5th edn. Wiley, Ames
223. Bacon NJ, Dernell WS, Ehrhart N et al (2007) Evaluation of primary re-excision after recent inadequate resection of soft tissue sarcomas in dogs: 41 cases (1999-2004). J Am Vet Med Assoc 230:548–554
224. Griffin MA, Culp WTN, Rebhun RB (2021) Canine and feline haemangiosarcoma. Vet Rec 189:e585
225. Szivek A, Burns RE, Gericota B et al (2012) Clinical outcome in 94 cases of dermal haemangiosarcoma in dogs treated with surgical excision: 1993-2007*. Vet Comp Oncol 10:65–73
226. U'Ren LW, Biller BJ, Elmslie RE et al (2007) Evaluation of a novel tumor vaccine in dogs with hemangiosarcoma. J Vet Intern Med 21:113–120
227. Konduri V, Halpert MM, Baig YC et al (2019) Dendritic cell vaccination plus low-dose doxorubicin for the treatment of spontaneous canine hemangiosarcoma. Cancer Gene Ther 26:282–291
228. Lucroy MD, Clauson RM, Suckow MA et al (2020) Evaluation of an autologous cancer vaccine for the treatment of metastatic canine hemangiosarcoma: a preliminary study. BMC Vet Res 16:447
229. Lindblad-Toh K, Wade CM, Mikkelsen TS et al (2005) Genome sequence, comparative analysis and haplotype structure of the domestic dog. Nature 438:803–819
230. Sutter NB, Ostrander EA (2004) Dog star rising: the canine genetic system. Nat Rev Genet 5:900–910
231. Patil SS, Gentschev I, Nolte I et al (2012) Oncolytic virotherapy in veterinary medicine: current status and future prospects for canine patients. J Transl Med 10:3
232. MacNeill AL, Weishaar KM, Seguin B et al (2018) Safety of an oncolytic Myxoma virus in dogs with soft tissue sarcoma. Viruses 10
233. Suter SE, Chein MB, von Messling V et al (2005) In vitro canine distemper virus infection of canine lymphoid cells: a prelude to oncolytic therapy for lymphoma. Clin Cancer Res 11:1579–1587
234. Barton KN, Paielli D, Zhang Y et al (2006) Second-generation replication-competent oncolytic adenovirus armed with improved suicide genes and ADP gene demonstrates greater efficacy without increased toxicity. Mol Ther 13:347–356
235. Laborda E, Puig-Saus C, Rodriguez-Garcia A et al (2014) A pRb-responsive, RGD-modified, and hyaluronidase-armed canine oncolytic adenovirus for application in veterinary oncology. Mol Ther 22:986–998
236. Autio KP, Ruotsalainen JJ, Anttila MO et al (2015) Attenuated Semliki Forest virus for cancer treatment in dogs: safety assessment in two laboratory Beagles. BMC Vet Res 11:170
237. LeBlanc AK, Naik S, Galyon GD et al (2013) Safety studies on intravenous administration of oncolytic recombinant vesicular stomatitis virus in purpose-bred beagle dogs. Hum Gene Ther Clin Dev 24:174–181
238. Smith BF, Curiel DT, Ternovoi VV et al (2006) Administration of a conditionally replicative oncolytic canine adenovirus in normal dogs. Cancer Biother Radiopharm 21:601–606
239. Hwang CC, Igase M, Sakurai M et al (2018) Oncolytic reovirus therapy: pilot study in dogs with spontaneously occurring tumours. Vet Comp Oncol 16:229–238
240. Naik S, Galyon GD, Jenks NJ et al (2018) Comparative oncology evaluation of intravenous recombinant oncolytic vesicular stomatitis virus therapy in spontaneous canine cancer. Mol Cancer Ther 17:316–326
241. Freytag SO, Barton KN, Brown SL et al (2007) Replication-competent adenovirus-mediated suicide gene therapy with radiation in a preclinical model of pancreatic cancer. Mol Ther 15:1600–1606
242. Lu Y, Zhang Y, Chang G et al (2013) Comparison of prostate-specific promoters and the use of PSP-driven virotherapy for prostate cancer. Biomed Res Int 2013:624632
243. Porrello A, Cardelli P, Spugnini EP (2004) Pet models in cancer research: general principles. J Exp Clin Cancer Res 23:181–193
244. MacNeill AL (2020) The potential of the combined use of targeted type I interferon pathway inhibitors and oncolytic viruses to treat sarcomas. Vet Comp Oncol 18:36–42
245. Favaudon V, Caplier L, Monceau V et al (2014) Ultrahigh dose-rate FLASH irradiation increases the differential response between normal and tumor tissue in mice. Sci Transl Med 6:245ra293
246. Montay-Gruel P, Petersson K, Jaccard M et al (2017) Irradiation in a flash: unique sparing of memory in mice after whole brain irradiation with dose rates above 100Gy/s. Radiother Oncol 124:365–369
247. Montay-Gruel P, Acharya MM, Petersson K et al (2019) Long-term neurocognitive benefits of FLASH radiotherapy driven by reduced reactive oxygen species. Proc Natl Acad Sci USA 116:10943–10951
248. Montay-Gruel P, Acharya MM, Goncalves Jorge P et al (2021) Hypofractionated FLASH-RT as an effective treatment against glioblastoma that reduces neurocognitive side effects in mice. Clin Cancer Res 27:775–784
249. Fouillade C, Curras-Alonso S, Giuranno L et al (2020) FLASH irradiation spares lung progeni-

tor cells and limits the incidence of radio-induced senescence. Clin Cancer Res 26:1497–1506
250. Levy K, Natarajan S, Wang J et al (2020) Abdominal FLASH irradiation reduces radiation-induced gastrointestinal toxicity for the treatment of ovarian cancer in mice. Sci Rep 10:21600
251. Bourhis J, Montay-Gruel P, Goncalves Jorge P et al (2019) Clinical translation of FLASH radiotherapy: Why and how? Radiother Oncol 139:11–17
252. Vozenin MC, De Fornel P, Petersson K et al (2019) The advantage of FLASH radiotherapy confirmed in mini-pig and Cat-cancer patients. Clin Cancer Res 25:35–42
253. Konradsson E, Arendt ML, Bastholm Jensen K et al (2021) Establishment and initial experience of clinical FLASH radiotherapy in canine cancer patients. Front Oncol 11:658004
254. Nolan MW, Kent MS, Boss MK (2019) Emerging translational opportunities in comparative oncology with companion canine cancers: radiation oncology. Front Oncol 9:1291
255. Liptak J, Forrest LJ (2013) Soft tissue sarcomas. In: Withrow SJ, Vail DM, Page RL (eds) Withrow & MacEwen's small animal clinical oncology. Elsevier Saunders, St. Louis, pp 369–374

Utilizing Comparative Oncology Approaches

Organizing and Conducting Comparative Oncology Clinical Trials

Amy LeBlanc, Christina Mazcko, Erika Berger, and Jessica Beck

1 Introduction and Overview

1.1 Why Conduct Comparative Oncology Clinical Trials?

Comparative oncology clinical trials refer to clinical studies conducted in privately owned companion animals, primarily dogs, with the purpose of advancing a therapeutic concept for human use [23, 40]. Such trials may result in the test article (drug, imaging agent, or device) being applicable and available for the care of the species involved but are generally not specifically designed to result in a new veterinary-specific drug or device approval.

Recognition of naturally occurring canine cancers as valued translational patient models for humans has been steadily growing over the last three decades. Canine comparative oncology trial data is increasingly recognized for its value in the human cancer drug development space. Examples of such trials have been highlighted and discussed in detail within several recent reviews [10, 17, 24, 64]. The earliest examples of comparative oncology trials were conducted by groups actively involved in osteosarcoma and mast cell tumor research, but quickly moved into other diseases and molecular targets as the concept gained traction [22, 29, 42, 46]. One of the best examples is the clinical studies of the liposomal form of Muramyl-TriPeptide-Phosphatidyl Ethanolamine (L-MTP-PE; L-mifamurtide, MEPACT®) conducted in dogs with osteosarcoma and other solid tumors, in which the efficacy of this agent in combination with cisplatin was shown in dogs and informed the ensuing studies in humans [33] More contemporary examples include trials that have evaluated experimental small molecule agents such as the selective inhibitor of nuclear export (SINE) verdinexor, the p97 inhibitor CB-5339, and the indenoisoquinoline class of topoisomerase-1 inhibitors, among others [4, 14, 27, 30, 31, 65, 67]. Studies evaluating agents such as ibrutinib, sirolimus, vemurafenib, sunitinib, and losartan also demonstrate the value of a comparative oncology trial to advance a novel antitumor concept through repurposed use of an FDA-approved and/or non-oncology drug [25, 26, 51–53, 59].

Comparative oncology trials have goals and objectives that are designed around drug development questions that are not adequately asked or answered within rodent studies and are deemed critical to optimizing development strategy for

A. LeBlanc (✉) · C. Mazcko · J. Beck
Comparative Oncology Program, Center for Cancer Research, National Cancer Institute, National Institutes of Health, Bethesda, MD, USA
e-mail: amy.leblanc@nih.gov

E. Berger
Frederick National Laboratory for Cancer Research in the Comparative Oncology Program, National Cancer Institute, National Institutes of Health, Bethesda, MD, USA

M. W. Nolan et al. (eds.), *Comparative Oncology*, https://doi.org/10.1007/978-3-032-04454-9_16

eventual human use. With that in mind, comparative oncology studies are not always feasible, tractable, or necessary. Ideally, canine data inform at least one (but often several) of the following critical information points in the conduct of subsequent human trials: a go/no-go decision; an optimal dose/schedule; elucidation of drug mechanism, including on-target, off-target, and on-tumor, off-tumor effects; optimal timing of PK/PD collections; or insight into responsive cancer histologies [11, 12, 41, 44]. Careful consideration of whether it is appropriate to acquire data from tumor-bearing pet dogs is needed; and when that data is generated, how it will be interpreted and incorporated into development strategy for that agent. The pet dog as a cancer patient does not equate to an informative or appropriate model for all human cancers, nor should one infer that tumors developing in the same site/location possess the same features and therapeutic vulnerabilities between species.

The main goal of comparative oncology clinical trials should be to first define the drug development and/or cancer biology questions that frame the context and objectives of the trial [24]. Are these questions that can't be sufficiently asked or answered in other cancer models? Has the relevant cancer biology been credentialed in the dog, and to what extent? Is a specific tumor type or histology necessary? Further, from the standpoint of cancer immunotherapy development, considerations may differ, particularly in the setting of target-specific vs. general immunotherapeutic strategies. The presence of an intact, educated immune system is a major advantage for the inclusion of pet dog data [1, 2, 9]. However, knowledge of the specific immune targets, and their expression and/or role in canine cancer immunobiology must be understood. Further, development of informative immunology assays with validated canine reagents should be incorporated to allow interpretation of the results and relation of the findings to known or suspected consequences of the same drug exposure in humans. Additional consideration should be given to the nature of the immunotherapy in question: is it relating to a specific immunologic target, or just leveraging the presence of a tumor that has developed in an immune-competent host? Is there a lack of available preclinical models or a specific aspect of drug mechanism that can't be sufficiently explored in a preclinical model? For such questions, comparative oncology trials provide opportunities for serial biological and clinical sample collection in a longitudinal setting. Further, new tools have become available in the last 3–5 years that support interpretation of data relating to correlative immunology, genomics, and circulating biomarkers. These include improved annotation of the canine genome, access to liquid biopsy techniques that leverage circulating tumor DNA, canine-specific transcriptional profiling tools, and increased availability of validated antibodies and other reagents [7, 8, 13, 18, 20, 28, 34, 45, 61–63, 69, 73].

1.2 Challenges Facing the Field

Despite significant and well-known advantages of the comparative oncology approach, key gaps in knowledge and challenges persist. A selected list of these challenges is outlined below:

- Credentialing of comparative biology: This is a key component of a successful comparative oncology trial. Rather than assuming human and canine cancers share the same driver/initiating events or therapeutic vulnerabilities, the investigative team must have knowledge of drug target(s) and an understanding of the correlative canine and human cancer biology. When detailed mechanisms and targets are unknown or not fully characterized, empiric validation of the approach can come from knowledge of the investigational agent drug class and/or purported mechanism of action (MOA) [4]. Specific knowledge of canine cancer biology and drug targets has been previously hindered by lack of large-scale genomic studies and canine-validated reagents for target detection and consequences (i.e., changes in downstream signaling) of target modulation. Recent efforts in this space have improved the overall landscape, but additional work is needed to expand this area to in turn support

additional comparative concepts to be considered.
- Enrollment: The comparative oncology space has expanded significantly in the last 5–8 years, with similar increasing demand for veterinary-specific oncology drugs. Competition for cases has necessitated expansion of the work from academic centers into large private practice groups that can participate in clinical trial activities. With this demand come issues relating to the workforce needed to conduct comparative oncology clinical trials and the need for protected time among veterinary clinicians and technical/support staff. Further, enrollment of pet dogs meeting a specific set of eligibility criteria cannot be predicted within a specific timeframe. While enrollment is facilitated by multi-center trial infrastructure, the timeline for completion of comparative oncology trials is not always congruent with that of a pharma-led drug development plan.
- Budget: Comparative oncology trials are costly in comparison to mouse/other preclinical species but are much less so than comparable human trials. In the planning phase of any trial, it is vitally important to ensure adequate budgeting for not just clinical management of animals, but for correlative studies that are key to interpreting study results, drug pharmacokinetics, tumor cytology/histopathology/immunohistochemistry, flow cytometry, or other assays that are valid in a dog-specific environment. Correlative studies that inform on the drug target(s) of interest and/or anticipated up- and downstream events are critical for interpretation of the clinical trial outcome. Additionally, funding to support pet owners through management of expected and unexpected adverse events should be included.
- Data sharing: This challenge is in part addressed through the National Cancer Institute's Integrated Canine Data Commons (ICDC), a node within the NCI's Cancer Research Data Commons environment [23]. The ICDC allows deposition of canine cancer datasets that span a variety of disciplines, including histopathology, imaging, genomics, and clinical data. As a publicly available repository, the ICDC facilitates access to and analysis of canine cancer datasets and encourages the comparisons between species.

2 Types of Comparative Oncology Clinical Trials

The design of comparative oncology clinical trials may borrow many elements from the classical phased approach to the registration of investigational new drugs for humans, but differ in many important ways. In addition, comparative oncology trials often do not neatly fit within a single phase, but rather may combine features of one or more phases, in order to maximize the value added by querying the pet dog. Below, a discussion of the classical phases of the investigational new drug pipeline is provided in the context of comparative oncology.

2.1 Phase 0 Trials

The classic phase 0 trial, also sometimes referred to as an exploratory or pre-phase I study, may investigate the agent's ability to accumulate within target lesions, show evidence of pharmacodynamic modulation, and demonstrate representative pharmacokinetic data [21]. These studies may also be used to choose a lead agent from a pool of chemically similar entities, especially if these entities perform equivocally in vitro or in vivo in rodent studies. The main draw of conducting such a study in human subjects is the collection of biologically rich data sets, such as blood samples, serial biopsies, and imaging data. However, they require that subtherapeutic doses (i.e., a dose unlikely to cause any toxicity) be given, and therefore, the chance of benefit to the patient approaches zero. In addition, the collection of such extensive serial data sets often requires the patient to submit to additional, sometimes invasive, tests without a meaningful chance of benefit from the agent.

2.2 Phase I Trials

A traditional phase I clinical trial is often referred to as "dose-finding" and its primary endpoint is the determination of a maximally tolerated dose (MTD). This is traditionally accomplished by treating cohorts of three individuals at progressively increasing doses of the experimental agent and monitoring for toxicity based upon standardized criteria, with tailoring for veterinary patients (Common Terminology and Criteria for Adverse Events [CTCAE; www.ctep.cancer.gov] [25, 26]). If a serious toxicity is seen, a cohort expansion is conducted, and if further serious toxicity is noted, the dose of the cohort below is considered the MTD. This is known as a 3 + 3 ("three-plus-three") design. Efficacy is not determined in these early phase trials.

2.3 Phase II Trials

The phase II trial is commonly known as an efficacy or activity trial. Here, the investigational agent is examined in the disease of interest for evidence of efficacy. Whether the investigational agent is superior or equivalent to the standard treatment is not examined, and thus, control groups or placebos are not utilized. These trials are larger than phase I trials, and enrollment is more limited to not only the disease but also the particular disease stage of interest. Therefore, the time commitment in the phase II trial is significantly higher than that of earlier phases. Because of the larger study population, rare adverse effects may be noted, and thus, safety continues to be an important secondary endpoint of phase II trials.

2.4 Phase III Trials

If an investigational agent shows efficacy in the disease of interest in its phase II trial, it can then progress to phase III, in which the agent is compared to either *placebo* (an inactive treatment) or no treatment, or to standard therapy. A placebo is only ethically used if no effective treatment is known. When an agent is compared to standard-of-care, it is important to define the goal of the trial: Is the intent to demonstrate *superiority*, that the investigational agent is better than the standard; *equivalence*, that the agent is materially similar to the standard; or *non-inferiority*, that the agent is not materially worse than the standard? In general, equivalence and non-inferiority are more forgiving standards; however, because the difference from the standard may be very small, a larger sample size is required to adequately power these trials.[1]

2.5 Unique Value of the Comparative Oncology Trial

One of the most valuable aspects of the well-designed comparative oncology trial is its ability to provide simultaneous insight into questions that traditionally must be asked in separate trials (Fig. 1). For instance, the comparative oncology trial is uniquely positioned to draw from many elements of the phase 0 trial, although rarely is it limited to *only* phase 0 activities. In particular, the pet dog's tolerance for serial biopsies and sample collection allows the accumulation of rich biologic data in the context of features of all phases. Thus, comparative oncology trials can provide insight into multiple investigational phases. Toxicity profiles, PK/PD relationships, efficacy, and head-to-head comparison of chemically equivalent compounds can all potentially be pursued in a well-designed and -funded pet dog study (Table 1).

The 3 + 3 design is a common choice for comparative oncology trials which are designed to query the acute and/or chronic toxicity profile of an agent. However, the canine 3 + 3 clinical trial is not limited to toxicity profiling; serial sampling, especially in the context of chronic drug exposure, can elucidate pharmacokinetic/pharmacodynamic relationships (a feature of phase 0

[1]For more information visit www.fda.gov/media/78504/download/; *Non-Inferiority Clinical Trials to Establish Effectiveness: Guidance for Industry.*

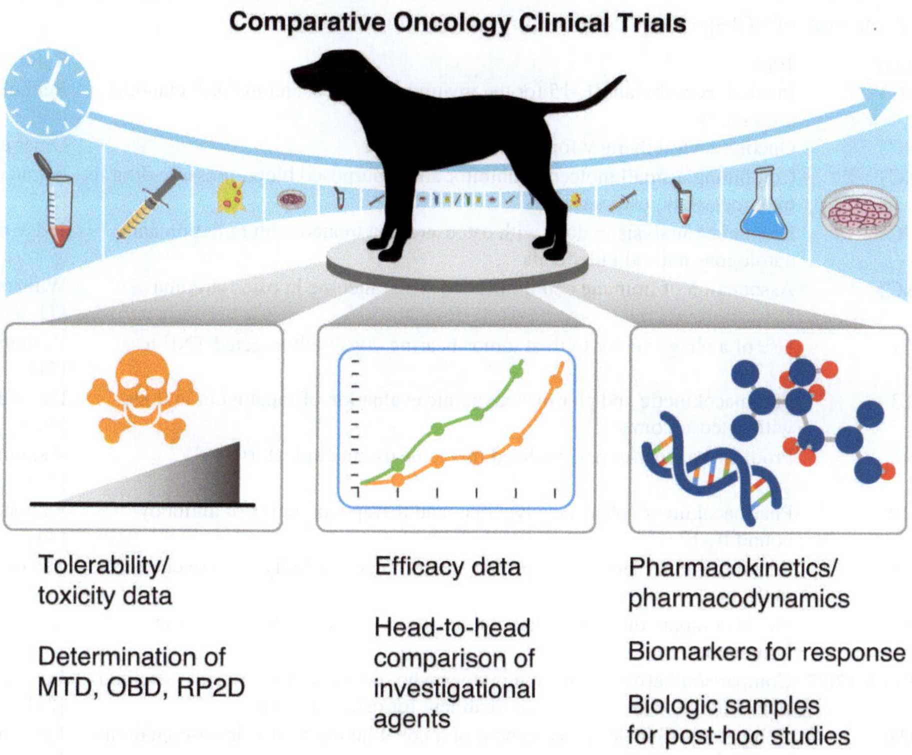

Fig. 1 Comparative oncology clinical trials conducted in pet dogs can provide a triad of data types within a single trial design, encompassing clinical data conducted in a longitudinal format, as well as correlative biologic data to enhance the translational value of such studies

trials), and because pet dogs may participate in clinical trials when treatment-naïve, efficacy signals (a traditional endpoint of phase II trials) may be seen outside the context of preexisting drug resistance.

Because the clinical course of some tumor types is accelerated in pet dogs compared to humans, efficacy of an agent can be determined in a shorter time. This may be particularly useful when an agent may show in vitro or in vivo preclinical efficacy in several seemingly unrelated malignancies. With properly credentialed biology in the equivalent canine tumor type, efficacy in one or more of the promising preclinical candidates can be further supported. Important considerations when examining efficacy in the comparative oncology context are the use of canine-appropriate endpoints and establishing whether a particular canine histology can be reasonably compared to a corresponding human histology.

2.6 Adaptive and Other Alternative Trial Designs

Because of the richness of correlative data that comparative oncology trials can provide (PK/PD, biomarker, etc.), they also lend themselves to adaptive designs of many types. An *adaptive* trial design is defined by the FDA as "a clinical trial design that allows for prospectively planned modifications to one or more aspects of the design based on accumulating data from subjects in the trial." This may be as simple as a planned interim analysis to examine the relationship between PK and PD modulation or an algorithm to define when the trial may be terminated prematurely in the face of clear futility or superiority. More recent adaptive designs employ a variety of formal statistical methods, such as in the case of *Bayesian* adaptive designs.

Table 1 A summary of NCI-sponsored comparative oncology clinical trials

Consortium	Topic	References
PRECINCT	Inhaled recombinant IL-15 for the treatment of osteosarcoma or melanoma metastases	Rebhun et al. [49]
PRECINCT	Oncolytic viral therapy for treatment of glioma	Omar et al. [37]
PRECINCT	Combining a small molecule inhibitor and repurposed blood pressure drug to treat metastatic osteosarcoma	Regan et al. [52]
PRECINCT	Biomarker analysis in dogs with osteosarcoma treated with radiation and autologous natural killer cells	Judge et al. [16]
PRECINCT	Association of immune cell infiltration with outcome in osteosarcoma	Withers et al. [71, 72]
COTC001	Use of a phage vector to treat tumor-bearing dogs with targeted TNF-α	Paoloni et al. [41]
COTC003	Pharmacokinetic and pharmacodynamic evaluation of rapamycin in dogs with osteosarcoma	Paoloni et al. [42]
COTC016	Proof-of-concept of personalized medicine use in clinical trials	Paoloni et al. [43]
COTC010	Pharmacokinetic, pharmacodynamic, and therapeutic index of antibody-bound IL-12	Paoloni et al. [44]
COTC018	Defining a pharmacokinetic profile and biological activity in a novel small molecule	Saba et al. [55]
COTC007b	Direct comparison of three novel topoisomerase I inhibitors in canine lymphoma	Burton et al. [4]
COTC020/021/022	Comparison between outcome in dogs who did and did not receive sirolimus in addition to standard-of-care treatment for osteosarcoma	LeBlanc et al. [27]
COTC028	Comparative oncology assessment of a novel inhibitor of valosin-containing protein in tumor-bearing dogs	LeBlanc et al. [27]

The oncology drug development landscape is increasingly dominated by individualized therapies—examples include small molecules, monoclonal antibodies, and engineered cellular therapies. These individualized therapies have necessitated refinement of the traditional phase III approach to include both (1) the variety of molecular changes present within a single tumor or histologic type, and (2) the similarity of molecular features across morphologically distinct malignancies. The resulting umbrella and basket trial designs address these situations.[2]

A *basket* trial design (Fig. 2a) utilizes a "histology-agnostic" approach that groups patients whose tumors have a particular feature or features, regardless of their tumor type. In theory, a basket design groups together patients most likely to benefit from a single targeted therapy together into the same group or "basket." In addition, basket designs can demonstrate a therapy's efficacy in several tumor types simultaneously. However, investigators should ensure that credentialed biology exists in all eligible histologies, and the pet dog is no exception.

In contrast, an *umbrella* clinical trial (Fig. 2b) groups a single tumor type under one "umbrella," and then subdivides it into groups, each based upon a common molecular feature. Each subgroup receives an experimental treatment targeted at their common feature, or in later phase trials may be randomized to receive either standard therapy or the experimental targeted agent. In general, umbrella trials also include a "standard" arm that allows participants without identified actionable features to receive standard-of-care therapy. This trial allows multiple targeted therapies to be directly compared to standard therapy, both within and without each subgroup, simultaneously. However, as with basket designs, credentialing the biology within the tumors and/or histology of interest is essential to a successful pet dog trial.

[2]For more information visit www.fda.gov/media/78495/download/; *Adaptive Designs for Clinical Trials of Drugs and Biologics: Guidance for Industry.*

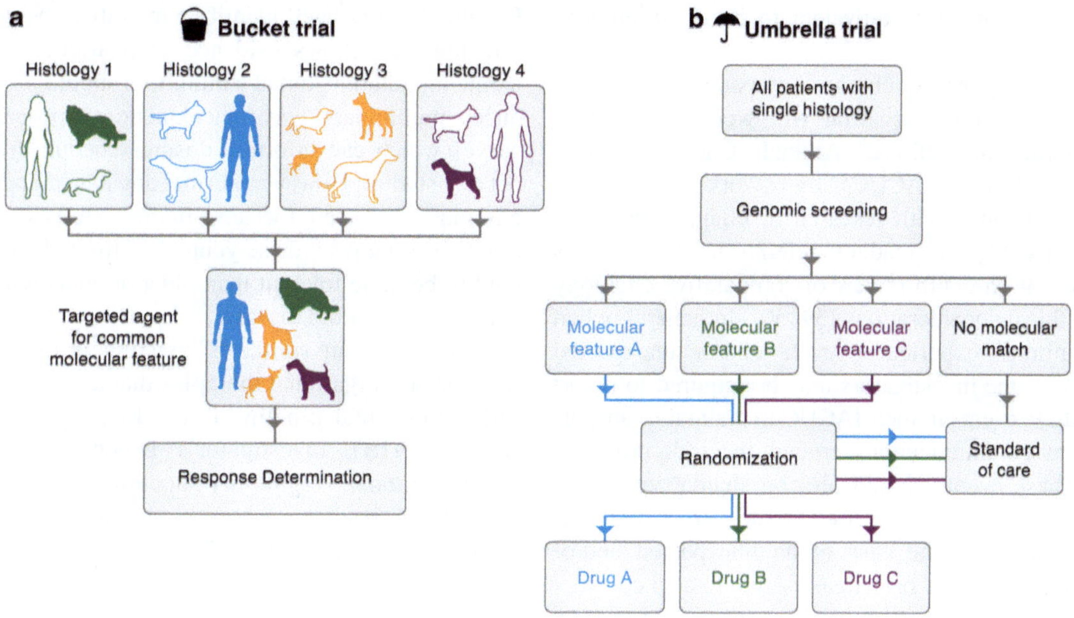

Fig. 2 (**a**) A basket trial enrolls patients whose tumors share a common molecular feature (*solid silhouettes*), regardless of their tumor type. (**b**) An umbrella trial enrolls patients with a single tumor type of interest and then subdivides them based upon molecular features (*Molecular Feature A/B/C*) common between their individual tumors

3 Organizing Clinical Trials: Logistical and Technical Aspects

In the same way that a well-planned pet dog trial can add invaluable correlated data to the investigation of a variety of research questions, a poorly planned trial will result in unusable or uninterpretable data while exposing client-owned animals to potential adverse events. Therefore, it is essential to carefully consider the organization and structure of a trial to ensure the data are able to answer the question or questions being asked of them. Many aspects of study design important in trials featuring human subjects are also important in trials of canine subjects. Careful consideration of these will improve study design both in respect to data collected and to the experience of the dog and their owner.

3.1 Regulatory Oversight Considerations

Comparative oncology trials are separate from veterinary registration trials, and do not aim to result in approval of a veterinary-specific drug or device. These research studies are not required to adhere to the Good Practices codes (Good Manufacturing, Laboratory, and Clinical Practices; GMP/GLP/GCP). GMP is not therefore required for the formulation of canine-specific research compounds/drugs, and studies in purpose-bred dogs are not required to adhere to GLP. However, it is best practice to work toward GCP guidelines when practical in the execution of pet dog trials to ensure quality data management. In addition, it may be beneficial to work with a veterinary pharmacologist or other professional with expertise in the formulation of veterinary drugs, as the canine species' tolerances for contaminants such as endotoxin, among others, are not equivalent to those of humans [17].[3]

Every institution enrolling patients on a comparative oncology trial will work within their home Institutional Animal Care and Use Committee (IACUC) framework to maintain compliance with research in client-owned animals [11]. The reader is referred to other sources for an in-depth review of comparative oncology ethical considerations [39, 50]. In general, when animals experience severe and/or unexpected AEs, the investigators may be required to report these events to their IACUC to maintain transparent communications around the trial progress. These events should also be shared with other investigators in the case of multi-site studies, particularly in the case of an unexpected and/or grade 5 event. Investigators should also consider the creation of a trial-specific Data Safety Monitoring Board (DSMB). The role of a DSMB is to act as an impartial source of guidance for the trial, with emphasis on the safety of the trial participants and attribution and grading of unexpected adverse events [11]. DSMB committees consist of a membership comprising knowledgeable veterinary oncologists and other subject matter experts who are not directly involved with the recruitment of the study to avoid conflicts of interest.

3.2 Data Required to Support the Comparative Oncology Trial

To give the best chance of IACUC approval, supporting data are needed to demonstrate a compound's preliminary safety in dogs at the dose or doses chosen for a trial. These data are primarily obtained in healthy, purpose-bred dogs. Such studies may or may not end with euthanasia, but should demonstrate that the proposed dose level(s) do not result in unacceptable toxicity. Ideally, the study will identify a tolerable dosing schedule that shows evidence of pharmacodynamic modulation, but at a minimum should produce preliminary pharmacokinetic exposure curves which can inform a dosing schedule for pet dog studies. However, normal dog data do not eliminate the need for dose-finding studies in tumor-bearing pets; these young healthy animals tend to be more tolerant than older animals who may have comorbid disease.

One important source of existing information for investigational therapies that are within a developmental pipeline is the Investigator's Brochure (IB). Investigator's Brochures are multifunctional, regulatory documents compiled by a study sponsor in preparation for human clinical trials. The IB is a compilation of confidential clinical and nonclinical data describing a variety of key aspects of the drug's physical, chemical, pharmaceutical, pharmacological, toxicological, and clinical properties. This document is regularly updated throughout the drug development process and is critical for initiating human clinical trials as it describes the rationale for drug dose/schedule/route of administration and patient safety monitoring procedures. Contained within the IB is a summary of laboratory animal data collected in preparation for a human clinical trial. If available to the veterinary investigator conducting a trial of the agent in pet dogs, these data can inform a starting dose/schedule and monitoring strategy that is harmonized with planned human clinical studies. Due to their comprehensive and confidential nature, IBs are not usually publicly available, but could be accessed through collaborative research agreements made between veterinary investigators and study sponsors.

3.3 Study Design Essentials

3.3.1 Identifying the Desired Trial Population

Considering what groups of dogs should be included in a comparative oncology trial is another important step of trial design.

[3]For more information visit https://www.fda.gov/drugs/pharmaceutical-quality-resources/current-good-manufacturing-practice-cgmp-regulations; *Current Good Manufacturing Practice Regulations.*

3.3.1.1 Demographics and Comorbid Disease

Generally, age restriction is not required; most pet dogs with cancer are middle-aged to older (6–11 years old); juvenile or young adult malignancy cases are seen but are the exception in canine oncology [47]. In some cases, determining whether a trial should only include neutered pets may be important. Many tumor-bearing pets have comorbidities of varying severity. Determining whether comorbid diseases may interact or interfere with the investigational agent can guide the definition of specific exclusion criteria. For example, a trial of a drug primarily excreted via the kidneys may wish to have more strict controls on renal function than one in which the investigational agent is processed exclusively by the liver. Trials of immune-active agents may wish to exclude dogs with comorbid autoimmune disease, such as primary immune-mediated hemolytic anemia or acquired myasthenia gravis, even if these diseases are well-controlled. The minimum weight of any pet enrolled on a trial must allow for collection of all desired research specimens, particularly blood sampling. In general, laboratory animal guidelines stipulate that no more than 10% of an animal's circulating blood volume be collected at a single time point, or if collecting serial samples, over a two-week period. A maximum weight may also need to be implemented based on drug supply availability and dosing requirements (number of capsules given at one time, volume of IV drug administration, etc.).

3.3.1.2 Disease and Stage

Along with demographic and general health history, histologic tumor diagnosis and disease stage are both important factors to consider. Does the trial need to include only one tumor type or histologic subtype, or can a group of tumor types or histologies be included? What about "all comers" trials? Are patients with metastatic disease permitted? If excluding patients with metastatic disease, understanding the natural history of the canine cancer or cancers included in the study is essential. In addition, the investigator must determine how the presence of metastatic disease will be determined. Can patients be pretreated, or must they be treatment-naïve? If pretreated patients are permitted, washout periods for chemotherapy, radiation therapy, and glucocorticoids should be considered at a minimum; the class of investigational agent (i.e., small molecule, immunotherapy) may dictate additional washout considerations. In addition, enrollment criteria should ensure that patient lesions for biopsy are of sufficient size, especially if serial biopsies are desired.

3.3.1.3 Identifying a Control Group

Control groups are important features of many clinical trials. The inclusion of a control group in a comparative oncology trial depends on the question or questions being asked of the resultant data. For example, in a trial in which the most important question is to identify a PK/PD relationship, a control group is unnecessary. A control group would also be unnecessary for a dose/schedule finding study. Even in trials asking efficacy-related questions, a control group may not be needed. However, there are many situations in which it is appropriate to include a control group. A control group may be a small cohort of healthy dogs if the only required samples are primarily noninvasive, and if healthy dogs represent an appropriate control. An appropriate control group may alternatively be dogs with cancer being treated with the current veterinary standard of care, if such standard is equivalent or at least comparable to the standard in human patients with the disease. Because prospectively enrolling such a group will both lengthen a trial (requiring additional enrollment) and raise associated costs, it is often appropriate to use historical control groups. When using historical controls, emphasis should be placed on groups that have received as standardized a treatment regimen as is possible. Historical control groups should be as recent as is available, and the group should be adequately powered. Data sharing resources such as the Integrated Canine Data Commons (ICDC), a project funded by the National Cancer Institute (NCI), can provide valuable datasets of historical patients with rich clinical and biological correlates which can serve as historical controls.

Generally, it is inappropriate to utilize a placebo treatment in dogs with cancer outside of veterinary pivotal registration trials; in limited circumstances, placebo treatment may be appropriate.[4]

3.3.2 Selecting Appropriate Endpoints

The NIH defines an *endpoint* as "an event or outcome [in a clinical trial] used to objectively measure the effect of a drug or other intervention being studied." Endpoints generally fall under one of three categories: biological, clinical, and humane. Biological endpoints denote biological samples collected in the trial. A trial may collect canine plasma to measure an investigational agent's pharmacokinetic properties; this is a biological endpoint. Clinical endpoints are statements of the goals of the trial. In a 3 + 3 dose-finding study, a clinical endpoint could be the toxicity profile of the investigational agent. Importantly, when defining a study's clinical endpoint, an investigator must account for the concept that euthanasia is an acceptable outcome in the tumor-bearing dog if the owner elects or circumstances warrant. Therefore, overall survival or related metrics may be inappropriate as their measurement can be biased by euthanasia. Investigators should instead consider surrogates such as progression-free survival or disease-free interval which are obtained more rapidly and avoid euthanasia bias. Finally, identification of humane endpoints is essential to the success of an ethical comparative oncology clinical trial. Humane endpoints are exit points or "relief valves" through which dogs who are not benefiting from the investigational therapy, or are experiencing adverse effects of the therapy, are released from the study to pursue a different treatment. Humane endpoints can encompass planned disease assessments, definition of *dose-limiting toxicity* (DLT) events, and regular clinical evaluation by veterinary investigators participating in the trial to ensure the health and comfort of patients. Furthermore, as is the case with human subjects, the owners (as proxy for their pet) retain the right to withdraw their pet from the study at any time.[5]

3.3.3 Correlative Assays and Biologic Sample Collection

Comparative oncology clinical trials offer opportunities to collect invaluable biospecimens. These samples can be interrogated to uncover new mechanisms of tumor sensitivity and identify predictive biomarkers with translational potential for human patients. A well-developed trial will include a thorough outline of the types and timing of sample collection during trial progression. Clear diagramming of a trial schema and use of well-written, thorough Standard Operating Procedures (SOPs) will assist veterinary investigators in their sample collection (Fig. 3). The ability of trial samples to inform cancer research hinges on the identification of appropriate biospecimens and application of suitable species-specific validated analyses.

From the initial biopsy to the collection of tissues at necropsy, histopathology is a critical component of all clinical trials. Formalin-fixed tissues collected at biopsy should be evaluated by a board-certified veterinary anatomic pathologist to confirm disease diagnosis and trial eligibility. Final diagnosis is based on the tumor's histologic appearance and may be supported by immunohistochemistry or histochemical stains. Depending on the trial, tumor grading can be completed and may parallel that described in physician medicine. Efforts to harmonize tumor classification and grading between human and canine patients continue to improve the translational value of canine clinical trials [3, 19, 58].

Following enrollment, multiple sample types are obtained from canine patients and vary based on the scientific question at hand. Commonly collected samples include tumor and non-tumor tissues, plasma, and whole blood. Laboratory work, including complete blood count (CBC), serum biochemical profile, urinalysis, imaging, and pharmacokinetic sampling of whole blood, is frequently used for clinical monitoring of dogs in

[4]For more information visit https://datacommons.cancer.gov/repository/integrated-canine-data-commons

[5]For more information visit: https://clinicalinfo.hiv.gov/en/glossary/clinical-endpoint

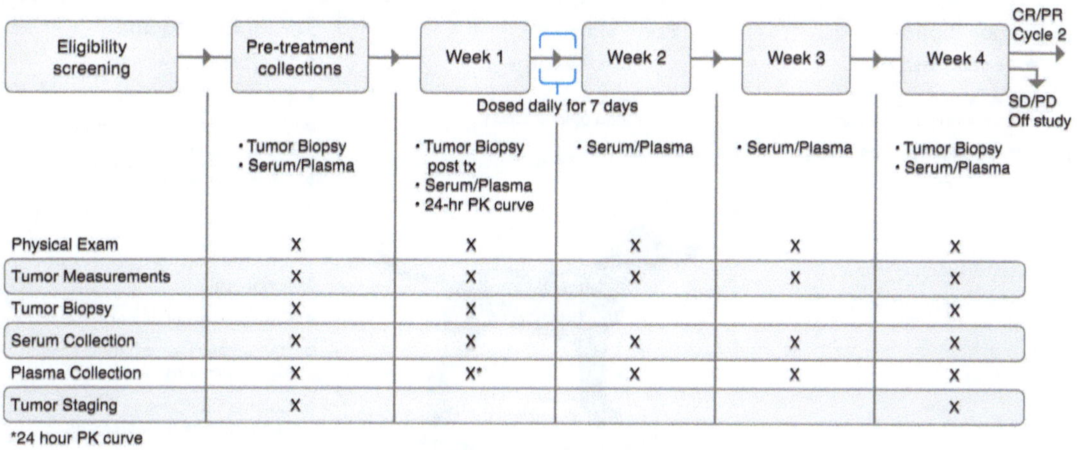

Fig. 3 A study schema presents a clear overview of essential trial information and, along with well-written, thorough standard operating procedures (SOPs), will assist veterinary investigators in their sample collection

trial (see Fig. 4) [4, 25, 26, 42, 43, 55]. Enrolled canine patients are repeatedly examined by veterinary oncologists and trial personnel during the progression of a clinical trial. This facilitates the collection of invaluable biospecimens including collection of pre- and posttreatment tissues. For example, serial tumor biopsies allow researchers to monitor T lymphocyte response to immunotherapeutics using immunohistochemistry or RNA expression of immune-related genes [16, 44]. Serial collection of non-tumor tissues through biopsy or postmortem exam has been used to gather critical understanding of treatment specificity which may hold relevance for acute treatment toxicities and potential chronic effects of cancer therapy [41, 55]. A critical feature of the tumor-bearing dog is its intact immune system which bears resemblance to the immune system in humans [1, 5, 9]. Different sample types can be evaluated to interrogate immune cell functions in canine patients. For example, fine needle aspiration of peripheral tumor-draining lymph nodes may elucidate the systemic immune response [44]. In addition, peripheral blood mononuclear cells (PBMCs) facilitate a variety of studies including ex vivo cytotoxicity or migration, flow cytometry, and RNA-seq while plasma samples are frequently used to assess treatment-associated cytokine production and its relevance to clinical response [16, 49, 52]. These types of studies highlight the value of the canine model for investigating antitumor immunity in cancer progression and treatment response [16, 71, 72].

Progression-free survival (PFS) is a critical outcome variable in canine trials. While clinical parameters, such as physical examination and imaging of metastases, are reliable indicators for PFS, autopsy offers a thorough examination of all tissues with histologic confirmation of suspected metastases. Compared to the diagnostic biopsy, autopsies offer access to larger volume samples including treatment-resistant primary and metastatic tumor tissue. Access to postmortem samples from human patients can be challenging which may be in part due to significant advances in medical diagnostics [6, 15, 60]. In canine patients, full necropsies are routinely completed, providing access to non-tumor and tumor tissues, including matched metastases. Compared to small antemortem tumor sampling, access to large tumors during autopsy can shed light on the spatial complexity and clonal evolution of a tumor through multi-region sampling. In addition, a postmortem examination permits the collection of multiple non-tumor samples, such as tumor-adjacent tissue and grossly normal organs, providing additional information about the tumor microenvironment and systemic effects of cancer and cancer therapy.

Determination of collected biospecimens and subsequent analyses is a critical component of

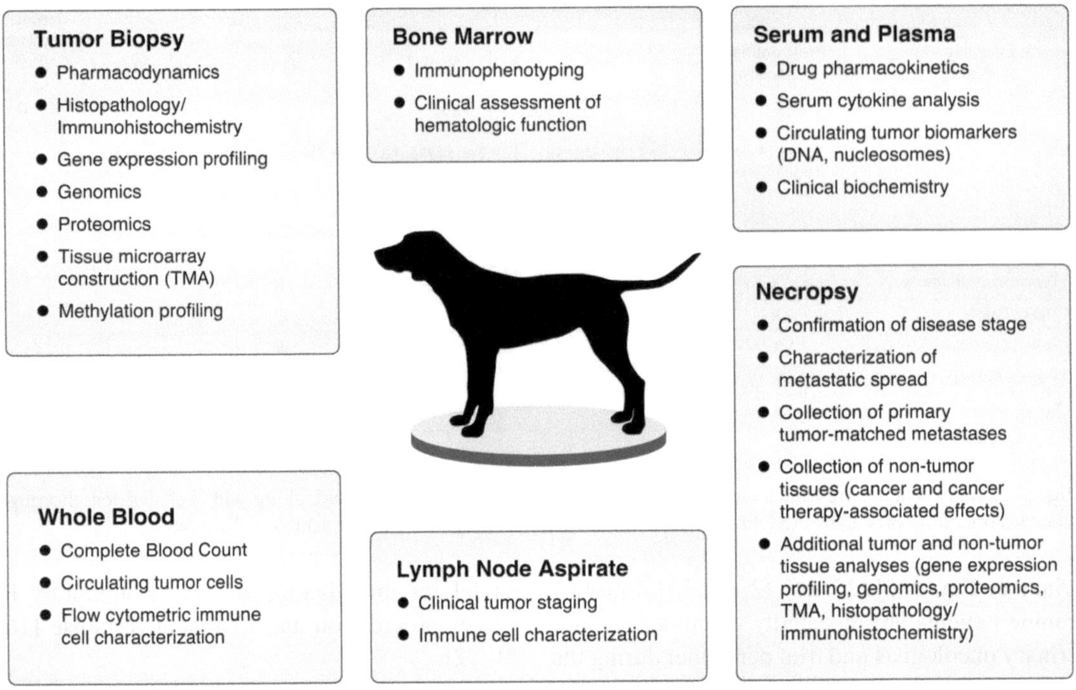

Fig. 4 Following enrollment, multiple sample types can be obtained from the same canine patient and lend themselves to an array of analyses based on the scientific question at hand

canine clinical trials that requires an immense amount of work but can yield tremendous data. Incorporating pathologist input on trial design helps ensure that the appropriate tissue samples are collected, processed, and stored. Standard operating procedures (SOP) should be implemented for all clinical trials. This ensures that all samples are collected following the same instructions. This is especially critical in a multi-institutional study where different groups will be collecting and processing samples. Before enrollment opens, it is important to know what type of samples will be collected and when; how they should be collected and stored; where they will be sent for analysis; and the timeline for shipment (overnight vs. batched). Participating sites would need to have the necessary equipment to process and store samples per the SOP. This information is critical to the study and should be in the SOP. It is recommended that the end user of the samples is involved in the SOP development to ensure they are receiving the samples that are the highest possible quality. The timing of sample collection should also be outlined in the study protocol. It is important to know which samples need to be shipped overnight and processed immediately. This will impact the overall study schedule and knowing what days of the week a patient can begin on study. Samples are typically collected prior to study test article administration to serve as a baseline and then at specific timepoints throughout the course of the study. A set window of time should be described in the protocol to allow for collections. For example, if collecting a pretreatment biopsy, an investigator may wish to specify that it occurs within 24 h of starting the drug administration. Samples collected during or post-administration should be at defined times (e.g., 30 min after beginning infusion; 4-h post-administration) to allow for uniformity across patient samples.

Higher incidence of certain cancer types in the dog provides for a significantly larger patient population which supports trial enrollment and biospecimen collection. While large trials with their associated sample repositories have clear benefits from a data perspective, they also offer unique challenges for sample storage and management particularly for frozen samples. Efforts to streamline sample collection include the preparation of trial kits which specify the samples to be taken and include the appropriate pre-labeled vials and storage media. If trial kits are not included, it is recommended that a detailed supply list (including vendors and catalog numbers) be provided. These methods can be further improved with an understanding of the subsequent analyses. For example, storage in RNA later and tissue-specific processing can enhance RNA extraction from frozen tissue aliquots [35]. In some cases, sending samples to a central location can help to improve processing and reduce batch effects. It is recommended to identify a sample tracking mechanism before beginning a clinical trial. A web-accessible system, such as the Labmatrix software platform, allows users to track samples from creation through exhaustion. It also facilitates a seamless transfer of samples between different users. The procurement of multiple sample types from the same patient allows for comprehensive assessment of treatment response and disease progression. In addition to informing the initial trial, these accumulated samples and data can support numerous post hoc studies which can, in turn, yield additional therapeutic targets to support future trial concepts.

3.3.4 Study Communications and Engaging Enrollment Sites

Even if the preclinical research for an investigational compound, imaging agent, or device is performed at a veterinary research institution, unless that institution also sees client-owned animals on a regular basis, investigators must engage with outside institutions to facilitate enrollment, data generation, and sample collection. This becomes increasingly true with larger studies: the more dogs to be enrolled, the more institutions must be engaged to ensure timely completion of enrollment.

The type of veterinary institution(s) engaged is also important. In the case of the tumor-bearing dog, the greatest concentration of potentially eligible dogs will likely occur at referral institutions where at least one board-certified veterinary oncologist is practicing. Smaller referral institutions are less likely to have the staff and equipment required for procedure-intensive trials or advanced sample processing (e.g., extraction of peripheral blood mononuclear cells from whole blood), although each institution must be examined separately. Each site engaged will need to have or be able to engage an established IACUC committee for protocol review and approval to ensure compliance with protocol and research standards. Existing consortia, such as the Comparative Oncology Trials Consortium (COTC; https://ccr.cancer.gov/comparative-oncology-program/consortium), Clinical and Translational Science Award (CTSA) One Health Alliance (COHA), the Duke/North Carolina State University Consortium for Canine Comparative Oncology (C3O), or the NCI-funded Pre-medical Cancer Immunotherapy Network for Canine Trials (PRECINCT; https://www.precinctnetwork.org/) can provide guidance to institutions prepared to conduct such trials. Another group of note is the Comparative Oncology Research Consortium (CORC), which represents a cooperative group of comparative oncology researchers and scientists with formal affiliation with an NCI Comprehensive Cancer Center (www.v.org/research/specialfunds/canine-comparative-oncology).

Comprehensive protocol review and good communication are critical for trials, particularly those that have open enrollment at multiple sites. It is recommended that a communication plan be put in place prior to a study opening. Typical methods include group emails or other communication applications such as Slack. It is also helpful to have final versions of the protocol, SOPs, and any protocol amendments available in a shared cloud-based location for ease of access. If the study is multi-institutional, it is critical to keep all sites aware of enrollment numbers and available spots. There is often a break in available enrollment spots during a dose escalation study, as the PI waits for patients to reach a certain time point. It is important to keep the study sponsor apprised of the progress of the study. This can often be accomplished with a monthly meeting to review the study reports.

3.3.5 Data Reporting and Statistical Considerations

When planning a comparative oncology trial, it is important to consider how the collected data will be reported. Two general schemas may be used: an intent-to-treat analysis or a per-protocol analysis. *Intent-to-treat* analysis includes all trial participants in the data analysis, whether or not they strictly adhered to trial protocol, completed the entire observation period, or even began treatment with the investigational agent. For example, in randomized trials, any patient that is randomized is included in an intent-to-treat analysis, regardless of what occurs after randomization. Conversely, a *per-protocol* analysis analyzes only patients who strictly adhered to and completed either the entire or at least a designated minimum portion (e.g., half the observation period) of the trial protocol. Intent-to-treat analysis is considered the gold standard of reporting which eliminates bias inherent in the per-protocol method and makes results more generalizable; however, per-protocol analysis has its place and can be used alongside intent-to-treat analyses to good effect. Excellent and detailed guidance about when and how to utilize these analysis strategies is presented by the Consolidated Standards of Reporting Trials (CONSORT). An updated veterinary-tailored reporting guidance, PetSORT, is also available to address the unique features and reporting requirements for client-owned pet populations [54, 56].

Additionally, before implementing a clinical trial, it is recommended that an electronic data capture platform is selected and designed. One example is REDCap (Research Electronic Data Capture), which is a user-friendly, secure web application for building and managing surveys and databases, and is commonly used for clinical trials. REDCap has the advantage of extensive customization options which lend its utility to many different types of studies. Once a study protocol is finalized, construction of the database can begin. Investigators and their teams should be trained on the database prior to enrolling their first patient.

3.3.6 Formulation of Investigational Agents

When conducting comparative oncology trials examining one or more investigational drugs, carefully considering the formulation to be used is essential. If the drug is intended for or is already being investigated in human patients, it is recommended that the same human formulation be utilized wherever possible. While potentially increasing expense, it ensures that any variance in PK or PD modulation in the dog may not be attributed to formulation variations. In the case of canine-specific research reagents, the compound may be given orally or intravenously, or more rarely intramuscularly or intratumorally. For orally administered agents, considerations include whether the powdered or liquid agent will be placed directly into a gelatin capsule (active pharmaceutical ingredient (API)-in-capsule), or whether a salt must be formulated and then placed in powdered form into a capsule (powder-in-capsule) or formulated into a pressed tablet. Thought should be given also to the dose size or sizes of capsules/tablets, as canine patients are of varying weights that can range from less than 3 kg to more than 65 kg at extremes. If the available dose sizes are too small, large dogs may have to take an unreasonable number of capsules/tablets per dose, which can cause gastrointestinal upset and even obstruction. If the available dose sizes are too large, smaller dogs will be unable to participate in the trial and the size of the eligible patient pool will be reduced. All agents must be free of contaminants just as they would for human studies. In particular, the dog is exquisitely sensitive to endotoxin, and the presence of even a small amount can cause severe adverse effects.[6]

3.4 Clinical Management of Patients on Trial

Veterinary oncology expertise is key to successful management of patients enrolled in comparative oncology clinical trials. Clinical data is

[6]For more information visit https://www.project-redcap.org/

routinely collected prior to, during, and after completion of the trial and includes physical exam findings and owner-reported historical data such as appetite, attitude at home, and/or the presence of specific clinical signs. If indicated, additional systems-specific instruments can be added to capture quality of life and performance metrics that are tailored for specific veterinary patients [32, 48, 57, 70].

3.4.1 Monitoring of Response

Staging of disease and confirmation of diagnosis is critical to patient eligibility determination. Review of original diagnostic material and associated reports (e.g., cytology or biopsy reports) can be considered alongside de novo procurement of tumor samples. This is particularly indicated in the case of historical disease progression/relapse, as comparative oncology trials often enroll both treatment-naïve and previously treated patients. Tumor staging, utilizing clinical imaging platforms congruent with human oncology (such as radiography, computed tomography, ultrasonography, magnetic resonance imaging) to determine response is often repeated during/after drug exposure according to trial endpoints and questions being asked within the trial schema. If repeated response measurements are taken, investigators should record "best response" and "overall response" to interpret the trajectory of response data.

Clinical imaging studies are often used to determine disease stage and monitor response to therapy. Whenever possible, it is advisable to standardize and ensure review of imaging studies by a board-certified veterinary radiologist. It could be noted that in the case of monitoring for pulmonary nodule progression, one should consider repeating thoracic radiographs in 3–4 weeks in the case of an equivocal or suspicious study and/or monitoring of small lesions (< 1.0 cm) in order to confirm disease progression. Recommendations for harmonized imaging standards have been developed to facilitate multicenter trials, specifically for brain tumors [38]. RECIST and lymphoma response guidelines have also been published to support standardization of response across enrolling centers [36, 68].

3.4.2 Adverse Events: Characterization and Management

Knowledge of the common presentation and natural course of the disease is important to management of these patients, as adverse events (AEs) that arise must be managed, described, and attributed appropriately. It is also important to communicate regularly with pet owners as some AEs are expected, while others can be unexpected. A list of expected adverse events should be listed in the informed consent that is signed by the pet owner and clinician before any study-related procedures occur. This is often the case in trials that are evaluating first-in-class agents and/or biologics. Updated standardized reporting guidelines, modeled on human Common Terminology and Criteria for Adverse Events (CTCAE), are available to assist in reporting and attribution of AEs observed in veterinary clinical trials [25, 26]. In general, these veterinary-specific CTCAE indicate that when a grade 2 event occurs, an intervention is needed to manage the event. Individual studies can define what grade and source of event (typically a grade 3 event) constitutes a dose-limiting toxicity (DLT). DLTs are important because when they occur, they may trigger a cohort expansion to more fully define the MTD for the agent under study. It is important to reconcile all adverse events that occur while on study. This is typically done between the study principal investigator (PI), the clinician team treating the patient, and possibly the study sponsor. During the reconciliation process, the grade should be confirmed based on the VCOG-CTCAE 2.0, or other AE reporting guidelines, and the attribution should be agreed upon. Standard attribution categories are as follows: Research, IND, Commercial, Disease, and Other. Each category is then given a score between 1 (unrelated) and 5 (definite). A detailed description can be found in the VCOG-CTCAE 2.0 [25, 26]. It is important to note that an event cannot be listed as "definite (5)" to more than one category, and it also cannot be listed as "unrelated (1)" in every category. As described above, standardized management of AEs is often included as part of a study protocol and is informed by the veterinary oncologists involved in the trial. As initiation of therapy is key to AE grading, it is advised to provide some prescriptive guidance for management of events that may occur to provide harmonization, particularly in the case of multicenter trials.

4 Conclusions

A conscientious investigator will ask several questions both before design, during the design phase, and before initiating a comparative oncology trial. Knowing the answers to these questions will ensure that the pet dog will be able to contribute valuable information to their effort in drug, imaging agent, or device development. Some important questions are outlined below:

What data need to be collected? Knowing this answer will allow the investigator to make informed choices of biological specimen collections and assays to evaluate those specimens.

Can the dog answer the question(s) being asked? Data and biological specimen collection in the dog should be driven by the investigator's ability to assess these valuable resources. Are assays available to evaluate the marker, interaction, or other processes in question? Have they been validated in the dog? Is the question being asked sufficiently specific to be viably answered? Can the question be answered with another model?

What value will the dog add to the research process? The investigator should imagine both positive and negative outcomes for a prospective pet dog trial, and what action(s) might be taken should these outcomes occur. The overarching goal of the comparative oncology trial is to impact the development of novel human therapies, devices, imaging agents, etc. Examples of possible outcomes and actions to be examined include: If a drug is found to have unacceptable toxicity in the dog, will development be halted? Has the trial been designed to sufficiently show a difference between the multiple compounds being examined? If one is shown to be superior (i.e., PK, PD modulation, toxicity profile), will the remaining compounds be retired? If the drug is not shown to be efficacious in the chosen canine tumor type, will the investigator be able to understand why? If the drug is efficacious, will the results be meaningful to physician-scientists treating the disease in human patients? If data, either positive or negative, derived from a pet dog trial cannot have meaning assigned to it, then no value is added, and such a trial should be reconsidered. However, if the investigator carefully designs and plans their comparative clinical trial, the dog can provide essential data unable to be generated in other model systems.

References

1. Amin SB, Anderson KJ, Boudreau CE et al (2020) Comparative molecular life history of spontaneous canine and human gliomas. Cancer Cell 37(2):243–257.e7
2. Ammons DT, MacDonald CR, Chow L, Repasky EA, Dow S (2023) Chronic adrenergic stress and generation of myeloid-derived suppressor cells: implications for cancer immunotherapy in dogs. Vet Comp Oncol. https://doi.org/10.1111/vco.12891. Epub ahead of print
3. Belluco S, Marano G, Baiker K et al (2022) Standardisation of canine meningioma grading: Inter-observer agreement and recommendations for reproducible histopathologic criteria. Vet Comp Oncol 20(2):509–520
4. Burton JH, Mazcko C, LeBlanc A et al (2018) NCI comparative oncology program testing of non-Camptothecin Indenoisoquinoline Topoisomerase I inhibitors in naturally occurring canine lymphoma. Clin Cancer Res. Published Online First. https://doi.org/10.1158/1078-0432.CCR-18-1498
5. Dow S (2020) A role for dogs in advancing cancer immunotherapy research. Front Immunol 17(10):2935
6. Duregon E, Schneider J, DeMarzo AM, Hooper JE (2019) Rapid research autopsy is a stealthy but growing contributor to cancer research. Cancer 125(17):2915–2919. https://doi.org/10.1002/cncr.32184
7. Favaro PF, Stewart SD, McDonald BR et al (2022) Feasibility of circulating tumor DNA analysis in dogs with naturally occurring malignant and benign splenic lesions. Sci Rep 12(1):6337. https://doi.org/10.1038/s41598-022-09716-6
8. Flory A, Kruglyak KM, Tynan JA et al (2022) Clinical validation of a next-generation sequencing-based

multi-cancer early detection "liquid biopsy" blood test in over 1,000 dogs using an independent testing set: The CANcer Detection in Dogs (CANDiD) study. PLoS One 17(4):e0266623. https://doi.org/10.1371/journal.pone.0266623
9. Gingrich AA, Reiter TE, Judge SJ et al (2021) Comparative immunogenomics of canine natural killer cells as immunotherapy target. Front Immunol 12:670309. https://doi.org/10.3389/fimmu.2021.670309
10. Gordon I, Khanna C (2010) Modeling opportunities in comparative oncology for drug development. ILAR J 51(3):214–220
11. Gordon I, Paoloni M, Mazcko C, Khanna C (2009) The Comparative Oncology Trials Consortium: using spontaneously occurring cancers in dogs to inform the cancer drug development pathway. PLoS Med 6(10). https://doi.org/10.1371/journal.pmed.1000161
12. Hansen K, Khanna C (2004) Spontaneous and genetically engineered animal models; use in preclinical cancer drug development. Eur J Cancer 40(6):858–880
13. Harris RA, Rout ED, Yoshimoto JA, Avery PR, Avery AC (2022) Using digital RNA counting to establish flow cytometry diagnostic criteria for subtypes of CD34+ canine acute Leukaemia. Vet Comp Oncol 20(3):710–719. https://doi.org/10.1111/vco.12825
14. Honigberg LA, Smith AM, Sirisawad M et al (2010) The Bruton tyrosine kinase inhibitor PCI-32765 blocks B-cell activation and is efficacious in models of autoimmune disease and B-cell malignancy. Proc Natl Acad Sci USA 107(29):13075–13080
15. Iacobuzio-Donahue CA, Michael C, Baez P, Kappagantula R, Hooper JE, Hollman TJ (2019) Cancer biology as revealed by the research autopsy. Nat Rev Cancer 19(12):686–697
16. Judge SJ, Yanagisawa M, Sturgill IR et al (2020) Blood and tissue biomarker analysis in dogs with osteosarcoma treated with palliative radiation and intra-tumoral autologous natural killer cell transfer. PLoS One 15(2):e0224775. https://doi.org/10.1371/journal.pone.0224775
17. Khanna C, London C, Vail D, Mazcko C, Hirschfeld S (2009) Guiding the optimal translation of new cancer treatments from canine to human cancer patients. Clin Cancer Res 15(18):5671–5677. https://doi.org/10.1158/1078-0432.CCR-09-0719
18. Kim J, Bae H, Ahn S et al (2021) Cell-Free DNA as a diagnostic and prognostic biomarker in dogs with tumors. Front Vet Sci 8:735682. https://doi.org/10.3389/fvets.2021.735682
19. Koehler JW, Miller AD, Miller CR et al (2018) A revised diagnostic classification of canine glioma: towards validation of the canine glioma patient as a naturally occurring preclinical model for human glioma. J Neuropathol Exp Neurol 77(11):1039–1054. https://doi.org/10.1093/jnen/nly085
20. Kruglyak KM, Chibuk J, McLennan L et al (2021) Blood-based liquid biopsy for comprehensive cancer genomic profiling using next-generation sequencing: an emerging paradigm for non-invasive cancer detection and management in dogs. Front Vet Sci 8:704835. https://doi.org/10.3389/fvets.2021.704835
21. Kummar S, Rubinstein L, Kinders R et al (2008) Phase 0 clinical trials: conceptions and misconceptions. Cancer J 14(3):133–137. https://doi.org/10.1097/PPO.0b013e318172d6f3
22. Kurzman ID, MacEwen EG, Rosenthal RC et al (1995) Adjuvant therapy for osteosarcoma in dogs: results of randomized clinical trials using combined liposome-encapsulated muramyl tripeptide and cisplatin. Clin Cancer Res 1(12):1595–1601
23. LeBlanc AK, Mazcko C (2020) Improving human cancer therapy through the evaluation of pet dogs. Nat Rev Cancer 20(12):727–742. https://doi.org/10.1038/s41568-020-0297-3
24. LeBlanc AK, Mazcko CN, Khanna C (2016) Defining the value of a comparative approach to cancer drug development. Clin Cancer Res 22(9):2133–2138
25. LeBlanc AK, Atherton M, Bentley RT et al (2021a) Veterinary cooperative oncology group-common terminology criteria for adverse events (VCOG-CTCAE v2) following investigational therapy in dogs and cats. Vet Comp Oncol 19(2):311–352. https://doi.org/10.1111/vco.12677
26. LeBlanc AK, Mazcko CN, Cherukuri A et al (2021b) Adjuvant Sirolimus does not improve outcome in pet dogs receiving standard-of-care therapy for appendicular osteosarcoma: a prospective, randomized trial of 324 dogs. Clin Cancer Res 27(11):3005–3016. https://doi.org/10.1158/1078-0432.CCR-21-0315
27. LeBlanc AK, Mazcko CN, Fan TM et al (2022) Comparative oncology assessment of a novel inhibitor of Valosin-containing protein in tumor-bearing dogs. Mol Cancer Ther 21(10):1510–1523. https://doi.org/10.1158/1535-7163.MCT-22-0167
28. Lenz JA, Assenmacher CA, Costa V et al (2022) Increased tumor-infiltrating lymphocyte density is associated with favorable outcomes in a comparative study of canine histiocytic sarcoma. Cancer Immunol Immunother 71(4):807–818. https://doi.org/10.1007/s00262-021-03033-z
29. London CA, Malpas PB, Wood-Follis SL et al (2009) Multi-center, placebo-controlled, double-blind, randomized study of oral toceranib phosphate (SU11654), a receptor tyrosine kinase inhibitor, for the treatment of dogs with recurrent (either local or distant) mast cell tumor following surgical excision. Clin Cancer Res 15(11):3856–3865. https://doi.org/10.1158/1078-0432.CCR-08-1860
30. London CA, Bear MD, McCleese J, Foley KP, Paalangara R, Inoue T et al (2011) Phase I evaluation of STA-1474, a prodrug of the novel HSP90 inhibitor ganetespib, in dogs with spontaneous cancer. PLoSOne 6(11):e27018
31. London CA, Bernabe LF, Barnard S, Kisseberth WC, Borgatti A, Henson M et al (2014) Evaluation of the novel, orally bioavailable selective inhibitor of nuclear export (SINE) KPT-335 in spontaneous canine cancer: results of a Phase I study. PLoS One 9(2):e87585

32. Lynch S, Savary-Bataille K, Leeuw B, Argyle DJ (2011) Development of a questionnaire assessing health-related quality-of-life in dogs and cats with cancer. Vet Comp Oncol 9(3):172–182. https://doi.org/10.1111/j.1476-5829.2010.00244.x
33. MacEwen EG, Kurzman ID, Rosenthal RC et al (1989) Therapy for osteosarcoma in dogs with intravenous injection of liposome-encapsulated muramyl tripeptide. J Natl Cancer Inst 81(12):935–938
34. Magee K, Marsh IR, Turek MM et al (2021) Safety and feasibility of an *in situ* vaccination and immunomodulatory targeted radionuclide combination immuno-radiotherapy approach in a comparative (companion dog) setting. PLoS One 16(8):e0255798. https://doi.org/10.1371/journal.pone.0255798
35. Nance R, Payal A, Sandey M et al (2020) A method for isolating RNA from canine bone. BioTechniques 68(6):311–317
36. Nguyen SM, Thamm DH, Vail DM, London CA (2015) Response evaluation criteria for solid tumours in dogs (v1.0): a Veterinary Cooperative Oncology Group (VCOG) consensus document. Vet Comp Oncol 13(3):176–183. https://doi.org/10.1111/vco.12032
37. Omar NB, Bentley RT, Crossman DK et al (2021) Safety and interim survival data after intracranial administration of M032, a genetically engineered oncolytic HSV-1 expressing IL-12, in pet dogs with sporadic gliomas. Neurosurg Focus 50(2):E5. https://doi.org/10.3171/2020.11.FOCUS20844
38. Packer RA, Rossmeisl JH, Kent MS et al (2018) Consensus recommendations on standardized magnetic resonance imaging protocols for multicenter canine brain tumor clinical trials. Vet Radiol Ultrasound 59(3):261–271. https://doi.org/10.1111/vru.12608. Erratum in: Vet Radiol Ultrasound 59(6):796
39. Page R, Baneux P, Vail D et al (2016) Conduct, oversight, and ethical considerations of clinical trials in companion animals with cancer: report of a workshop on best practice recommendations. J Vet Intern Med 30(2):527–535. https://doi.org/10.1111/jvim.13916
40. Paoloni M, Khanna C (2008) Translation of new cancer treatments from pet dogs to humans. Nat Rev Cancer 8:147–156
41. Paoloni MC, Tandle A, Mazcko C et al (2009) Launching a novel preclinical infrastructure: comparative oncology trials consortium directed therapeutic targeting of TNFalpha to cancer vasculature. PLoS One 4:e4972
42. Paoloni MC, Mazcko C, Fox E (2010) Rapamycin pharmacokinetic and pharmacodynamic relationships in osteosarcoma: a comparative oncology study in dogs. PLoS One 5(6):e11013
43. Paoloni M, Webb C, Mazcko C et al (2014) Prospective molecular profiling of canine cancers provides a clinically relevant comparative model for evaluating personalized medicine (PMed) trials. PLoS One 9(3):e90028. https://doi.org/10.1371/journal.pone.0090028
44. Paoloni M, Mazcko C, Selting K et al (2015) Defining the pharmacodynamic profile and therapeutic index of NHS-IL12 immunocytokine in dogs with malignant melanoma. PLoS One 10(6):e0129954. https://doi.org/10.1371/journal.pone.0129954
45. Prouteau A, Denis JA, De Fornel P et al (2021) Circulating tumor DNA is detectable in canine histiocytic sarcoma, oral malignant melanoma, and multicentric lymphoma. Sci Rep 11(1):877. https://doi.org/10.1038/s41598-020-80332-y
46. Pryer NK, Lee LB, Zadovaskaya R et al (2003) Proof of target for SU11654: inhibition of KIT phosphorylation in canine mast cell tumors. Clin Cancer Res 9(15):5729–5734
47. Rafalko JM, Kruglyak KM, McCleary-Wheeler AL et al (2023) Age at cancer diagnosis by breed, weight, sex, and cancer type in a cohort of more than 3,000 dogs: determining the optimal age to initiate cancer screening in canine patients. PLoS One 18(2):e0280795. https://doi.org/10.1371/journal.pone.0280795
48. Rassnick KM, Bailey DB, Kamstock DA et al (2021) Survival time for dogs with previously untreated, peripheral nodal, intermediate- or large-cell lymphoma treated with prednisone alone: the Canine Lymphoma Steroid Only trial. J Am Vet Med Assoc 259(1):62–71. https://doi.org/10.2460/javma.259.1.62
49. Rebhun RB, York D, Cruz SM et al (2022) Inhaled recombinant human IL-15 in dogs with naturally occurring pulmonary metastases from osteosarcoma or melanoma: a phase 1 study of clinical activity and correlates of response. J Immunother Cancer 10:e004493. https://doi.org/10.1136/jitc-2022-004493
50. Regan D, Garcia K, Thamm D (2018) Clinical, pathological, and ethical considerations for the conduct of clinical trials in dogs with naturally occurring cancer: a comparative approach to accelerate translational drug development. ILAR J 59(1):99–110. https://doi.org/10.1093/ilar/ily019
51. Regan DP, Coy JW, Chahal KK et al (2019) The angiotensin receptor blocker losartan suppresses growth of pulmonary metastases via AT1R-independent inhibition of CCR2 signaling and monocyte recruitment. J Immunol 202(10):3087–3102. https://doi.org/10.4049/jimmunol.1800619
52. Regan DP, Chow L, Das S et al (2022) Losartan blocks osteosarcoma-elicited monocyte recruitment, and combined with the kinase inhibitor toceranib, exerts significant clinical benefit in canine metastatic osteosarcoma. Clin Cancer Res 28(4):662–676. https://doi.org/10.1158/1078-0432.ccr-21-2105
53. Rossman P, Zabka TS, Ruple A et al (2021) Phase I/II trial of vemurafenib in dogs with naturally occurring, *BRAF*-mutated urothelial carcinoma. Mol Cancer Ther 20(11):2177–2188. https://doi.org/10.1158/1535-7163.MCT-20-0893
54. Ruple A, Sargeant JM, Selmic LE, O'Connor AM (2023) The standards of reporting randomized

trials in pets (PetSORT): methods and development processes. Front Vet Sci. https://doi.org/10.3389/fvets.2023.1137774
55. Saba C, Paoloni M, Mazcko C et al (2016) A comparative oncology study of Iniparib defines its pharmacokinetic profile and biological activity in a naturally-occurring canine cancer model. PLoS One 11(2):e0149194. https://doi.org/10.1371/journal.pone.0149194
56. Sargeant JM, Ruple A, Selmic LE, O'Connor AM (2023) The standards of reporting trials in pets (PetSORT): explanation and elaboration. Front Vet Sci. https://doi.org/10.3389/fvets.2023.1137781
57. Schmutz A, Spofford N, Burghardt W, De Meyer G (2022) Development and initial validation of a dog quality of life instrument. Sci Rep 12(1):12225. https://doi.org/10.1038/s41598-022-16315-y
58. Simpson RM, Bastian BC, Michael HT et al (2014) Sporadic naturally occurring melanoma in dogs as a preclinical model for human melanoma. Pigment Cell Melanoma Res 27(1):37–47. https://doi.org/10.1111/pcmr.12185. Epub 2013 Nov 21
59. Smith MR (2015) Ibrutinib in B lymphoid malignancies. Expert Opin Pharmacother 16(12):1879–1887. https://doi.org/10.1517/14656566.2015.1067302
60. Spunt SL, Vargas SO, Coffin CM et al (2012) The clinical, research, and social value of autopsy after any cancer death: a perspective from the Children's Oncology Group Soft Tissue Sarcoma Committee. Cancer 118(12):3002–3009. https://doi.org/10.1002/cncr.26620
61. Tanvetthayanont P, Yata T, Boonnil J, Temisak S, Ponglowhapan S (2022) Validation of droplet digital PCR for cytokeratin 19 mRNA detection in canine peripheral blood and mammary gland. Sci Rep 12(1):13623. https://doi.org/10.1038/s41598-022-17493-5
62. Tawa GJ, Braisted J, Gerhold D et al (2021) Transcriptomic profiling in canines and humans reveals cancer specific gene modules and biological mechanisms common to both species. PLoS Comput Biol 17(9):e1009450. https://doi.org/10.1371/journal.pcbi.1009450
63. Terrell J, Bougoussa M, Butera T (2022) Evaluation of plasma nucleosome concentrations in dogs with a variety of common cancers and in healthy dogs. BMC Vet Res 18(1):329. https://doi.org/10.1186/s12917-022-03429-8
64. Thamm DH (2019) Canine cancer: strategies in experimental therapeutics. Front Oncol 15(9):1257. https://doi.org/10.3389/fonc.2019.01257
65. Thamm DH, Vail DM, Kurzman ID et al (2014) GS-9219/VDC-1101--a prodrug of the acyclic nucleotide PMEG has antitumor activity in spontaneous canine multiple myeloma. BMC Vet Res 10:30. https://doi.org/10.1186/1746-6148-10-30
66. Vail DM, MacEwen EG (2000) Spontaneously occurring tumors of companion animals as models for human cancer. Cancer Investig 18:781–792
67. Vail DM, Thamm DH, Reiser H et al (2009) Assessment of GS-9219 in a pet dog model of non-Hodgkin's lymphoma. Clin Cancer Res 15(10):3503–3510
68. Vail DM, Michels GM, Khanna C et al (2010) Response evaluation criteria for peripheral nodal lymphoma in dogs (v1.0)–a Veterinary Cooperative Oncology Group (VCOG) consensus document. Vet Comp Oncol 8(1):28–37. https://doi.org/10.1111/j.1476-5829.2009.00200.x
69. Wang C, Wallerman O, Arendt ML et al (2021) A novel canine reference genome resolves genomic architecture and uncovers transcript complexity. Nat Commun Biol 4(1):185. https://doi.org/10.1038/s42003-021-01698-x
70. Weiske R, Sroufe M, Quigley M et al (2020) Development and evaluation of a caregiver reported quality of life assessment instrument in dogs with intracranial disease. Front Vet Sci 18(7):537. https://doi.org/10.3389/fvets.2020.00537
71. Withers SS, Skorupski KA, York D et al (2019a) Association of macrophage and lymphocyte infiltration with outcome in canine osteosarcoma. Vet Comp Oncol 17(1):49–60. https://doi.org/10.1111/vco.12444
72. Withers SS, York D, Choi JW et al (2019b) Metastatic immune infiltrates correlate with those of the primary tumour in canine osteosarcoma. Vet Comp Oncol 17(3):242–252. https://doi.org/10.1111/vco.12459
73. Wu K, Rodrigues L, Post G et al (2023) Analyses of canine cancer mutations and treatment outcomes using real-world clinico-genomics data of 2119 dogs. NPJ Precis Oncol 7(1):8. https://doi.org/10.1038/s41698-023-00346-3

Clinical Investigation for Developing Imaging Technology

Brian Flesner, Maureen Griffin, and Amy LeBlanc

1 Introduction

Comparative oncology studies have clearly established roles in cancer biology investigation and drug development [1]. However, comparative approaches have also played a vital role in the development of imaging technologies, including research related to hardware and devices and imaging agents. Pet dogs, in particular, with their longstanding role in biomedical research and comparable body size to humans, add significant complementary value to data collected in conventional research species, such as rodents and pigs [2–4]. Additional features of spontaneous canine cancers, such as naturally co-evolving tumors and associated stroma, the presence of an intact educated immune system, and the natural development of tumor-associated vasculature and necrosis, have significant advantages over traditional laboratory animal systems used for imaging modality development and validation [5].

B. Flesner (✉)
Department of Clinical Sciences & Advanced Medicine, University of Pennsylvania School of Veterinary Medicine, Philadelphia, PA, USA

Mission Veterinary Emergency & Specialty, Mission, KS, USA
e-mail: bflesner@ardentanimalhealth.com

M. Griffin
Department of Clinical Sciences & Advanced Medicine, University of Pennsylvania School of Veterinary Medicine, Philadelphia, PA, USA

A. LeBlanc
Comparative Oncology Program, Center for Cancer Research, National Cancer Institute, National Institutes of Health, Bethesda, MD, USA

Cancer imaging plays a key role in the practice of both veterinary and physician oncology. In modern veterinary practice, several imaging modalities are routinely used for cancer detection, staging, and monitoring both during and after therapy. These include, but are not limited to, standard two-dimensional radiography, fluoroscopy, endoscopy, planar/single-photon nuclear scintigraphy, ultrasonography, computed tomography (CT), and magnetic resonance imaging (MRI) [6]. More recently, additional sophisticated techniques such as positron emission tomography (PET), both alone and fused with CT, have entered specialty veterinary practices and academic centers [7]. A variety of imaging agents, such as the radiopharmaceuticals ^{99m}Tc, ^{18}F-FDG, and ^{123}I, are used in veterinary cancer imaging [8–10]. Standard intravenous and *per os* contrast agents, such as barium, iohexol (iodine-based), and gadolinium, are often used in combination with these imaging platforms [11–13]. Indeed, the veterinary cancer patient will often undergo the same or similar imaging studies as their human counterparts during cancer diagnosis and management.

Access to such imaging technology within the context of modern veterinary oncology practice creates opportunities for comparative studies and clinical trials that leverage access to both

M. W. Nolan et al. (eds.), *Comparative Oncology*, https://doi.org/10.1007/978-3-032-04454-9_17

sophisticated molecular imaging techniques and spontaneous veterinary cancers, with the intent to use the knowledge gained from these studies to inform human cancer care. Veterinary patients benefit from participation in such clinical studies as access to high-level care often accompanies participation in the trial itself. Additionally, knowledge gained from comparative cancer imaging studies naturally benefits the veterinary community through the dissemination of data, refinement of techniques, and development of experience.

Imaging studies designed to evaluate agents or platforms destined for human use may require access to areas of hospitals or research facilities that are restricted from animals. Further, the use of radioactive substances in companion animals requires careful and early planning with the institutional radiation safety office and staff to maintain compliance with local and state regulations that govern the use of radioactive materials. A series of reviews covers these topics and offers guidance for those interested in exploring ways to use advanced imaging approaches for comparative studies [14, 15]. As most animal imaging studies require anesthesia and/or deep sedation for patient positioning and data collection, particularly for kinetic or intra-operative studies, how this may impact the findings should be considered when designing the study. Anesthesia and sedation may impact blood flow through lowering of systemic blood pressure and cardiac output, as well as cause respiratory depression and poor ventilation. Support of the patient through careful monitoring of vital signs and provision of mechanical ventilation should be considered. Urinary catheters can assist with collection of radioactive urine for storage until decay occurs and disposal is appropriate.

2 Areas of Active Exploration in Comparative Cancer Imaging

Successful comparative cancer imaging studies hinge on the definition of the scientific questions to be asked within the trial design. Careful consideration of these questions, the structure/design of the trial, and the data that is generated within is warranted to ensure that the conduct of the study is both ethical and likely to enhance and/or inform the forward progress of the approach. Conversely, comparative oncology studies in general also have the power and potential to generate data that can halt the forward progress of an approach that is unlikely to have future success in patients. Both outcomes have value to the cancer research community. Such questions can be broadly classified into the following categories.

2.1 Optimization and Alignment with Human Imaging Standards

2.1.1 PET and PET/CT

It is important to benchmark the performance of imaging modalities utilized in veterinary cancer patients against the standards employed in physician-based oncology before the approach can be widely recommended as a research or practice tool. The best example of this approach is the study of ^{18}F-FDG utilizing PET and PET/CT in companion animals (mainly cats and dogs) with cancer. In human patients, ^{18}F-FDG PET/CT is the most common modality used for detection, disease staging, and often monitoring tumor response [16–18]. Although it is not a cancer-specific technique, it is widely used across a variety of tumor types. The first studies of ^{18}F-FDG PET established that many common canine cancers, in addition to some infectious/inflammatory disease processes, can be detected and characterized in a similar manner [19–21].

Underpinning these early studies was the recognition that, as with any new technology, it was necessary to first demonstrate imaging agent performance in clinically normal animals, and to explore biodistribution and imaging characteristics of various approaches that are commonplace in the practice of human oncology. For example, the initial studies of ^{18}F-FDG utilizing PET and PET/CT in clinically normal cats [22] and dogs [23, 24] helped lay the groundwork for understanding the avidity of canine cancers for this key imaging agent and to understand the landscape of physiologic uptake and common artifacts. The feasibility of this approach and the technical aspects of PET radiopharmaceuticals in privately owned pets were explored and reported, with an emphasis on shared equipment/facilities, radiation safety, and radiation exposure to veterinary staff. As access and expertise with ^{18}F-FDG PET/CT grew, additional reports of its use in tumor staging, disease monitoring, and prognostication appeared in the veterinary literature [9, 25, 26]. Experience with other PET radiopharmaceuticals such as ^{18}FLT, ^{18}F-MISO, ^{64}Cu-ATSM, and ^{124}I has also been reported to showcase the similarities between canine and human cancers and determine performance characteristics that further establish the comparative link between the two species (Fig. 1) [27–31].

Collective expertise across the veterinary community with PET radiopharmaceuticals, along with increased access to PET cameras and established guidelines for managing radioactive waste in companion animals, has helped develop PET imaging to become an emerging offering available at both veterinary academic and private referral centers [9]. The recent creation of a network of veterinary schools actively using PET/CT technology, within the NCI's Comparative Oncology Trials Consortium (COTC) [32], enables the inclusion of molecular imaging endpoints into multicenter comparative oncology trials, enhancing their translational value and broadening the menu of opportunities for stakeholders seeking to leverage this type of technology within a harmonized clinical trial infrastructure [33].

2.1.2 Sentinel Lymph Node Mapping

The determination of lymph node status has become an important aspect of staging. This procedure can inform treatment recommendations and provide prognostic information in many malignant solid tumors experienced by both human and veterinary oncology patients. However, patterns of lymphatic drainage have been shown to be highly variable. Routine techniques such as palpation, radiography, ultrasonography, and even advanced imaging modalities including CT and MRI have substantial limitations in detecting lymph node metastasis or determining the nodes at greatest risk for metastasis. In patients without definitive evidence of nodal metastatic disease, identification of sentinel lymph nodes (SLN), the first lymph nodes to drain a tumor and thus the most likely to harbor metastasis, is now considered standard of care [34]. Not only does SLN mapping accurately predict the nodal metastatic disease burden of a patient, it also avoids unnecessary lymph node bed dissection, which carries potential for morbidity (Fig. 2).

Multiple SLN mapping techniques exist in a preoperative and/or intraoperative setting. All involve injection of an imaging agent into the peritumoral (or potentially tumoral) tissues with subsequent imaging (real-time or serial) to trace the agent from the tumor through lymphatics to the first draining lymph node(s). Methods of SLN mapping, including lymphoscintigraphy, indirect radiographic lymphography, indirect CT lymphography, contrast-enhanced ultrasound (CEUS), vital dye (colorimetric) mapping, and near-infrared (NIR) fluorescence imaging, have now been translated and applied to multiple tumor types in canine patients, such as superficial solid tumors, mammary tumors, anal sac tumors, head/neck tumors, and mast cell tumors [35–44]. Both human and canine studies have demonstrated that a combination of SLN mapping techniques provides optimal results [37, 45]. Overall, the evidence to support SLN mapping procedures for lymph node staging is substantial in humans, and this evidence base is growing in veterinary medicine. Novel tumor types, such as anal sac tumors unique to veterinary patients, also lend support for improved SLN mapping applications [42]. A recent study in dogs with oral tumors demonstrated the value of SLN mapping with indirect computed tomography lymphangiography (ICTL) followed by targeted lymph node biopsy as an alternative to extensive neck dissection for tumor staging. Of 39 dogs, the SLN was detected with ICTL in 38 (97% of cases), with histopathologic confirmation of metastasis in 13 dogs [46]. Importantly, ICTL imaging features alone did not predict metastasis, so cytologic or

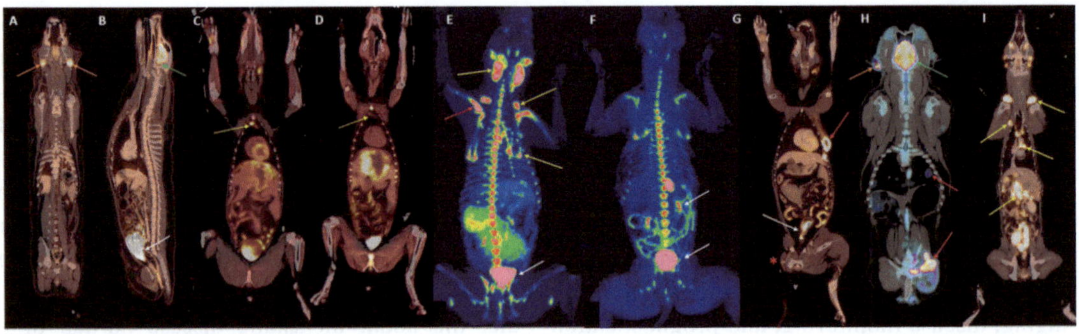

Fig. 1 Composite of PET and fusion PET/CT images of healthy dogs and dogs with neoplasia imaged with commonly used tracers, 18F-FDG and 18F-FLT. (**a**) Healthy dog coronal view, 18F-FDG. Note normal uptake in mandibular salivary glands (orange arrows). (Image courtesy of Dr. Lynn Griffin—Colorado State University). (**b**) Normal dog sagittal view, 18F-FDG. Note normal uptake in brain (green arrow) and normal clearance through urinary bladder (white arrow). (Image courtesy of Dr. Lynn Griffin—Colorado State University). (**c**) Dog with hepatocellular carcinoma, 18F-FDG. Reactive retrosternal lymph node is evident with FDG (yellow arrow). (Image courtesy of Drs. LeBlanc and Vail, from Vail, LeBlanc, Jeraj 2020). (**d**) Same dog as in **b**, with hepatocellular carcinoma, 18F-FLT. Note the increased tumor conspicuity with FLT particularly when discerning tumor borders from surrounding hepatic parenchyma. A reactive retrosternal lymph node is not evident with FLT (yellow arrow). (Image courtesy of Drs. LeBlanc and Vail, from Vail, LeBlanc, Jeraj 2020). (**e**) Dog with lymphoma, 18F-FLT. Uptake in the peripheral nodes (yellow arrows) and bone marrow (red arrow). Normal clearance through urinary bladder (white arrow). (Image courtesy of Drs. Lawrence and Vail, from Lawrence 2009). (**f**) Same dog as in **e**. with lymphoma, 3 weeks following the final dose of chemotherapy, 18F-FLT. The lymph nodes were small on CT with minimal FLT uptake on PET. Normal clearance in kidneys and bladder (white arrows). (Image courtesy of Drs. Lawrence and Vail, from Lawrence 2009). (**g**) Dog with previously amputated osteosarcoma (hindquarter amputated, red asterisk), 18F-FDG. Development of subcutaneous metastasis (red arrow). Normal bladder clearance (white arrow). (Image courtesy of Dr. Lynn Griffin—Colorado State University). (**h**) Dog with pelvic carcinoma (red arrow, presumed metastatic) of unknown primary, with additional avid left pulmonary nodule (red arrow), 18F-FDG. Note normal uptake in brain (green arrow) and probable ear uptake from chronic otitis (orange arrow). (Image courtesy of Dr. Lynn Griffin—Colorado State University). (**i**) Dog with lymphoma, 18F-FDG. Note peripheral and central lymphadenopathy (yellow arrows). (Image courtesy of Dr. Lynn Griffin—Colorado State University)

histopathologic sampling is still recommended for fully informed clinical decision-making.

With regard to future investigations of lymph node staging, SLN mapping remains to be evaluated in many canine and human tumor types to determine optimal methods and techniques. In addition, although SLN mapping has proven effective in identifying the lymph node(s) at greatest risk for subclinical metastatic disease for subsequent sampling and diagnosis, the potential effect on outcomes with the removal of metastatic lymph nodes in an early metastatic setting is largely unknown in companion animals. Multi-institutional, large-scale, collaborative studies will be ideal to answer these questions. In addition, future efforts to develop NIR imaging agents may prove beneficial for lymph node staging as well, with the goal of developing targeted agents that effectively differentiate metastatic from non-metastatic lymph nodes for subsequent extirpation.

2.2 Evaluation and Validation of Novel Imaging Agents, Platforms, and Protocols

2.2.1 Novel PET Radiopharmaceuticals and Chemistry

Several studies in dogs have explored the performance of new PET imaging agents for hallmark features of solid tumors, including hypoxia, proliferation, angiogenesis, metabolism, and apoptosis [30, 33, 47]. Further, multi-tracer protocols that interrogate several aspects of cancer biology

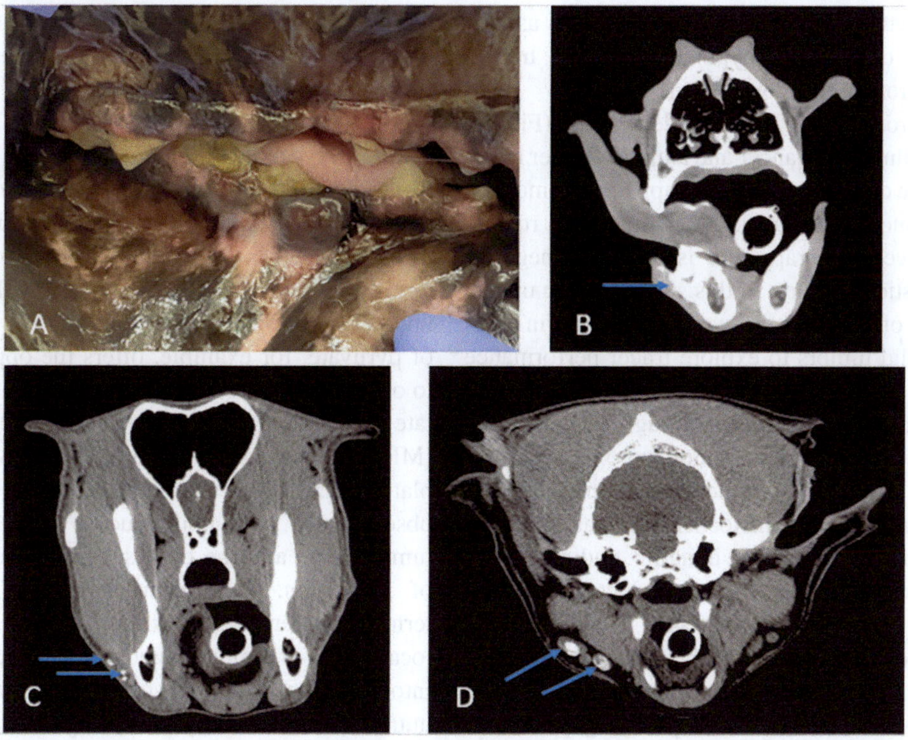

Fig. 2 Sentinel lymph node mapping with indirect CT lymphography in a dog with residual oral malignant melanoma and scar following prior cytoreduction. All CT images are 1 min following peritumoral contrast injection with 1 ml iohexol 350 mg/ml diluted with 1 ml sterile saline. (**a**) Gross image demonstrating location of oral malignant melanoma (soft tissue component) and scar on the right mandibular gingival margin and buccal mucosa. (**b**) Arrow pointing to iodinated contrast accumulation around the tumor subsequent to peritumoral contrast injection. (**c**) Arrows pointing to enhancing lymphatic vessels draining the tumor en route to the sentinel lymph node(s). (**d**) Arrows pointing to two enhancing right mandibular lymph nodes (dorsal and ventral) that retain normal size, shape, and margination. These lymph nodes are considered the sentinel lymph nodes in this indirect CT lymphography study

have been combined before, during, and after directed cancer treatment to elucidate changes within tumor tissue and allow individual tracer performance characteristics to be linked to treatment response.

While most PET imaging agents are administered intravenously as intact radionuclides attached to a specific targeting molecule or antibody, recent advances to in vivo pre-targeting based on the inverse electron demand Diels-Alder (IEDDA) click ligation have shown promise. A study performed in dogs with suspect osteosarcoma revealed that decoupling radionuclides from their targeting molecules/antibodies and relying on "click chemistry" may be an attractive strategy to mitigate healthy tissue uptake or toxicity. Dogs received bone-targeting trans-cyclooctene (TCO-BP) intravenously 1 h prior to the administration of a ^{64}Cu-labeled tetrazine (Tz) ligand. The methodology followed that (1) the TCO-BP molecule would accumulate in areas of high bone turnover and be cleared from circulation prior to (2) ^{64}Cu-SarAr-Tz administration, which would then "click" ligate with the TCO-BP, allowing for positron emission imaging [48]. This work supports the clinical translation of IEDDA-based pre-targeting imaging for human studies.

Another area where comparative cancer imaging can serve in a translational role is the head-to-head assessment of imaging agents to determine which has superior performance in a spontaneous tumor setting. One recent example is the assessment of the hypoxia PET tracers ^{18}F-fluoromisonidazole (FMISO) and ^{18}F-fluoroazamycin-arabinoside (FAZA) (Fig. 3). As a hallmark of cancer and a major barrier to the effective delivery of radiotherapy and chemotherapy, tumor hypoxia plays an important role in resistance to therapy and is a known negative prognostic indicator. In this study, kinetic uptake studies of both tracers were conducted in dogs with solid tumors to explore tracer performance metrics and to inform on optimal timepoints for static timepoint imaging. Although not performed in this particular trial, tumor hypoxia measurements using oxygen electrodes and/or tissue staining for immunohistochemical markers could be used to validate the imaging findings. Such measurements have been conducted in other studies of the hypoxia agents ^{64}Cu-ATSM and ^{18}F-misonidazole. Again, the clinically relevant lesions and naturally co-evolving components of canine solid tumors fill an important gap between murine preclinical studies and human clinical trials by providing an experimental system that bridges the induced disease model to the human cancer patient [30, 49].

2.2.2 HyperPET

Combined PET and MRI techniques, particularly those employing hyperpolarized ^{13}C substrates, have informed beyond what can be observed in terms of tumor metabolic activity with ^{18}FDG uptake. Hyperpolarized carbon 13 (^{13}C) labeling of pyruvate, for example, offers the opportunity to observe the interconversion of pyruvate to lactate when magnetic resonance spectroscopy (MRS) is performed using a fused MRI/PET platform [50]. With simultaneous ^{18}FDG PET, the observer can map both glucose uptake within tumor tissue and the downstream consequences of glycolysis. This form of hybrid imaging, termed HyperPET, provides powerful spatial localization of tumor metabolism and key insights into how specific tumor types generate and utilize nutrients. In one study of 17 dogs, a significant correlation between ^{18}FDG uptake and

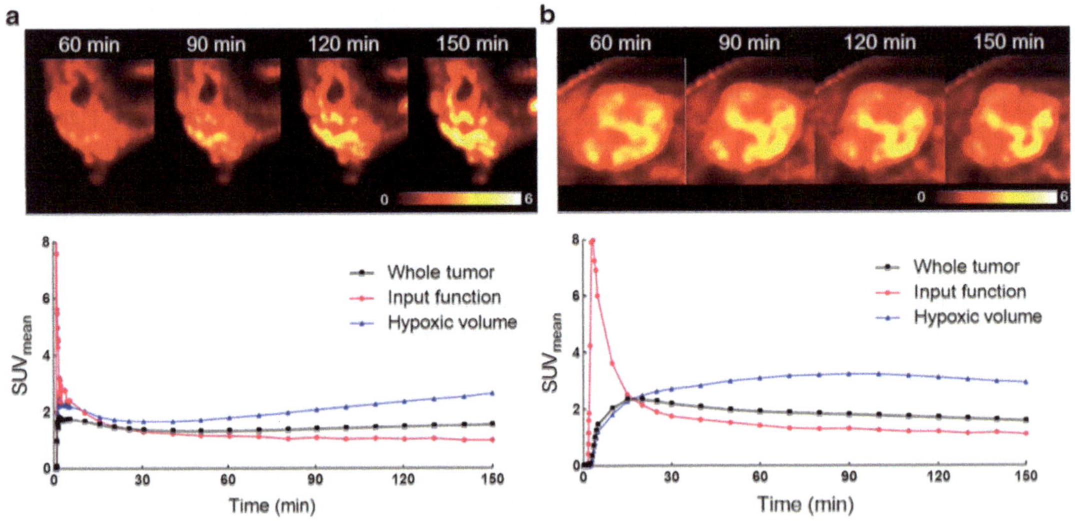

Fig. 3 Representative PET images of canine spontaneous hypoxic tumors (top) obtained in the 60-, 90-, 120-, and 150-min timeframes after radiotracer injection and time-activity curves (bottom). (**a**) [18F]FMISO PET scan of mammary gland carcinoma (dog 2). (**b**) [18F]FAZA PET scan of fibrosarcoma in thoracic wall (dog 9). [18F]FAZA showed acceptable consistency of hypoxic volume between 120- and 150-min timeframes. (Credit given to: Choen S, Kent MS, Chaudhari AJ, Cherry SR, Krtolica A, Zwingenberger AL. Kinetic Evaluation of the Hypoxia Radiotracers [^{18}F]FMISO and [^{18}F]FAZA in Dogs with Spontaneous Tumors Using Dynamic PET/CT Imaging. Nucl Med Mol Imaging. 2023 Feb;57(1):16–25. doi: 10.1007/s13139-022-00780-4. Epub 2022 Oct 11. PMID: 36643946; PMCID: PMC9832187. Link to License: https://creativecommons.org/licenses/by/4.0/legalcode). Changes made: none

pyruvate-to-lactate conversion was noted for 11 sarcoma patients, providing a method for metabolic phenotyping that may have applications for treatment planning and therapeutic monitoring [51]. The technology was also applied using combined [^{68}Ga]Ga-NODAGA-RGD-PET with hyperpolarized [1-^{13}C]pyruvate-MRS imaging to describe patterns of overlapping tumor angiogenesis and energy metabolism in 11 dogs with a variety of solid tumors (Fig. 4) [47]. Such efforts to simultaneously profile hallmark processes in spontaneous canine cancers have the potential to inform the clinical translation of hyperpolarized PET to human patients and provide new insights into therapy planning.

2.2.3 Near-Infrared Imaging

Nonradioactive agents may also be useful for cancer imaging, especially in the perioperative setting. A major challenge of surgical oncology involves the identification and removal of all neoplastic tissues to eliminate or minimize postoperative residual disease while concurrently preserving normal tissues to reduce morbidity. As the full extent of neoplastic disease may not be readily discernible on preoperative imaging or intraoperative visualization and palpation, intraoperative imaging may play an important role in the detection and removal of these tissues. Whereas nonspecific intraoperative NIR imaging agents, such as indocyanine green, accumulate in many human and canine tumor tissue types via the enhanced permeability and retention effect, false negatives (i.e., lack of fluorescence of neoplastic tissues) are possible, and the nonspecific nature of these imaging agents can also result in false positive findings (i.e., fluorescence of nonneoplastic tissues) [52–55]. Alternatively, targeted NIR fluorescent probes that selectively activate or bind substances overexpressed by tumor tissues allow for optimized detection of neoplastic tissues and their margins relative to nonneoplastic tissues [56–60]. Studies utilizing spontaneously occurring tumors in dogs as translational models of human cancer have demonstrated that NIR imaging can accurately detect tumors, tumor margins, and residual local disease in primary lung tumors, sarcomas, and mammary tumors (Fig. 5) [52, 53, 61–64]. In addition, a recent study demonstrated the successful clinical translation of a cathepsin-activated probe from its use in canine pulmonary tumors to human patients with pulmonary tumors [65]. This study highlights the effectiveness of the canine spontaneous neoplasia model in the evaluation of targeted NIR agents for subsequent use in humans with cancer.

With regard to the future uses of NIR imaging in both human and veterinary oncology patients, areas of needed improvement and study include methods to reduce background fluorescence (autofluorescence and off-target binding) with targeted imaging agents to improve specificity, enhancement of imaging depth of penetration, development of agents and imaging techniques that allow detection of micrometastasis and microscopic residual disease, and development of flexible endoscopic NIR-capable systems for greater utility of this imaging modality within organ systems. In addition, though targeted NIR agents have resulted in clinically significant surgical oncology benefits in people, such as the detection of occult or synchronous lesions, data is still lacking regarding any relationship to survival benefit. The canine spontaneous disease model may prove useful in this assessment.

2.3 Development of Molecular Imaging Approaches

Imaging studies conducted in pet dogs have elucidated drug mechanisms of action and/or assisted in the prediction of therapeutic responses, with clear translatability to humans. Ideally, the imaging agent is linked mechanistically to the therapeutic strategy being tested, as in the case of ^{18}FLT imaging in dogs receiving GS9219 therapy and in dogs undergoing ^{124}I PET scans, allowing more accurate dosimetry of ^{131}I for thyroid carcinoma (Fig. 6) [31, 66]. However, in other cases, molecular imaging with nonspecific metabolic agents such as ^{18}F-FDG showed the spectrum of responses for other investigational agents [67]. Additionally, ^{18}F-FDG PET imaging may also impart information on cancer patients' quality of

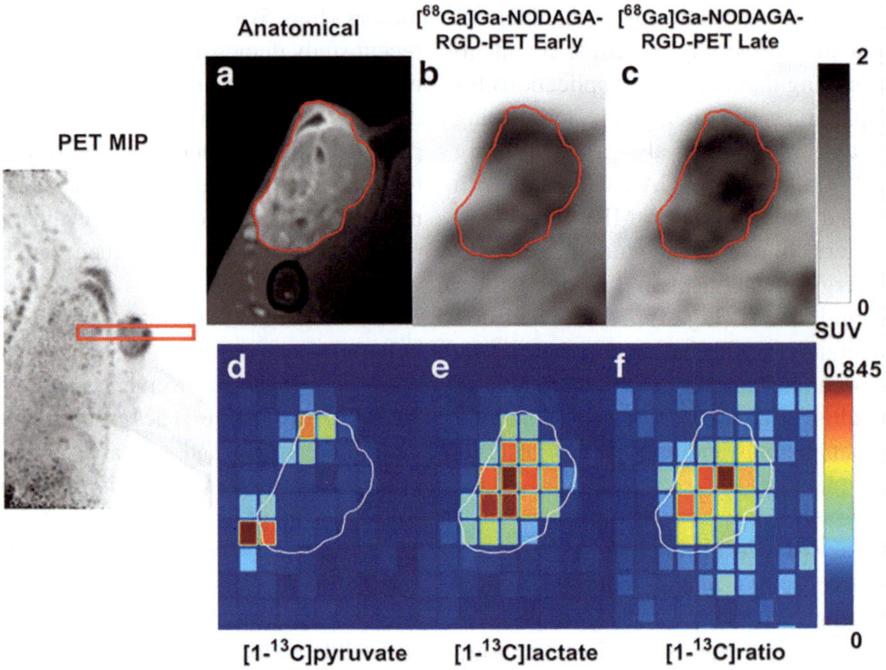

Fig. 4 Example of hyperPET images with a soft tissue sarcoma adjacent to humerus. Far left is an RGD-PET MIP showing the tumor location and ^{13}C-MRSI slice (red box). Panels (**a–f**) show imaging in the plane of the ^{13}C-MRSI. Gd-enhanced T1-weighted anatomical MRI with tumor region of interest (ROI) outlined in red (**a**), along with [^{68}Ga]Ga-NODAGA-RGD PET uptake images at 7 (**b**) and 53 min (**c**). Panels **d–f** show false-color images of metabolite distribution for [1-^{13}C]pyruvate (**d**), for [1-^{13}C]lactate (**e**), and ratio of [1-^{13}C]lactate to total ^{13}C (**f**) signal as determined by ^{13}C-MRSI. (Credit given to: Clemmensen A, Hansen AE, Holst P, Schøier C, Bisgaard S, Johannesen HH, Ardenkjær-Larsen JH, Kristensen AT, Kjaer A. [^{68}Ga]Ga-NODAGA-E[(cRGDyK)]$_2$ PET and hyperpolarized [1-^{13}C] pyruvate MRSI (hyperPET) in canine cancer patients: simultaneous imaging of angiogenesis and the Warburg effect. Eur J Nucl Med Mol Imaging. 2021 Feb;48(2):395–405. doi: 10.1007/s00259-020-04881-0. Epub 2020 Jul 3. PMID: 32621132; PMCID: PMC7835292. Link to License: https://creativecommons.org/licenses/by/4.0/legalcode). Changes made: none

life (QOL), specifically the degree of response and improvement of cancer-related pain. In human medicine, ^{18}F-FDG PET has been used to evaluate pain severity or predict improvement in pain for patients receiving palliative radiation for bone metastases [68–70]. Again using the comparative naturally occurring model of canine osteosarcoma, pre- and post-treatment ^{18}F-FDG PET scans showed an objective reduction in SUV_{max} and increased tumor uniformity after dogs received standard bisphosphonate and palliative radiation therapy [71]. While using ^{18}F-FDG is understood to be nonspecific to cancer and related cancer-induced pain, novel targeted radionuclides are being developed to target pain receptors and the multifactorial causes of cancer-induced pain to improve patient QOL (Fig. 7) [72]. This offers another avenue to use dogs as a translational large animal model to improve both canine and human health.

3 The Future of Comparative Cancer Imaging

3.1 New Imaging Platforms (Total-Body PET)

While PET is highly sensitive for tomographic imaging of cancer's protein pathways and interactions, it has been an inherently inefficient process. Historical scanners have a limited field of view (FOV), typically 25 cm or less, which only allows portions of the body to be scanned at one time. This

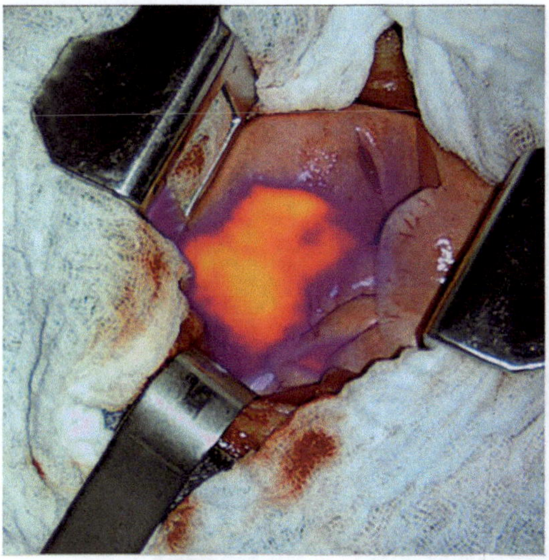

Fig. 5 Intraoperative near-infrared (NIR) image demonstrating fluorescence of a canine primary pulmonary tumor following IV injection of VGT-309 (Vergent Bioscience), a cathepsin-targeted quenched activity-based probe, using a Vision Sense (Iridium, Medtronic) NIR imaging system. (*Image courtesy of David E. Holt, BVSc, DACVS)

results in serial scans being used for full-body evaluations, negating the ability to evaluate radiotracer distribution in the entire body in real time [73]. To address this issue, a collaborative group led by researchers at the University of California-Davis, University of Pennsylvania, and industry partners developed total-body PET imaging scanners named uEXPLORER (UC Davis) and PennPET EXPLORER (Penn) [74, 75]. These scanners have several advantages, including shorter scan durations with less activity and no compromise in image quality. Specific to the PennPET, the axial FOV is 64 cm, and the scanner contains three rings, compared to one ring in standard PET scanners. These three rings allow a sensitivity of 55 kcps/MBq, approximately nine-fold greater than the sensitivity of a single ring [76]. Patient imaging studies in these EXPLORERs allow high-resolution time-activity curves of major organs and vasculature circulation, with low sampling noise; dynamic scans lend a key tool in PET kinetic studies. With both of the EXPLORER institutions housing veterinary schools, a natural segue evaluating veterinary patients seems appropriate and forthcoming.

3.2 Contrast Agents and Contrast-Enhanced Ultrasound (CEUS)

Canine tumors, with their naturally co-evolving tumor, stroma, neovasculature, and microenvironment, are the ideal proving ground for novel contrast agents. Such studies enable the exploration of variable infusion protocols, wash-in/wash-out kinetics, and specificity for tumors vs. normal tissues [77]. Further, the dogs' physical size and clinically relevant lesion dimensions support the use of the same imaging hardware set (i.e., whole-body CT scanner or ultrasonography probe) that would be used for human studies.

B-mode ultrasonography is a widespread imaging modality used in primary tumor assessment and staging of both companion animals and people. However, important limitations of this modality involve the inability to consistently differentiate benign from malignant lesions, determine the underlying etiology of a mass, or consistently identify small lesions or lesions within tissues of similar echotexture. Contrast-enhanced ultrasonography (CEUS) utilizes an ultrasonographic microbubble contrast agent that can be injected intravenously with subsequent interrogation of the structure of interest for enhancement and vascular properties that can be used to aid in diagnosis (Fig. 8). CEUS has been widely utilized in humans for multiple diagnostic purposes, and applications in veterinary oncology are being developed. For example, CEUS evaluation of the enhancement pattern of canine hepatic masses and nodules during multiple phases (arterial, portal, and parenchymal) has demonstrated a high level of accuracy in differentiating benign from malignant disease [78, 79]. In addition, studies in dogs with spontaneous neoplasms have demonstrated a potential use of CEUS in differentiating benign vs. malignant adrenal tumors (with one study reporting an accuracy of 92%), characterizing focal splenic lesions as benign vs. malignant, and differentiating between an exocrine vs. endocrine origin of pancreatic tumors [80–83]. As CEUS becomes more widely used and studied in veterinary medicine, additional information regarding tumor type differentiation, disease stage, and prognosis

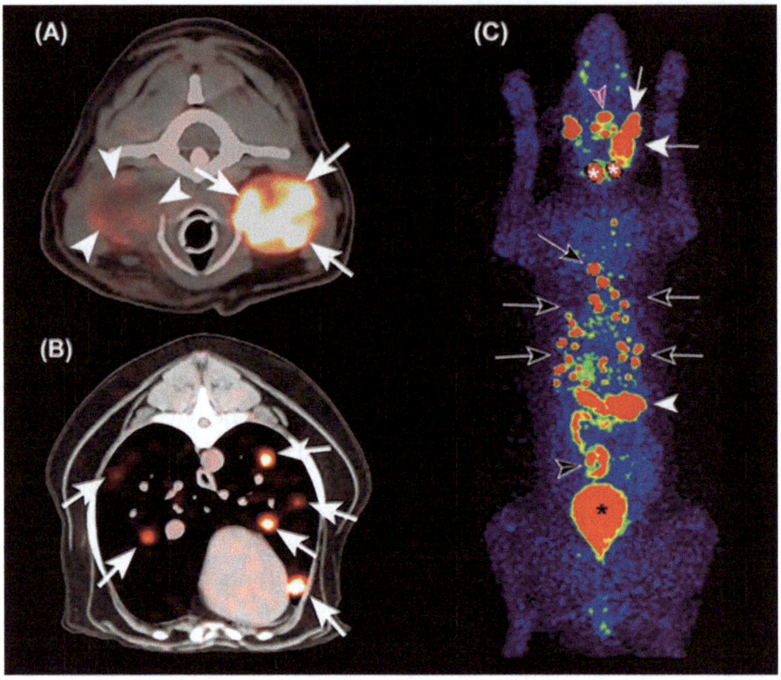

Fig. 6 Metastatic basihyoid ectopic thyroid carcinoma. Panels (**a**) and (**b**) are fused PET/CT transverse images and panel (**c**) is a dorsal plane maximum intensity projection. **a**, Severely enlarged but only mildly and heterogeneously avid metastatic right medial retropharyngeal lymph node (arrowheads). The left medial retropharyngeal lymph node is also severely enlarged, but is strongly and much more homogenously avid compared with the right (arrows). **b**, Multiple variably avid metastatic pulmonary nodules (arrows). **c**, Basihyoid ectopic thyroid carcinoma (pink arrowhead), metastatic left medial retropharyngeal lymph node (white arrows), normal thyroid gland (white asterisks), pulmonary metastasis (black arrows), normal gastric avidity (white arrowhead), physiologic colonic avidity (black arrowhead), and normal urinary bladder avidity (black asterisk). Patient imaged in sternal recumbency. (Color figure can be viewed at wileyonlinelibrary.com)

may be possible to obtain from this imaging modality, with potential translation to human oncology patients. In addition, important applications for CEUS in interventional oncology have recently been documented in humans. For instance, CEUS has improved guidance of biopsy procurement and ablation therapy and has been used to determine treatment response following ablation and embolization procedures [84–86]. As interventional oncology procedures (e.g., embolization of hepatic and prostatic tumors) become more common in veterinary patients, it will be important to develop accurate, minimally invasive, and affordable methods to document responses to treatment, provide prognostic information, and help guide recommendations for adjuvant therapy. CEUS may play an important role in this capacity.

3.3 Immunotherapeutic Imaging

Immunotherapy of cancer is a growing and important field. The contributions of comparative oncology in this setting are reflected in several recent publications and federally funded initiatives. Imaging support to immunotherapeutic comparative oncology trials presents a new frontier for therapy and imaging. Commercially available imaging agents such as ^{18}FDG and ^{18}FLT have the potential to inform immunotherapy treatment decisions, when used in combination to generate an FDG/FLT uptake ratio, termed the imaging immune response (IMR) ratio [33]. In this context, ^{18}FDG is used as a surrogate for therapy-induced tumor-associated inflammation. At the same time, tumor uptake of thymidine is measured through FLT uptake and

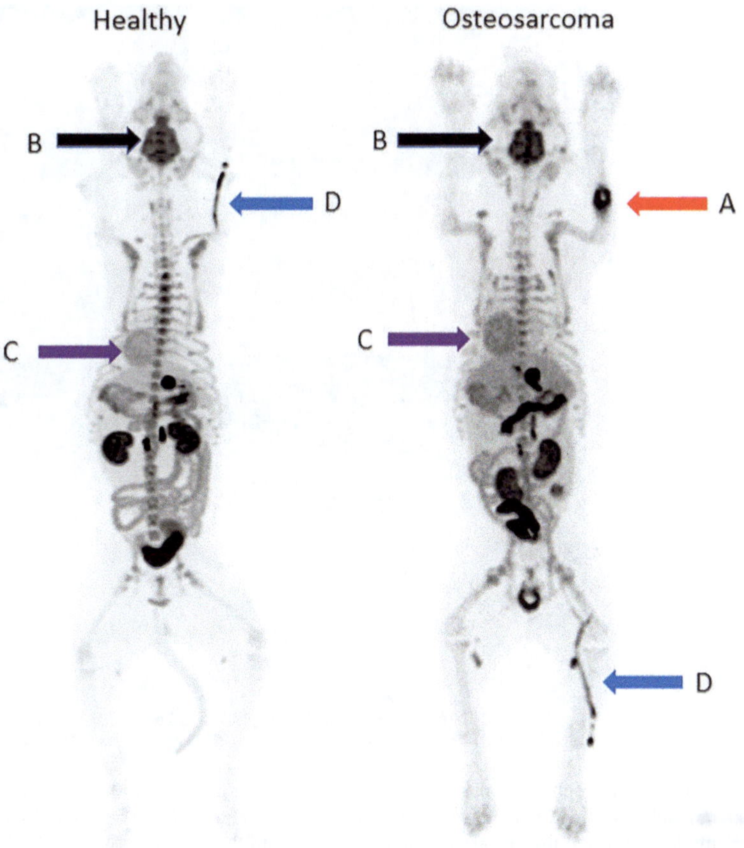

Fig. 7 Normal, healthy dog and a dog with osteosarcoma were imaged with 18F-FTC-146 PET, a novel pain/cancer radionuclide for the Sigma-1 receptor. Similar to humans, normal uptake was noted in the brain (**b**, black arrow) and heart (**c**, purple arrow). Vascular attachment (**d**, blue arrow) is associated with the injection port. In the dog with osteosarcoma (tumor noted with **a**, red arrow), a proximal ulnar lesion was noted. (Dogs were imaged at the University of Missouri and images were provided by BK Flesner)

serves as an indirect indicator of tumor response to treatment. Clinical validation of this approach is underway and could serve as an important advance in cancer immunotherapy.

3.4 Theranostics and Radiomics

Theranostics (therapy + diagnostics) refers to the creation of companion imaging and therapeutic molecules that share a specific target in diseased cells or tissues. Nuclear theranostics allows for the imaging of specific disease targets, such as cell surface proteins, that can guide the delivery of a therapeutic radioactive payload [87]. These agents can also provide information about the detection of potential targets within a patient's tumor and normal tissues, generating an estimation of likely response and/or toxicity. An existing example in veterinary oncology is the use of radiopharmaceuticals for scintigraphic imaging of thyroid tumors (i.e., with ^{99m}Tc or ^{123}I), which informs the use and allows the prescription of an appropriate dose of therapeutic iodine (^{131}I).

Antibody-based imaging agents designed specifically as reporters for cell surface antigens in dogs have been developed and present an exciting frontier for tumor-specific imaging that could be linked to novel therapeutic options such as antibody-drug conjugates [88, 89]. Challenges for further development of this field in veterinary cancer imaging are the need for canine-reactive antibodies and/or antibody fragments to localize radiopharmaceuticals to tumor cells and methods to overcome the physical/structural hurdles associated with the penetration of large molecules into the tumor mass.

Immuno-radiotherapy is an exciting new approach that leverages external beam radiotherapy, immunocytokine therapy, and targeted radionuclides in a combinatorial theranostic protocol. This approach was assessed in both the

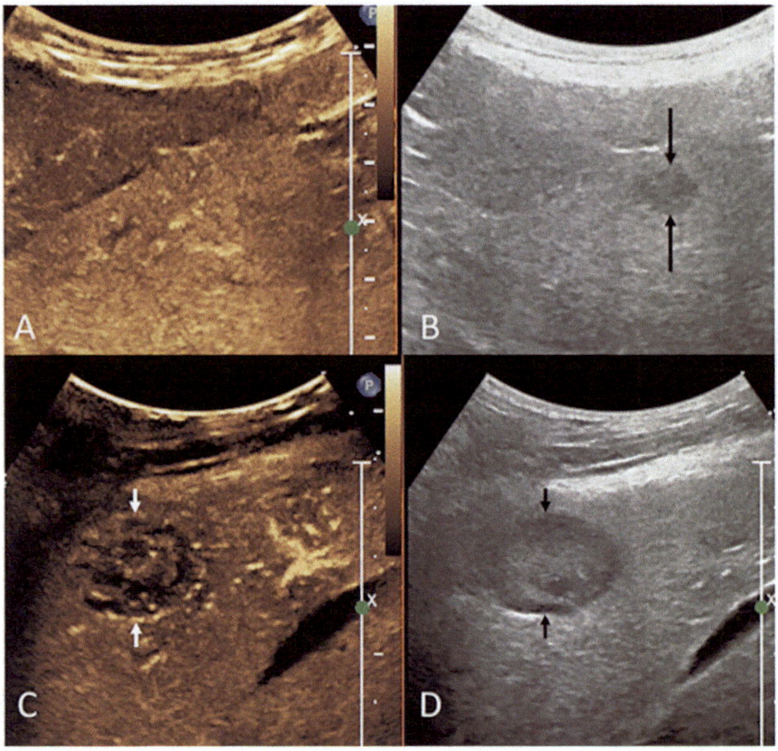

Fig. 8 Contrast-enhanced ultrasound (CEUS) of benign (**a**, **b**) and malignant (**c**, **d**) liver nodules in two dogs. The B-mode ultrasound images are on the right (**b**, **d**) and the CEUS images are on the left (**a**, **b**). The images were obtained at approximately 2 min (**a**, **b**) and 3.5 minutes (**c**, **d**) following IV contrast injection. The contrast microbubbles are within both macroscopic and microscopic vasculature, allowing for assessment of lesion perfusion. **a, b**, The hypoechoic liver nodule seen on B-mode (long black arrows) is not visible on the CEUS image, as the nodule is isoperfused relative to the surrounding liver parenchyma. This is a benign enhancement pattern, and this dog was diagnosed with vacuolar hepatopathy. **c, d**, The mixed hypoechoic and hyperechoic nodule seen on B-mode (short black arrows) is predominately hypoperfused on the CEUS image (short white arrows) as compared to the surrounding liver parenchyma, aside from some very small intralesional vessels. This hypoperfusion is known as "washout," which is a term describing the temporal perfusion of nodules relative to adjacent normal liver. Malignant nodules often display washout as they have lower portal venous/hepatic sinusoidal blood flow compared to normal liver. This dog was diagnosed with hepatic metastasis from an intestinal carcinoma. (*Image courtesy of Jennifer A. Reetz, DVM, DACVIM (LAIM), DACVR)

combined and component settings in a comparative oncology trial of dogs with advanced solid malignancies (Fig. 9) [90]. This work demonstrated the feasibility of the approach, validating the application of paired $^{86}Y/^{90}Y$ theranostics for tumor imaging and therapy and the use of tumor biopsy specimens to validate the immunologic consequences of treatment.

Radiomics refers to the extraction of a large number of shape and/or textural features from image data that may aid in clinical decision-making beyond the standard assessment provided by a radiologist. Such features can be analyzed using statistical packages such as R-studio to create predictive mathematical models with potential clinical value, particularly when assessed in the context of histologic diagnosis, tumor stage, and other patient factors. The technique has been applied in a limited setting thus far, using CT and MRI datasets from dogs with hepatic, lung, and brain tumors [91–93]. This is a growing field in veterinary oncology with the potential for new Artificial Intelligence/Machine Learning (AI/ML) techniques to be assessed in dogs, with an eye toward comparative clinical translation to humans. To date, AI/ML techniques have been applied to two-dimensional radiography and computed tomographic (CT) images from dogs, digitized whole-slide images from histopathology samples from dogs with a variety of cancer types, and through the use of a handheld device to collect thermal data from superficial malignancies in dogs [94–104]. This reflects the rapid growth of these investigations in human medicine and demonstrates how this field can provide a new dimension of comparative prognostic/predictive biomarkers. Undoubtedly, this will be an area of significant growth as the availability of publicly available datasets increases and the application of AI/ML percolates through the cancer research community.

3.5 Collaborations and Harmonization Strategies

Despite these advances, molecular imaging of naturally occurring canine cancers continues to be an underutilized opportunity in cancer research and drug development. This is largely due to a

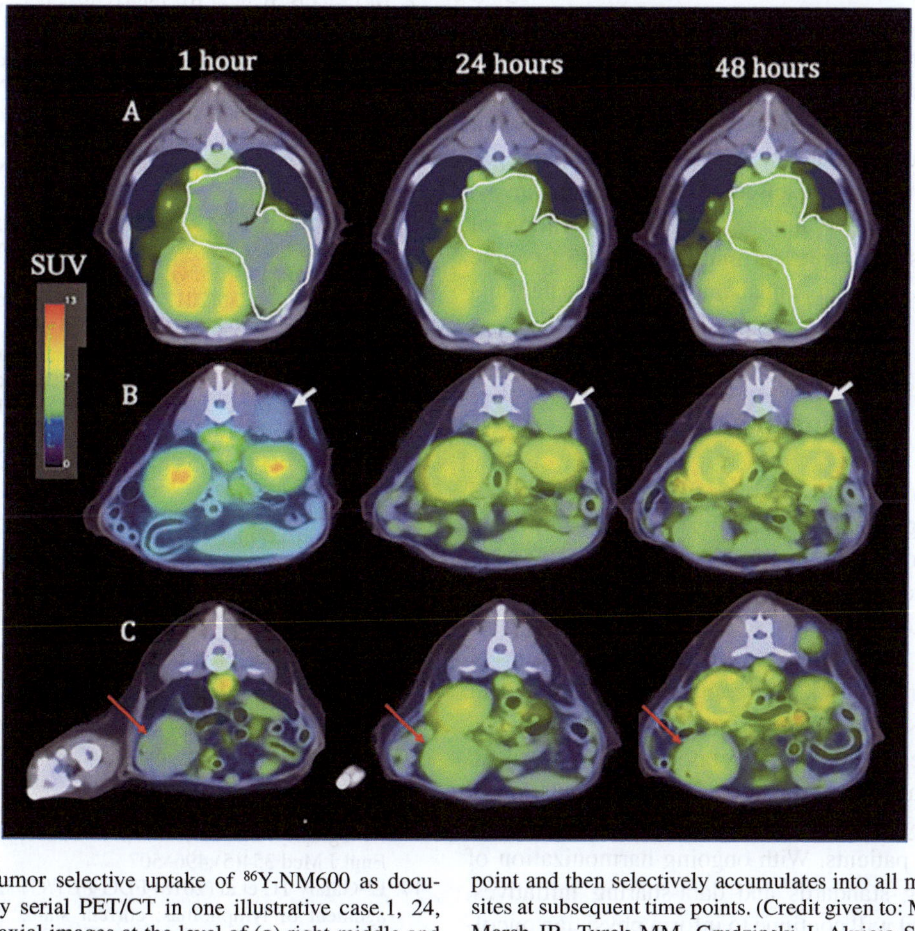

Fig. 9 Tumor selective uptake of ^{86}Y-NM600 as documented by serial PET/CT in one illustrative case.1, 24, and 48 h axial images at the level of (**a**) right middle and caudal lung lobe melanoma metastasis (outlined in white); (**b**) right epaxial muscle melanoma metastasis (white arrow) that was used as the index tumor for external beam radiation therapy and intratumoral hu14.18-IL2 immunocytokine to create an in situ vaccination; (**c**) jejunal melanoma metastasis (red arrow). Note that ^{86}Y-NM600 is primarily in the vascular compartment at the 1 h time point and then selectively accumulates into all metastatic sites at subsequent time points. (Credit given to: Magee K, Marsh IR, Turek MM, Grudzinski J, Aluicio-Sarduy E, Engle JW, et al. (2021) Safety and feasibility of an *in situ* vaccination and immunomodulatory targeted radionuclide combination immuno-radiotherapy approach in a comparative (companion dog) setting. PLoS ONE 16(8): e0255798. https://doi.org/10.1371/journal.pone.0255798. Link to License: https://creativecommons.org/licenses/by/4.0/legalcode). Changes made: none)

lack of harmonized imaging standards and uniform access to equipment, personnel, and radiopharmaceuticals or other imaging agents that are not commercially available. Recent efforts to create harmonized imaging standards for multicenter clinical trials have been addressed through NCI-led consortiums such as the Comparative Brain Tumor Consortium [105, 106]. On a broader scale, increased awareness and continuity among molecular imaging researchers is being addressed through the formation of the NCI PET/CT consortium and other federally funded comparative oncology trials networks (PRECINCT). Access to canine cancer imaging data is available through the public-facing NCI Integrated Canine Data Commons, which contains imaging data with correlative clinical and genomic/histopathologic data [5]. Ongoing efforts to populate the ICDC with multiple types of canine cancer datasets will support new investigations into radiomics and the integration of datasets that represent multiple facets of canine cancers, further enhancing their translational value.

4 Conclusions

The comparative approach to the development of imaging agents and platforms adds significant value to the discovery and translational process for novel anticancer strategies. With careful consideration of the key scientific questions, experimental goals and objectives, and inclusion of appropriately selected companion animal cancer patients, powerful studies can be designed and executed in this space. Pet dogs, in particular, fill important experimental gaps in the translation of imaging technology between rodent models and human patients. With ongoing harmonization of imaging standards and data-sharing initiatives, this field will continue to inform physician oncology while also benefiting veterinary oncology practice. Exciting new opportunities in the fields of radiomics, theranostics, and the application of artificial intelligence/machine learning algorithms provide new frontiers for this aspect of comparative oncology.

References

1. Paoloni M, Khanna C (2008) Translation of new cancer treatments from pet dogs to humans. Nat Rev Cancer 8(2):147–156
2. Axiak-Bechtel SM et al (2015) Preclinical imaging and treatment of cancer: the use of animal models beyond rodents. Q J Nucl Med Mol Imaging 59(3):303–316
3. LeBlanc AK (2014) Cancer and comparative imaging. ILAR J 55(1):164–168
4. Thamm DH (2019) Canine cancer: strategies in experimental therapeutics. Front Oncol 9:1257
5. LeBlanc AK, Mazcko CN (2020) Improving human cancer therapy through the evaluation of pet dogs. Nat Rev Cancer 20(12):727–742
6. Wisner ER, Pollard RE (2004) Trends in veterinary cancer imaging. Vet Comp Oncol 2(2):49–74
7. LeBlanc AK, Daniel GB (2007) Advanced imaging for veterinary cancer patients. Vet Clin North Am Small Anim Pract 37(6):1059–1077. v-i
8. Daniel GB, Neelis DA (2014) Thyroid scintigraphy in veterinary medicine. Semin Nucl Med 44(1):24–34
9. Randall EK (2016) PET-computed tomography in veterinary medicine. Vet Clin North Am Small Anim Pract 46(3):515–533. vi
10. McGuire AR et al (2017) What is your diagnosis? J Am Vet Med Assoc 251(3):273–275
11. Ridgway RL, Suter PF (1979) Clinical and radiographic signs in primary and metastatic esophageal neoplasms of the dog. J Am Vet Med Assoc 174(7):700–704
12. Holland M (1993) Contrast agents. Vet Clin North Am Small Anim Pract 23(2):269–279
13. Constant C et al (2016) Gadoxetate disodium (GD-EOB-DTPA) contrast enhanced magnetic resonance imaging characteristics of hepatocellular carcinoma in dogs. Vet Radiol Ultrasound 57(6):594–600
14. LeBlanc AK, Morandi F (2014) Invited review–off-site PET imaging programs: challenges and opportunities. Vet Radiol Ultrasound 55(1):109–112
15. LeBlanc AK, Peremans K (2014) PET and SPECT imaging in veterinary medicine. Semin Nucl Med 44(1):47–56
16. Juweid ME, Cheson BD (2006) Positron-emission tomography and assessment of cancer therapy. N Engl J Med 354(5):496–507
17. El-Galaly TC et al (2018) FDG-PET/CT in the management of lymphomas: current status and future directions. J Intern Med 284(4):358–376
18. Hillner BE et al (2008) Impact of positron emission tomography/computed tomography and positron emission tomography (PET) alone on expected management of patients with cancer: initial results from the National Oncologic PET Registry. J Clin Oncol 26(13):2155–2161

19. LeBlanc AK et al (2009) 18FDG-PET imaging in canine lymphoma and cutaneous mast cell tumor. Vet Radiol Ultrasound 50(2):215–223
20. Grobman M et al (2018) (18) F-FDG-PET/CT as adjunctive diagnostic modalities in canine fever of unknown origin. Vet Radiol Ultrasound 59(1):107–115
21. Frank I, Mann K, Duerr F (2019) Fluorine-18-fluoro-2-deoxy-d-glucose PET-CT aids in detection of soft-tissue injuries for dogs with thoracic or pelvic limb lameness. Vet Radiol Ultrasound 60(5):575–585
22. LeBlanc AK et al (2009) Normal thoracic and abdominal distribution of 2-deoxy-2-[18F]fluoro-D-glucose (18FDG) in adult cats. Vet Radiol Ultrasound 50(4):436–441
23. Lee MS et al (2010) Characterization of physiologic 18F-FDG uptake with PET-CT in dogs. Vet Radiol Ultrasound 51(6):670–673
24. LeBanc AK et al (2008) Thoracic and abdominal organ uptake of 2-deoxy-2-[18F]fluoro-D-glucose (18FDG) with positron emission tomography in the normal dog. Vet Radiol Ultrasound 49(2):182–188
25. Crooks C, Randall E, Griffin L (2021) The use of fluorine-18-fluorodeoxyglucose-positron emission tomography/computed tomography as an effective method for staging in dogs with primary appendicular osteosarcoma. Vet Radiol Ultrasound 62(3):350–359
26. Willcox JL et al (2021) Evaluation of accuracy for (18) F-FDG positron emission tomography and computed tomography for detection of lymph node metastasis in canine oral malignant melanoma. Vet Comp Oncol 19(3):463–472
27. Caldwell JH et al (1995) Comparison of fluorine-18-fluorodeoxyglucose and tritiated fluoromisonidazole uptake during low-flow ischemia. J Nucl Med 36(9):1633–1638
28. Rowe JA et al (2019) Relative skeletal distribution of proliferating marrow in the adult dog determined using 3′-deoxy-3′-[(18) F]fluorothymidine. Anat Histol Embryol 48(1):46–52
29. Hansen AE et al (2012) Multimodality functional imaging of spontaneous canine tumors using 64Cu-ATSM and 18FDG PET/CT and dynamic contrast enhanced perfusion CT. Radiother Oncol 102(3):424–428
30. Maitz CA et al (2022) Paired 18F-Fluorodeoxyglucose (18F-FDG), and 64Cu-Copper(II)-diacetyl-bis(N(4)-methylthiosemicarbazone) (64Cu-ATSM) PET scans in dogs with spontaneous tumors and evaluation for hypoxia-directed therapy. Radiat Res 197(3):253–260
31. Shumway KL et al (2022) Biodistribution and image characteristics of (124) I-positron emission tomography in dogs with neuroendocrine neoplasia. Vet Radiol Ultrasound 63(3):298–305
32. Gordon I et al (2009) The Comparative Oncology Trials Consortium: using spontaneously occurring cancers in dogs to inform the cancer drug development pathway. PLoS Med 6(10):e1000161
33. Vail DM, LeBlanc AK, Jeraj R (2020) Advanced cancer imaging applied in the comparative setting. Front Oncol 10:84
34. Leong SP et al (2022) Cancer microenvironment and genomics: evolution in process. Clin Exp Metastasis 39(1):85–99
35. Beer P et al (2018) The role of sentinel lymph node mapping in small animal veterinary medicine: a comparison with current approaches in human medicine. Vet Comp Oncol 16(2):178–187
36. Fournier Q et al (2021) Contrast-enhanced ultrasound for sentinel lymph node mapping in the routine staging of canine mast cell tumours: a feasibility study. Vet Comp Oncol 19(3):451–462
37. Wan J et al (2021) Determining agreement between preoperative computed tomography lymphography and indocyanine green near infrared fluorescence intraoperative imaging for sentinel lymph node mapping in dogs with oral tumours. Vet Comp Oncol 19(2):295–303
38. Beer P, Rohrer-Bley C, Nolff MC (2022) Near-infrared fluorescent image-guided lymph node dissection compared with locoregional lymphadenectomies in dogs with mast cell tumours. J Small Anim Pract 63(9):670–678
39. Brissot HN, Edery EG (2017) Use of indirect lymphography to identify sentinel lymph node in dogs: a pilot study in 30 tumours. Vet Comp Oncol 15(3):740–753
40. Randall EK et al (2020) The development of an indirect computed tomography lymphography protocol for sentinel lymph node detection in head and neck cancer and comparison to other sentinel lymph node mapping techniques. Vet Comp Oncol 18(4):634–644
41. Soultani C et al (2017) Assessment of sentinel lymph node metastasis in canine mammary gland tumors using computed tomographic indirect lymphography. Vet Radiol Ultrasound 58(2):186–196
42. Majeski SA et al (2017) Indirect computed tomographic lymphography for iliosacral lymphatic mapping in a cohort of dogs with anal Sac gland adenocarcinoma: technique description. Vet Radiol Ultrasound 58(3):295–303
43. Grimes JA et al (2017) Indirect computed tomography lymphangiography with aqueous contrast for evaluation of sentinel lymph nodes in dogs with tumors of the head. Vet Radiol Ultrasound 58(5):559–564
44. Worley DR (2014) Incorporation of sentinel lymph node mapping in dogs with mast cell tumours: 20 consecutive procedures. Vet Comp Oncol 12(3):215–226
45. Ishiguro K et al (2020) Sentinel lymph node biopsy with preoperative CT lymphography and intraoperative indocyanine green fluorescence imaging for N0 early tongue cancer: a long-term follow-up study. J Craniomaxillofac Surg 48(3):217–222
46. Goldschmidt S et al (2023) Contrast-enhanced and indirect computed tomography lymphangiography accurately identifies the cervical lymphocenter at

risk for metastasis in pet dogs with spontaneously occurring oral neoplasia. PLoS One 18(3):e0282500
47. Clemmensen A et al (2021) [(68)Ga]Ga-NODAGA-E[(cRGDyK)](2) PET and hyperpolarized [1-(13)C] pyruvate MRSI (hyperPET) in canine cancer patients: simultaneous imaging of angiogenesis and the Warburg effect. Eur J Nucl Med Mol Imaging 48(2):395–405
48. Maitz CA et al (2022) Pretargeted PET of osteodestructive lesions in dogs. Mol Pharm 19(9):3153–3162
49. Bruehlmeier M et al (2005) Measurement of tumor hypoxia in spontaneous canine sarcomas. Vet Radiol Ultrasound 46(4):348–354
50. Gutte H et al (2015) Simultaneous hyperpolarized (13)C-pyruvate MRI and (18)F-FDG-PET in cancer (hyperPET): feasibility of a new imaging concept using a clinical PET/MRI scanner. Am J Nucl Med Mol Imaging 5(1):38–45
51. Hansen AE et al (2018) Combined hyperpolarized (13)C-pyruvate MRS and (18)F-FDG PET (hyperPET) estimates of glycolysis in canine cancer patients. Eur J Radiol 103:6–12
52. Holt D et al (2014) Intraoperative near-infrared imaging can distinguish cancer from normal tissue but not inflammation. PLoS One 9(7):e103342
53. Holt D, Singhal S, Selmic LE (2020) Near-infrared imaging and optical coherence tomography for intraoperative visualization of tumors. Vet Surg 49(1):33–43
54. Favril S et al (2018) Clinical use of organic near-infrared fluorescent contrast agents in image-guided oncologic procedures and its potential in veterinary oncology. Vet Rec 183(11):354
55. Favril S et al (2020) Fluorescence-guided surgery using indocyanine green in dogs with superficial solid tumours. Vet Rec 187(7):273
56. Singhal S, Nie S, Wang MD (2010) Nanotechnology applications in surgical oncology. Annu Rev Med 61:359–373
57. Madajewski B et al (2012) Intraoperative near-infrared imaging of surgical wounds after tumor resections can detect residual disease. Clin Cancer Res 18(20):5741–5751
58. van Dam GM et al (2011) Intraoperative tumor-specific fluorescence imaging in ovarian cancer by folate receptor-α targeting: first in-human results. Nat Med 17(10):1315–1319
59. Behbahaninia M et al (2013) Intraoperative fluorescent imaging of intracranial tumors: a review. Clin Neurol Neurosurg 115(5):517–528
60. Pysz MA, Gambhir SS, Willmann JK (2010) Molecular imaging: current status and emerging strategies. Clin Radiol 65(7):500–516
61. Holt D et al (2015) Intraoperative near-infrared fluorescence imaging and spectroscopy identifies residual tumor cells in wounds. J Biomed Optics 20(7):076002
62. Keating JJ et al (2017) Intraoperative near-infrared fluorescence imaging targeting folate receptors identifies lung cancer in a large-animal model. Cancer 123(6):1051–1060
63. Newton A et al (2020) Intraoperative near-infrared imaging can identify canine mammary tumors, a spontaneously occurring, large animal model of human breast cancer. PLoS One 15(6):e0234791
64. Zelken JA, Tufaro AP (2015) Current trends and emerging future of indocyanine green usage in surgery and oncology: an update. Ann Surg Oncol 22(3):1271–1283
65. Kennedy GT et al (2022) A Cathepsin-targeted quenched activity-based probe facilitates enhanced detection of human tumors during resection. Clin Cancer Res 28(17):3729–3741
66. Vail DM et al (2009) Assessment of GS-9219 in a pet dog model of non-Hodgkin's lymphoma. Clin Cancer Res 15(10):3503–3510
67. Leblanc AK et al (2012) Preliminary evaluation of serial (18) FDG-PET/CT to assess response to toceranib phosphate therapy in canine cancer. Vet Radiol Ultrasound 53(3):348–357
68. Tahara T et al (2016) Fluorodeoxyglucose uptake on positron emission tomography is a useful predictor of long-term pain control after palliative radiation therapy in patients with painful bone metastases: results of a single-institute prospective study. Int J Radiat Oncol Biol Phys 94(2):322–328
69. Adli M et al (2013) FDG PET uptake as a predictor of pain response in palliative radiation therapy in patients with bone metastasis. Radiology 269(3):850–856
70. Zhao F et al (2015) FDG-PET predicts pain response and local control in palliative radiotherapy with or without systemic treatment in patients with bone metastasis from non-small-cell lung cancer. Clin Lung Cancer 16(6):e111–e119
71. Flesner BK et al (2021) A pilot study of cancer-induced bone pain using validated owner questionnaires, serum N-telopeptide concentration, kinetic analysis, and PET/CT. Front Vet Sci 8:637195
72. Cipriano PW et al (2018) Successful treatment of chronic knee pain following localization by a sigma-1 receptor radioligand and PET/MRI: a case report. J Pain Res 11:2353–2357
73. Cherry SR et al (2017) Total-body imaging: transforming the role of positron emission tomography. Sci Transl Med 9(381)
74. Zhang X et al (2020) Total-body dynamic reconstruction and parametric imaging on the uEXPLORER. J Nucl Med 61(2):285–291
75. Karp JS et al (2020) PennPET explorer: design and preliminary performance of a whole-body imager. J Nucl Med 61(1):136–143
76. Pantel AR et al (2020) PennPET explorer: human imaging on a whole-body imager. J Nucl Med 61(1):144–151
77. Ghaghada KB et al (2016) Computed tomography imaging of solid tumors using a liposomal-iodine contrast agent in companion dogs with naturally occurring cancer. PLoS One 11(3):e0152718

78. Kanemoto H et al (2009) Characterization of canine focal liver lesions with contrast-enhanced ultrasound using a novel contrast agent-sonazoid. Vet Radiol Ultrasound 50(2):188–194
79. Nakamura K et al (2010) Contrast-enhanced ultrasonography for characterization of canine focal liver lesions. Vet Radiol Ultrasound 51(1):79–85
80. Bargellini P et al (2016) Use of contrast-enhanced ultrasound in the differential diagnosis of adrenal tumors in dogs. J Am Anim Hosp Assoc 52(3):132–143
81. Nakamura K et al (2010) Contrast-enhanced ultrasonography for characterization of focal splenic lesions in dogs. J Vet Intern Med 24(6):1290–1297
82. Pey P et al (2014) Use of contrast-enhanced ultrasonography to characterize adrenal gland tumors in dogs. Am J Vet Res 75(10):886–892
83. Vanderperren K et al (2014) Description of the use of contrast-enhanced ultrasonography in four dogs with pancreatic tumours. J Small Anim Pract 55(3):164–169
84. Malone CD et al (2020) Contrast-enhanced US for the interventional radiologist: current and emerging applications. Radiographics 40(2):562–588
85. Eisenbrey JR et al (2018) Sensitization of hypoxic tumors to radiation therapy using ultrasound-sensitive oxygen microbubbles. Int J Radiat Oncol Biol Phys 101(1):88–96
86. Gummadi S, Eisenbrey JR, Lyshchik A (2018) Contrast-enhanced ultrasonography in interventional oncology. Abdom Radiol (NY) 43(11):3166–3175
87. Gomes Marin JF et al (2020) Theranostics in nuclear medicine: emerging and re-emerging integrated imaging and therapies in the era of precision oncology. Radiographics 40(6):1715–1740
88. Fu Y et al (2022) Anti-GD2 antibody for radiopharmaceutical imaging of osteosarcoma. Eur J Nucl Med Mol Imaging 49(13):4382–4393
89. Fazekas-Singer J et al (2017) Development of a radiolabeled caninized anti-EGFR antibody for comparative oncology trials. Oncotarget 8(47):83128–83141
90. Magee K et al (2021) Safety and feasibility of an in situ vaccination and immunomodulatory targeted radionuclide combination immuno-radiotherapy approach in a comparative (companion dog) setting. PLoS One 16(8):e0255798
91. Wanamaker MW et al (2021) Classification of neoplastic and inflammatory brain disease using MRI texture analysis in 119 dogs. Vet Radiol Ultrasound 62(4):445–454
92. Able H et al (2021) Computed tomography radiomic features hold prognostic utility for canine lung tumors: an analytical study. PLoS One 16(8):e0256139
93. Shaker R et al (2021) Machine learning model development for quantitative analysis of CT heterogeneity in canine hepatic masses may predict histologic malignancy. Vet Radiol Ultrasound 62(6):711–719
94. Dank G et al (2023) A pilot study for a non-invasive system for detection of malignancy in canine subcutaneous and cutaneous masses using machine learning. Front Vet Sci 10:1109188
95. Müller TR, Solano M, Tsunemi MH (2022) Accuracy of artificial intelligence software for the detection of confirmed pleural effusion in thoracic radiographs in dogs. Vet Radiol Ultrasound 63(5):573–579
96. Li S et al (2020) Pilot study: application of artificial intelligence for detecting left atrial enlargement on canine thoracic radiographs. Vet Radiol Ultrasound 61(6):611–618
97. Adrien-Maxence H et al (2022) Comparison of error rates between four pretrained DenseNet convolutional neural network models and 13 board-certified veterinary radiologists when evaluating 15 labels of canine thoracic radiographs. Vet Radiol Ultrasound 63(4):456–468
98. Boissady E et al (2020) Artificial intelligence evaluating primary thoracic lesions has an overall lower error rate compared to veterinarians or veterinarians in conjunction with the artificial intelligence. Vet Radiol Ultrasound 61(6):619–627
99. Banzato T et al (2021) Automatic classification of canine thoracic radiographs using deep learning. Sci Rep 11(1):3964
100. Burti S et al (2022) A machine learning-based approach for classification of focal splenic lesions based on their CT features. Front Vet Sci 9:872618
101. Patkar S et al (2023) Deep domain adversarial learning for species-agnostic classification of histologic subtypes of osteosarcoma. Am J Pathol 193(1):60–72
102. Choi BK et al (2023) Can CT texture analysis parameters be used as imaging biomarkers for prediction of malignancy in canine splenic tumors? Vet Radiol Ultrasound 64(2):224–232
103. Rai T et al (2022) Deep learning for necrosis detection using canine perivascular wall tumour whole slide images. Sci Rep 12(1):10634
104. Zuraw A, Aeffner F (2022) Whole-slide imaging, tissue image analysis, and artificial intelligence in veterinary pathology: an updated introduction and review. Vet Pathol 59(1):6–25
105. Packer RA et al (2018) Consensus recommendations on standardized magnetic resonance imaging protocols for multicenter canine brain tumor clinical trials. Vet Radiol Ultrasound 59(3):261–271
106. LeBlanc AK et al (2016) Creation of an NCI comparative brain tumor consortium: informing the translation of new knowledge from canine to human brain tumor patients. Neuro-Oncology 18(9):1209–1218

Integrating Comparative Oncology into the Translational Workflow

Suzanne Bartholf DeWitt, Heather L. Gardner, Nicole Cantor, Nicole Levine, Isabelle McMullen, Joanne Tuohy, Beatrice Schleupner, Veronica Colmenares, William C. Eward, and Jason A. Somarelli

1 Introduction

1.1 Cancer as a Disease of Multicellularity

The classic definition of cancer is a disease in which cells grow uncontrollably and with the potential to invade or spread to other parts of the body. While this definition is accurate, it is also true that cancer, at its essence, is a disease of multicellularity in which a genetically and/or epigenetically distinct cell takes on the properties of a single-celled organism from within a multicellular organism. The emergence of cancer is so intimately connected to multicellularity that almost all multicellular organisms have cancer or cancer-like phenomena wherein cells no longer contribute to normal tissue or organ functions, but instead, they divide uncontrollably to form invasive local tumors and metastases [1]. Viewing cancer as a feature that is inexorably linked to multicellularity presents an opportunity to discover fundamental properties of cancer, uncover potentially actionable mechanisms of cancer protection, and evaluate new treatments in nonhuman models of cancer, such as companion animals. Herein, we focus on the use of studies in companion animals as a means to facilitate the translation of novel therapies for humans and other animals with cancer.

1.2 Cancers Exhibit Distinct Similarities and Differences Across Species

Biomedical research commonly relies on the use of model organisms for fundamental discoveries of disease processes. Naturally occurring canine cancers have become increasingly recognized as a tractable model system in which to better

S. B. DeWitt
Department of Pathology, Duke University Medical Center, Durham, NC, USA

H. L. Gardner
Cummings School of Veterinary Medicine, Tufts University, North Grafton, MA, USA

N. Cantor
School of Osteopathic Medicine, Campbell University, Lillington, NC, USA

N. Levine · B. Schleupner · W. C. Eward
Department of Orthopaedics, Duke University Medical Center, Durham, NC, USA

I. McMullen
College of Veterinary Medicine, North Carolina State University, Raleigh, NC, USA

J. Tuohy
Virginia-Maryland College of Veterinary Medicine, Virginia Polytechnic Institute and State University, Roanoke, VA, USA

V. Colmenares
Department of Medicine, University of Louisville, Louisville, KY, USA

J. A. Somarelli (✉)
Department of Medicine, Duke University Medical Center, Durham, NC, USA
e-mail: jason.somarelli@duke.edu

M. W. Nolan et al. (eds.), *Comparative Oncology*, https://doi.org/10.1007/978-3-032-04454-9_18

understand and treat canine and human cancers. As with any model system, recognizing the strengths and weaknesses of the model is critical to ensuring that questions are answered using the best approach available. While cancer exhibits many phenotypic and genetic similarities across species, differences in disease biology and treatment approaches can have major impacts on (1) how knowledge about cancer in one species is compared to another species and (2) how this knowledge is subsequently translated into clinical settings for different species. The power of comparative oncology is grounded in an understanding of the similarities and differences between cancer across species and leveraging the strengths to answer scientific questions that would be challenging to address in other model systems or in people.

The clinical and genetic differences in cancer across species highlight the ways in which we can use cancer in one species to understand cancer in another. Striking parallels exist between several human tumors and their canine counterparts [2]. For example, appendicular osteosarcoma is the most common bone tumor in large and giant breed dogs. By contrast, appendicular osteosarcoma in children occurs less frequently (<1000 cases/year in people and > 35,000 cases/year in dogs). In dogs, surgery to control the local disease and chemotherapy prolong disease progression, with most dogs experiencing disease progression with metastasis to the lungs within 6–8 months [3]. Many children are likewise treated with surgery and chemotherapy, with approximately 30% of patients developing metastasis to the lungs and having poor clinical outcomes. Osteosarcoma in both species exhibits similar complex genetic alterations, including mutations in *TP53* and frequent copy number changes impacting *MYC*. The many parallels between canine and human osteosarcoma provide a unique opportunity to use veterinary clinical settings to advance therapies, leveraging the increased frequency of disease occurrence and more rapid progression to improve the speed of testing novel therapeutic interventions. Despite these similarities, however, there are also differences in the genetic changes observed between canine and human osteosarcoma. For example, *SETD2* and *DMD* structural variants and copy number loss are common in canine osteosarcoma, but are not observed in human osteosarcoma [4, 5]. These differences must be considered carefully when designing studies in which individual genetic mutations are key to the translation of findings across species, such as for precision oncology and targeted therapy approaches.

As molecular/targeted therapies become more common, evaluation of shared genetic mutations across multiple tumor histologic classifications can provide insight into potential activity and adverse events associated with the use of novel therapies. For example, mast cell tumors are one of the most common skin tumors in dogs, but the most closely related disease in people (systemic mastocytosis) is a distinct disease process. However, canine mast cell tumors have frequent mutations in *KIT,* [6, 7] resulting in persistent activation and signaling. *KIT* mutations are common in human cancers, particularly gastrointestinal stromal tumors (GIST) [8]. Therefore, *KIT*-mutant canine mast cell tumors can be used to evaluate the activity of KIT-targeted agents prior to further drug development and clinical trials in people [9, 10].

2 Translational Studies in Comparative Oncology

While the cancer research community has produced many successes, there remains a high failure rate for the translation of new discoveries into approved therapies [11]. To improve this failure rate for approvals of novel cancer treatments, many researchers have turned their attention to novel preclinical models, such as patient-derived organoids and humanized mouse models. Similarly, there has also been an increase in the number of studies examining the similarities of cancers across species, particularly for pet dogs with naturally occurring cancers. In contrast to mouse models, the study of pet dogs with cancer allows for the investigation of spontaneously occurring tumors in the context of an intact immune system. Additionally, dogs share a more similar body size and environment with humans. For example, dogs have a shorter lifespan and often a more rapid disease progression than humans, both of which can expedite translation of novel treatments [4]. Below, we highlight examples of comparative translational studies across the treatment landscape of cancer, from surgical interventions to novel immunotherapies and precision oncology platforms.

2.1 Surgical Studies

Surgical resection is a mainstay treatment for many solid tumors, and investigations of new procedures to more effectively remove tumor tissue and decrease the risk of recurrence are aided by comparative oncology approaches. For example, the discovery and characterization of cathepsin-cleavable fluorescent probes to detect residual disease following surgical resection by Mito et al. [12] provided the foundation for further studies using fluorescent probes in mouse models of soft tissue sarcoma to identify intraoperative tumor beds and detect residual cancerous tissue and disease recurrence. Following the success of fluorescent cancer detection in mouse models, cathepsin-activated probes were utilized in canines prior to a wide resection of naturally occurring soft tissue sarcoma [13]. Similar to the mouse model studies, fluorescence was higher in diseased tissue, and nine of the 10 canines had negative margins following histopathology, suggesting that cathepsin can be successfully utilized during surgical operations to pinpoint residual malignant tissue.

Subsequent work led to the development of the cathepsin activatable fluorescent probe, LUM015. LUM015 was tested in mouse models of soft tissue sarcoma in which mice were injected with LUM015 that was coupled to a laser ablation system to target fluorescent tissue in the margins and avoid neurovascular structures [14]. A similar prospective clinical trial found that LUM015 could be injected into canines with soft tissue sarcoma or mast cell tumors to detect malignant tissue during surgery. Approximately 92% of the 101 biopsies from these procedures indicated that LUM015 correctly distinguished cancerous from normal tissue [15]. LUM015 was also evaluated in a phase 1 trial of human soft tissue sarcoma and breast cancer patients (NCT01626066), demonstrating a favorable safety profile with tumor-specific signal in ex vivo cancer tissues from these patients [16]. This platform has recently received FDA approval for use in the surgical intervention of adults with breast cancer.

2.2 Small Molecule and Drug Studies

One of the benefits of studies in canines is the ability to perform first-in-kind studies. These early in vivo drug studies aid in the development of novel agents through assessment of pharmacodynamics and pharmacokinetics, particularly when species-specific differences in pharmacological endpoints are carefully considered [17]. Canines are attractive models of human disease because of the ability to administer treatments in a way that mimics those used in people, resulting in more relevant pharmacokinetic/pharmacodynamic and adverse event profiles as compared to rodent models. This is particularly important in the evaluation of cancer drugs, where knowledge of drugs that will induce nausea and vomiting is important but cannot be assessed using murine models. While these studies make critically important contributions to Food and Drug Administration (FDA) approvals, thoughtful trial design that considers human and canine cancer as a single entity with similar biology can further capitalize on the full potential of cross-species studies to (1) better understand mechanisms of action, [18–20], (2) develop and assess correlative biomarkers, [21, 22] or (3) evaluate therapeutic efficacy throughout all stages of human preclinical and clinical studies [23–27]. Below, we highlight examples in which the comparative approach has facilitated the translation of novel therapeutic agents.

Standard cytotoxic chemotherapy has had little success in the treatment of metastatic osteosarcoma. Among the many difficulties in treating lung metastases, achieving sufficient doses to induce cancer cell death within the lung metastatic microenvironment is a challenge. One approach to overcome this challenge has been to use aerosolized versions of chemotherapy to achieve higher concentrations at the site of metastatic disease in the lungs. To test this approach, 20 canines with osteosarcoma were enrolled in a study of aerosolized gemcitabine. After the death of the canines, lung and metastatic tissues were obtained for sampling [23]. Minimal airway toxicity was observed in these canines, and there was a marked increase in necrosis within the metastatic foci appreciated among the treatment group. Success in these preclinical trials provided the rationale for a phase 1 study of aerosol gemcitabine in patients with solitary tumors and pulmonary metastases, with a planned enrollment for 44 patients with lung metastases from solid tumors to assess the maximum tolerated dose and toxicity of aerosol gemcitabine.

The use of comparative approaches in the development of novel targeted therapies is further exemplified by the translation of losartan, an angiotensin receptor inhibitor, for the treatment of metastatic osteosarcoma. Preclinical studies in canine osteosarcoma cell lines and in vivo models of metastasis in mice demonstrated blockade of monocyte recruitment, which supported a phase 1 clinical trial in dogs [28] and a subsequent ongoing phase 1 clinical trial (ClinicalTrials.gov Identifier: NCT03900793) in people with osteosarcoma.

Several multi-targeted kinase inhibitors blocking the tyrosine kinase receptor KIT have also been evaluated in dogs with KIT-mutant mast cell tumors as a model of KIT-driven human malignancies, such as GIST (reviewed in [29]). Toceranib phosphate (Palladia(R), Zoetis) was initially developed alongside a similar drug candidate (sunitinib; Sutent(R)). Prior to the clinical development of sunitinib, toceranib was evaluated in dogs with cutaneous mast cell tumors, which commonly have activating internal tandem duplications in KIT. The clinical studies in dogs helped characterize the side effect profile and PD/PK relationships associated with dosing schedule and activity of toceranib prior to moving forward with early-phase clinical studies of sunitinib in people. Sunitinib subsequently received FDA approval after its demonstrated efficacy in advanced renal cell carcinoma and drug-resistant GIST in people. Toceranib was co-developed with sunitinib and FDA-approved for the treatment of cutaneous mast cell tumors in dogs.

2.3 Evaluation of Novel Immuno-oncology Agents

As with targeted therapies, canine comparative approaches have helped provide insights into the development and translation of novel immuno-oncology agents (reviewed in [30]). The use of canines to evaluate novel immuno-oncology therapies provides multiple advantages over rodent models. Canine cancers arise spontaneously within the context of a fully intact immune system. By contrast, studies in rodent models often rely on genetically engineered models that are induced to develop rapidly in the absence of immune system surveillance from the time of oncogenesis. Canines also share our environments, while most rodent systems occur within germ-free environments (reviewed in [30]). However, while these features are attractive for the discovery of new immunotherapies, these studies can also be hampered by the need to (1) better understand and characterize the canine immune system and (2) improve our suites of analytical tools and immunotherapies for canines.

One early example of immunotherapy development in canines was with liposomal muramyl tripeptide phosphatidylethanolamine (L-MTP-PE), a synthetic liposomal analog of MTP, an immunogenic portion of mycobacterium [31]. This work began in rodent models, [32, 33] then preclinical canine models, [34–37] followed by canine, [38, 39] and human clinical trials [40, 41]. These studies led to the approval of L-MTP-PE in Europe for the treatment of metastatic osteosarcoma. Another immunomodulatory therapy tested across multiple species is the intratumoral injection of complete Freund's adjuvant (CFA). CFA is a potent immune stimulant, which consists of heat-killed *Mycobacterium tuberculosis*, mineral oil, and surfactant. Carroll *et al.* evaluated the use of this drug in mouse, dog, and horse patients with promising success across multiple cancer types [42]. A phase 1 human clinical trial demonstrated significant immune infiltration of tumors on post-treatment biopsy in five of eight patients [42].

2.4 Personalized Medicine Approaches in Comparative Oncology

Similar to population-level studies, precision oncology approaches in dogs with cancer can provide insights prior to the initiation of human clinical studies. Historically, the primary challenge has been the limited availability of advanced genetic/genomic tools and reagents required for this work. Over the past five years, however, the rapid rise in multi-omic characterization of canine tumors and more complete builds of the canine reference genome have facilitated this process. The development of a cross-species platform to develop new patient-derived models of cancer for drug discovery combining high-throughput small-molecule screens with patient-derived models of cancer from both canines and humans led to the discovery of combined proteasome inhibition and protein trafficking inhibition (XPO1 inhibitors) as a promising combination therapy for osteosarcoma [43]. Application of this platform to a canine patient with leiomyosarcoma pinpointed proteasome inhibitors as a lead candidate for personalized therapy; however, treatment of the patient led to a heterogeneous clinical response, with some metastatic lesions responding, others exhibiting stable disease, and others progressing on therapy [44]. Genomic analysis of these multiple sites and the patient-derived models revealed extensive heterogeneity in mutational profiles across the different tumors within this single patient, underscoring the need to develop patient-derived models that can capture intra-patient heterogeneity. These studies are also time- and cost-intensive. Further development of these platforms that couple organoid technology [45–47] with longitudinal and single-cell or rare-cell sampling [48–50] may improve the speed, cost-effectiveness, and accuracy of these platforms to truly pave the way for precision oncology-guided therapy in canine and human patients.

3 Current Limitations for Maximizing Benefits of Comparative Oncology

The field of comparative oncology represents a unique framework in which to enhance our understanding of cancer; however, despite this promise, key gaps remain that have prevented the broader applicability of these approaches. These gaps include (1) a need for greater funding and infrastructural support to perform canine trials, (2) enhanced integration across the veterinary/human translational oncology landscape, and (3) improved tools to study non-model organisms at sufficient breadth and depth.

3.1 Increased Support for Canine Clinical Trials

With nearly 80 million pet dogs owned in the United States (https://www.avma.org/resources-tools/reports-statistics/us-pet-ownership-statistics) and over four million cancer diagnoses in dogs each year, [51] there is ample opportunity to further integrate studies of companion animals into human cancer research and translational oncology. To this end, the National Cancer Institute's (NCI) Comparative Oncology Program (COP) was created in 2003 to provide grant opportunities and support to fund cancer studies in animals [52]. Beyond these foundational efforts, there remains a substantial need for the cancer research community to be educated on the value and appropriate use of comparative approaches to studying cancer. Similarly, the additional One Health concepts on a broader scale, including comparative immuno-oncology, evolutionary biology, and comparative genomics, to medical training and science curricula will help future physicians and scientists to (1) understand cancer dynamics across the entire disease process and the selection pressures that lead to disease progression and treatment resistance, [1, 53] and (2) gain the tools and knowledge to properly leverage comparative approaches.

3.2 Greater Integration and Collaboration in the Scientific Community

Continued integration of research collaborations between human physicians, PhD researchers, and veterinarians will continue to speed the progress of cancer research. While this is relatively easier in regions co-localized with veterinary schools, on a broader scale, active membership and participation in organizations/societies with common research interests will enable the growth of comparative oncology studies. Transdisciplinary approaches that foster collaboration between medical professionals can be further promoted at the institutional level. For example, the Clinical and Translational Science Award One Health Alliance (COHA; https://www.ctsaonehealthalliance.org/about) consists of veterinary schools partnered with medical schools through a Clinical and Translational Science Institute. COHA supports the integration of human and animal medical studies through efforts in biobanking, clinical trials, education and training, and support of meetings and collaboration that include clinician-scientist training workshops and Good Clinical Practice training modules for veterinary studies. Similarly, consortia like the Comparative Oncology Consortium (https://dukecancerinstitute.org/news/consortium-canine-comparative-oncology) exemplify the collaborative institutional frameworks that can be created across institutions to capitalize on the opportunities provided by studying cancer across species. In addition, some universities provide courses for both students in the College of Veterinary Medicine and the College of Medicine, allowing students to learn with and from their peers in other medical fields. Increasing the prevalence of transdisciplinary classes required for both medical school students and veterinary school students can foster communication and relationships between the two professions, leading to a more streamlined and comprehensive approach to cancer research.

3.3 Improving Tools to Study Cancer in Non-model Organisms and Companion Animals

Enhancements in molecular and genomics toolkits and cancer databases have facilitated deeper insights into cancer across species. These resources have helped illuminate cancer risk across species, [54, 55] pinpoint potential driver genes and pathways in canine cancer and other species, [56] and identify cancer protective mechanisms that may have relevance to human cancer [57–59]. Resource and tool development should consider every stage of the study process, including sample acquisition, storage, shipping, sample quality control, culture and growth methods, molecular and bioengineering reagents and tools, novel real-time imaging strategies, analysis reagents (e.g., capture baits, sequencing panels, species agnostic platforms), databases, and easy-to-use analysis pipelines. From an informatics perspective, computational analysis tools often need to be modified to work in nonhuman/nonrodent species, and these tools and data require rigorous benchmarking in dogs. Historically, tools designed for the analysis of canine cancers relied only on a single reference genome, but this has since changed with the release of several new high-quality dog reference genomes, which will help address many of the limitations of the previous canine reference genome [60].

The development and launch of animal health databases have increased access to animal cancer studies. For example, the American Veterinary Medical Association (AVMA) Animal Health Studies Database (AAHSD) was created in 2016 to serve as a running archive of past and present veterinary clinical trials [61]. The AAHSD accepts publications of studies performed in all species and disciplines and provides some standardization, as the information required largely mirrors the requirements for listing on ClinicalTrials.gov, and all listed studies are reviewed for authenticity [62]. Similarly, the VCS website's clinical trials page provides another resource for investigating cancer clinical trials being performed in animals. This webpage provides links to the AAHSD and to information on trials being conducted across the United States at university veterinary schools and other specialty hospitals as an organized effort to provide access to information on clinical trials [62].

In addition to data availability on clinical trials, availability of genomics data in canine cancer continues to improve. The National Cancer Institute invested nearly $5.5 million to launch the Integrated Canine Data Commons (ICDC) in 2020 with the goal of furthering research on human cancers using canines as a comparative model [63]. The ICDC provides cloud-based public access to canine cancer data from studies performed through NCI programs, including the COP and the NCI Cancer Moonshot℠-funded Cancer PRE-medical Cancer Immunotherapy Network Canine Trials (PRECINCT) [64]. This tool facilitates access to high-powered cloud computing and analysis through Seven Bridges Cancer Genomics Cloud (https://datacommons.cancer.gov/repository/integrated-canine-data-commons). Studies submitted to the ICDC are subjected to review by the Data Governance Advisory Board to be granted inclusion in the ICDC. Additional regulations and expectations have been established by the ICDC to improve consistency in data and terminology [65].

Jaguar Health Canine Cancer established Take C.H.A.R.G.E (Canine Health and ReGistry Exchange) Registry and Cancer Care Index in 2022, the first-of-its-kind canine cancer database that aids in tracking the occurrence and prevalence of canine cancer [66]. Take C.H.A.R.G.E allows dog owners and veterinary clinics to upload medical records of dogs with cancer at no cost, resulting in an assessment of more than 35,000 canine medical records in the first year. Take C.H.A.R.G.E was established to provide data on the incidence and prevalence of canine cancer. The Take C.H.A.R.G.E's Scientific Advisory Board (SAB) is dedicated to supporting the COP by improving the continuity and availability of canine cancer data. A major directive of the SAB is establishing and encouraging the adoption of a consistent canine cancer diagnostic coding system that aligns with the recently published Veterinary International Classification of Diseases for Oncology Canine Tumors First Edition (Vet-ICD-O-canine-1), which is based on the most recent human cancer coding system, ICD-O-3.2 [67].

The recent emergence of open-access medical records and clinical trial databases will aid in improving transdisciplinary access to cancer data and will increase awareness of the potential for advancement in cancer research through comparative oncology. The increased participation of veterinary clinics and increased use of these databases by researchers, along with standardization of medical record entry and appropriate training in data entry standards, are important next steps in furthering our study of cancer through spontaneous cancers in animals.

4 Conclusion

The phenotypic, genetic, and clinical similarities of cancer across species provide a unique opportunity to leverage naturally occurring cancers in dogs to fill knowledge gaps and advance cancer research for the benefit of both people and animals. Continued integration and optimization of approaches using dogs and other animals with cancer will help optimize clinical drug development and our understanding of cancer biology.

Bibliography

1. Aktipis CA, Boddy AM, Jansen G et al (2015) Cancer across the tree of life: cooperation and cheating in multicellularity. Philos Trans R Soc Lond Ser B Biol Sci 370(1673). https://doi.org/10.1098/rstb.2014.0219
2. Breen M, Modiano JF (2008) Evolutionarily conserved cytogenetic changes in hematological malignancies of dogs and humans–man and his best friend share more than companionship. Chromosom

Res 16(1):145–154. https://doi.org/10.1007/s10577-007-1212-4
3. LeBlanc AK, Mazcko CN, Cherukuri A et al (2021) Adjuvant Sirolimus does not improve outcome in pet dogs receiving standard-of-care therapy for appendicular osteosarcoma: a prospective, randomized trial of 324 dogs. Clin Cancer Res 27(11):3005–3016. https://doi.org/10.1158/1078-0432.CCR-21-0315
4. LeBlanc AK, Mazcko CN (2020) Improving human cancer therapy through the evaluation of pet dogs. Nat Rev Cancer 20(12):727–742. https://doi.org/10.1038/s41568-020-0297-3
5. Sarver AL, Mills LJ, Makielski KM et al (2023) Distinct mechanisms of PTEN inactivation in dogs and humans highlight convergent molecular events that drive cell division in the pathogenesis of osteosarcoma. Cancer Genet 276–277:1–11. https://doi.org/10.1016/j.cancergen.2023.05.001
6. London CA, Kisseberth WC, Galli SJ, Geissler EN, Helfand SC (1996) Expression of stem cell factor receptor (c-kit) by the malignant mast cells from spontaneous canine mast cell tumours. J Comp Pathol 115(4):399–414. https://doi.org/10.1016/s0021-9975(96)80074-0
7. Preziosi R, Morini M, Sarli G (2004) Expression of the KIT protein (CD117) in primary cutaneous mast cell tumors of the dog. J Vet Diagn Invest 16(6):554–561. https://doi.org/10.1177/104063870401600610
8. Lasota J, Miettinen M (2006) KIT and PDGFRA mutations in gastrointestinal stromal tumors (GISTs). Semin Diagn Pathol 23(2):91–102. https://doi.org/10.1053/j.semdp.2006.08.006
9. London CA, Gardner HL, Rippy S et al (2017) KTN0158, a humanized anti-kit monoclonal antibody, demonstrates biologic activity against both normal and malignant canine mast cells. Clin Cancer Res 23(10):2565–2574. https://doi.org/10.1158/1078-0432.CCR-16-2152
10. London CA, Malpas PB, Wood-Follis SL et al (2009) Multi-center, placebo-controlled, double-blind, randomized study of oral toceranib phosphate (SU11654), a receptor tyrosine kinase inhibitor, for the treatment of dogs with recurrent (either local or distant) mast cell tumor following surgical excision. Clin Cancer Res 15(11):3856–3865. https://doi.org/10.1158/1078-0432.CCR-08-1860
11. Paul SM, Mytelka DS, Dunwiddie CT et al (2010) How to improve R&D productivity: the pharmaceutical industry's grand challenge. Nat Rev Drug Discov 9(3):203–214. https://doi.org/10.1038/nrd3078
12. Mito JK, Ferrer JM, Brigman BE et al (2012) Intraoperative detection and removal of microscopic residual sarcoma using wide-field imaging. Cancer 118(21):5320–5330. https://doi.org/10.1002/cncr.27458
13. Eward WC, Mito JK, Eward CA et al (2013) A novel imaging system permits real-time in vivo tumor bed assessment after resection of naturally occurring sarcomas in dogs. Clin Orthop Relat Res 471(3):834–842. https://doi.org/10.1007/s11999-012-2560-8
14. Lazarides AL, Whitley MJ, Strasfeld DB et al (2016) A fluorescence-guided laser ablation system for removal of residual cancer in a mouse model of soft tissue sarcoma. Theranostics 6(2):155–166. https://doi.org/10.7150/thno.13536
15. Bartholf DeWitt S, Eward WC, Eward CA et al (2016) A novel imaging system distinguishes neoplastic from normal tissue during resection of soft tissue sarcomas and mast cell tumors in dogs. Vet Surg 45(6):715–722. https://doi.org/10.1111/vsu.12487
16. Whitley MJ, Cardona DM, Lazarides AL et al (2016) A mouse-human phase 1 co-clinical trial of a protease-activated fluorescent probe for imaging cancer. Sci Transl Med 8(320):320ra4. https://doi.org/10.1126/scitranslmed.aad0293
17. Lawrence J, Cameron D, Argyle D (2015) Species differences in tumour responses to cancer chemotherapy. Philos Trans R Soc Lond Ser B Biol Sci 370(1673). https://doi.org/10.1098/rstb.2014.0233
18. Pang LY, Argyle DJ (2009) Using naturally occurring tumours in dogs and cats to study telomerase and cancer stem cell biology. Biochim Biophys Acta 1792(4):380–391. https://doi.org/10.1016/j.bbadis.2009.02.010
19. Pazzi KA, Kraegel SA, Griffey SM, Theon AP, Madewell BR (1996) Analysis of the equine tumor suppressor gene p53 in the normal horse and in eight cutaneous squamous cell carcinomas. Cancer Lett 107(1):125–130. https://doi.org/10.1016/0304-3835(96)04359-5
20. van der Weyden L, Brenn T, Patton EE, Wood GA, Adams DJ (2020) Spontaneously occurring melanoma in animals and their relevance to human melanoma. J Pathol 252(1):4–21. https://doi.org/10.1002/path.5505
21. Giuliano A (2021) Companion animal model in translational oncology; feline oral squamous cell carcinoma and canine oral melanoma. Biology (Basel) 11(1). https://doi.org/10.3390/biology11010054
22. Monjazeb AM, Kent MS, Grossenbacher SK et al (2016) Blocking indolamine-2,3-dioxygenase rebound immune suppression boosts antitumor effects of radio-immunotherapy in murine models and spontaneous canine malignancies. Clin Cancer Res 22(17):4328–4340. https://doi.org/10.1158/1078-0432.CCR-15-3026
23. Rodriguez CO, Crabbs TA, Wilson DW et al (2010) Aerosol gemcitabine: preclinical safety and in vivo antitumor activity in osteosarcoma-bearing dogs. J Aerosol Med Pulm Drug Deliv 23(4):197–206. https://doi.org/10.1089/jamp.2009.0773
24. Paoloni M, Mazcko C, Selting K et al (2015) Defining the pharmacodynamic profile and therapeutic index of NHS-IL12 immunocytokine in dogs with malignant melanoma. PLoS One 10(6):e0129954. https://doi.org/10.1371/journal.pone.0129954
25. Deville J-L, Ravaud A, Maruzzo M et al (2020) 265 Phase 1b study of Avelumab + M9241 (NHS-IL12) in patients with advanced solid tumors: interim analysis results from a urothelial carcinoma (UC)

dose-expansion cohort. In: Regular and young investigator award abstracts. BMJ, pp A163.1–A1A163. https://doi.org/10.1136/jitc-2020-SITC2020.0265
26. Patel DM, Foreman PM, Nabors LB, Riley KO, Gillespie GY, Markert JM (2016) Design of a phase I clinical trial to evaluate M032, a genetically engineered HSV-1 expressing IL-12, in patients with recurrent/progressive glioblastoma multiforme, anaplastic astrocytoma, or gliosarcoma. Hum Gene Ther Clin Dev 27(2):69–78. https://doi.org/10.1089/humc.2016.031
27. Omar NB, Bentley RT, Crossman DK et al (2021) Safety and interim survival data after intracranial administration of M032, a genetically engineered oncolytic HSV-1 expressing IL-12, in pet dogs with sporadic gliomas. Neurosurg Focus 50(2):E5. https://doi.org/10.3171/2020.11.FOCUS20844
28. Regan DP, Chow L, Das S et al (2022) Losartan blocks osteosarcoma-elicited monocyte recruitment, and combined with the kinase inhibitor Toceranib, exerts significant clinical benefit in canine metastatic osteosarcoma. Clin Cancer Res 28(4):662–676. https://doi.org/10.1158/1078-0432.CCR-21-2105
29. Gardner HL, Fenger JM, London CA (2016) Dogs as a model for cancer. Annu Rev Anim Biosci 4:199–222. https://doi.org/10.1146/annurev-animal-022114-110911
30. Park JS, Withers SS, Modiano JF et al (2016) Canine cancer immunotherapy studies: linking mouse and human. J Immunother Cancer 4:97. https://doi.org/10.1186/s40425-016-0200-7
31. Kleinerman ES, Erickson KL, Schroit AJ, Fogler WE, Fidler IJ (1983) Activation of tumoricidal properties in human blood monocytes by liposomes containing lipophilic muramyl tripeptide. Cancer Res 43(5):2010–2014
32. Sugimoto M, Germain RN, Chedid L, Benacerraf B (1978) Enhancement of carrier-specific helper T cell function by the synthetic adjuvant, N-acetyl muramyl-L-alanyl-D-isoglutamine (MDP). J Immunol 120(3):980–982
33. Fidler IJ, Sone S, Fogler WE, Barnes ZL (1981) Eradication of spontaneous metastases and activation of alveolar macrophages by intravenous injection of liposomes containing muramyl dipeptide. Proc Natl Acad Sci USA 78(3):1680–1684. https://doi.org/10.1073/pnas.78.3.1680
34. Shi F, MacEwen EG, Kurzman ID (1993) In vitro and in vivo effect of doxorubicin combined with liposome-encapsulated muramyl tripeptide on canine monocyte activation. Cancer Res 53(17):3986–3991
35. Kurzman ID, Shi F, MacEwen EG (1993) In vitro and in vivo canine mononuclear cell production of tumor necrosis factor induced by muramyl peptides and lipopolysaccharide. Vet Immunol Immunopathol 38(1-2):45–56. https://doi.org/10.1016/0165-2427(93)90112-h
36. Smith BW, Kurzman ID, Schultz KT, Czuprynski CJ, MacEwen EG (1993) Muramyl peptides augment the in vitro and in vivo cytostatic activity of canine plastic-adherent mononuclear cells against canine osteosarcoma cells. Cancer Biother 8(2):137–144. https://doi.org/10.1089/cbr.1993.8.137
37. Kurzman ID, Shi F, Vail DM, MacEwen EG (1999) In vitro and in vivo enhancement of canine pulmonary alveolar macrophage cytotoxic activity against canine osteosarcoma cells. Cancer Biother Radiopharm 14(2):121–128. https://doi.org/10.1089/cbr.1999.14.121
38. MacEwen EG, Kurzman ID, Rosenthal RC et al (1989) Therapy for osteosarcoma in dogs with intravenous injection of liposome-encapsulated muramyl tripeptide. J Natl Cancer Inst 81(12):935–938. https://doi.org/10.1093/jnci/81.12.935
39. Kurzman ID, MacEwen EG, Rosenthal RC et al (1995) Adjuvant therapy for osteosarcoma in dogs: results of randomized clinical trials using combined liposome-encapsulated muramyl tripeptide and cisplatin. Clin Cancer Res 1(12):1595–1601
40. Kleinerman ES, Gano JB, Johnston DA, Benjamin RS, Jaffe N (1995) Efficacy of liposomal muramyl tripeptide (CGP 19835A) in the treatment of relapsed osteosarcoma. Am J Clin Oncol 18(2):93–99
41. Chou AJ, Kleinerman ES, Krailo MD et al (2009) Addition of muramyl tripeptide to chemotherapy for patients with newly diagnosed metastatic osteosarcoma: a report from the Children's Oncology Group. Cancer 115(22):5339–5348. https://doi.org/10.1002/cncr.24566
42. Carroll CSE, Andrew ER, Malik L et al (2021) Simple and effective bacterial-based intratumoral cancer immunotherapy. J Immunother Cancer 9(9). https://doi.org/10.1136/jitc-2021-002688
43. Somarelli JA, Rupprecht G, Altunel E et al (2020) A comparative oncology drug discovery pipeline to identify and validate new treatments for osteosarcoma. Cancers (Basel) 12(11). https://doi.org/10.3390/cancers12113335
44. Rao SR, Somarelli JA, Altunel E et al (2020) From the clinic to the bench and back again in one dog year: how a cross-species pipeline to identify new treatments for sarcoma illuminates the path forward in precision medicine. Front Oncol 10:117. https://doi.org/10.3389/fonc.2020.00117
45. Inglebert M, Dettwiler M, Hahn K et al (2022) A living biobank of canine mammary tumor organoids as a comparative model for human breast cancer. Sci Rep 12(1):18051. https://doi.org/10.1038/s41598-022-21706-2
46. Sato Y, Elbadawy M, Suzuki K et al (2023) Establishment of an experimental model of canine malignant mesothelioma organoid culture using a three-dimensional culture method. Biomed Pharmacother 162:114651. https://doi.org/10.1016/j.biopha.2023.114651
47. Elbadawy M, Usui T, Mori T et al (2019) Establishment of a novel experimental model for muscle-invasive bladder cancer using a dog bladder cancer organoid culture. Cancer Sci 110(9):2806–2821. https://doi.org/10.1111/cas.14118

48. Chmielewska M, Łosiewicz K, Socha P, Mecik-Kronenberg T, Wasowicz K (2013) The application of circulating tumor cells detecting methods in veterinary oncology. Pol J Vet Sci 16(1):141–151. https://doi.org/10.2478/pjvs-2013-0022
49. Marconato L, Facchinetti A, Zanardello C et al (2019) Detection and prognostic relevance of circulating and disseminated tumour cell in dogs with metastatic mammary carcinoma: a pilot study. Cancers (Basel) 11(2). https://doi.org/10.3390/cancers11020163
50. Wright TF, Brisson BA, Belanger CR et al (2023) Quantification of circulating tumour cells over time in dogs with appendicular osteosarcoma. Vet Comp Oncol. https://doi.org/10.1111/vco.12918
51. Schiffman JD, Breen M (2015) Comparative oncology: what dogs and other species can teach us about humans with cancer. Philos Trans R Soc Lond Ser B Biol Sci 370(1673). https://doi.org/10.1098/rstb.2014.0231
52. National Cancer Institute. Comparative Oncology Program | Center for Cancer Research. National Cancer Institute Comparative Oncology Program. Accessed 10 Mar 2023. https://ccr.cancer.gov/comparative-oncology-program
53. Vincent MD (2010) The animal within: carcinogenesis and the clonal evolution of cancer cells are speciation events sensu stricto. Evolution 64(4):1173–1183. https://doi.org/10.1111/j.1558-5646.2009.00942.x
54. Vincze O, Colchero F, Lemaître J-F et al (2022) Cancer risk across mammals. Nature 601(7892):263–267. https://doi.org/10.1038/s41586-021-04224-5
55. Nair NU, Cheng K, Naddaf L et al (2022) Cross-species identification of cancer resistance-associated genes that may mediate human cancer risk. Sci Adv 8(31):eabj7176. https://doi.org/10.1126/sciadv.abj7176
56. Gunady EF, Ware KE, Hoskinson Plumlee S et al (2022) Exome sequencing of hepatocellular carcinoma in lemurs identifies potential cancer drivers: a pilot study. Evol Med Public Health 10(1):221–230. https://doi.org/10.1093/emph/eoac016
57. Trivedi DD, Dalai SK, Bakshi SR (2023) The mystery of cancer resistance: a revelation within nature. J Mol Evol 91(2):133–155. https://doi.org/10.1007/s00239-023-10092-6
58. Schraverus H, Larondelle Y, Page MM (2022) Beyond the lab: what we can learn about cancer from wild and domestic animals. Cancers (Basel) 14(24). https://doi.org/10.3390/cancers14246177
59. Seluanov A, Gladyshev VN, Vijg J, Gorbunova V (2018) Mechanisms of cancer resistance in long-lived mammals. Nat Rev Cancer 18(7):433–441. https://doi.org/10.1038/s41568-018-0004-9
60. Wang C, Wallerman O, Arendt M-L et al (2021) A novel canine reference genome resolves genomic architecture and uncovers transcript complexity. Commun Biol 4(1):185. https://doi.org/10.1038/s42003-021-01698-x
61. Murphey DE (2019) The AVMA animal health studies database. Top Companion Anim Med 37:100361. https://doi.org/10.1016/j.tcam.2019.100361
62. AVMA. AAHSD Study search. Animal Health studies database. Accessed 13 June 2023. https://ebusiness.avma.org/aahsd/study_search.aspx
63. Pot D, Worman Z, Baumann A, Pathak S, Beck R, Beck E, et al (2024) NCI cancer research data commons: cloud-based analytic resources. Cancer Res 84(9):1396–1403. https://doi.org/10.1158/0008-5472.CAN-23-2657
64. National Cancer Institute. NCI-Funded Canine Immunotherapy Trials Network Treats Pet Dogs to Study Cancers Common to Humans | News & Events | DCTD. Accessed 13 June 2023. https://dctd.cancer.gov/NewsEvents/20190327_canine_immunotherapy.htm
65. Naess K (1961) Noradrenaline and transmission in sympathetic ganglia. Nord Med 66:1723–1724. Danish
66. Jaguar Health Announces Launch of the First U.S. Canine Cancer Registry and Canine Cancer Care Index | Jaguar Health, Inc. Accessed 10 Mar 2023. https://jaguarhealth.gcs-web.com/news-releases/news-release-details/jaguar-health-announces-launch-first-us-canine-cancer-registry
67. Poleshchuk IS (1961) On the diagnosis and treatment of postoperative gastrocolic fistula. Vestn Khir Im I I Grek 87:76–78. Russian

MIX
Papier aus verantwortungsvollen Quellen
Paper from responsible sources
FSC® C105338

If you have any concerns about our products,
you can contact us on
ProductSafety@springernature.com

In case Publisher is established outside the EU,
the EU authorized representative is:
Springer Nature Customer Service Center GmbH
Europaplatz 3, 69115 Heidelberg, Germany

Printed by Libri Plureos GmbH
in Hamburg, Germany